Postgraduate Gynecology

System requirement:

- **Windows XP or above**
- **Power DVD player (Software)**
- **Windows media player 10.0 version or above (Software)**

Accompanying DVD ROM is playable only in Computer and not in DVD player.

Kindly wait for few seconds for CD to autorun. If it does not autorun then please do the following:

- Click on my computer
- Click the **CD/DVD drive** and after opening the drive, kindly double click the file **Jaypee**

Postgraduate Gynecology

B Presannakumari MD DGO
Former Professor of Obstetrics and Gynecology
Medical College, Thiruvananthapuram, Kerala, India

Senior Consultant in Obstetrics and Gynecology
Sree Uthradum Thirunal General Hospital
Thiruvananthapuram, Kerala, India

JAYPEE BROTHERS MEDICAL PUBLISHERS (P) LTD

Kochi • St Louis (USA) • Panama City (Panama) • London (UK) • New Delhi • Ahmedabad
Bengaluru • Chennai • Hyderabad • Kolkata • Lucknow • Mumbai • Nagpur

Published by
Jitendar P Vij
Jaypee Brothers Medical Publishers (P) Ltd

Corporate Office
4838/24 Ansari Road, Daryaganj, **New Delhi** - 110002, India, Phone: +91-11-43574357, Fax: +91-11-43574314

Registered Office
B-3 EMCA House, 23/23B Ansari Road, Daryaganj, **New Delhi** - 110 002, India
Phones: +91-11-23272143, +91-11-23272703, +91-11-23282021
+91-11-23245672, Rel: +91-11-32558559, Fax: +91-11-23276490, +91-11-23245683
e-mail: jaypee@jaypeebrothers.com, Website: www.jaypeebrothers.com

Offices in India

- **Ahmedabad**, Phone: Rel: +91-79-32988717, e-mail: ahmedabad@jaypeebrothers.com
- **Bengaluru**, Phone: Rel: +91-80-32714073, e-mail: bangalore@jaypeebrothers.com
- **Chennai**, Phone: Rel: +91-44-32972089, e-mail: chennai@jaypeebrothers.com
- **Hyderabad**, Phone: Rel:+91-40-32940929, e-mail: hyderabad@jaypeebrothers.com
- **Kochi**, Phone: +91-484-2395740, e-mail: kochi@jaypeebrothers.com
- **Kolkata**, Phone: +91-33-22276415, e-mail: kolkata@jaypeebrothers.com
- **Lucknow**, Phone: +91-522-3040554, e-mail: lucknow@jaypeebrothers.com
- **Mumbai**, Phone: Rel: +91-22-32926896, e-mail: mumbai@jaypeebrothers.com
- **Nagpur**, Phone: Rel: +91-712-3245220, e-mail: nagpur@jaypeebrothers.com

Overseas Offices

- **North America Office, USA,** Ph: 001-636-6279734, e-mail: jaypee@jaypeebrothers.com, anjulav@jaypeebrothers.com
- **Central America Office, Panama City, Panama,** Ph: 001-507-317-0160, e-mail: cservice@jphmedical.com
  Website: www.jphmedical.com
- **Europe Office, UK,** Ph: +44 (0) 2031708910, e-mail: info@jpmedpub.com

Postgraduate Gynecology

First Edition: **2011**

ISBN: 978-93-5025-082-2

Typeset at JPBMP typesetting unit
Printed at Ajanta Offset & Packagings Ltd., New Delhi

Dedicated to the fond memory of my beloved brother

Twin brother Bhasi nice and warm
Born to teachers wise and calm
Amid the charm of rice and palm
Always to needy ice and balm

Friend indeed when in need
Beloved teacher to kids plenty
Refrains not from sharing views
Rich and vast his range and depth

Learning is earning he did view
Yearning for learning anything new
As you drain, so you gain
Vidyadhan, the treasure supreme

When values turn valueless
Dishonour is high 'honour'
Perversion is the 'right' version
Disorder the new order

Then love and concern incarnate
Find just and truth do alienate
Peace in life shifts farther remote
Heaven calls them not too late

To shine a new star among the stars!

Contributors

B Presannakumari MD DGO
Former Professor of Obstetrics and Gynecology
Medical College, Thiruvananthapuram, Kerala, India
Senior Consultant in Obstetrics and Gynecology
Sree Uthradum Thirunal General Hospital
Thiruvananthapuram, Kerala, India

K Jayakrishnan MD DGO DNB
Consultant Reproductive Medicine
KJK Hospital
Fertility Research Centre
Nalanchira, Thiruvananthapuram,
Kerala, India
kjkhospital@vsnl.com, kjkhospital@gmail.com
www.kjkhospital.com

Madhu KN MD
Paul's Hospital
Kochi, Kerala, India

NS Sreedevi MD DGO
Former Professor and HOD
Department of Obstetrics and Gynecology
Medical College Kozhikode
Calicut, Kerala, India

PG Paul MBBS DGO
Director, Endoscopic Surgeon
Paul's Hospital, Kochi, Kerala, India

Sareena Gilvaz MBBS MD DGO
Associate Professor and HOD,
Department of Obstetrics and Gynecology
Jubilee Mission Medical College
Trichur, Kerala, India

Sejal Naik MD
Department of Gynecology Endoscopy
Paul's Hospital
Kochi, Kerala, India

Preface

Medical education around the world is rapidly expanding and there is an adequate need for the development of women's health education. The Council on Graduate Medical Education's (COGME) Fifth Report on Women and Medicine states that "changes in undergraduate and graduate medical education, in addition to continuing medical education, are needed to address adequately the comprehensive health needs of women." The objective of this book is to be an invaluable resource for the medical practitioners, who step into the field of gynecology. This book proposes them to have a systematic study of the subject, for empowering them with the knowledge and skills required for the practice of gynecology. Keeping this in mind, the best efforts have been made into this work to make it pleasant for the readers.

At-a-Glance Outline Format

Chapters are introduced with a non-formal statement that sets the tone for developing the core idea. They are then structured into subtopics and are further divided into small and discrete sections to which the reader's attention is sought.

Concise Points in Boxes

Concise, high-yield subject matter is provided in boxes, to enhance the study experience of the students.

Flow Charts

Flow charts give easy understanding of evaluation and management protocols in a student-friendly manner.

Evidence-based Management Approach

The practicing obstetrician-gynecologist should be equipped today with a far richer armamentarium than ever before. This is in part due to sheer expansion in knowledge and technology and in part due to the conditionality of evidence-based practice. Evidence-based practice is gaining momentum and where possible it is in the interest of both the clinician and the patient to subscribe to these rules as they support the better traditions of medical care. In order to be successful, the clinician should be able to sift through evidence and make decisions considering the patient's socioeconomic background, attitudes and believes.

Work-out of Real-time Clinical Scenarios

A unique feature of this book is the work-out of real-time clinical scenarios, giving explanations as to how to arrive at a rational clinical diagnosis and management. This helps the students understand the topic in a better way, equipping them to manage the patients themselves.

Usage of Latest Technologies in Gynecology

Imaging modalities like ultrasonography, CT, MRI and PET-scan, have developed in a big way in the recent times. The usage of these imaging modalities is discussed in appropriate situations in the various chapters. Though most of the imaging modalities are rightly under the purview of the radiologist, every student and specialist in obstetrics-gynecology ought to have proficiency in ultrasonography. In numerous clinical emergency situations like ectopic gestation, as well as in the routine diagnosis of uterine and ovarian pathologies, the obstetrician-gynecologist will be better placed to perform, interpret and decide on emerging issues. Thus, sonography has become an essential part of any specialist training. Explanations on the techniques, tips and interpretations of ultrasonography have been detailed in a separate chapter. The obstetrician-gynecologist should acquire the knowledge and skills in the field of ultrasonography so much so that it evolves as an essential armamentarium for diagnosis and management by themselves.

The author believes that the guiding philosophy behind the book would naturally justify its existence. It is felt that the postgraduate students, who are the specialists of tomorrow to whom it attempts to reach out, would find the book accessible to them and that the dealing of the subject is appropriate to their requirements.

Online Access

www.obsgynec.com
Students can log onto the above site for contacting the author for posting their queries.

B Presannakumari

Acknowledgments

To the Almighty for His Blessings

At the fag end of 32 years of my clinical career, I realized that something was missing. Pondering over it, it struck me that it is my urge to compile the knowledge that I have acquired over the years of dedicated work. When I ventured into it, volumes of help came pouring from my colleagues, teachers, students and my family members. My dream came true due to their collective efforts. I am indebted to them for extending me their time and support to make this book a reality.

First and foremost, I would like to thank all my teachers for the foundation they helped to lay in shaping my career.

Special thanks to Dr Aasams Jacob for translating the contents and the tables into the digital format. I would like to thank him for his perseverance and commitment.

I would like to thank Dr Vivek Krishnan, Dr Divya Nambiar and Dr Megha Jayaprakash who also helped in typing the contents. I would like to appreciate the sincere efforts of Dr Lekshmi Ammal and Dr Deepti B in the proofreading of the draft of the book. Special thanks to Dr Sreekala MD, for helping me in editing the chapter on PCOS. I would like to appreciate the brilliant efforts of the artists, Dr Renjit Nair and Dr Lekshmi Vijai. I would like to thank Mr Nishanth Rajan for securing the required copyright permissions from the international organizations like FIGO, ASRM and AJOG.

Special thanks to Dr Hafeez Rehman MD (Sunrise Hospitals, Kochi) for contributing many video clips on endoscopic surgery for the DVD. Also, thanks to Dr Beena Guhan MD, DGO, Dr Sumangala Devi, MD, DGO and Dr Jyothy Chandran, MD, DGO (Medical College, Calicut) for providing a number of excellent clinical pictures.

I would like to express my heartfelt gratitude to my brother Bhasi's friend, Prof Mukundan K, who has penned the poem in the fond memory of my brother.

I would like to thank all my family for their love and support. This book would not have been possible but for the great sacrifice from my husband Dr Sivanandan who is a physician and Ex-Major, Indian Army. He committed himself to the fulfillment of the book by benevolently accepting and adjusting to the loneliness created by my unavailability. I could not have been what I am today but for my late parents who were teachers. I remember them at this juncture with great love and affection.

I would like to thank the following for copyrights

1. Giedre Liepyte, Administration Assistant, FIGO—the International Federation of Gynecology and Obstetrics, FIGO "Staging and classification of gynecological malignancies and treatment recommendations"
2. Mitzi Mize, Director of Communications, Eleanor Nicoll, Public Affairs Manager, American Society for Reproductive Medicine
3. Kerry Parker, Rights Assistant, Elsevier Limited (for American Journal of Obstetrics and Gynecology)

I thank M/s Jaypee Brothers Medical Publishers (P) Ltd. for their whole-hearted cooperation in bringing out this book.

And most of all, thanks to all of my patients for helping me to bring this book to life.

Contents

DVD Contents

Basic Surgical Skills

Basic surgical skills form the basis of gynecologic surgery as in any other specialty. Video clips on these skills are provided in a manner which is easy to follow.

Surgical Procedures

High-definition video clips, demonstrating steps of most of the major gynecologic surgeries including endoscopic surgeries, are given in the DVD. Aspiring students can easily learn surgical skills with the help of the DVD.

1 Surgical Anatomy

B Presannakumari

Surgical procedures in gynecology are continuously evolving, demanding knowledge of the anatomy of unfamiliar areas. Understanding anatomy, especially of the pelvis, perineum, abdominal wall and thigh is crucial to the gynecologic surgeon not only for performing difficult surgical procedures like Wertheim's hysterectomy, radical vulvectomy etc but also for routine surgical procedures. The traditionally described anatomy may have individual variations. There can be differing patterns of blood vessels between individuals. Knowledge of congenital anomalies of the genitourinary system which occur in 10% of individuals would prove beneficial in diagnosing and managing them as well as in preventing complications while encountering them during surgical procedures. Distortion of pelvic anatomy associated with endometriosis, pelvic inflammatory disease, previous pelvic surgery as well as adnexal and uterine masses predispose to injuries to ureter, bladder, rectum, pelvic vessels and nerves. Delineating anatomy in these situations helps in preventing visceral injuries to a great extent. Evolution of newer surgical techniques like laparoscopic surgery demands understanding anatomy in a different perspective.

1.1 THE BONY PELVIS

The bony pelvis protects the pelvic viscera as well as provides support by its connections with the muscles and connective tissues of the pelvis. The bony pelvis is formed by the sacrum and coccyx posteriorly and the two innominate bones anterolaterally. The ilium, ischium and pubis together form the hip bone. These three meet at the acetabulum, which is a cup shaped structure into which the femoral head fits. The ischial spine separates the greater sciatic notch from the lesser sciatic notch. In the normal position, the cervix is suspended at the level of the ischial spine. The bony pelvis is divided into an upper false pelvis and a lower true pelvis by the plane of the pelvic brim. The pelvic organs occupy the true pelvis. The pelvic brim is formed by the upper margin of the pubic symphysis anteriorly, iliopectineal line (arcuate line) laterally and the sacral promontory posteriorly. The pelvic cavity is a curved canal like the joint of a drain-pipe, the anterior wall being much shorter than the posterior wall. In the standing position, the pelvic inlet is at about 60° with the horizontal plane while the plane of the outlet is almost horizontal (15-20° with the horizontal).

The sacrum is formed by the fusion of 5 sacral vertebrae and 4 coccygeal vertebrae. The sacral promontory has surgical importance to the gynecologist. The anterior longitudinal ligament is a thick ligament made of dense connective tissue seen in the anterior aspect of the 1st sacral vertebra. In sacral colpopexy, the vaginal apex is fixed to the anterior longitudinal ligament of the first sacral vertebra. It should be kept in mind that the middle sacral artery, a branch of the aorta and the pelvic plexus are encountered in this site. The aortic bifurcation takes place above the sacral promontory at the lower border of the 4th lumbar vertebra. Even though the level of umbilicus can have individual variation, the aortic bifurcation is usually at the level of umbilicus which should be remembered while introducing the primary trochar during laparoscopy.

Through the anterior sacral foramina exits the anterior rami of the corresponding sacral nerves and vessels. The lumbo-sacral plexus lies over the piriformis, which is seen in the posterolateral aspect of the pelvic cavity.

Striated muscles within the investing fascia cover the posterolateral and inferior walls of the pelvis. Posterolaterally, the muscles are the piriformis which arises from the ventral surface of the sacrum. Its tendon exits through the greater sciatic foramen to get inserted to the greater trochanter. It is a lateral rotator of the thigh. Laterally, the obturator internus muscle overlies the ilium, ischium and obturator membrane. Its tendon exits from the pelvis through the lesser sciatic foramen and gets inserted on to the greater trochanter. It is also an external rotator of the thigh. Parietal fascia which is a part of endopelvic fascia covers these muscles. Through its fascial connection to the visceral fascia, the pelvic viscera are indirectly attached to the bony pelvis.

1.1.1 The Ligaments of the Bony Pelvis (Fig. 1.1)

The *sacrotuberous ligament* stretches from the sacrum to the ischial tuberosity. The *sacrospinous ligament* extends from the ischial spine to the lower anterior aspect of the sacrum. The ligament is closely related to the coccygeus muscle which also stretches from the spine to the sacrum. In sacrospinous colpopexy, the vaginal wall is fixed to this ligament. The ligament is approached by dissecting between the rectum and the vagina upwards and backwards. Palpation of the ischial spine helps in identifying the ligament. The

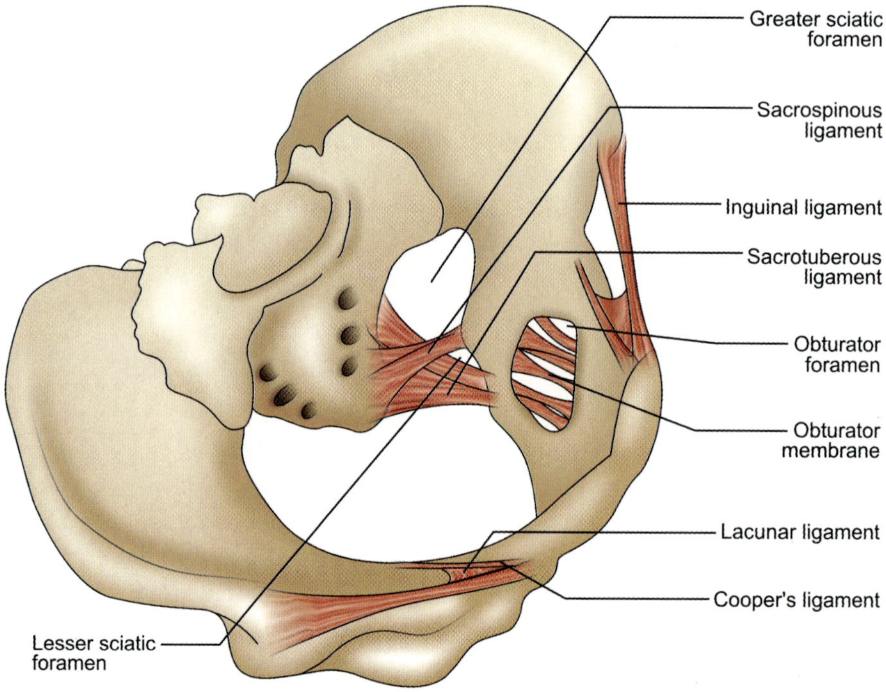

Fig. 1.1: The bony pelvis showing ligaments

ligament can be felt stretching from the spine medially and is widened as it goes medially. Bites from this ligament should be taken at about 2 finger breadths medial to the ischial spine in order to avoid injuries to the pudendal vessels and nerve which passes from behind the ligament and the spine. The inferior gluteal artery which goes posteriorly between the coccygeus muscle and the piriformis can also get injured.

Inguinal ligament: The inguinal ligament is formed by the folded lower edge of the aponeurosis of the external oblique muscle. It stretches between the anterior superior iliac spine and the pubic tubercle. Inferiorly it fuses with the fascia lata. Medially it forms the *lacunar ligament*. Below the inguinal ligament, the femoral vein, artery and the femoral nerve emerges into the thigh. The femoral vessels carry along with it an extension of the fascia, the femoral sheath. Medial to the vein is the femoral canal and lateral to the femoral vein is the femoral artery. The femoral nerve escapes to the thigh and lies outside the femoral sheath.

Lacunar ligament: Lacunar ligament is a triangular ligament which is formed by the deep fibres of the medial end of the inguinal ligament. The sharp lateral edges of the lacunar ligament lies in close apposition to the femoral canal.

Cooper's ligament: The Cooper's ligament is also known as the pectineal ligament. This is the fibrous tissue which stretches along the pectineal line. It is a thickening of the periosteum of the pubic bone. Medially it merges with the lacunar ligament. In Burch colposuspension, the paravaginal and the paraurethral fascia are attached to the Cooper's ligament.

1.2 THE VISCERAL FASCIA AND LIGAMENTS

1.2.1 Pelvic Connective Tissue

Pelvic cellular tissue fills the space between the peritoneum above and the pelvic diaphragm below. This extraperitoneal pelvic cellular tissue condensation forms the ligaments which has a role in supporting the pelvic viscera especially the uterus. Even though visceral connective tissue is continuous and interdependent, De Lancey described three levels of connective tissue support (Fig. 1.2).

Level I—Cervical and upper vaginal support: The cervix and the upper vagina are attached to the pelvic side wall by condensations of visceral pelvic connective tissue called uterosacral and cardinal ligaments (Mackenrodt's ligament).

The *Mackenrodt's ligament* (Cardinal ligament) primarily consists of perivascular connective tissue. It extends from the cervix and the upper vagina to the pelvic side wall. The ureter passes through a tunnel in this ligament during its course from behind forwards to the bladder. At this point the ureter is 1.5-2 cm lateral to the cervix. While clamping the ligament during hysterectomy, injury to the ureter should be avoided by applying the clamp close to the cervix. In type III hysterectomy the ureter is dissected from the ureteric tunnel and the Mackenrodts ligament is clamped and cut lateral to the ureter.

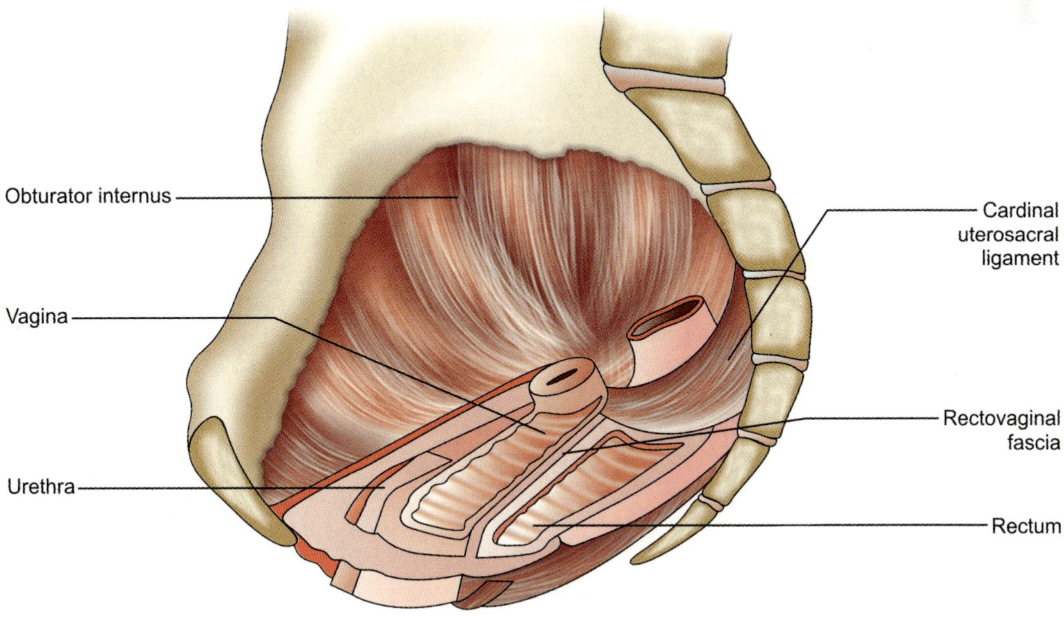

Fig. 1.2: Sagittal view of female pelvis showing the relation of pelvic viscera to endopelvic fascial attachments

Uterosacral ligaments attach the cervix to a broad area of the second and third piece of the sacrum and form the lateral boundaries of the posterior cul-de-sac.

Pelvic cellular tissue on either side of the cervix which harbors the uterosacral and the cardinal ligaments is called the parametrium. The parametrium continues caudally as paracolpos around the vagina.

Level II—Mid-vaginal support: Arcus Tendineus Fascia Pelvis (ATFP) stretches from the pubis to the ischial spine. The anterior vaginal wall is supported by the attachment of the pubovesicocervical fascia to the ATFP. The so called pubovesicocervical fascia is actually the adventitia of the vaginal wall which is made of collagen and elastin and separates the vagina from the bladder and urethra. It should be correctly named as vaginal adventitia. Laterally, this vaginal adventitia is attached to the ATFP and levator ani. The attachment to the levator ani is responsible for bladder neck elevation during increased intra-abdominal pressure. Failure of midvaginal support results in cystocele, rectocele and stress urinary incontinence. Detachment of the fascia from the ATFP results in lateral cystocele. Defects in the middle portion of the fascia results in midline cystocele. Fascial defect at the level of the urethro-vesical junction results in descent of the bladder neck and stress urinary incontinence. The layer of connective tissue intervening between the rectum and vagina is the rectovaginal septum originally described as Denonvillier's fascia. This fascia is attached inferiorly to the perineal body.

Level III—Distal vaginal support: Anteriorly the vagina is attached to the urethra. Laterally it is attached to the pubovaginalis muscle and perineal membrane and posteriorly to the perineal body. In women where perineal body is deficient due to previous obstetric trauma, it can result in gaping introitus and fecal incontinence.

1.2.2 Muscles

The muscles of the pelvis (Figs 1.3 to 1.5) include those of the lateral wall of the pelvis and the pelvic floor. The pelvic floor muscles form an important support for the pelvic viscera. The pelvic diaphragm is the most important structure supporting the pelvic contents. This is a funnel shaped fibromuscular structure composed of the levator ani and the coccygeus muscles along with its covering fasciae.

Levator Ani

The levator ani is the most important support for the pelvic viscera. The muscle complex with its superior and inferior fascial coverings forms the pelvic diaphragm. The urethra, vagina and the anal canal passes through the levator ani which supports these structures. Levator ani is in a constant state of contraction. The tone of contraction will be adjusted depending upon the changes in the intra-abdominal pressure. This helps in reducing the strain on the ligaments which support the pelvic viscera. The muscle originates from the posterior wall of the pubic bone and the tendinous arch (white line) which extends from the pubis to the ischial spine, on the medial side of the obturator internus muscle. The levator ani muscle ends in the vaginal wall, wall of the anal canal, central tendon of the perineum, anococcygeal ligament and coccyx. The muscle includes the pubococcygeus, puborectalis and the iliococcygeus.

The iliococcygeus arise from the arcus tendineus fascia and the ischial spine. The muscle of one side joins that of the other side in the anococcygeal raphi and thus the coccyx.

The puborectalis is the portion of levator ani which arises from either side of pubic bone and form a U-shaped sling behind the ano-rectal junction. It aids in defecation and maintains fecal continence.

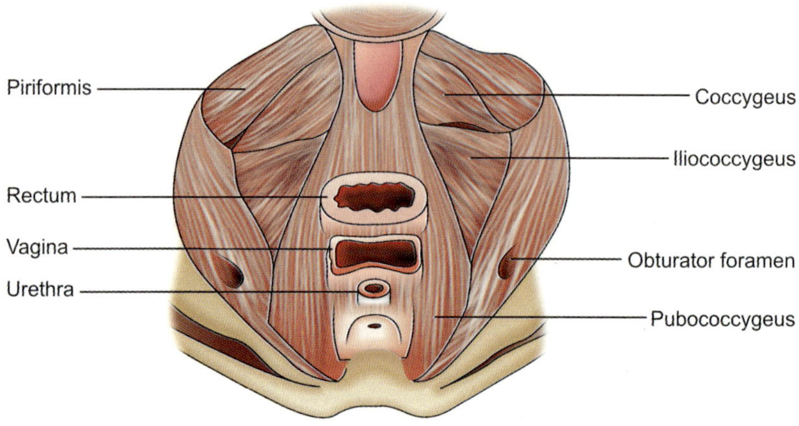

Fig. 1.3: View of the pelvic floor from above showing the relation of the muscles of the pelvic floor to the pelvic viscera and pelvic bone

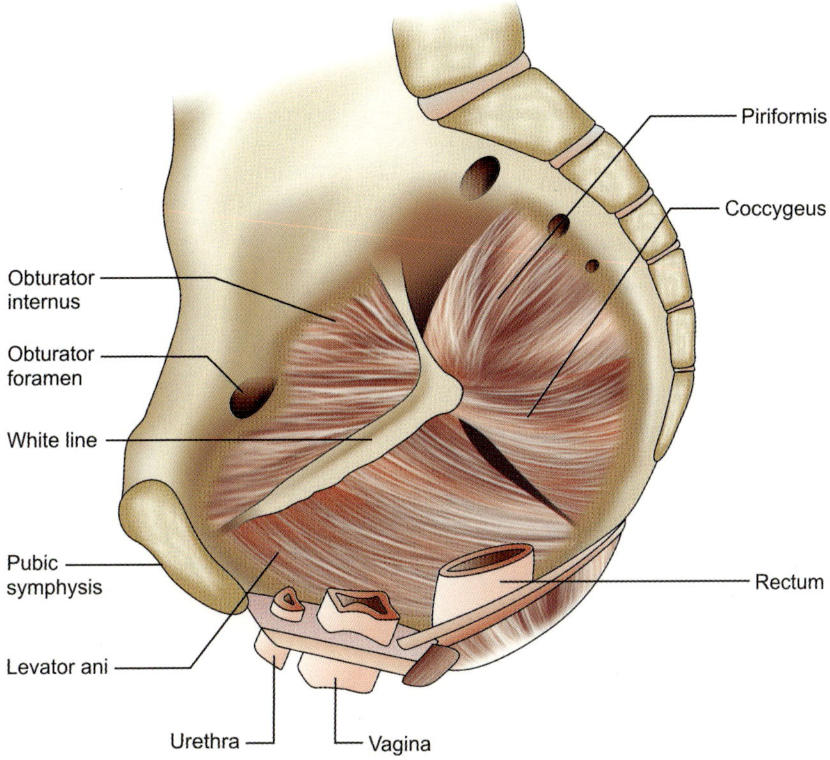

Fig. 1.4: Section of the pelvis showing the muscles of the pelvic floor and side wall

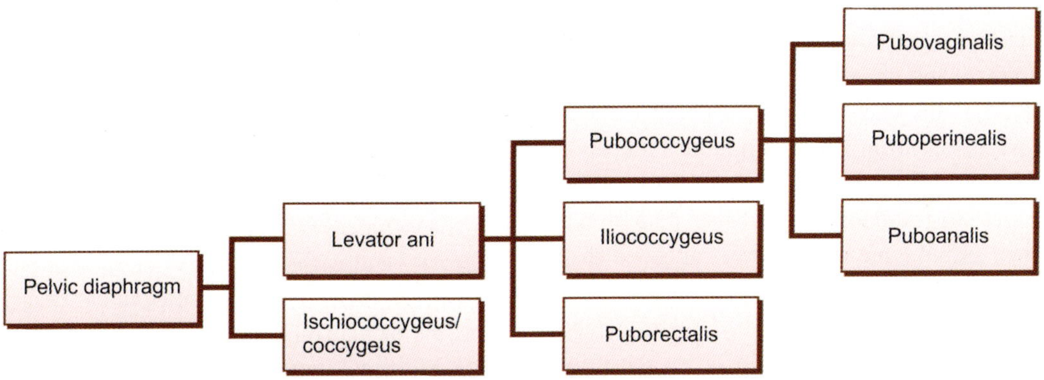

Fig. 1.5: The components of the pelvic diaphragm

By contracting it compresses the anal canal and obliterates it. The nerve supply is by separate branches of S3 and S4. This is called the inferior rectal nerve. In posterior colpoperineorrhaphy, the muscle is plicated in the midline. This procedure is criticized recently as it is alleged to cause dyspareunia.

The pubococcygeus can be divided into pubovaginalis, puboperinealis and puboanalis. Pubovaginalis elevates the vagina during increased intra-abdominal pressure. There is no direct attachment to the urethra, but contractions of pubovaginalis during increase in intra-abdominal pressure elevate the urethra and helps maintain continence. The puboperinealis are the fibres which are attached to the perineal body. The puboanalis is attached to the anal canal between the external and the internal anal sphincter. Contraction of this portion of the muscle causes elevation of the anal canal and helps to close it during increased intra-abdominal pressure and keeps the urogenital hiatus closed.

The Levator Plate

The levator plate lies between the anus and the coccyx and is formed by the tendinous portion of the iliococcygeus muscle. The rectum, upper vagina and the uterus rest on this. When the levator plate is normally supported, it lies in a horizontal position. When the woman is standing, the upper vagina and rectum rests on it. Injuries to levator plate, the commonest cause being child birth, leads to sagging of levator plate and widening of the genital hiatus (Refer Pelvic Organ Prolapse). The levator muscle is supplied by separate branches of S2,4 and 5 whereas the external anal sphincter and the urethral sphincter are supplied by the pudendal nerve. This explains the reason why several women with significant prolapse do not have incontinence and vice versa.

Coccygeus

The coccygeus muscle originates from the ischial spine and the sacrospinous ligament to get inserted to the lateral margin of the 5th sacral vertebra and the coccyx.

1.3 UROGENITAL DIAPHRAGM (PERINEAL MEMBRANE)

The perineal membrane is the fibromuscular connective tissue sheet that stretches between the ischiopubic rami to the distal urethra and vagina. Thus it supports the distal vagina and urethra by indirectly attaching to the bony pelvis. Above this sheet of fibromuscular tissue lies the urogenital sphincter complex. The urogenital sphincter complex consists of the rhabdosphincter and two strap muscles,- the compressor urethrae and urethrovaginal sphincter. The compressor urethrae and the urethrovaginal sphincter were originally named as the deep transverse perineal muscle. The muscle originates from the ischiopubic rami and is supplied by S2,3,4 (pudendal nerve).

Sphincter urethrae (rhabdosphincter) also arise from the medial aspect of ischiopubic rami and get attached to the lower half of the urethra and the vagina. It is a voluntary compressor of the urethra. It is also supplied by the pudendal nerve. The urogenital diaphragm reinforces the pelvic diaphragm. It is intimately related to the vagina and urethra below the level of the levator ani.

1.4 THE PERINEUM

The perineum is the lower most part of the trunk between the buttocks. It is diamond shaped and it extends from the lower margin of the pubic symphysis anteriorly, to the tip of the coccyx posteriorly and the ischial tuberosities laterally. This space can be divided into an anterior urogenital triangle and a posterior anal triangle by an imaginary line extending between the ischial tuberosities which pass across the perineal body.

The Urogenital Triangle

The external genital structures, the vulva and the urethral openings are situated in the urogenital triangle. Behind these external structures lie the superficial and the deep perineal spaces.

1.4.1 The Superficial Perineal Space

This space lies between the deep fascia of the perineum and the perineal membrane. The superficial perineal muscles, the bulb of the vestibule and the vestibular glands occupy this space. The bulbospongiosus muscle extends from the perineal body posteriorly to the dorsal aspect of the clitoris. It is a sphincter of the vagina. The bulb of the vestibule is a 3 cm long highly vascular structure surrounding the vestibule and located under the bulbocavernosus muscle. The muscle compresses the vestibular bulb (Fig. 1.6).

The ischiocavernosus muscle originates from the ischial tuberosity and gets inserted to the ischiopubic rami.

The superficial transverse perineal muscle originates from the ischial tuberosity and is inserted to the perineal body. Pudendal nerve supplies all these muscles.

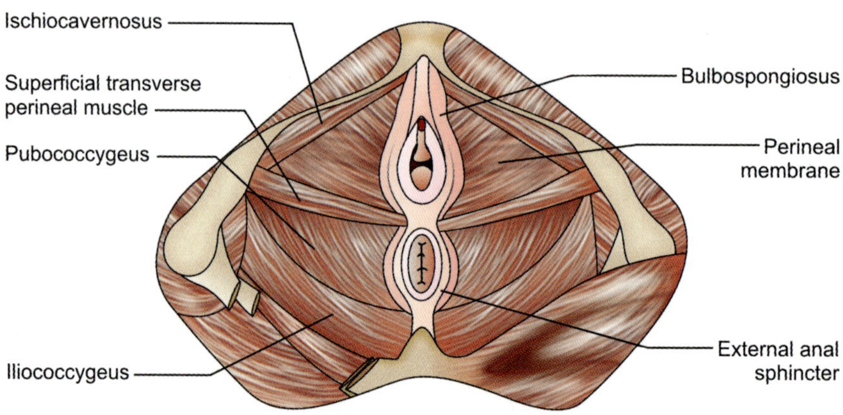

Fig. 1.6: Pelvic diaphragm viewed from below showing superficial perineal muscles and the perineal membrane

Laterally the ischiorectal fossa intervenes between the pelvic diaphragm and the bony pelvis. The fossa on one side is continuous with that of the other side through the posterior aspect. Hence pus from one ischiorectal fossa can track to the opposite side.

The Greater Vestibular Glands (Bartholin's Gland)

These glands are situated one on either side of the vestibule behind the posterior end of the bulb of the vestibule. The glands drain through a duct into the vestibule at a point which corresponds to the junction of the posterior 1/3rd and the anterior 2/3rd of the labia minora. The opening is situated between the hymen and the labia minora. Mediolateral episiotomy should always start from the midline and proceed laterally. If the initial cut is a bit lateral, it may injure the Bartholin's gland duct and the bulb of the vestibule which can cause primary hemorrhage, hematoma formation, gaping of episiotomy wound as well as infection.

1.4.2 Deep Perineal Space

The deep perineal space lies above the level of the urogenital diaphragm. Urogenital sphincter complex which lies above the perineal membrane consists of

1. The external urethral sphincter which surrounds the middle 1/3rd of the urethra
2. The compressor urethrae which arches across the ventral aspect of the urethra
3. The urethrovaginal sphincter which surrounds the ventral aspect of the urethra and terminate in the lateral wall of the vagina.

1.4.3 Perineal Body (Central Tendon of the Perineum)

The perineal body is a pyramidal structure which lies posterior to the lower 1/3rd of the vagina with its apex cephalad. It is formed by the decussation of the superficial muscles of the perineum, the bulbospongiosus, the external anal sphincter, the anterior fibres of levator ani and the superficial transverse perineal muscle. Tearing or stretching of the perineal body during child birth interferes with the support of the lower part of the posterior vaginal wall leading to prolapse and/or fecal incontinence. Hence, tearing of muscles of the perineal body during child birth should be properly repaired.

1.4.4 Blood Supply

The perineum is supplied by the pudendal artery which is the terminal branch of the internal iliac artery. The venous drainage is by the corresponding vein to the internal iliac vein.

1.4.5 Lymphatic Drainage

Superficial and deep compartments drain to the internal iliac group of nodes. Lymphatics of the perineal structures including the lower part of anal canal, vagina and urethra drain to the inguinal lymph nodes. Lymph from the upper part of these viscera drains superiorly into the pelvis.

1.4.6 Nerve Supply

The cutaneous innervation of the vulva is by the branches of the ilioinguinal, genital branch of the genitofemoral and perineal branch of the lateral femoral cutaneous nerve of thigh. The pudendal nerve supplies the muscles of the superficial and deep perineal compartments.

1.4.7 Imaging of the Pelvic Floor

Magnetic resonance imaging can image the levator ani muscle. But the recent introduction of 4D imaging of the pelvic floor muscles has largely replaced MRI.

1.5 THE PELVIC URETER

The gynecologic surgeon should be thorough with the anatomy of the urinary tract due to its close proximity with the ovary, uterus and vagina.

The ureter is 25-30 cm long half of which is in the abdomen and the rest in the pelvis. After emerging from the renal pelvis it courses downward retroperitoneally over the psoas muscle. It enters the pelvis over the bifurcation of the common iliac vessels (Fig.1.7). It then passes postero-medially along the anterior border of the greater sciatic notch in the ovarian fossa and then anteriorly and forwards below the uterine artery. During its course anteromedially, the ureter lies in the substance of the Mackenrodt's ligament (ureteric tunnel) which is about 1.5-2 cm lateral to the cervix. Emerging from the ligament it is in relation to the anterolateral aspect of the vagina (vaginal vault).

The left ureter is more extensively related to the vault than the right due to the dextrorotation of the uterus; the reverse can also happen when the uterus is levorotated. On entering the bladder the ureter courses for about 1.5 cm in the muscular wall of the bladder. The two ureteric openings are about 5 cm apart in a distended bladder and 2.5 cm apart in a non-distended bladder. The blood vessels supplying the ureter are branches from the common iliac, internal iliac, uterine and the vesical arteries which form a plexus in the connective tissue covering of the ureter.

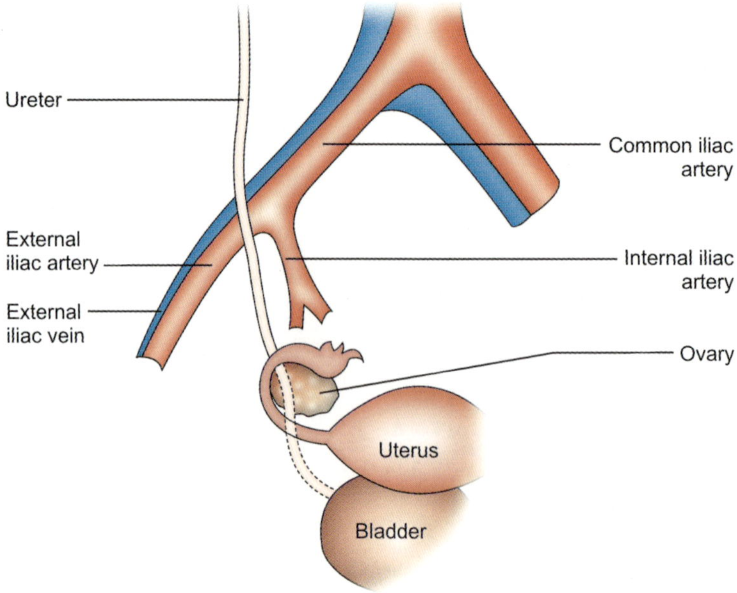

Fig. 1.7: Course of the pelvic ureter

During pelvic surgery the ureter can be identified as it crosses the pelvic brim over the bifurcation of the common iliac. The presence of peristalsis, absence of pulsations and the characteristic feel of quill help in identification of the ureter. When the ureter is caught with the finger and thumb and slipped, it will go with a snap sound which is characteristic. During internal iliac artery ligation the ureter should be identified at the pelvic brim and peritoneum lateral to the ureter should be incised at the level of bifurcation of the common iliac vessels. The ureter with the attached peritoneum should be reflected medially to expose the internal iliac vessels. This will help preserve the blood supply to the ureter.

The ureter is at risk of injury while clamping the infundibulo-pelvic ligament and while clamping and cutting uterine vessels during hysterectomy. The risk of injury is more especially when the anatomy is distorted. In severe endometriosis and in situations where ovarian tumor or fibroid burrows retroperitoneally, the ureter will not be seen in its normal position. In these instances the ureter should be identified by palpation. In severe endometriosis with extensive pelvic adhesions, difficulty in identification of the ureter should be anticipated. Preoperative stenting of the ureter preferably with an illuminated stent would help in identification.

During uterosacral ligament fixation of the vault, the sutures taken higher up are likely to involve the pelvic ureter. Hence cystoscopy should be performed during the procedure to exclude ureter ligation by looking for the ureteric reflux.

Wertheim's hysterectomy necessitates extensive dissection of the ureter predisposing to direct injury, avascular necrosis and fistula formation later on. To avoid this, the ureter should be identified from the pelvic brim and the attachment of the ureter to the medial peritoneal flap should be maintained up to the level of the uterosacral ligament. Afterwards, the ureter needs to be dissected from the Mackenrodt's ligament by opening the roof of the ureteric tunnel. Bleeding from vessels at this point should be meticulously controlled and inadvertent attempts to arrest hemorrhage by blind clamping should be avoided.

During hysterectomy for cervical fibroid, the ureter is likely to be injured because of its close proximity. Identification of the ureter would be easy if hysterectomy is preceded by myomectomy. Broad ligament fibroids will also displace the ureter laterally and can be very close to the tumor. Opening the leaf of the broad ligament will help removal of the fibroid without injuring the ureter.

During vaginal hysterectomy, bladder injury can occur while separating the bladder from the cervix. The portion injured will be near the trigonal area where the ureters traverse through the bladder wall. Suturing should be done after inserting ureteric catheters, lest the portion of the ureter in the bladder wall be likely to be incorporated in the suture.

1.6 THE PELVIC VISCERA

The relations of the pelvic viscera can be understood in the sagittal and coronal sections of the pelvis (Figs 1.8 and 1.9). The vagina extends from the vestibule to the uterus. The

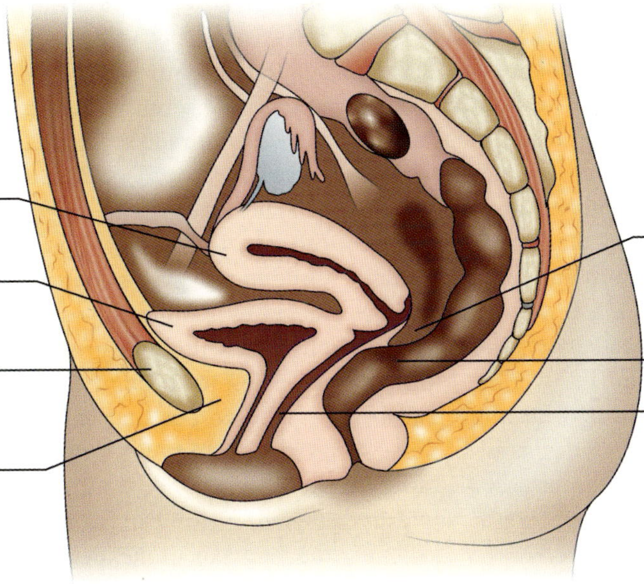

Fig. 1.8: Sagittal section through female pelvis

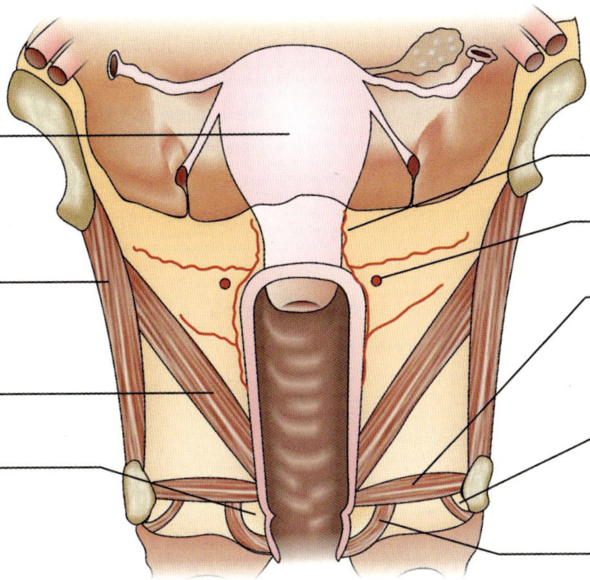

Fig. 1.9: Diagrammatic coronal section through pelvis and perineum

upper vagina is almost horizontal in the standing position and rests on the levator plate. The vaginal wall is composed of the following three layers:

1. **Vaginal epithelium:** The vaginal epithelium is composed of non-stratified squamous epithelium without glands and hence the term vaginal mucosa is a misnomer. The epithelium has transverse ridges formed by the underlying muscular layer. The epithelium is sensitive to estrogen. Under estrogenic influence it undergoes proliferation and maturation in the reproductive period and later atrophy in the post menopausal period with absent or marked reduction of rugae.
2. **Muscle wall:** Outer to the epithelium is the muscular wall of the vagina constituted by the inner circular and outer longitudinal layer.

3. **Adventitia:** The portion of the endopelvic fascia covering the muscular wall of the vagina is the outermost covering of the vagina. Anteriorly, there is no definite supporting layer of endopelvic fascia between the vagina and bladder or urethra. However, thickening of the fascia, the Denonvillier's fascia is seen between the vagina and the rectum above the level of the perineal body.

The upper vagina is supplied by the cervical branches of the uterine; the midvagina by the vaginal artery, a branch of the internal iliac artery and the lower 1/3rd by the pudendal artery and the middle rectal artery. There is a rich anastamosis of vessels supplying the vagina. Multiple vaginal lacerations with uncontrolled bleeding, can be tackled by ligating the internal iliac arteries, as all the vessels supplying the vagina originate from the internal iliac artery.

The upper vagina is innervated by the presacral plexus and the lower vagina by the pudendal nerve.

1.6.1 Uterus

The uterus consists of the uterine body (corpus) and the cervix. The portion of the corpus above the attachment of the round ligament is the fundus. Between the body of the uterus and the cervix is the isthmus. The uterine corpus is covered by peritoneum which is closely adherent to the underlying myometrium of the body of the uterus. Anteriorly, it covers the isthmus and gets reflected (Fig. 1.10) on to the dome of the bladder—uterovesical fold of peritoneum. The uterovesical fold of peritoneum is loosely attached to the isthmus of the uterus with intervening areolar tissue. In abdominal hysterectomy, this loose fold of peritoneum is incised and the urinary bladder with the peritoneum is separated from the cervix before clamping the uterine arteries. Posteriorly, the peritoneum is closely attached to the lower uterine segment, the cervix and the upper vagina and then gets reflected on to the rectosigmoid.

The size of the uterus depends upon the age and reproductive status. The body to cervix ratio is 1:1 in childhood; after puberty, the size of the uterine body increases and the corpus to cervix ratio become 3:1 in the child bearing age group. After menopause the cervix atrophies and become flushed with the vaginal vault.

The corpus and cervix are not usually in the same vertical plane. When the corpus is anteriorly angled with the cervix, it is anteflexion and when it is posteriorly angled, it is retroflexion. The long axis of the vagina and the long axis of the uterus are also not in the same vertical plane. When the long axis of uterus is directed anteriorly, it is anteversion and when it is posteriorly directed, it is retroversion.

1.6.2 Fallopian Tube

The fallopian tubes are tubular structures extending from the cornua laterally. It represents the unfused ends of the Mullerian duct. They usually measure about 10cms in length. The fallopian tube can be differentiated into four regions:

1. **Interstitium:** This is the narrowest portion of the tube and the lumen measures <1 mm in diameter. It is the intramuscular portion of the fallopian tube and starts

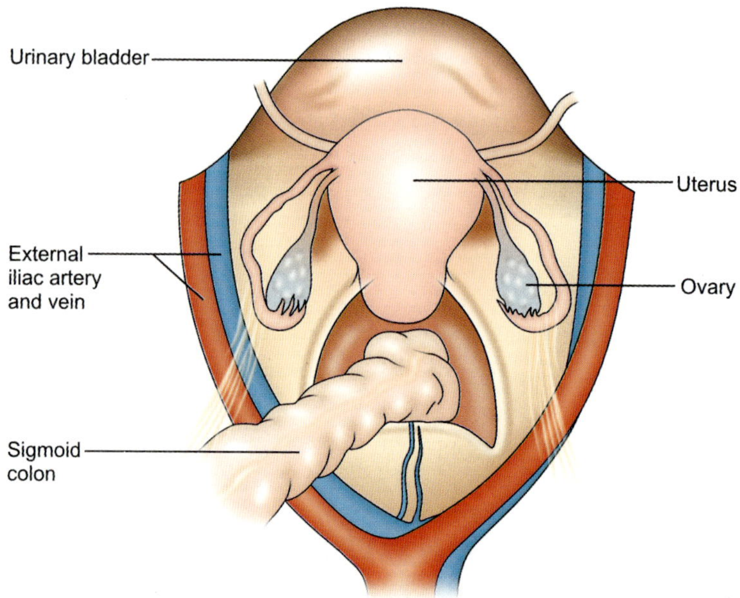

Fig. 1.10: Pelvic viscera viewed through the laparoscope

from the tubal ostia. The direction of the interstitial portion of the tube varies in different individuals.

2. **Isthmus:** This is the narrow segment of the tube which is close to the uterine wall. In female sterilization, the fallope ring or the Hulka clip should be inserted in this region of the tube as failure rate will be less and the chance of successful recanalisation better. This is because recanalisation can be done without luminal disparity if tubotubal anastamosis is done in the isthmial region of the tube.
3. **Ampulla:** This is the longest portion of the tube and is broader than the isthmial region. Fertilization usually takes place in the ampullary region of the tube. This is a common site for ectopic pregnancies.
4. **Infundibulum/fimbrial region:** This is the funnel shaped portion of the tube which opens into the peritoneal cavity. It has numerous finger-like projections which aid in ovum pick up. One fimbria, the fimbria ovarica, is longer and extends to the ovary.

The tube is lined by ciliated columnar epithelium which, along with the peristaltic movement helps in the transport of ovum, sperm and zygote. The muscular wall of the tube consists of inner circular and outer longitudinal layers. The peritoneum of the broad ligaments covers the fallopian tube and is called the mesosalpinx.

The fallopian tube is supplied by uterine and ovarian arteries which form an arterial arcade in the mesosalpinx parallel and below the tube.

1.6.3 Ovaries

The ovaries are situated between the pelvic side wall and the uterus in the ovarian fossa. The double fold of peritoneum which attaches the ovary to the pelvic side wall is the infundibulopelvic ligament. The ovarian artery, which is a branch of the aorta enters the ovary through this ligament. Hence while doing ovariotomy, the pedicle should be carefully ligated especially in the presence of an ovarian tumor where the vessel will be enlarged. The fold of peritoneum which attaches the ovary to the posterior leaf of the broad ligament is called the mesovarium. The medial end of the ovary is attached to the upper and posterolateral aspects of the uterus with the help of the ovarian ligament which is developed from the gubernaculum of the ovary.

The size of the ovary varies with age and functional status. The ovarian size is less in women who are on medication for ovulation suppression and more in those who are on ovulation induction. The normal ovary in the child bearing age group measures 4 × 3 × 2 cm. On cut section the ovarian substance can be differentiated into outer cortex and inner medulla. The cortex harbors the follicles. The medulla which is only a small portion of the ovary near the hilar region is composed of fibromuscular tissue and blood vessels. The peritoneum of the mesovarium is continuous with the outer covering of the ovary which is made up of cuboidal low columnar epithelium.

1.6.4 Urinary Bladder

The urinary bladder occupies the anterior compartment of the pelvis. It is located behind the pubic bone anterior to the cervix and the vagina. The parietal peritoneum gets reflected from the anterior abdominal wall to the dome of the bladder. From the dome of the bladder the peritoneum is reflected on to the isthmus of the uterus. The wall of the bladder which is close to the vagina and cervix is called the trigone of the bladder. During vaginal hysterectomy, the bladder can get injured while separating it from the cervix. Since the portion injured can be near to the ureteral orifice, suturing the bladder defect can occlude the intramuscular portion of the ureter. Hence ureteric stenting is mandatory during the repair of such defects (Figs 1.11 and 1.12).

Retroperitoneal Spaces

The space between the peritoneum of the pelvis above, the pelvic diaphragm below and the bony pelvis on the sides can be divided into potential spaces by the pelvic viscera and the ligaments. These are described below.

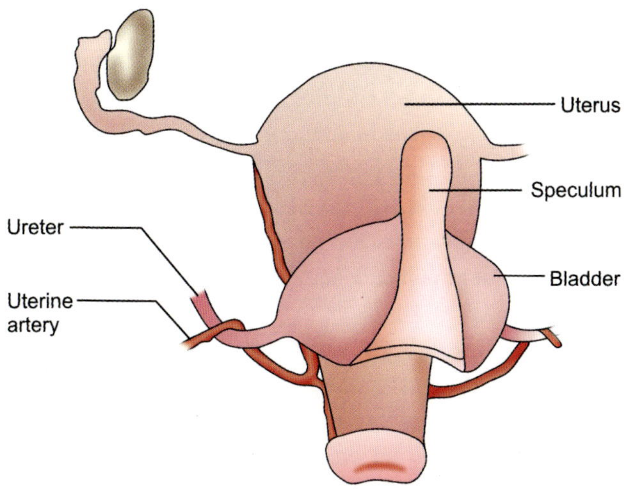

Fig. 1.11: Diagram showing speculum retracting the bladder from the cervix after cutting the vesicocervical ligament during vaginal hysterectomy. As the bladder is pushed and retracted, the ureter will be away from the uterine artery which can be clamped close to the cervix to avoid injury to the ureter

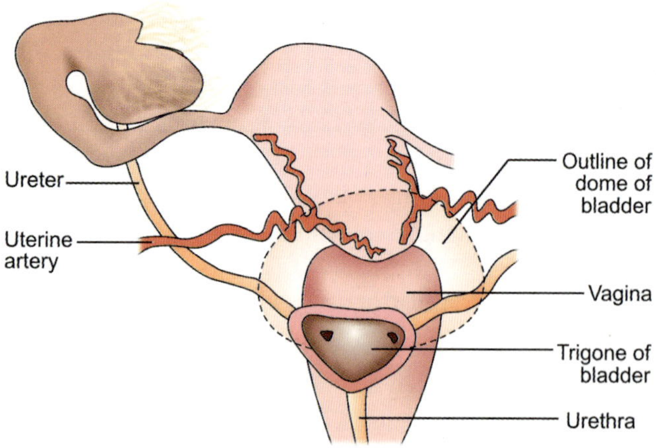

Fig. 1.12: Diagram showing the relation of trigone and dome of the bladder to the vagina and cervix

Prevesical Space (Cave of Retzius)

This is the space between the anterior surface of the bladder and pelvic surface of the pubic bone. It is filled with loose fatty tissue- the retropubic pad of fat. The space is limited inferiorly by the pubourethral ligaments which pass to the lower part of the bladder. Superiorly the space is continuous with the loose extra peritoneal tissue which extends up to the anterior abdominal wall to the level of the umbilicus. Because of this anatomy, the bladder can expand superiorly between the anterior abdominal wall and its peritoneum, up to the level of umbilicus.

In Burch colposuspension the cave of Retzius is entered by separating the bladder and urethra from the pubic symphysis. The medial part of the inguinal ligament, the lacunar ligament and the iliopectineal ligament are identified. The lateral fornix of the vagina is pushed from below and three series of bites are taken from the vaginal adventitia lateral to the bladder, urethrovesical junction and upper urethra and anchored to the iliopectineal ligament with non absorbable or delayed absorbable sutures. Lateral to the lacunar ligament the femoral canal and the femoral vein will be seen and care should be taken not to injure the vein.

While doing TVT insertion for stress urinary incontinence, the ends of the tape are inserted on either side of the mid urethra and traversed through the retropubic space upwards to emerge on either side of the midline about 2.5 cm apart. As the tape is passed through the retropubic space the urinary bladder can be inadvertently injured. However keeping close to the pubic bone will avoid such occurrence. While the tape emerges through the lower abdomen, the inferior epigastric vessels are likely to be injured, which can be avoided by keeping the distance between the emergences of the tape at 2.5 cm.

The trans-obturator tape is maneuvered to emerge through the obturator membrane lateral to the ischio-pubic rami. More lateral and upward steering of the tape can injure the obturator neurovascular bundle.

Paravesical Space

Paravesical space lies between the pelvic diaphragm laterally, the bladder pillar medially, endopelvic fascia inferiorly and the lateral umbilical ligament superiorly.

Vesicovaginal Space

Vesicovaginal space is the space lying between the bladder anteriorly and vagina posteriorly.

Rectovaginal Space

Rectovaginal space lies between the rectum and the vagina and extends from the superior border of the perineal body to the peritoneum of the pouch of Douglas. The rectovaginal septum forms the upper and anterior wall of the space. The rectal wall forms the posterior boundary.

Para-rectal Space

Pararectal spacc is bound by the levator ani laterally and medially by the fascia covering the rectum (rectal pillar).

Retro-rectal Space

This space lies between the rectum anteriorly and the anterior aspect of the sacrum posteriorly.

Presacral Space

Presacral space is the superior extension of the retrorectal space. The middle sacral vessels and hypogastric plexus lies in the loose areolar tissue of the space. In presacral neurectomy, the space is opened. Care should be taken not to injure the presacral vessels during the procedure.

1.7 BLOOD VESSELS OF THE PELVIS

The blood vessels supplying the pelvis are shown in Figure 1.13. The pelvic organs are supplied by the branches of the internal iliac artery. The common iliac artery bifurcates into external and internal iliac arteries over the sacroiliac joint. The external iliac artery courses over the psoas muscle, into the thigh behind the inguinal ligament and is in line with the common iliac artery. The internal iliac artery turns sharply medially and downwards and divides into anterior

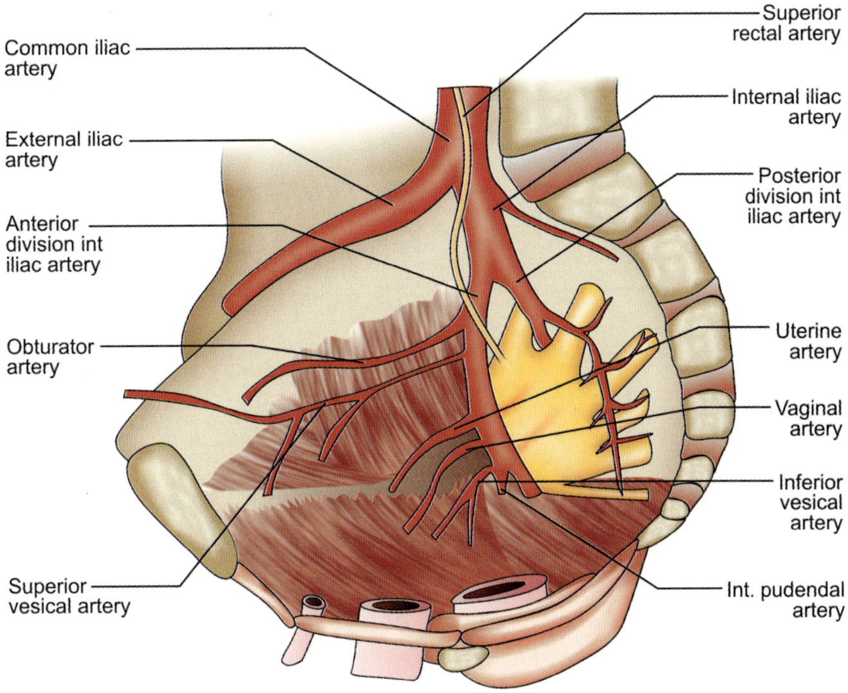

Fig. 1.13: Blood vessels of the pelvis

and posterior branches. The posterior division escapes through the greater sciatic foramen into the gluteal region to supply the gluteus muscle. The anterior division supplies the pelvic viscera and gives off the following branches.

The obturator is the initial branch of the anterior division. It courses through the pelvic side wall along with the obturator nerve and escapes through the obturator fossa. The obturator group of nodes are in relation to the vessel in the obturator fossa. During pelvic lymphadenectomy the obturator node should be removed carefully since serious hemorrhage can be encountered at this site.

The other branches are the uterine, vesical, vaginal, inferior gluteal and the internal pudendal.

Uterine Artery

The uterine artery arises as a branch of the anterior division of the internal iliac artery. It supplies the uterine body, the uterine cervix, the fallopian tubes, and the upper part of the vagina. It gives off two main branches as it crosses anterior to the ureter (Fig. 1.14). From its origin, the uterine artery crosses the ureter anteriorly in the broad ligament before branching at the level of the uterus. One of the major branches passes superiorly over the uterus in a tortuous manner within the broad ligament until it reaches the region of the ovarian hilum where it anastomoses with branches of the ovarian artery. Another branch descends over the uterus to supply the cervix and anastomoses with the branches of the vaginal artery to form two median longitudinal vessels, the azygos arteries of the vagina, which descend anterior and posterior to the vagina. Although there are anastomoses with the ovarian and vaginal arteries, the dominance of the uterine artery is indicated by its marked hypertrophy during pregnancy.

Each uterine artery gives off numerous branches which are also tortuous. These enter the uterine wall, divide and run circumferentially as groups of anterior and posterior arcuate arteries. The branches narrow as they approach the midline and hence the midline of the uterus is less vascular. The left and right arterial arteries anastomose across the midline and unilateral ligation can be performed without serious effects. The arcuate arteries give off radial branches, which pass centripetally through the deeper myometrial layers to reach the endometrium. Terminal branches in the uterine muscle called helicine arterioles are also tortuous. From the arcuate arteries many helical arteriolar rami pass into the endometrium. In the proliferative phase of menstrual cycle, helical arterioles are less prominent, whereas they grow in length and caliber, becoming even more tortuous in the secretory phase.

1.8 NERVE SUPPLY TO THE PELVIC VISCERA

The pelvic viscera are supplied by sympathetic and parasympathetic nerve plexus. The ovaries and fallopian

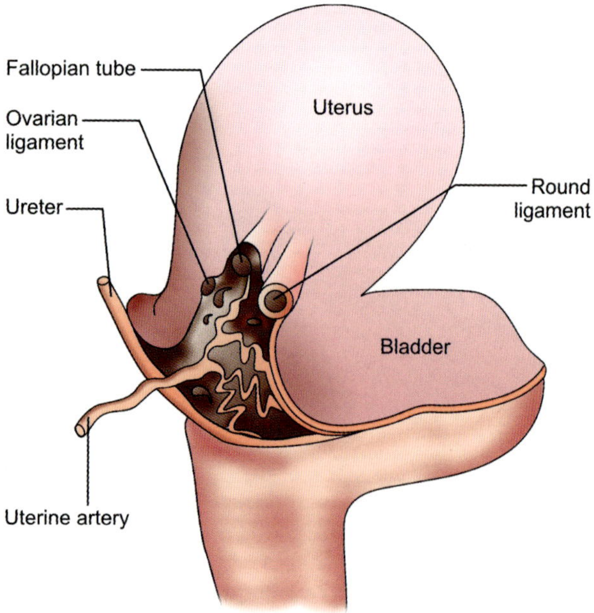

Fig. 1.14: Relation of uterine artery to the ureter. Note the tortuosity typical of the uterine artery

tubes are supplied by the ovarian plexus which originate from the aortic plexus and accompany the ovarian vessels. Thus the parasympathetic supply to the ovary and lateral part of the fallopian tube is from the vagus nerve. The uterine nerve supply comes from the superior hypogastric plexus which lies in the areolar tissue over the 5th lumbar vertebra and sacral promontory. The plexus is in close relation to the presacral artery and is constituted by 2-3 incompletely fused nerve trunks. It is formed of post ganglionic fibres from higher sympathetic ganglia and sacral sympathetic trunk along with visceral afferents. The superior hypogastric plexus thus formed divides into two nerve trunks named as the hypogastric nerves. These nerves proceed to the inferior hypogastric plexus which are located in the pelvic side wall in relation to the internal iliac vessels. The parasympathetic supply to the pelvic organs is from S2,3,4 segments which joins the inferior hypogastric plexus. Thus the inferior hypogastric plexus carries both sympathetic and parasympathetic nerves to the bladder, urethra, rectum, uterus, vagina, clitoris and vestibular bulbs. These nerve fibers are distributed along the blood vessels which supply these organs. The sensory afferent fibers from these organs course through the same pathway.

In presacral neurectomy, a portion of the presacral nerve is dissected and removed at the region of the sacral promontory. Care should be taken to avoid injury to the presacral artery. Presacral neurectomy can interfere with bladder and bowel function as the nerve supplies these organs as well. Hence the alternative procedure advocated is resection of a portion of uterosacral ligament so that interference with bladder and bowel function can be prevented.

1.9 LYMPHATIC DRAINAGE OF THE PELVIS AND THE PERINEUM

Lymphatic Drainage of the Uterus and Cervix

The important group of nodes draining the uterus and adnexa are:

1. Internal iliac
2. External iliac
3. Common iliac
4. Sacral group
5. Inguinal group
6. Pre and para-aortic group

The internal iliac group of nodes: These are found surrounding the internal iliac artery and its branches. They lie in the adipose tissue in between its main branches. The largest and most numerous lie on the lateral pelvic wall, but may be found adjacent to the viscera.

The external iliac group of nodes: They are around 8-10 nodes usually arranged in lateral, anterior and medial groups. The medial group drains the upper vagina and cervix uteri.

Common iliac nodes: Four to six nodes arranged in medial, lateral and intermediate group. Grouped around the artery one or two are found inferior to the aortic bifurcation, anterior to the fifth lumbar vertebra and sacral promontory.

Sacral nodes: This group of nodes found along the medial and lateral sacral vessels, one group in the obturator canal along the obturator artery.

Pre aortic nodes: Lies anterior to the abdominal aorta and receive efferents from the common iliac group of nodes.

1.10 ANTERIOR ABDOMINAL WALL

The muscles of the abdominal wall are:

1. **Rectus abdominis:** The muscle arises from the pubic symphysis and its superior ramus and gets inserted on to the anterior surface of the xiphisternum and the cartilage of 5th-7th ribs.
2. **External oblique muscles:** It originates from the outer surface of 5th-12th rib and is directed downwards , forwards and medially to get inserted on to the iliac crest and pubic tubercle and the free inferior border forms the inguinal ligament.
3. **Internal oblique muscles:** Originates from the anterior 2/3rd of iliac crest and inguinal ligament and gets inserted on to the inferior border of the 10th-12th rib.

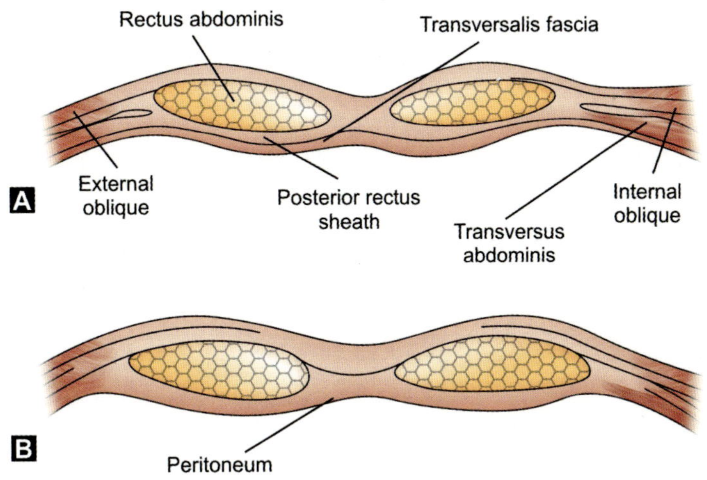

Figs 1.15A and B: Transverse section through the anterior abdominal wall. (A): above the arcuate line (B): below the arcuate line

4. **Transversus abdominis:** Originate from the lower 6 ribs, thoracolumbar fascia, iliac crest and lateral 1/3rd of inguinal ligament. It joins the aponeurosis of the internal oblique and forms the linea alba. The inferior fibres join with the internal oblique forming the conjoint tendon which forms the roof and posterior wall of inguinal canal.
5. **Pyramidalis:** It is a small triangular muscle seen medial and anterior to the lower part of the rectus muscle above the pubic symphysis.

The Rectus Sheath (Figs 1.15A and B)

The aponeuroses of the external oblique, internal oblique and the transverses abdominis join together at the lateral border of rectus muscle and splits into anterior and posterior sheath to enclose the rectus muscle. The two layers fuse in the midline to form the linea alba. Below the arcuate line, all three layers are anterior to the rectus muscle. Hence below the arcuate line the rectus sheath is applied to the transversalis fascia and the peritoneum.

The inferior epigastric vessel (Fig. 1.16) which originates from the external iliac runs superiorly between the peritoneum and the muscle layers of the abdominal wall. It is vulnerable to damage by accessory trocar while performing laparoscopic surgery. Because of its deeper location it cannot be trans-illuminated, but can be identified by locating the lateral umbilical ligament intra-abdominally. The artery will be seen lateral to the lateral umbilical ligament. Hence the accessory trocar entry should be either medial to the lateral umbilical ligament or far lateral to it.

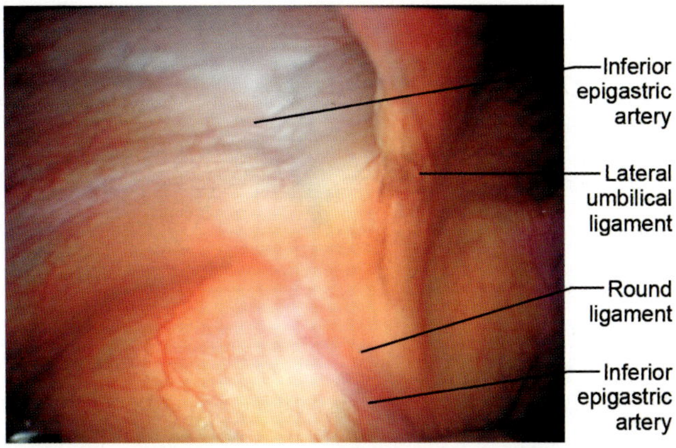

Fig. 1.16: Laparoscopic view of inferolateral anterior abdominal wall showing the relation of inguinal canal, inferior epigastric artery and lateral umbilical ligament. The lateral umbilical ligament is formed by the obliterated umbilical artery which lies medial to the inferior epigastric artery

In low transverse incisions, it can be injured if the extent of the incision goes far laterally.

1.11 CONCLUSION

Understanding relevant anatomy is a must for all gynecologic surgeons. Learning anatomy should be an ongoing process which should begin while assisting experienced surgeons and should be periodically reviewed by dissecting cadaveric specimens when newer techniques are adopted. The surgeon should be able to identify the different structures by their characteristic appearance and feel because distortion of anatomy can be encountered very often. Complications of surgery can be prevented to a great extent if the surgeon is thorough with the anatomy and is able to identify the different structures by their nature.

2 Embryology of the Female Genital Tract and its Congenital Anomalies

B Presannakumari

2.1 INTRODUCTION

Knowledge of the embryology of the female genital tract forms the basis for understanding its congenital defects as well as for correcting such defects. Defects in the genital tract are seen in 10% of female infants.

2.2 DEVELOPMENT OF THE UTERUS (FIGS 2.1 AND 2.2A TO C)

There is a close relation between the reproductive tract and the urinary tract during the early intra-uterine life. Both develop from a common mesodermal ridge which runs along either side of the midline in the posterior abdominal wall. At the 5th embryonic week, the nephrogenic cord develops from the mesoderm and forms the urogenital ridge and mesonephric duct. The mesonephros is an oval structure seen on either side of the midline. Two pairs of genital ducts develop in male as well as female individuals, which are known as the Wolffian ducts or the mesonephric ducts and the Mullerian ducts or the paramesonephric ducts respectively. The uterus, fallopian tubes and most of the vagina are derived from the mullerian duct. These ducts are formed as a result of invagination of the mesothelium of the coelomic cavity in the ventral part of the intermediate cell mass. Under the influence of gonadal hormones, further development of para-mesonephric and mesonephric ducts occur. In the absence of anti mullerian factor, the para-mesonephric duct develops into the uterus, cervix and the upper vagina. The cephalic ends of the duct remain separate and form the fallopian tubes. The middle portion runs ventral to the mesonephric duct, towards the midline and meets that

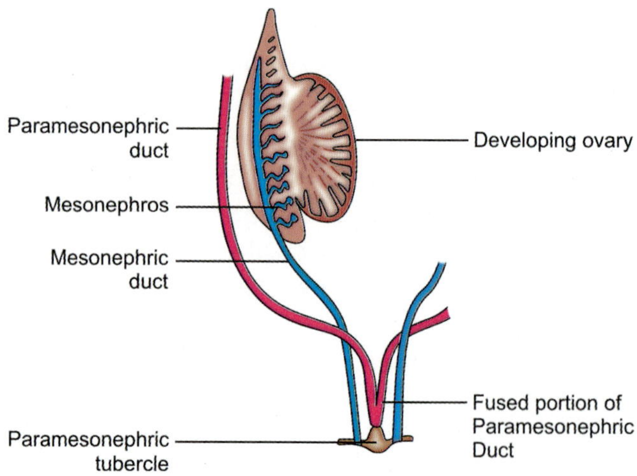

Fig. 2.1: The development of the uterus.The mullerian ducts and the mesonephric ducts are seen. The developing ovary is seen medial to the mesonephros

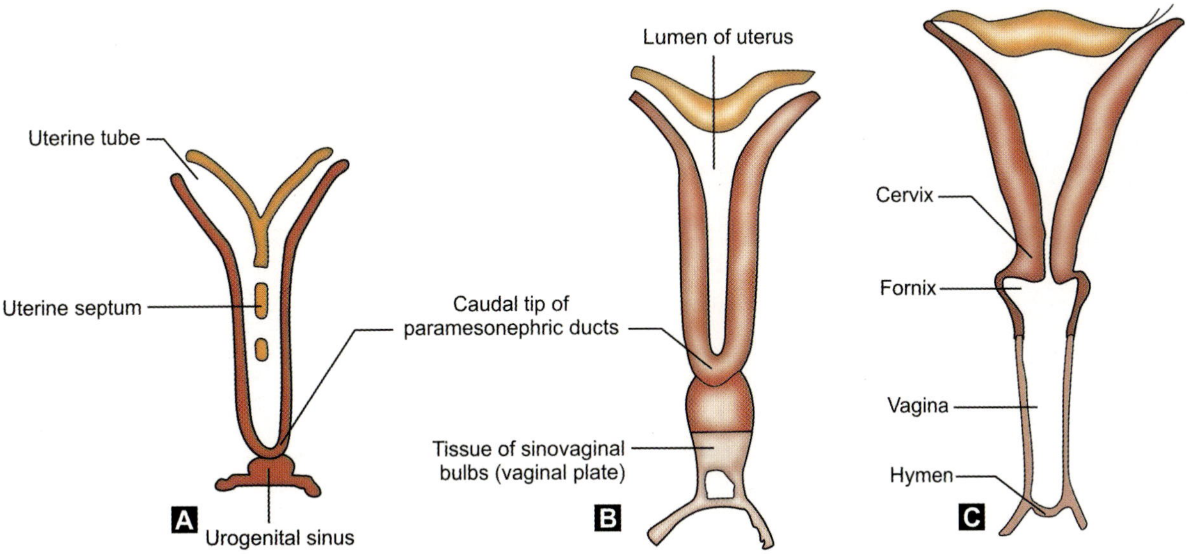

Figs 2.2A to C: Formation of the uterus and vagina. (A) 9 weeks. Note the disappearance of the uterine septum. (B) At the end of the third month. Note the tissue of the sinovaginal bulbs. (C) Newborn. The fornices and the upper portion of the vagina are formed from the fused lower end of paramesonephric duct, and the lower portion of the vagina is formed from the sinovaginal bulbs

of the opposite side. As the ovary descends to the pelvis, the fused portion forms the uterus, cervix and the upper vagina. Along the length of fusion, a midline septum will be present initially, which later disappears at about the 20th week of intrauterine life. The uterus can be identified as early as the end of the 3rd month. In the early stages of development, the uterus is bicornuate. The upper ends of the un-fused Mullerian duct form the abdominal ostia of the fallopian tubes. The Wolffian structures regress due to lack of testosterone. Remnants of these persist in the female as epoophoron and paroophoron.

The mesenchyme surrounding the Mullerian duct forms the muscular part of the uterus, the myometrium and its peritoneal covering forms the perimetrium. As the Mullerian ducts come to the midline it draws a peritoneal fold along with it medially .This fold becomes the broad ligament of the uterus. The fallopian tube will occupy its upper border and the ovary lies on its posterior surface. The formation of the uterus and broad ligaments divide the pelvic cavity into a posterior utero-rectal pouch and an anterior utero-vesical pouch.

The tip of the combined ducts projects into the posterior wall of the urogenital sinus forming the paramesonephric or the Mullerian tubercle. The upper end of the mesonephric duct forms the definitive kidney. When there is unilateral aplasia or hypoplasia of the Mullerian duct it can be associated with renal aplasia of the same side. The kidney develops at a lower level than the gonads and ascends in later fetal life. Failure to ascend would result in pelvic kidney.

An outgrowth from the lower end of the mesonephric duct develops into the ureter.

2.3 DEVELOPMENT OF THE VAGINA AND VULVA (FIGS 2.2A TO C)

The part of the hindgut caudal to the attachment of the allantoic diverticulum is called the cloaca. By the 7th week, these parts are separated from each other by the formation of the urorectal septum (Figs 2.3 and 2.4), which later gives rise to the perineal body. The ventral sub division is called primitive urogenital sinus and the dorsal part, the primitive rectum. Extension of the urogenital sinus to the cloacal membrane occurs. An ectodermal anal pit forms and meets the anorectal canal which later canalizes to form the anal canal.

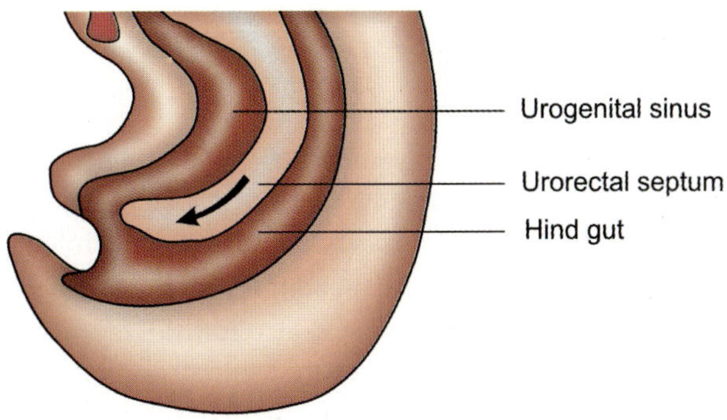

Fig. 2.3: Development of the urorectal septum which separates the bladder and the vagina from the rectum and anal canal

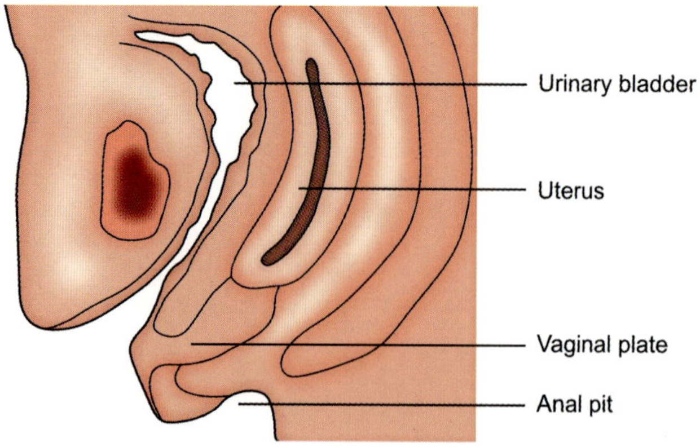

Fig. 2.4: The non-canalized stage in the development of the vagina. The anorectal canal is near the anal pit, but has not reached it

The vagina develops from two sources; the lower ends of the uterovaginal canal and the pelvic portion of the urogenital sinus. In the region where the utero-vaginal canal reaches the pelvic portion of the urogenital sinus, the endoderm of the urogenital sinus will be stimulated to form two outgrowths named the sino-vaginal bulbs. Later, a solid vaginal plate is formed, which is derived partly from the mesoderm of utero-vaginal canal (Mullerian tubercle) and partly from the sinovaginal bulbs. This plate then proliferates and elongates in both directions. Finally, vagina is formed by canalization of vaginal plate, which begins from the upper portion and then extends caudally forming the vaginal introitus. The canalization will be complete by 20 weeks of gestation.

The upper three quarters of the vagina develops from the fused mullerian ducts and the lower quarter from the sino-vaginal bulbs. The hymen represents the remnant of the fused sino-vaginal bulbs and the mullerian tubercle (the vaginal plate). The epithelium of the vagina and the portio-vaginalis of cervix are derived from an up growth of the urogenital sinus.

The vulva is developed from the urogenital sinus.

2.4 DEVELOPMENT OF THE EXTERNAL GENITALIA (FIG. 2.5)

Simultaneous with the development of the internal duct system, the external genitalia develops. The urinary tract and the genital tract open between the genital folds, by canalization of the urogenital membrane. Paired genital folds develop on either side of the urogenital membrane. Proliferation of tissue outer to the genital folds develops into the genital swellings. The genital tubercle which develops in the midline anteriorly forms the clitoris, the genital folds form labia minora and the genital swellings, the labia majora. In the male, the genital tubercle develops into glans, the genital folds into penis and urethra, and the genital swellings into scrotum. Virilization of external genitalia depends on the production of dihydrotestosterone. In the absence of dihydrotestosterone, even a male fetus will have female type of external genitalia as it is the neutral norm.

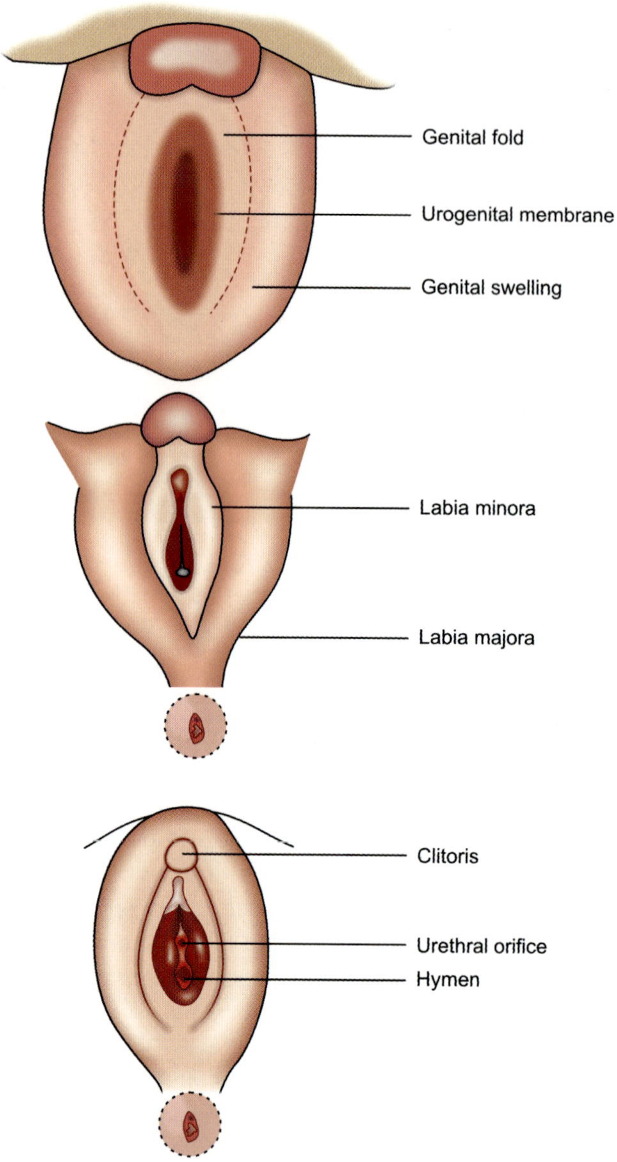

Fig. 2.5: Development of female external genitalia

2.5 DEVELOPMENT OF THE OVARIES

The sex of the embryo is determined at the time of fertilization. Ovary develops at a later stage in the development of an embryo with 46,XX chromosome compliment and no Y chromosome *(Sexual differentiation is dealt with in the chapter on Primary amenorrhea).* The morphological differentiation of the ovary starts 2 weeks later than the development of the testis. The ovarian development occurs from three sources; the coelomic epithelium of the genital ridge, the mesenchyme of the genital ridge and the germ cells which migrate from the yolk sac through the dorsal mesentery. The genital ridges are formed by the thickening of the coelomic epithelium on the medial side of the mesonephros, which occurs at about the 6th week of intrauterine life. Very soon it develops a mesentery of its own, called meso-ovarium, attached to the intermediate cell mass. The infundibulopelvic fold passes upwards from the upper pole of the ovary and it contains the ovarian vessels and nerves. Ovarian vessels arising from the abdominal aorta indicate the lumbar position of the upper part of genital ridge. The genital fold of ovary passes from its lower pole to the internal abdominal ring below. The part of the genital fold proximal to its interfusion with Mullerian duct becomes the ovarian ligament while the distal portion becomes the round ligament.

Cords of cells, the sex cords or medullary cords proliferate from the germinal epithelium and grow into the underlying mesoderm. Primordial germ cells, formed in the yolk sac migrate along the dorsal mesentery to the genital ridges and give rise to oocytes. The sex cords become broken up into small masses. The cells of each mass surround one primordial germ cell or oocyte to form the primordial follicle. The surrounding mesenchyme becomes the stroma. The ovary descends from its original lumbar position, so that at term it lies at the level of the pelvic brim.

The 1st meiotic division of the oocyte begins by the 20th week of intra-uterine life, but gets arrested in the prophase until ovulation occurs. The 2nd meiotic division occurs only at fertilization when the sperm penetrates the zona pellucida. The fetal ovaries contain 7 million follicles at the 20th week of intra uterine life, which later degenerate and reduce to 2 million follicles at birth. Of these 300 to 400 ovulate during the life span of a woman.

2.6 DEVELOPMENTAL ABNORMALITIES OF THE MULLERIAN DUCT

A large variety of developmental abnormalities can occur ranging from total non development of the Mullerian duct to different varieties of lateral fusion defects or incomplete canalization due to dys-regulation of mullerian duct development. Each anomaly is distinctive; some are common while others are very rare. There can be different combinations of the anomalies of the uterus, vagina and vulva. Moreover mullerian anomalies can be associated with anomalies of other systems, commoner being those of urinary and skeletal systems.

2.6.1 Incidence

The incidence reported by Grimbiz[1] et al is 4.3% among fertile women, 3-6% among infertile women and 5-10% among women who had recurrent abortion.This shows that mullerian anomalies cause recurrent abortion rather than infertility.

2.6.2 Associated Anomalies

Approximately 1/3rd of women who have complete vaginal agenesis will have associated renal anomalies. The renal anomalies reported include unilateral renal agenesis, unilateral or bilateral pelvic kidney, horseshoe kidney and a variety of patterns of urethral hypoplasia or duplication. Women with partial vaginal agenesis also may have associated urinary tract anomalies.

Associated skeletal anomalies are seen to occur in about 12% of women. The skeletal anomalies include anomalies of vertebral column, limbs or ribs. Other rare associated anomalies include congenital cardiac anomalies, absence of a digit or syndactyly.

2.6.3 Etiology of Mullerian Anomalies

The exact etiology of Mullerian anomaly is not known. The possibility of a genetic background is being studied. The etiological factors suggested are the following.

1. Inappropriate Mullerian inhibiting factor production.
2. Regional deficiency of estrogen receptor.
3. Teratogenic insult during 37th to 41st day.
4. Sporadic gene mutation.

Depending upon the type of Mullerian anomaly and the other associated anomalies, the presentation can vary. If there is associated obstruction of bladder or bowel, the condition will be noticed even in the newborn period. Children with obstruction to the menstrual flow usually present at puberty as cryptomenorrhea. Patients with anomalies of the vulva and presence of incomplete vaginal septum usually present in adulthood due to coital problems. Presence of lateral fusion defects can cause infertility, repeated abortions, retained placenta or malpresentations.

The true incidence of anomalies is difficult to estimate.

Women with Mullerian duct anomalies have higher incidence of infertility, repeated abortions, preterm labor, fetal growth retardation, fetal malpresentations and retained placenta. Hence identification of anomalies and treatment with surgical correction is important. By imaging, the surgically correctable types can be distinguished from uncorrectable types.

2.6.4 Classification of Uterovaginal Anomalies (Fig. 2.6)

Previously uterovaginal anomalies were classified based on clinical findings. The understanding of embryology has enabled classification on an embryologic basis. The American Fertility Society has classified these anomalies into VII types which are shown in Table 2.1. Mullerian anomalies can result from abnormality of lateral fusion of the two mullerian ducts or abnormality of vertical fusion (abnormal fusion between the down-growing mullerian duct and the up-growing derivative of the urogenital sinus). The American Fertility Society classification is just a framework; not all anomalies will fit neatly into one of its classes. Moreover innumerable anomalies may be encountered in practice.

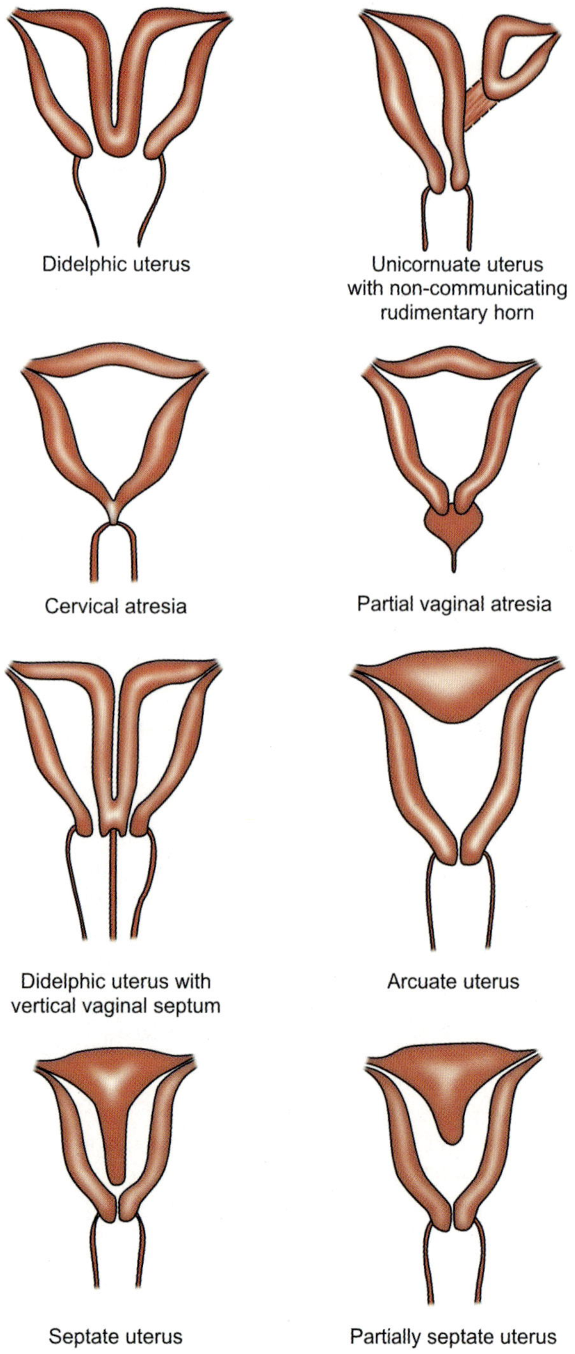

Fig. 2.6: Common types of uterine anomalies

Table 2.1: American Fertility Society classification of mullerian anomalies

Category	*Anomaly*
Class I	**Segmental, Mullerian agenesis-hypoplasia**
	A. Vaginal
	B. Cervical
	C. Fundal
	D. Tubal
	E. Combined anomalies
Class II	**Unicornuate**
	A. Communicating
	B. Non-communicating
	C. No cavity
	D. No horn
Class III	**Didelphis**
Class IV	**Bicornuate**
	A. Complete (division down to internal os)
	B. Partial
Class V	**Septate**
	A. Complete (septum to internal os)
	B. Partial
Class VI	**Arcuate**
Class VII	**Diethylstilbestrol related**

Adapted with permission from the American Fertility Society Classification of Mullerian anomalies Fertil Steril 1988;49:944.

Appropriate description of the defect helps to direct treatment and is especially important, given the distinct differences in interventions between the different anomalies.

Meyer-Rokitansky-Kuster-Hauser Syndrome (Congenital Absence of the Uterus and Vagina)

The most commonly encountered abnormality in the development of the uterus and vagina is congenital absence of the uterus and vagina, known as *Meyer-Rokitansky-Kuster-Hauser syndrome*. These girls will have normal karyotype and normally developed ovaries as well as normal secondary sexual characteristics. They usually present in adolescence with complaints of not having attained menarche. They may also have associated skeletal or urologic abnormalities. The former include rudimentary vertebral bodies, supernumerary vertebrae, syndactyly, or absence of a digit. The usual renal anomalies are unilateral renal agenesis, bilateral/unilateral pelvic kidney, horse shoe kidney, hydronephrosis, hydroureter and a variety of ureteral duplication. Rarely congenital heart disease and inguinal hernias can be associated with the syndrome. A genetic basis is being investigated for the syndrome. It is postulated that the etiology may be teratogenic insult during the development of Mullerian duct (37th-41st gestational days).

Disorders of Lateral Fusion

Lateral fusion defects can be divided into symmetric and asymmetric groups and are further subdivided into obstructive and nonobstructive categories, based on whether they result in obstruction to menstrual flow. These defects occur by means of arrests in different stages of mullerian duct development. In general, the arrested stages include incomplete fusion of the caudal mullerian ducts, failed septum resorption, and defective development of all or part of a duct.

Symmetric lateral non fusion results in the following types of anomalies:

1. Didelphic uterus
2. Septate uterus
3. Bicornuate uterus
4. T shaped uterus (DES exposure *in utero*)
5. Arcuate uterus

In didelphic uterus, there will be two separate uterine bodies and two separate cervices, which will be widely placed. In septate uterus the cavity will be divided into two by a midline septum, which can be complete or partial. Rarely, the cervix may also be septate but the two cervical canals will be close together. The complete septum in the uterus might extend to the introitus as a longitudinal vaginal septum.

In bicornuate uterus there will be separation of the cavity as well as the uterine wall. Bicornuate uterus can also be partial or complete (Figs 2.7A and B). In the complete forms there will be separation up to the level of the internal os. In the partially bicornuate uterus the separation will be incomplete.

Uterus didelphis, septate uterus and bicornuate uterus can be associated with partial or complete longitudinal vaginal septum. The T shaped uterus may be hypoplastic and irregular and is usually seen associated with diethyl stilbestrol exposure in utero. The arcuate uterus refers to the presence of a small septum in the uterine fundus with no clear separation of the uterine cavities.

When there is *asymmetric* disorder of lateral fusion, it results in obstruction. Unilateral mal-development of the Mullerian duct will be invariably associated with absence of ipsilateral kidney.

The following are the usual types of asymmetric anomalies:

1. Unicornuate uterus and a non-communicating horn having functioning endometrium.
2. Unilateral obstruction of a cavity of a double uterus.
3. Unilateral obstruction of septate vagina.

Disorders of Vertical Fusion

Defective vertical fusion between the Mullerian duct component and the urogenital sinus component can result in disorders characterized by an atretic portion of the vagina. The length of this atretic portion can vary from a large segment of the vagina to a thin obstructive membrane. These types of anomalies can also be of the obstructive or non obstructive type. In the obstructive type the atretic portion will be complete resulting in collection of menstrual effluent

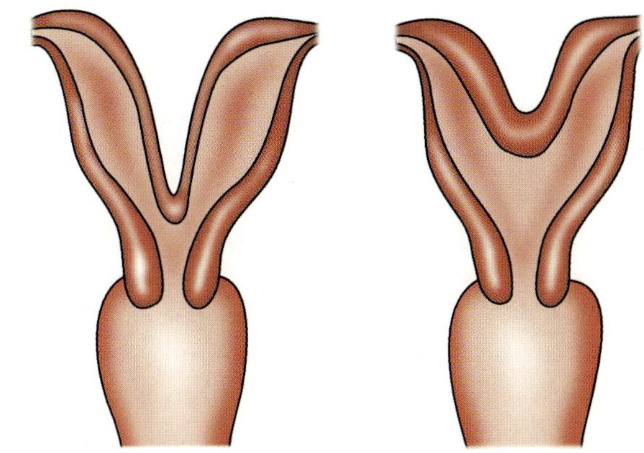

Fig. 2.7A: Complete and partial bicornuate uterus

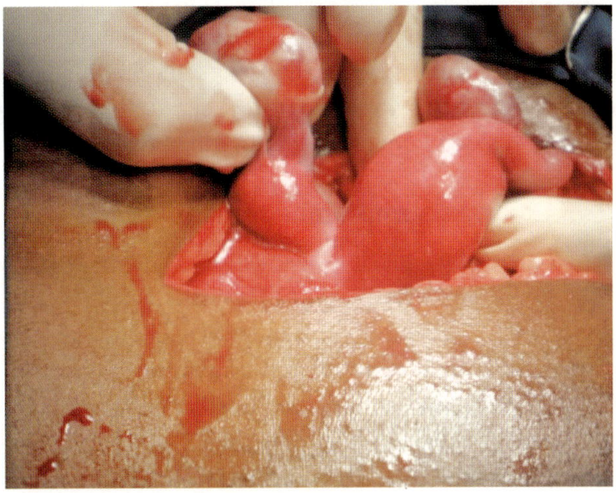

Fig. 2.7B: Partial bicornuate uterus with under developed right horn in a lady who presented with primary infertility

in the portion cephalad. In the non obstructive type, there can be patent regions through which menstrual blood can come out, so that these patients will present with coital problems or infertility.

Vaginal Atresia

When the atretic portion is thin, it can result in a transverse vaginal septum, which can vary in thickness and can be at any level in the vagina (Fig. 2.13). Lodi reported that 46% occur in the upper vagina, 40% in the mid-vagina and 14% in the lower vagina. The lower surface is covered by squamous epithelium. The upper surface is usually covered with columnar epithelium which will be converted to squamous epithelium after correction. In the neonatal period, infants with this type of septum can develop collection of mucous or even blood due to the withdrawal of maternal hormones following delivery.

Abnormalities of Cervical Development

Abnormalities of development of the cervix include cervical dysgenesis and agenesis.

Cervical agenesis denotes non-development of the cervix while cervical dysgenesis is abnormally developed cervix. This can be of different types. The cervical tissue may be present in varying proportions with non developed cervical canal.

Isolated abnormality of cervical development (Class Ib) is rare and usually occurs in association with complete or partial vaginal agenesis. Abnormalities of cervical development also include defects involving the length, width, and/or size of the cervix.

Abnormalities of Fallopian Tube Development

Isolated abnormality of fallopian tube development is rarely encountered. These abnormalities include fallopian tube duplication, absent muscular layer, ectopic location, luminal atresia, and absent ampulla with blind fimbrial end.

2.6.5 Diagnosis and Management

Uterine anomalies causing obstruction to menstrual flow cause symptoms shortly after menarche and hence will present early. The typical presentation is with cyclical lower abdominal pain followed by retention of urine resulting from obstruction to the urethra caused by haematocolpos. Adolescents in the pubertal age group presenting with cyclical lower abdominal pain and retention of urine should raise the suspicion of haematocolpos. At times, on evaluation of anomalies of the urinary tract, uterine anomalies may be diagnosed. Anomalies which do not cause obstruction to the menstrual flow may go unnoticed but will be diagnosed on routine ultrasound examination. In the antenatal period presence of uterine anomaly can be suspected by the abnormal uterine shape with or without associated mal-presentation. On occasions, the anomaly happens to be diagnosed while routinely examining the adnexa during cesarean section. If the fallopian tube and ovary are not seen on one side, it could be a bicornuate uterus with the non-pregnant horn deep in the pelvis. Hence in such situations it is mandatory that a rudimentary horn and adnexa be looked for in the pelvis. Rarely these women will present with dysmenorrhea or menorrhagia. Women having septate vagina can present with coital problems. If a perforated septum is located higher up in the vagina, it can cause infertility even in the absence of cryptomenorrhea or coital problems.

Most patients with uterine anomalies are able to conceive but may have repeated abortions, preterm labour or cesarean section for an abnormal presentation like breech or transverse lie and retained placenta. Uterine anomaly is found to exist in 10% of women with recurrent abortions. Early second trimester abortion is characteristically associated with uterine anomalies. The cause of abortion may be abnormal implantation of the placenta on the poorly vascularized septum, inadequate space for fetal growth or associated cervical incompetence. The obstetric outcome in patients with didelphic uterus will be better than those with septate uterus. Even though these patients are prone for abortions and preterm labor, the subsequent pregnancies will reach more maturity.

Anomalies like didelphic uterus can be diagnosed by speculum examination. The two cervices can be clearly identified. Didelphic uterus can be associated with longitudinal vaginal septum. Women with perforated transverse vaginal septum will not have cryptomenorrhea and will be presenting later in life with coital problem or infertility. The septum will be quite obvious on inspection.

Diagnostic Imaging

Most anomalies can be diagnosed by TVS. Septate uterus can be imaged in the semi-axial plane by the transvaginal probe. There will not be myometrial separation, but the two uterine cavities will give an owl's eye appearance (picture provided in the chapter on ultrasound). Ultrasound examination should preferably be performed in the secretory phase for better delineation of the endometrial cavities. The two uterine bodies of bicornuate uterus can also be made out by TVS. If there is doubt, 3D ultrasound is a very effective tool for the diagnosis. A sensitivity of 93% and a specificity of 100% have been achieved with 3 D ultrasound in experienced hands.[2] Unicornuate uterus should be suspected by the fusiform shape of the uterus as well as by finding the deviation of the uterine body to one side of the pelvis. 3D ultrasound will help confirm the diagnosis. Mullerian agenesis can be diagnosed by the absence of uterus and presence of ovaries on imaging. Laparoscopy is not necessary for the diagnosis.

MRI for the diagnosis of uterine anomaly has greatly been replaced by 3D ultrasound. However, complicated asymmetric anomalies can be convincingly diagnosed only by MRI.[3] MR imaging is reported to have 100% accuracy in diagnosing mullerian anomalies.

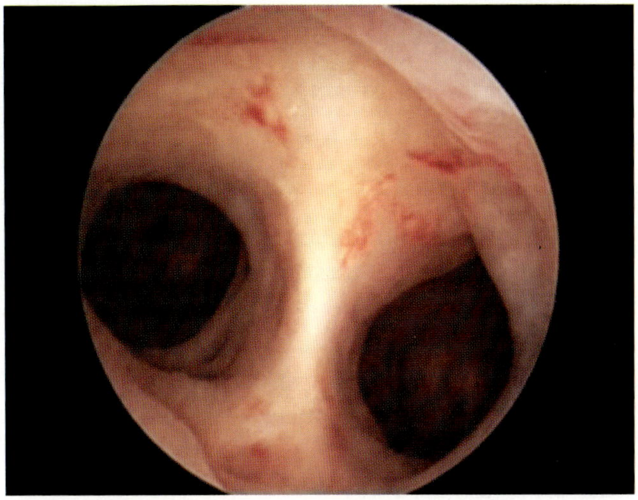

Fig. 2.9: Hysteroscopic picture showing uterine septum

Hysterogram

Anomalies like septate uterus and bicornuate uterus can be diagnosed by hysterogram. However distinction between the two cannot be made out by hysterogram as both will show two uterine cavities. The angle between the long axes of the uterine cavities will be less than 90° in septate uterus and more than 90° in bicornuate uterus as well as in septate uterus having thick vaginal septum[4] (Figs 2.8A and B).

Hysteroscopy

Hysteroscopy is helpful in diagnosing as well as treating uterine septum (Fig. 2.9). However, hysteroscopy will not help to differentiate between septate and bicornuate uterus. The septum can be resected by hysteroscopy where as bicornuate uterus needs resection of myometrium from the outer aspect through an abdominal approach. The differentiation should be made out by prior ultrasound examination, preferably 4 D or by MR imaging before attempting hysteroscopic resection.

Laparoscopy

With the advent of high resolution ultrasound, especially 4 D US, and magnetic resonance imaging, laparoscopy for

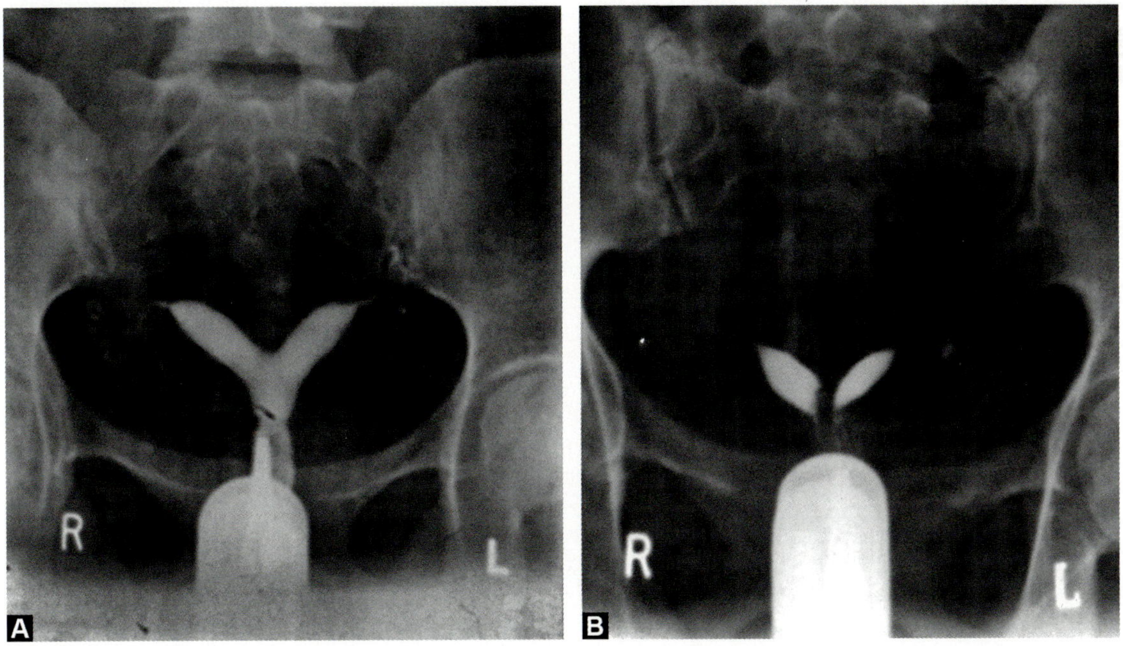

Figs 2.8A and B: Hysterosalpingogram showing wide angle between the two cavities(A), suggestive of bicornuate uterus and uterus didelphys showing two uterine cavities and cervical canals (B)

diagnostic purpose is seldom necessary. The role of laparoscopy is for excluding perforation while performing hysteroscopic septal resection or for the resection of rudimentary uterine horn.

Surgical Correction

Anomalies producing obstruction require immediate surgical correction to relieve the obstruction so that retrograde flow of menstrual blood with its consequent effects is prevented. Anomalies which do not cause obstruction may also need surgical correction to improve coital function or as a treatment for infertility or repeated abortion.

Management of Disorders of Vertical Fusion

MRKH syndrome: Counseling of the patient and the parents should be given sufficient importance as the information about the anomaly will be emotionally shocking especially to the parents. Coital problems and infertility are the two important issues which should be addressed. The option of gestational surrogacy should also be discussed. By means of surrogacy these individuals can become 'genetic parents'. The management mainly includes creating artificial vagina which previously used to be done a few months before marriage. However, there can be problems due to improper healing. Hence it is advisable to time the surgery at about 17-20 years of age when the girl will be physically as well as emotionally mature enough to understand the procedure as well as the need for using the vaginal form to maintain the newly created vagina patent.

Creating a new vagina is a surgically easy procedure in this situation since the uterus is not functioning. Several surgical and non-surgical methods are described for the creation of a new vagina. The non-surgical procedure involves the use of dilators (Frank, 1938).

Artificial vagina can be created by several surgical methods

1. *William's vulvo-vaginoplasty (Fig. 2.10)*[9]: This procedure is technically simple and avoids the serious complication of injury to bladder, urethra or rectum. A horse-shoe shaped incision is made in the vulva along the medial side of the labia majora to the level of the external urethral meatus. Then sufficient skin is mobilized to form the new vagina. The inner skin margins are sutured together. Then the subcutaneous layers are approximated with a second layer of sutures. The external skin margin is sutured as a last procedure. The patient is advised bed rest with continuous bladder drainage for 1 week.
2. *Abbe-Wharton-McIndoe operation*: This is the most popular operation presently resorted to for creating an artificial vagina. Here, the space between the bladder and the rectum is dissected to a sufficient depth. Care should be taken not to injure the urethra or the bladder anteriorly and the rectum and anal canal posteriorly. Scarring and constriction of the space can be prevented by regular use of a sponge in the dissected space. Bleeding from granulation tissue is a later complication. This can be prevented by using a split-thickness skin graft after dissection of the space and keeping a mould to prevent constriction of the newly formed vagina. Instead of skin graft, amniotic membrane homograft may be used.

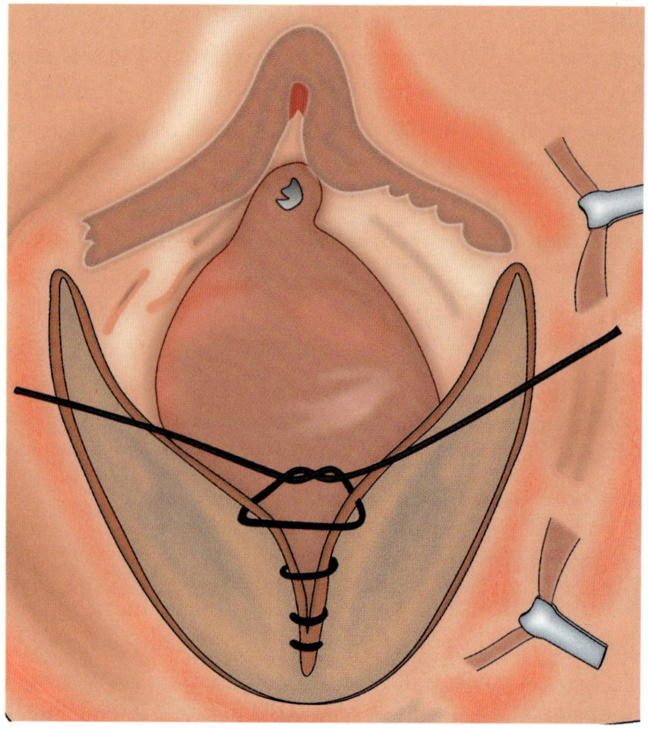

Fig. 2.10: William's vulvovaginoplasty. 3-0 polyglycolic acid sutures are used for suturing the inner and outer skin margins

3. *Bowel vaginoplasty*: In bowel vaginoplasty, sigmoid colon grafts are made use of to form a neovagina. Through laparotomy or laparoscopy, a loop of the sigmoid is dissected along with its mesentery and the loop is brought to the introitus. Since the procedure is complicated it is not resorted to at present.

Hematocolpos: Atresia of the vagina (Figs 2.11 and 2.12) in the presence of a functioning uterus results in haematocolpos when the girl attains puberty. The typical clinical presentation of haematocolpos is urinary retention and cyclical abdominal pain, in the pubertal age group. The haematocolpos will present as a cystic mass in the hypogastrium. The cystic mass can be appreciated anterior to the rectum by rectal examination.

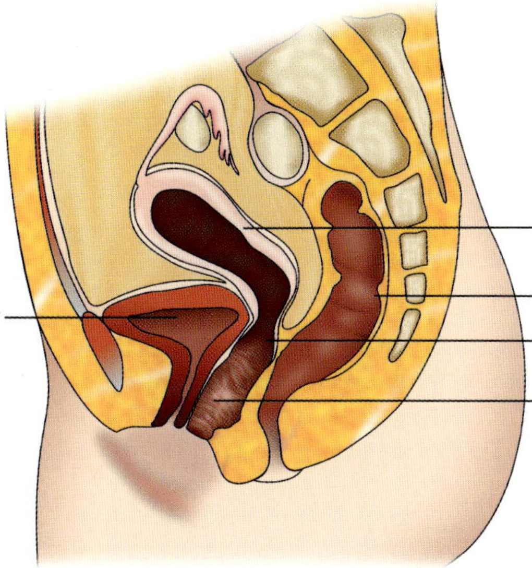

Fig. 2.11: Atresia of the lower 2/3rd of vagina resulting in hematocolpos

The lower extent depends upon the length of the atretic portion of the vagina. Thin septum lower down or imperforate hymen can cause a bulge in the introitus. The extent of haematocolpos can be made out by imaging. Unless the condition is kept in mind, it can be mistaken for an ovarian cyst. Associated hematometra and hematosalpinx can be present, which can also be made out by ultrasound.

Rarely, atresia of the vagina presents in the neonatal period or infancy. Collection of mucus can form a large mass which can cause compression of the urinary bladder, rectum and ureters. Since the septum is placed high in the vagina, there may not be a bulge in the vulva. Excision of the septum is required as an emergency procedure as greatly enlarged hydrocolpos can cause obstruction to the ureter, bladder or rectum. The child should be followed up for vaginal stenosis.

Occasionally, a small tract or two small tracts can be present in the atretic portion of the vagina on either side, which will allow menstrual blood to escape out in varying amounts so that the presentation can vary. Sometimes there may not be obstruction to menstrual flow at all so that the woman presents with coital difficulty if the septum is lower down. If the septum is higher, coital problems may not occur but she may present with inability to conceive.

Vaginal atresia can be associated with congenital vesicovaginal fistula. In such a situation, the girl presents with cyclical hematuria.

For relieving the acute pain associated with hematocolpos, needle aspiration under ultrasound guidance followed by continuous use of combination oral contraceptive can be resorted to. Counseling prior to the procedure is important. The girl should be mature enough to understand the importance of keeping the neovagina patent after surgical correction. The anomaly should be corrected without much delay, as long standing haematocolpos can lead to hematometra and development of pelvic endometriosis.

Surgical Correction of Vaginal Atresia

The space between the urethra and bladder anteriorly and the rectum and anal canal posteriorly can be easily dissected out so that the bulging hematometra can be reached. A catheter in the bladder and a finger in the rectum will help identify these structures so as to prevent injuring them. The hematometra should be differentiated from the bladder anteriorly and the rectum posteriorly and can be confirmed by aspiration with a needle. Continuity can be established with the upper vagina by cutting the intervening tissue. The collected blood will get drained. Reconstructing the vagina after the excision of a thin septum is easier. In most situations the vaginal epithelium will be greatly stretched and redundant and can be mobilized so that after dissection the upper and lower vagina can be anastomosed. In the case of atretic lower vagina, after the dissection of the space the redundant upper vagina can be advanced to the introitus and sutured. If the atretic portion is too long to be anastomosed, an acrylic vaginal mould which has a central hole for the escape of collected menstrual blood can be kept in the vagina so that gradual epithelialization occurs. The mould should be worn in the vagina for 4-6 months so that epithelialization will be complete. After dissecting the space

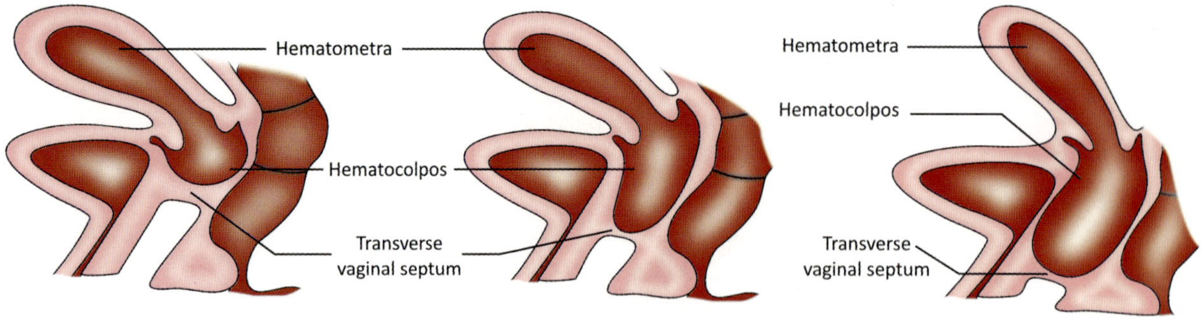

Fig. 2.12: Different positions of transverse vaginal septum causing complete obstruction to menstrual flow producing hematocolpos and hematometra. 1. Transverse vaginal septum 2. Hematometra 3. Hematocolpos

and draining the menstrual fluid, if the patency of the space is not maintained it can result in stenosis and complete obstruction to menstrual flow. A repeat procedure has a higher risk of injury to the bladder, urethra or rectum. As an alternative to using a mould, the raw area can be covered with a split thickness skin graft which is sutured to the vaginal wall.

Management of Disorders of Lateral Fusion

Disorders of lateral fusion can cause anomalies which can be of obstructed or non-obstructed types.

Non-obstructed Type

These anomalies can be of different types as discussed earlier. It could be septate uterus, bicornuate uterus or didelphic uterus.

Uterine anomalies are not the sole cause of primary infertility. However, if no other cause of infertility is identified in the presence of uterine anomaly, it is prudent to surgically correct the anomaly. Repeated abortions and preterm deliveries can be caused by uterine anomalies. 5-10% of repeated abortions are estimated to be due to uterine anomalies.

Surgical correction of uterine septum: The procedure adopted previously was John's metroplasty. In this method the septum with the overlying myometrium is excised as a wedge and the myometrium is repaired with polyglactin 910 (vicryl). Care should be taken to avoid transecting the intramural portion of the tube by confining to the midline of the uterine corpus.

The present management of uterine septum is by transcervical resection through hysteroscope.[5] The decrease in the spontaneous abortion rate reported is from 88 to 5.9% after hysteroscopic **metroplasty**. Hysteroscopic resection avoids the disadvantages of laparotomy and uterine scar. The use of preoperative GnRH is resorted to by some surgeons for proper visualization. If GnRH is not being given, the surgery should be timed in the immediate post menstrual phase. Laparoscopic guidance is preferable to exclude perforation of the uterus during the procedure. The septum is approached through the hysteroscope and cut with the help of a knife or with wire loop electrode till both the ostia can be visualized in the same field. Transcervical lysis can also be done for complete septum extending to the level of the external os. After resection, a few weeks should be given before attempting conception to allow the endometrium to grow. Vaginal delivery can be attempted as the myometrium is not incised

Surgical correction of bicornuate uterus: Repeated pregnancy loss is an indication for unification of bicornuate uterus.[6] The procedure adopted for unification is Strassmann metroplasty. In complete bicornuate uterus, there will be a band of tissue seen coursing between the two uterine hemicorpora, attached to the bladder anteriorly and rectosigmoid posteriorly.This should be cut initially taking care not to injure the rectum or bladder. The medial side of both the cornua should be incised till the cavity is seen. The upper end should not be near the interstitial portion of the tube. The myometrium is repaired inserting the sutures in such a way that the final suture line is in the sagittal plane. Care should be taken to avoid postoperative adhesion formation by meticulous handling of tissues and continuous irrigation with heparinized saline.

Cervical encirclage: Cervical incompetence is common among women who have uterine anomalies. If there is evidence of cervical incompetence, cervical encirclage should be performed. Encirclage need not be done if there is no evidence of cervical incompetence.

Uterus didelphys: Uterus didelphys is the anomaly which is most commonly associated with complete or partial longitudinal vaginal septum. The septum should be excised as it can cause problems with coitus. Unification of didelphic uterus should better be avoided, as the cervix will be widely separated and unification will be technically difficult and can cause more harm than good.

Arcuate uterus: The arcuate uterus is characterized by a near complete resorption of the uterovaginal septum at the region of the uterine fundus. In the original Buttram and Gibbons classification, the arcuate uterus was subclassified with the bicornuate uterus. In the classification by the American Fertility Society, the arcuate uterus is classified as a separate entity because it can be distinguished from a bicornuate uterus on the basis of its complete fundal unification. Both poor and good obstetric outcomes have been reported among women with arcuate uterus.

It has been proposed that reproductive outcome can be predicted by calculating the ratio between the height of the fundal indentation and the distance between the lateral apices of the horns on the basis of HSG findings. A ratio of less than 10 is not anticipated to have an adverse pregnancy outcome. Hysteroscopic correction may be considered in selected patients with recurrent pregnancy loss if no other cause has been identified.

Unicornuate uterus: The uterus can be unicornuate with or without a rudimentary horn on the other side. Isolated unicornuate uterus is seen in 35%, associated rudimentary horn without endometrium in 33% and associated horn with endometrium is seen in 32%. Those who have rudimentary horn with functioning endometrium will present right from menarche with severe dysmenorrhea. Women with unicornuate uterus[7] are reported to have poor obstetric outcome. Heinonen reported a miscarriage rate of 34.4%, preterm delivery rate of 43.3%, and the live birth rate of 54.2% among such women. The reduced capacity of the uterus, inability to expand sufficiently during pregnancy and abnormal blood supply are thought to be the causes for abortion and preterm labor. Abnormal presentations are more common among women with unicornuate uterus. Pregnancy can occur in the non communicating rudimentary horn by transperitoneal migration of sperm or ovum from the opposite side. Rupture of the rudimentary horn pregnancy can result in massive intra-abdominal hemorrhage and shock. The diagnosis can be made by ultrasound before rupture and the horn can be excised.[8]

Associated renal anomalies are found to be as high as 40%. The commonest anomaly encountered is absence of kidney on the abnormal side.

Nothing much can be done to improve the pregnancy outcome in women who have unicornuate uterus. Cervical incompetence, if diagnosed can be managed by cervical encirclage.

Disorders of Lateral Fusion with Obstruction

Defective fusion can result in a variety of asymmetric types of anomalies.

Unicornuate uterus with non-communicating uterine horn and functional endometrium: In this type, a unicornuate uterus will be seen on one side and a hypoplastic horn on the other. In the presence of functioning endometrium in the hypoplastic horn, hematometra can occur and the individual might present with severe dysmenorrhea. As regular menstruation can occur from the other side, cryptomenorrhea might go unnoticed. Rarely the rudimentary horn may have a small communication with the uterine cavity of the developed horn, in which case retrograde menstruation and resultant pelvic endometriosis can occur.

Unilateral obstruction of the cavity of a septate uterus: In few women with septate uterus, one cavity will be obstructed with collection of menstrual blood inside. The treatment is excision of the septum with reconstruction of the cavity. Ultrasound guided needle aspiration followed by hysteroscopic septal excision avoids laparotomy and opening the myometrium.

Double uterus with obstructed hemi-vagina: One-half of the vagina in a woman who has didelphic uterus and septate vagina can be obstructed at the outlet so that menstrual blood can get collected in the obstructed half. Menstruation continues through the patent vagina. The woman usually will present with severe dysmenorrhea and para-vaginal mass which could be hematocolpos or hematometra. MR imaging should be done to delineate the abnormality and to exclude associated renal anomalies like absent kidney or pelvic kidney. Management involves excision of the septum. After opening the hematocolpos the blood can be removed by suction. This can be done as a 2 stage procedure as described by Haddad. 2-3 cm of the septum is excised and the hematocolpos can be drained. About a month later the septum can be excised in the post menstrual period.

Abnormalities of Cervical Development

Cervical agenesis denotes non development of the cervix while cervical dysgenesis is abnormally developed cervix.

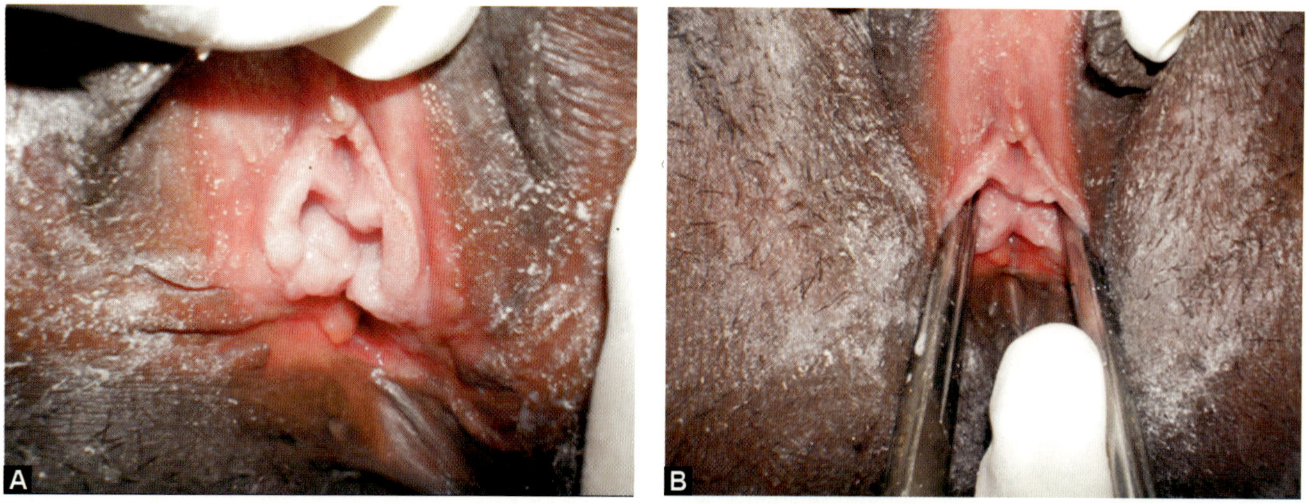

Figs 2.13A and B: External genitalia showing perineal anus and longitudinal vaginal septum. The septum is not extending up to the vulval outlet. The two forceps are seen in the two hemivagina

This can be of different types. The cervical tissue may be present in varying proportions with non developed cervical canal.

Cervical agenesis and dysgenesis are infrequent congenital anomalies. It is usually associated with atresia of the vagina also. The presentation is like haematocolpos, with complaints of cyclical lower abdominal pain and a mass in the hypogastrium on examination, due to the presence of hematometra. Distinction from agenesis of vagina alone is difficult as the dilated uterine cavity and cervix in isolated vaginal agenesis is difficult to differentiate from the dilated uterine cavity in cervical agenesis. Ultrasound and MRI will help in differentiating these two situations. Such differentiation is important as cervical agenesis is difficult to correct whereas if the cervix is normal vagina can be reconstructed.

When a normally developed uterus is present and the cervix and vagina are not developed, the management is challenging. It is difficult to make a satisfactory cervical canal which can be kept patent to allow normal menstruation to occur. Several methods have been tried. Even though a satisfactory tract may be established to allow menstrual blood to escape, cervical glandular epithelium cannot be created. Endometriosis can still occur due to retrograde menstruation. Endometriosis can also occur along the newly created track. Recurrent pelvic infection is a reported complication of such procedure and might necessitate hysterectomy. If a satisfactory cervical tract cannot be established, hysterectomy is the only option. The decision for hysterectomy should be taken sufficiently early so that the ovaries are not affected by pelvic infection or endometriosis and can be retained. These individuals can have their genetic offspring by growing their ovum in a host uterus. Individuals with a well formed cervical body can be expected to conceive after cervical reconstruction. Hence careful selection is important before cervical reconstruction.

Abnormalities in the Development of the Vulva

Abnormal development of the perineum can result in perineal anus or vaginal anus (Figs 2.13A and B). In instances like intrauterine androgen exposure as well as in adreno-genital syndrome, a female fetus can develop virilization of external genitalia. The male external genitalia development is dependent on the presence of dihydrotestosterone. In the absence of Dihydrotestosterone or androgen receptors virilization will not occur as in 5 α reductase deficiency or testicular feminization syndrome, in which case the genetically male individual will have female type of external genitalia at birth and will be reared as female.

Unusual Combination of Mullerian Anomalies

Rarely unusual combinations of vertical and transverse fusion defects or combination of mullerian anomalies with ano-rectal anomalies can be encountered. Disorder of vertical fusion can be associated with disorder of lateral fusion (Figs 2.14A and B). Didelphic uterus might co-exist with transverse vaginal septum causing haematocolpos and hematometra. Septate vagina may be associated with perineal anus. An effort should be done to define the abnormality clinically as well as by imaging (if necessary by MRI) before venturing for surgical correction.

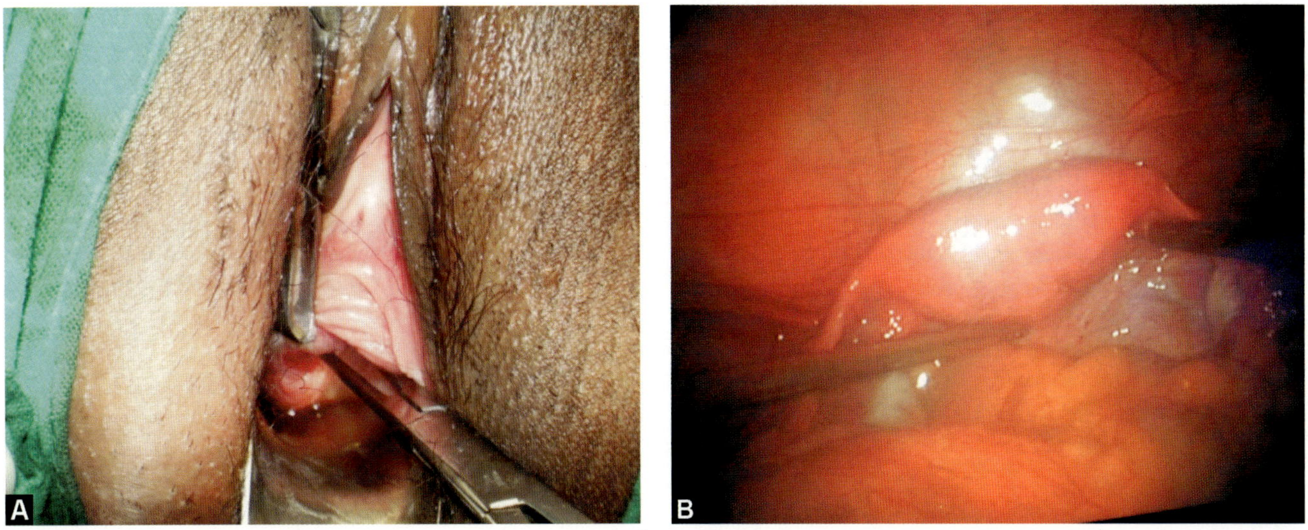

Figs 2.14A and B: Speculum examination showing transverse vaginal septum with central hole (A). Patient presented with primary infertility. Her uterus was partially bicornuate (B). She had polycystic ovarian disease also

2.7 CONCLUSION

The genital tract and the urinary tract develop from a common paraxial mesoderm. Hence anomalies of the genital tract can be associated with renal anomalies. Knowledge about the development of the female genital tract and the urinary tract is important in understanding the congenital defects of both the systems. The female genital tract develops from the fused paramesonephric or the Mullerian duct. The Wolffian duct which develops into the male internal genitalia degenerates in the female. In the male foetus, the mullerian duct degenerates under the influence of the Anti-Mullerian factor produced by the testis. The male external genitalia and duct system develops under the influence of androgen. In the presence of androgens, even a female foetus will develop male type external genitalia. In the absence of androgen or its receptor, the external genitalia of the genetically male foetus will be of the female type, as it is the neutral norm and does not need estrogen for its development. Mullerian duct anomalies encompass a wide spectrum of clinical and imaging findings. Recurrent abdominal pain in a pubertal girl who has secondary sexual development appropriate for the age should raise the suspicion of cryptomenorrhea. In the presence of anomalies which cause asymmetric obstruction, hematometra and haematocolpos can occur despite regular menstruation. Genital tract anomalies should be looked for in women who present with recurrent miscarriage. These may rarely be a cause of infertility. While many of the anomalies will be diagnosed initially at HSG or two-dimensional US, further, three-dimensional US will often be required for a definitive diagnosis. Currently MR imaging is the study of choice for the diagnosis of complicated mullerian anomalies because of its high accuracy and detailed elaboration of utero-vaginal and ovarian anatomy. Laparoscopy and hysteroscopy are to be reserved for women, who need interventional therapy, and should not be resorted to solely for diagnostic purpose. Precise imaging characterization is essential, for planning treatment. Proper treatment planning is very important in the successful management of these anomalies, especially the complicated ones. Hysteroscopic septal resection is the treatment of choice for women with septate uterus who have had recurrent miscarriage. Unification is better avoided in uterus didelphys due to the ineffective unification of the cervix. Women with lateral fusion defects are prone for cervical incompetence in pregnancy. Cervical encirclage is indicated only if there is evidence of incompetence. With proper delineation of the defect and resorting to correct surgical method whenever necessary, fertility as well as coital function can be restored in most situations.

REFERENCES

1. Grimbizis GF, Camus M, Tarlatzis BC, Bontis JN, Devroey P. Clinical implications of uterine malformations and hysteroscopic treatment results. Hum Reprod Update. Mar-Apr 2001;7(2):161-74. [Nahum GG. Uterine anomalies. How common are they, and what is their distribution among subtypes? J Reprod Med. Oct 1998;43(10):877-87.
2. Wu MH, Hsu CC, Huang KE. Detection of congenital mullerian duct anomalies using three-dimensional ultrasound. J Clin Ultrasound 1997; 25:487-92.

3. Pellerito JS, McCarthy SM, Doyle MB, Glickman MG, DeCherney AH. Diagnosis of uterine anomalies: relative accuracy of MR imaging, endovaginal ultrasound, and hysterosalpingography. Radiology 1992; 183:795-800.
4. Yoder IC, Hall DA. Hysterosalpingography in the 1990s. AJR Am J Roentgenol 1991; 157:675-83.
5. DeCherney AH, Russell JB, Graebe RA, Polan ML. Resectoscopic management of mullerian fusion defects. Fertil Steril 1986; 45:726-8.
6. Strassmann EO. Fertility and unification of double uterus. Fertil Steril 1966; 17:165-76.
7. Heinonen PK. Unicornuate uterus and rudimentary horn. Fertil Steril 1997;68:224.
8. Fedele L, Bianchi S, Agnoli B, Tozzi L, Vignali M. Urinary tract anomalies associated with unicornuate uterus. J Urol 1996; 155:847-8.
9. Rock JA. Surgery for anomalies of the Müllerian ducts. In: Thompson JD, Rock JA, TeLinde's operative gynecology. 9th ed. Philadelphia, PA: JB Lippincott, 2003.

3

Urinary Incontinence

B Presannakumari

3.1 INTRODUCTION

Urinary incontinence is the inability to control the leakage of urine and is a common problem in women than in men. Even though urinary incontinence is not life-threatening, it is a distressing symptom which can severely compromise the quality of a woman's life. Majority of women who have symptoms do not care to seek medical advice because they consider it as an inevitable part of child birth and ageing. To deal with the problem, most of them rely on absorbent pads or changes in lifestyle. Some women may feel ashamed or depressed or may even avoid social or work events. They think that nothing can be done to correct it. After appropriate investigations if the correct surgical or medical therapy is resorted to, most women can be cured and the condition of the rest can be improved.

3.2 EPIDEMIOLOGY

The prevalence of incontinence in women is reported to vary from 9 to 72%. Largest of the prevalence studies have found an overall prevalence of 25% among community-dwelling women, aged 20 years or over (Hunskaar, 2002). Mild leakage affects most women at some time in their lives. Severe leakage is less common. There is an association with increasing age, childbirth, obesity, presence of lower urinary tract symptoms and decreased mobility.

3.3 DEFINITION

Urinary incontinence is the inability to control the leakage of urine from the bladder. It may vary in severity from minor leaks or dribbles of urine, or frequent wetting of cloths to worrisome total incontinence. For a few, incontinence means both urinary and fecal incontinence—the uncontrollable loss of stools.

The International Continence Society (ICS) defines incontinence as a symptom, sign and as an urodynamic finding separately.[1]

The *symptom* of urinary incontinence is "the complaint of any involuntary leakage of urine". This is perceived by the patient or the care giver.

The *sign* of incontinence is that observed by the physician by simple means (during physical examination as an observation of the loss of urine while coughing or straining) or by the use of the pad test, from the symptom score or voiding diary.

Incontinence established by urodynamic study reflects the definitive pathophysiologic condition that is causing the incontinence. When the incontinence cannot be documented by an urodynamic observation, it may be presumed by clinical documentation.

These definitions present logical problems that invalidate its use in biomedical research. As definition and medical decision are different concepts, this does not necessarily affect the potential utility of the problem assessment aspect[2] when used in everyday clinical practice.

3.4 CLASSIFICATION OF INCONTINENCE (FIGS 3.1 AND 3.2)

Incontinence of urine can be urethral or extra-urethral. Urethral incontinence is caused by an abnormality of the bladder, urethra or both. Bladder abnormalities that cause incontinence include detrusor overactivity and low bladder compliance. Urethral abnormalities include urethral hypermobility and intrinsic sphincter deficiency. Extra-urethral incontinence is caused by an ectopic ureter or urinary fistula. It is the observation of urine leakage through channels other than the urethra.

3.5 RELEVANT ANATOMICAL BASIS

3.5.1 Applied Anatomy of Lower Urinary Tract

Urinary bladder is a hollow musculo-membranous sac which holds urine and eliminates it at convenient intervals. When filled, bladder has the capacity of approximately 500 ml and assumes an ovoid shape. The empty bladder is tetrahedral, having a superior surface with the apex at the urachus, two infero-lateral surfaces, and a posterior surface or base with bladder neck at the lowest point.

The superior surface of bladder is covered by peritoneum. With distension, the bladder rises out of the true pelvis and separates the peritoneum from the anterior abdominal wall. When the bladder is full, it is therefore possible to perform suprapubic cystostomy without risking entry into the peritoneal cavity. Posteriorly, the peritoneum is reflected on to the uterus forming the vesico-uterine pouch and then on to the anterior surface of the uterine body, closely adhering to the myometrium. Posteriorly the peritoneum gets reflected from the uterus on to the rectum forming the recto-uterine pouch. The vagina and uterus intervene between the bladder and rectum, so that the base of the bladder and urethra rest on the anterior vaginal wall.

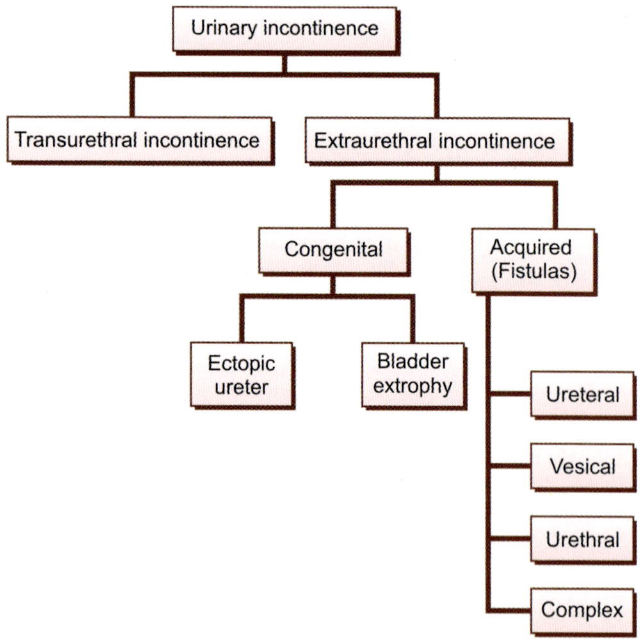

Fig. 3.1: Classification of incontinence

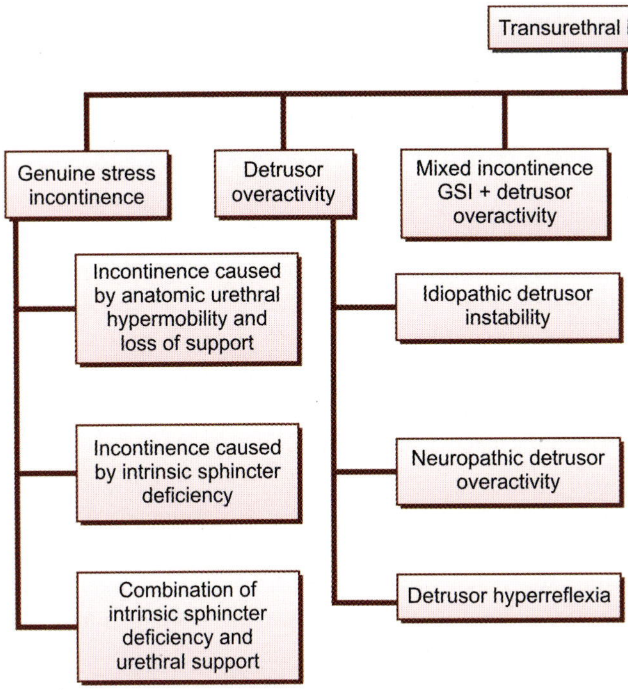

Fig. 3.2: Classification of transurethral incontinence

3.5.2 Urethral Sphincter

The normal adult female urethra measures 4-5 cm. The sphincter mechanism of the urethra (Fig. 3.3) consists of an intrinsic sphincter and an extrinsic sphincter.

The intrinsic sphincter has two components—the thin internal sphincter which is a continuation of the detrusor muscle and a thick external sphincter which consists of striated muscle fibers (rhabdo sphincter). Contraction of longitudinal smooth muscle stabilizes the urethra and allows force generated by circular elements to occlude the lumen. In the urethral wall, striated muscle forms a rhabdosphincter that is separate from the peri-urethral skeletal muscle of the pelvic floor. The rhabdosphincter, which is responsible for urethral closure at rest is horse shoe shaped and extends from the proximal urethra distally. It is thicker anteriorly and thins out as it goes laterally. It is almost deficient posteriorly. The main bulk of the rhabdosphincter is in the middle third of the urethra.

Extrinsic sphincter consists of striated periurethral part of levator ani which is situated at a level of about 2-3 cm above the external urethral meatus. This extrinsic sphincter gives an additional closure mechanism when there is an increase in the intra-abdominal pressure. The extrinsic sphincter along with the intrinsic sphincter maintains continence by developing a sufficient positive closure pressure.

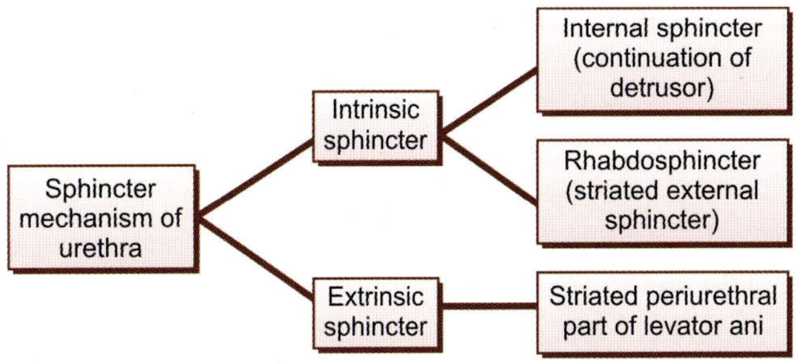

Fig. 3.3: Sphincteric mechanism at the bladder neck

The principles of sphincter function are:

1. Watertight apposition of urethral lumen
2. Compression of the wall around the lumen
3. Structural support to keep proximal urethra from moving during increase in intra-abdominal pressure
4. A means of compensating for abdominal pressure changes
5. Neural control.

Urethra maintains a water-tight seal mainly by the following factors:

1. Wall tension or external compression
2. Inner wall softness
3. Filler material beneath the mucosa that helps to deform the mucosal folds into apposition

4. Lining mucus provides the stickiness that enables coaptation of the mucosal folds.

External compression of the urethral lumen is achieved by:

1. Smooth and striated muscle tone and its phasic contractions.
2. Elastic and viscoelastic properties of the extracellular matrix.
3. Mechanical factors related to transmission of abdominal pressure.

3.5.3 Innervation

The detrusor muscle is innervated by parasympathetic nerves from S 2, 3 and 4. Sympathetic supply is from T10-L2. Visceral afferent fibers travel along the thoracolumbar and sacral afferent nerves and convey sensation of bladder distention. Stretch receptors carry impulses to the spinal segment S2, 3 and 4 (Fig. 3.4).

3.5.4 Histology and Structure of Bladder and Urethra

The urinary bladder is lined by urothelium, which is transitional epithelium 6-cells thick. The inner surface is smooth when full and contracts into folds when the bladder is empty. Below the urothelium is the fibro- elastic connective tissue layer called lamina propria. The muscular bladder wall, the detrusor is a syncitium of large branching interlacing bundles. This meshwork is ideally suited for its synchronous contraction to empty the spherical bladder.

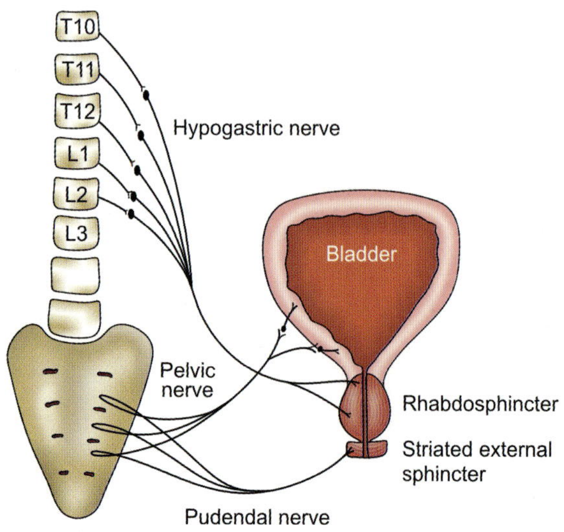

Fig. 3.4: Innervation of the bladder and urethra

Near the bladder neck, the detrusor muscle is clearly separable into inner longitudinal, middle circular and outer longitudinal layers. They converge down and pass down the urethra as the inner smooth muscle sphincter.

The longitudinally arranged abundant collagen and elastin of urethral stroma also contributes to continence. The vascular filling of lamina propria provides coaptation of mucosa. Since estrogen maintains urethral blood flow and thus coaptation of the urethra, its deficiency can contribute to stress incontinence.

The periurethral external striated sphincter has got the pelvic floor still external to it. The additional muscle structures in the distal sphincter include compressor urethrae and urethrovaginal sphincter. With variations in intra-abdominal pressure, continence is maintained by various mechanisms. Bladder neck and proximal urethra are located above the pelvic floor. Hence when intra abdominal pressure raises an equal amount of pressure is transmitted to the proximal urethra raising the urethral resistance. A guarding reflex involving an active contraction of striated extrinsic sphincter can transiently help continence. However this was contradicted by DeLancey[3] in his article stating that "during cough, urethral closure pressure increase and compress the urethra supporting it like a hammock, rather than the upper urethra being intra-abdominal".

3.6 PHYSIOLOGY OF MICTURITION

From the functional and anatomic perspective, the lower urinary tract is considered to have two parts the urinary bladder as reservoir and the bladder outlet as sphincter mechanism. Incontinence can occur when there is a dysfunction of bladder as in detrusor overactivity, impaired compliance or dysfunction of sphincter as in intrinsic sphincter deficiency and urethral support defect (hypermobility).

Micturition is a complex series of finely tuned and integrated neuromuscular events that involve anatomic and neurologic mechanisms. The bladder stores urine, and contracts to empty urine normally under voluntary control.

3.6.1 Bladder Filling

The bladder is a low-pressure system that expands to accommodate increasing volumes of urine without an appreciable rise in pressure. The bladder muscle (the detrusor) remains inactive during bladder filling, without involuntary contractions. Normally bladder fills at a rate of 1-2 drops every 2 seconds. When the bladder is being filled at this rate, the detrusor pressure remains nearly constant because of a special property of bladder known as accommodation. This is due to the highly compliant structure of the bladder wall, the viscoelastic properties based on the composition by smooth muscles, collagen, elastin and the transitional epithelium.

During the filling stage, proprioceptive afferent impulses from the stretch receptors within the bladder are carried via the pelvic nerves to the dorsal sacral roots of S2, 3, 4. These impulses are carried to the cerebral cortex through the lateral spinothalamic tract. When the bladder has filled to a certain volume of about 200-250 ml, fullness is registered by stretch receptors. The first desire to void will be appreciated at this point. As the bladder further fills, these impulses increase, but micturition is inhibited consciously depending on the social circumstances. During this period there will be voluntary pelvic floor contraction, which increases urethral pressure preventing the involuntary escape of urine. Voiding starts when the detrusor pressure overcomes the urethral pressure.

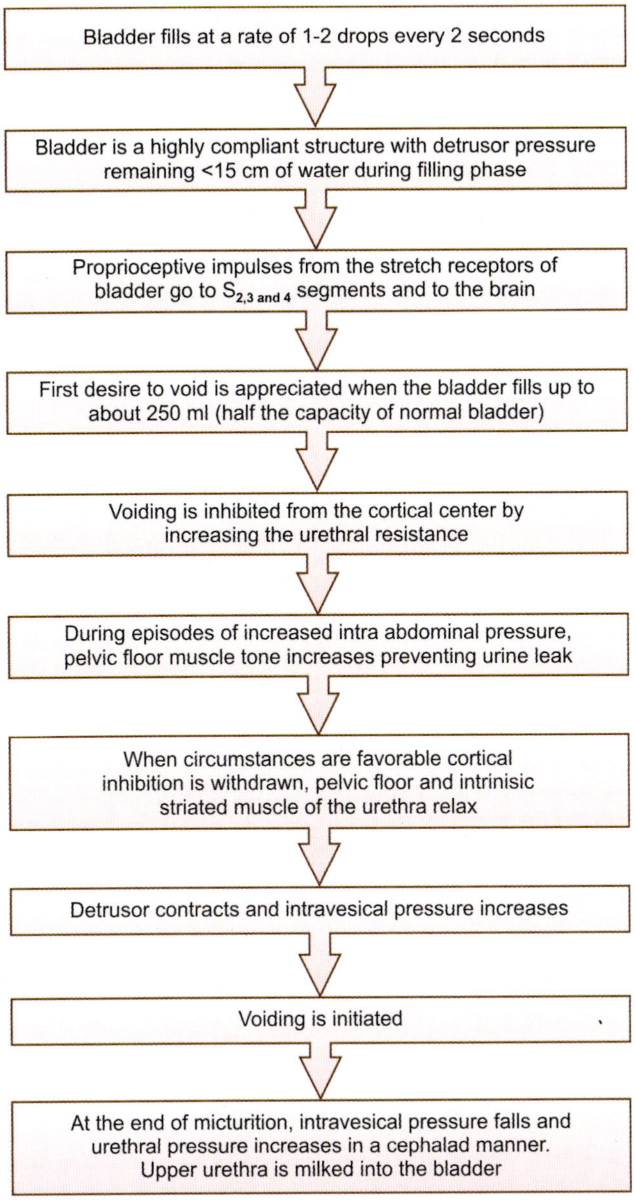

3.6.2 Bladder Emptying

Voiding is accomplished by micturition reflex. It is normally under voluntary control and is organized by the pontine micturition center. It requires integration and modulation by the sacral micturition center dealing with parasympathetic and somatic components as well as the thoracolumbar sympathetic components. The high level intense vesical afferent activity for micturition is carried by pelvic nerves, which produce activation of the sacral parasympathetic pathways (bladder contraction and sphincter relaxation) and inhibition of the sympathetic (bladder neck relaxation) and somatic (external striated sphincter relaxation) pathways.

The expulsion phase consists of an initial relaxation of the urethral sphincter followed by contraction of the bladder. This micturition reflex is controlled by the cerebral cortex. Voiding commences when the circumstances are appropriate. There is voluntary relaxation of the pelvic floor causing marked fall in intraurethral pressure. The inhibitory influences from the cortex are suppressed allowing discharge of parasympathetic impulses from S2,3,4 segments to the pelvic nerves causing detrusor contraction. This raises the detrusor pressure to a level not more than 60 cm of water. Normal voiding is accomplished by voluntary relaxation of the pelvic floor and urethra, which decreases the urethral pressure, accompanied by sustained contraction of the detrusor muscle, leading to voiding. Interruption of micturition can be achieved by contraction of the extrinsic striated muscle of the pelvic floor, which brings about an increase in the urethral pressure to exceed the intravesical pressure and the flow of urine is stopped. When the bladder empties at the end of micturition, the pelvic floor and intrinsic striated muscle of the urethra contract and any urine which is left in the proximal urethra will be milked back into the bladder. As the urethra closes off, subconscious inhibition of the sacral micturition centre is reinstituted and the bladder again enters the filling phase.

The storage function is dependent on:

1. The spinal reflexes that activate sympathetic and somatic pathways to the bladder outlet
2. Tonic inhibitory influence from the brain that suppresses excitatory parasympathetic outflow to the bladder. The

low level afferents of bladder distention is carried in pelvic nerves leading to sympathetic stimulation of bladder outlet smooth muscles and pudendal outflow to external urethral sphincter. Sympathetic stimulation also inhibits the bladder musculature and transmission in the bladder parasympathetic ganglia.

The spinal reflex pathway producing these responses represents guarding reflexes for continence.

Urethra to bladder reflexes: Barrington made a landmark contribution to the progress of neurourology in 1931. He reported that urine flow or mechanical stimulation of the urethra with a catheter could excite afferent nerves which in turn facilitate reflex bladder contraction. This urethra to bladder reflex could promote complete bladder emptying. This may be an explanation why stress incontinence and urge incontinence often occur together in women. Stress induced leakage of urine into the urethra can stimulate afferents and induce detrusor contractions. Surgical cure of stress incontinence in women with mixed incontinence has resolved urge incontinence in half of the patients.

3.7 PATHOPHYSIOLOGY OF INCONTINENCE

Alterations in any of the physiological control mechanisms may result in abnormalities in emptying or urinary incontinence or both. Thus the pathophysiology of major causes of incontinence can be:

1. A fall in urethral pressure associated with a rise in intra-vesical pressure can cause incontinence. This occurs in detrusor instability.
2. Abnormal rise in detrusor pressure in the bladder filling phase. This occurs due to decreased compliance of the bladder. Decreased compliance can occur following pelvic radiation and chronic inflammatory conditions like tuberculosis.
3. When the urethral sphincter is insufficient to maintain tone, it can result in incontinence due to intrinsic sphincter deficiency even if there is no displacement of urethra. This can occur after menopause and after radiotherapy or surgery.
4. When there is lack of urethral support, the bladder neck and proximal urethra descend to a lower level. During periods of increased intra abdominal pressure like coughing or sneezing, the normal increase in the intra-urethral pressure does not occur. This results in stress incontinence.

3.8 TYPES OF TRANSURETHRAL INCONTINENCE (TABLE 3.1)

3.8.1 Stress Urinary Incontinence

Stress urinary incontinence is one of the most common types of incontinence. It is the involuntary loss of urine occurring with a transient rise in intra-abdominal pressure as in coughing, laughing and sneezing. Leakage occurs when the pressure in the bladder is greater than the pressure in the urethra. This leak can also happen when a woman walks, runs, exercises or lifts something heavy. It is more prominent when the bladder is full. It is caused by a defect in the support of bladder neck and proximal urethra or by a weak sphincter. Physical changes resulting from pregnancy, childbirth and menopause can result in stress incontinence.

International Continence Society (ICS) Definitions of SUI

The symptom: The symptom is the complaint of involuntary leakage during situations of increased intra-abdominal pressure, such as on exertion, sneezing or coughing. Women who complain of urine leak may not have genuine stress incontinence (GSI) documented in urodynamic studies. It can sometimes be urgency precipitated by cough which might have been overlooked.

The sign: The sign is the observation of involuntary urine loss from the urethra synchronous with exertion, sneezing or coughing. The mere leakage of urine during exertion does not mean that the patient has clinical problem of GSI. According to ICS, incontinence exists when urine loss becomes a social problem.

Urodynamic stress incontinence: Urodynamic stress incontinence is noted during urodynamic testing (filling cystometry) and is defined as involuntary leakage of urine with increase in abdominal pressure in the absence of a detrusor contraction.

Table 3.1: Types of transurethral incontinence

Types of transurethral incontinence
Stress urinary incontinence
Urge urinary incontinence
Mixed incontinence
Functional incontinence
Postmicturition dribble
Overflow incontinence
Temporary urinary incontinence

3.8.2 Urge Urinary Incontinence (UUI)

When there is a sudden, intense desire to urinate, followed by an involuntary loss of urine, it is urge incontinence. The feeling of urge is due to unstable bladder contractions which may give a warning of only a few seconds to a minute to reach the toilet. Urgency need not always end in incontinence. With urge incontinence, the patient may also need to urinate often, resulting in frequency. When she needs to wake up several times at night for voiding, it is nocturia.

Urge incontinence can be provoked by hearing the sound of water running or after drinking a small quantity of liquid. In some women, even simply changing the position from sitting to standing may cause leakage of urine.

Urge incontinence can also be caused by urinary tract infection or by anything that irritates the bladder. It can also be caused by bowel problems or damage to the nervous system associated with multiple sclerosis, Parkinson's disease, Alzheimer's disease, stroke or injury. In urge incontinence, the bladder is said to be hyper-reflexic or "overactive bladder"—the bladder contracts even when it is not full.

ICS Definition of UUI

The symptom: The symptom is the complaint of an involuntary leakage accompanied by or immediately preceded by urgency.

The sign: The sign is the observation of involuntary loss of urine from the urethra that is accompanied by or immediately preceded by urgency.

Detrusor overactivity incontinence: Detrusor overactivity incontinence is incontinence related to an involuntary detrusor contraction during urodynamic testing.

3.8.3 Mixed Incontinence

Women with a combination of stress urinary incontinence and urge incontinence, occurring together is said to have mixed incontinence. This combination may cause more urine to leak than either type alone. It is more common in older women.

ICS Definition of Mixed Incontinence

The complaint of involuntary leakage of urine associated with urgency and also with exertion effort, sneezing or coughing.

3.8.4 Continuous Incontinence

Continuous urinary incontinence is continuous leakage of urine which occurs when there is a fistula. It is actually extra urethral incontinence.

3.8.5 Functional Incontinence

Older adults experience incontinence simply because a physical or mental impairment prevents them from making it to the toilet in time. For example, a person with severe arthritis may not be able to reach a toilet quick enough. Women with degenerative brain disease and dementia may not plan well enough to make a timely trip to the toilet. This type of incontinence is called functional incontinence. Sometimes drugs and urinary infection can cause temporary functional incontinence called transient incontinence.

3.8.6 Postmicturition Dribble

Postmicturition dribble is the complaint of involuntary loss of urine immediately after passing urine. This occurs in the presence of urethral diverticulum.

3.8.7 Overflow Incontinence

Overflow incontinence is not a symptom or condition but rather a term used to describe leakage of urine associated with urinary retention. Incontinence will be in the form of frequent or constant dribble of urine. Retention can result from a bladder outlet obstruction or a non-contractile bladder.

3.8.8 Temporary Urinary Incontinence

Certain foods and drinks can cause temporary urinary incontinence. Alcoholic drinks have a diuretic effect. It causes the bladder to fill quickly, triggering an urgent and sometimes uncontrollable desire to urinate (urgency). In addition, alcohol can temporarily impair the ability to recognize the need to urinate and answer that need in a timely manner.

Over-hydration: Drinking a lot of water or other beverages, particularly in a short period of time, increases the urine output, overfills the bladder, and may result in an occasional leak.

Under-hydration: In women with urge incontinence, there is a tendency to limit fluid intake to reduce the number of urge episodes and needs to void. This can result in collection of concentrated urine in the bladder. The concentrated waste products thus collected can irritate the bladder provoking urge incontinence.

Caffeine: Caffeine has a diuretic action. Caffeine, tea, carbonated drinks, citrus fruits, spicy foods and artificial sweeteners are bladder irritants. They may worsen urge incontinence.

Drugs: Certain medications are known to alter urinary tract function. Sedative-hypnotics such as diazepam may cause confusion and can interfere with the ability to control bladder function, especially in old age.

Diuretics such as hydrochlorothiazide used in treating hypertension in elderly may worsen incontinence by increasing the volume of urine.

There are several drugs that have an action on the bladder as a side effect. They include antihistaminics, antidepressants and antispasmodics. They have got an anticholinergic action, and impair the detrusor contractility, leading to overflow incontinence.

Sympatholytic agents like clonidine, phenoxybenzamine and tamsulosin may cause or worsen stress urinary incontinence by decreasing the urethral closure pressure.

Sympathomimetics like ephedrine, pseudoephedrine, phenylephrine (common in anti-cold tablets), and tricyclic antidepressants such as imipramine increase bladder outlet resistance and cause overflow incontinence.

Use of ACE inhibitor drugs like captopril, enalapril for control of hypertension in women with stress incontinence will result in chronic cough and worsening of incontinence.

Constipation: The rectum and bladder shares many of the same nerves. Hard, impacted stool in the rectum can cause these nerves to be overactive and trigger urine frequency. Constipation and painful anal conditions cause functional retention of urine and may result in overflow incontinence.

3.9 GENUINE STRESS INCONTINENCE (GSI)

There are several names used to describe stress incontinence like urethral sphincter incontinence, urodynamic stress incontinence and genuine stress incontinence. Genuine stress incontinence is a cystometric diagnosis defined as "the involuntary loss of urine that occurs when, in the absence of a detrusor contraction the intravesical pressure exceeds the maximum urethral pressure".[4]

3.9.1 Pathophysiology of Genuine Stress Incontinence

Effective closure of the urethra is important in continence. Anything which interferes with the urethral closure mechanisms can cause incontinence. The urethra remains closed during episodes of increased intra-abdominal pressure. Urethra remains closed in the filling phase by several extrinsic and intrinsic factors.

Intrinsic Factors

- α adrenergic sympathetic tone
- Striated urethral sphincter
- Mucosal coaptation
- Submucosal venous plexus
- Internal urethral sphincter

Extrinsic Factors

- The support of the bladder neck and urethra by the endopelvic fascial integrity.
- The levator ani muscle which helps to support the upper urethra and bladder neck.
- The reflex contraction of the pelvic muscle complex when there is an increase in the intra-abdominal pressure.

3.9.2 Factors Causing Stress Incontinence

The two important factors causing stress incontinence are:

1. Descent of the Bladder Neck

The upper urethra is normally supported by the endopelvic fascia and levator ani muscle. The most important factor in the maintenance of continence during rise in abdominal pressure is the urethral support. The loss of structural urethral support results in descent of the bladder neck and urethra leading to urethral hyper mobility and stress urinary incontinence. Normally bladder neck and proximal urethra are located in a high retro-pubic position above the pelvic floor. Abdominal pressure is transmitted equally to both bladder and urethra. During stress, when there is descent of urethra, the urethra attains a low level below the pelvic floor and the rise in abdominal pressure is transmitted unequally, thereby the bladder pressure exceeds urethral pressure resulting in stress induced urine loss.

2. Intrinsic Sphincter Deficiency

Intrinsic sphincter deficiency is an intrinsic malfunction of the urethral sphincter, regardless of the descent. Normal urethra is intended to remain closed, no matter what the degree of stress or rotational descent is. This is why many women with rotational descent remain continent. Deficient sphincteric mechanism is characterized by an open bladder neck and proximal urethra at rest. Urethral hypermobility and intrinsic sphincter deficiency may coexist in some patients.

3.9.3 Risk Factors

Sex: Women are more likely than men to have stress incontinence. Pregnancy and childbirth, menopause, and normal female anatomy account for this difference. Partial denervation of the pelvic floor, descent of the bladder neck etc may be the reasons for the development of incontinence after vaginal delivery.

Age: Except in infancy, incontinence is not a normal phenomenon at any age. Ageing can lead to associated weakening of pelvic support, sphincter tone and changes in bladder wall resulting in reduced volume and compliance. All these predispose to incontinence.

Obesity: Obesity predisposes to stress incontinence by increasing the abdominal pressure over the bladder and by weakening the pelvic floor.

Smoking: Smoking predisposes to chronic cough which can contribute to the development of stress incontinence and worsening of the existing incontinence. Smokers are also at risk of developing overactive bladder.

Renal diseases: Renal diseases with high urine output can predispose to incontinence.

3.9.4 Evaluation of Patients with Incontinence

History

A thorough history is important in the evaluation of urinary incontinence. The clinician should try to identify the risk factors and should try to find out whether there is any cause for transient incontinence from the history. The patient should be thoroughly interrogated to elicit the type and character of incontinence, exacerbating and alleviating factors and the use of chronic medications. Whether symptoms are acute or chronic, their progression, severity and their impact on quality of life should be assessed. Enquiry about symptoms related to prolapse should also be made.

It is difficult to arrive at a diagnosis of the type of incontinence from the history alone but a careful history will often determine the etiology. In stress urinary incontinence, sudden leakage of urine occurs with activities that increases the intra-abdominal pressure, like coughing, sneezing, laughing, exercise, rising up from the sitting position, etc. It is common in women after childbirth and menopause. The woman should be asked whether the leak is a few drops or is severe enough to saturate the outer cloth, whether protective pads need to be worn, do pads become saturated, how often they are changed; all indicating the severity of incontinence. Some women are not aware of incontinence while urine leaks. They just find themselves wet, often referred to as unconscious incontinence. Incontinence associated with a powerful urge to void goes in favor of urge incontinence. But according to a study by James et al (1999) GSI cannot be diagnosed from history alone.[5]

The distinction from urge incontinence is important in that, urge incontinence may result from underlying pathological processes like cystitis, neurogenic bladder or bladder outlet obstruction with loss of bladder compliance. They are more amenable to medical management. Diseases involving storage phase or filling phase cause irritative bladder symptoms like frequency, urgency and nocturia and need detailed enquiry. How long the patient can wait comfortably between urination or how often she voids during day and night indicates frequency. The cause of frequent voiding like urgency, convenience or an attempt to prevent incontinence should be sorted out. In urge incontinence, how long the patient can postpone micturition after feeling urgency should be noted. Sometimes incontinence is positional, occurring only in some position of the patient like sitting or lying down.

Diseases affecting the emptying phase can cause obstructive urinary symptoms. Voiding difficulty also should be elicited in the history as it is important in planning treatment. Voiding difficulty can be in the form of trouble starting the stream (hesitancy), need to strain for voiding, poor flow or post micturition dribble. Combination of urgency, frequency and dysuria suggest urinary tract infection. It may be a psychosocial reaction to stress or can be rarely due to neoplasia. *Persistence of such symptoms necessitates cystourethroscopic examination.*

Overflow incontinence also called paradoxical incontinence, is secondary to chronic retention and high residual volume. Here the bladder is chronically distended and never empties completely. It develops over a length of time and the patient gives history of incomplete emptying. The urine may dribble out in drops or small amounts and is likely to occur at night when the patient sleeps.

Continuous incontinence is commonly due to genito-urinary fistula. An ectopic ureter entering the urethra or genital tract can cause continuous incontinence with a normal voiding in between.

Nocturnal enuresis is the incontinence that occurs during sleep. It is normal in children up to 3 years of age, but may persists in 15% of children at 5 years and in 1% at 15 years of age. Usually children will not have any urological abnormality when investigated.

The causes of functional or transient incontinence occurring in old age can be remembered by the mnemonic suggested by Resnick, DIAPPERS- Delirium, Infection (urinary tract infection), Atrophic vaginitis or urethritis, Psychological, Pharmacological, Excessive production of urine, Restricted mobility, and Stool impaction.[6]

History of any neurological conditions that are known to affect the bladder and sphincter function like spinal cord injury, myelodysplasia, stroke, Parkinsonism, diabetes and multiple sclerosis should be elicited. A history of double vision, muscular weakness, poor coordination, tremor, numbness, and tingling sensation are important. History of surgery like vaginal surgery, abdomino-perineal resection for carcinoma of the rectum or hysterectomy may be associated with incontinence due to urinary fistula. Radiation therapy can affect bladder capacity, compliance and urethral coaptation.

Detailed history of the use of drugs which can affect lower urinary tract function like anti-hypertensives, sedatives, and antidepressants should be taken. Diuretic drugs worsen incontinence by increasing urine production. α blockers decrease urethral pressure and can lead to stress incontinence. ACE inhibitors can cause chronic cough which can precipitate incontinence. Sedatives can produce confusion in elderly patients and can lead to incontinence.

History should also include prolonged obstructed labor, number of vaginal deliveries and any hormone replacement therapy.

The physician should also elicit the extent to which the symptoms affect the quality of life. *If the complaint is minimal and does not affect social or professional life, aggressive surgical treatment should be avoided.* An assessment of the extent or severity of symptoms can be used as a baseline for assessing response to treatment. Enquiry should be made about the urinary frequency. A frequency of more than 7 voids/day should be taken as abnormal. Even though frequency depends upon habit and fluid intake, it forms a part of initial evaluation. The patient should be asked to keep a urinary diary for at least 3-5 days. It should contain the volume and time of each void, the precipitating factors and whether it is associated with urgency or not. The diary can be used to assess the severity of incontinence and to find out its relationship to precipitating factors. This record is used in the follow-up of patients who are under bladder retraining program.

Causes of transient incontinence in old age (DIAPPERS)

- Delirium
- Infection
- Atrophic vaginitis/urethritis
- Psychological
- Pharmacological
- Excessive urine production
- Restricted mobility
- Stool impaction

Physical Examination

General examination

The patient's appearance and gait as she enters the room should be observed. Limping gait, abnormal movements or abnormalities of speech point towards an underlying neurological disorder. The general fitness of the patient, as well as her mobility, mental status etc should be assessed to make out the fitness to undergo surgical procedures, which is important in planning management. A younger patient who is otherwise healthy, whose incontinence affects her professional or social life needs an aggressive treatment irrespective of the amount of urine leak, compared to a frail, very elderly lady with severe incontinence.

Neurological examination

Focused neurological examinations to make out the integrity of sacral innervations include assessment of genital and peri-anal sensation, anal sphincter tone and bulbocavernosus reflex (BCR). BCR is checked by stroking the clitoris and feeling the anal sphincter or perineal muscles for contraction.

Examination of the genitalia and pelvis

The genitalia should be inspected for atrophy, excoriation or erythema due to wetting. If the patient has significant incontinence there will be skin changes in the vulva. A thorough examination should be done to assess the pelvic support and function. Speculum examination should be done to inspect the vaginal walls to assess the degree of vaginal wall descent or prolapse of the uterus. Uterine and adnexal pathology should be excluded by bimanual examination.

Examination should be carried out in the lithotomy position with the bladder comfortably full. The patient should be asked to cough or strain in an attempt to reproduce stress incontinence. If no incontinence is demonstrated in a patient with history of stress incontinence, repeat the examination in standing position. Ask the patient to stand with one foot raised over a foot stool, and look for incontinence again while coughing or performing valsalva.

Urethral support can be evaluated by inspecting the vagina overlying the urethra and bladder neck. The method is subjective and hence the inference is prone for individual variation. The precise way is to do a radiological assessment. As a substitute the Q-tip test is introduced.

Investigations (Table 3.2)

The Q-tip Test (Figs 3.5A and B)

The Q-tip test is done to make out bladder neck descent. The test is done with the patient in the dorsal lithotomy position. A long cotton swab is lubricated with sterile jelly

Table 3.2: Investigations in genuine stress incontinence

Preliminary	*Investigations*
Q-Tip test	To assess bladder neck descent
Midstream specimen of urine for routine examination and culture	To exclude urinary tract infection
Urinary Diary (for 3-5 days)	To assess the frequency of urine leak and to find out its relation to other symptoms and fluid intake
Post void residual urine	To exclude voiding dysfunction
Ultrasound	To assess residual volume
Pad test	To quantify the urine leak
Basic Urodynamics	
Uroflowmetry	To assess urine flow rate so as to exclude associated voiding problems
Cystometry	To measure pressure volume relationships of the bladder so as to exclude detrusor overactivity
Special Investigations	
Ambulatory urodynamics	To assess pressure changes in bladder during natural filling and voiding
Video cystourethrography (previous surgery failure, suspicion of mixed incontinence or has unusual symptoms)	To assess bladder and urethral morphology, presence of diverticulum, vesico-ureteric reflux, vesico-vaginal fistula
Urethral pressure profilometry (previous surgery failure)	To measure urethral function (urethral instability or relaxation)
Cystourethroscopy (history of hematuria or recurrent UTI)	To assess bladder mucosa and urethral lumen

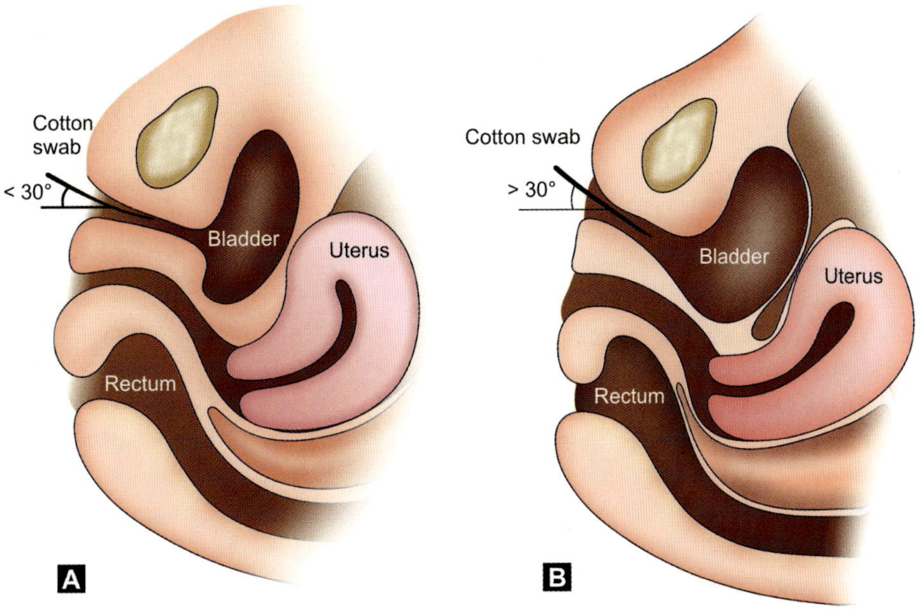

Figs 3.5A and B: Q tip test: (A) Normal angle of the cotton swab in the urethra with the horizontal (<30°). (B) Bladder neck descent resulting in >30° angle

and introduced through the urethra into the bladder. The swab is then withdrawn until definite resistance is felt when the inner end is at the urethro-vesical junction. The angle the Q-tip makes with the horizontal is measured. The angle is again measured with the patient straining. If the angle which the Q-tip makes with the horizontal is more than 30° while at rest or while straining, urethral hypermobility is thought to exist.[7] Presence of urethral hypermobility was thought to be a factor which determines the type of corrective surgery. Those who have hypermobility can be taken up for colposuspension and those who do not have it can be preferred for sling surgery. But this contention has not been convincingly proved in studies. Even though bladder neck descent is seen in women with stress urinary incontinence, it is not the sole pathophysiology in all women having incontinence. Moreover all women with bladder neck descent need not have incontinence. A simple test to differentiate between urethral hyper mobility and intrinsic sphincter deficiency as the cause for incontinence is clinical examination by elevating the urethra and supporting it with the use of an open ring forceps or a long artery clamp kept in the vagina, with the two arms placed in the two lateral vaginal fornices. The woman whose problem is bladder neck descent will not have incontinence, whereas if the problem is intrinsic sphincter deficiency, the woman will continue to leak even after the bladder neck is elevated. Bonney's test which involves obstruction to the bladder neck region will anyway stop urine leak, irrespective of the pathophysiology of stress incontinence and hence is not advised at present. Urethral hypermobility can be assessed more correctly by radiologic studies–bead-chain cystourethrography and voiding cystometrogram.

Midstream Urine Examination

Urinary symptoms like urgency, frequency etc can occur in urinary tract infection. Treatment of urinary infection will alleviate these symptoms. Hence it is important to exclude urinary tract infection in all women presenting with incontinence. Mid stream urine should be examined microscopically for pus cells. Urine should also be cultured and sensitivity tested. Invasive investigations should be started only after treating urinary tract infection if it is present.

Urinary Diary

Urinary diary is a reliable method of assessing the severity of incontinence. Urinary diary is a record of the fluid intake and output of the patient. Documentation is better than recall from memory. The patient should record the time, number and amount of leakage of urine, the quantity, quality and time of fluid intake. The diary should be maintained for a minimum of 5 days. Frequency due to overdrinking as well as the severity and frequency of urine leakage can be made out from the diary. The disadvantage of urinary diary is that the cause of the leakage cannot be determined. The diary is useful in the follow-up of a patient who is on a bladder retraining program.

Post Void Residual Urine

Post void residual urine should be assessed in all women presenting with lower urinary symptoms suggestive of incontinence, voiding dysfunction or urinary tract infection. Instead of catheterising to estimate the residual urine, a non-invasive method of assessing the residual urine volume by ultrasound should be resorted to. The normal residual urine can be <50 ml. Measurement of a catheterized sample is more accurate than ultrasound measurement.[8]

Ultrasound

Ultrasound is presently the investigation of choice for assessing residual volume. It avoids catheterization and the associated risk of urinary infections. Ultrasound can be used for the measurement of bladder wall thickness which is a predictor of detrusor overactivity (thickness >5 mm).

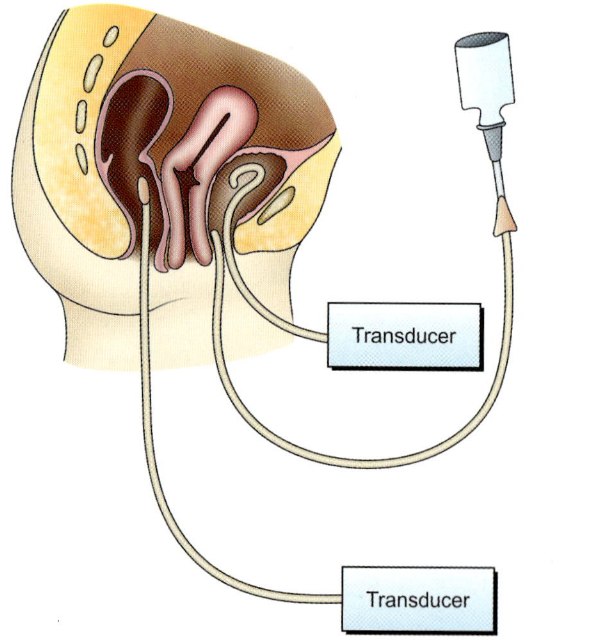

Fig. 3.6: Filling cystometry (multi channel). Pressure catheters are seen in the bladder and rectum. The filling catheter is seen in the bladder. Total bladder pressure, rectal (abdominal) pressure and subtracted detrusor pressure can be recorded

Presently the role of 3-dimensional ultrasound is being investigated for assessing the volume of rhabdosphincter. The rhabdosphincter is reported to be smaller in women with GSI.

The Pad Test

The pad test gives a measurement of leaked urine. The International Continence Society recommends a one hour pad test after 500 ml fluid load. The woman is asked to wear a weighed sanitary towel and drink 500 ml of water. After resting for 15 minutes she is asked to perform gentle exercises like walking or climbing steps. She is then asked to do more provocative exercises like running, walking, etc. The pad is weighed after one hour. An increase in weight of more than one gram is considered significant. An extended pad test for a period of 24 hours will give a better estimate of urine leakage. It is better to do a pad test for all women presenting with incontinence to know the severity of the symptom.

Uroflowmetry

This is a noninvasive investigation to establish the presence of voiding problems. The woman is asked to pass urine into the equipment which makes a graphic record of the flow. The normal recording gives a bell-shaped curve. The peak flow rate is 15 ml/sec for a voided volume of 150 ml. If the flow rate is less than normal the patient is likely to develop voiding difficulties in the postoperative period following surgery for incontinence. Even though noninvasive, this is not routinely done for women who are clinically suspected of having stress urinary incontinence.

Cystometry (Figs 3.7 to 3.10)

Cystometry is the most commonly performed urodynamic investigation. It is the investigation to find out the pressure volume changes in the bladder. Cystometry helps to differentiate between urge incontinence, stress incontinence, mixed incontinence as well as voiding difficulties. The investigation need not be done for all women presenting with incontinence. In a small group of women, when the clinical diagnosis of pure stress incontinence can be clearly made, cystometry need not be done. It should be done in the following situations:

1. When clinical features are not typical of either stress incontinence or urge incontinence.
2. When mixed incontinence is suspected.
3. It is ideal to exclude detrusor overactivity by cystometry before resorting to surgical procedures to treat stress incontinence.
4. It is a must before a repeat procedure. If urge incontinence is missed in a patient who has mixed incontinence and surgical correction is done for stress incontinence the patient will have severe urge incontinence postoperatively, a point which should be discussed with the patient before surgery.
5. When there are symptoms suggestive of voiding dysfunction.

Procedure

Filling cystometry (Fig. 3.6): In filling cystometry, only the pressure changes in the bladder is measured. Since the bladder pressure is affected by several factors, the most important being abdominal pressure, multichannel cystometry is preferred.

Multichannel cystometry: In multichannel cystometry the bladder pressure and the intra-abdominal pressure are measured. The intra-abdominal pressure is subtracted from the bladder pressure to get the detrusor pressure. Initially the woman is asked to void into a flow meter to measure urine flow rate. The residual volume is then measured. To measure bladder pressure, a fluid filled line which is attached to an external pressure transducer is introduced into the bladder. The intra-abdominal pressure is measured by placing a similar catheter covered with a rubber finger into the rectum to indirectly measure the intra-abdominal pressure. The bladder is filled with a 12 F catheter at a rate of 10-100 ml/minute. The detrusor pressure is calculated by subtracting the abdominal pressure from the intravesical pressure. Normally this bladder filling will not

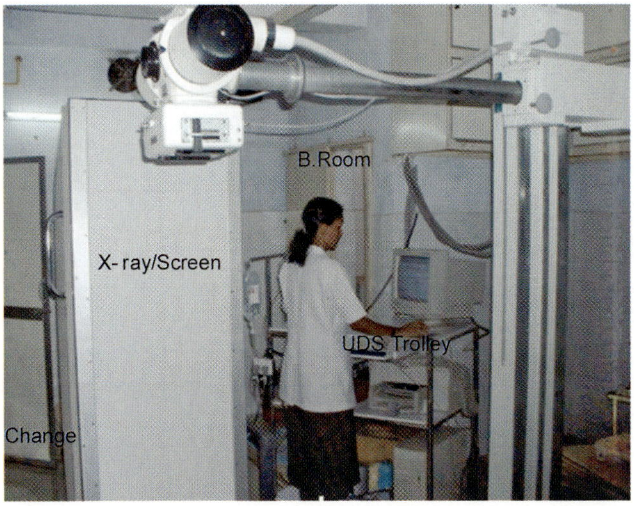

Fig. 3.7: Set-up for urodynamics. Urodynamic pump, computer and printer are seen. The X-ray unit for taking cystogram is also seen. *Courtesy: Specialist Hospital, Kochi*

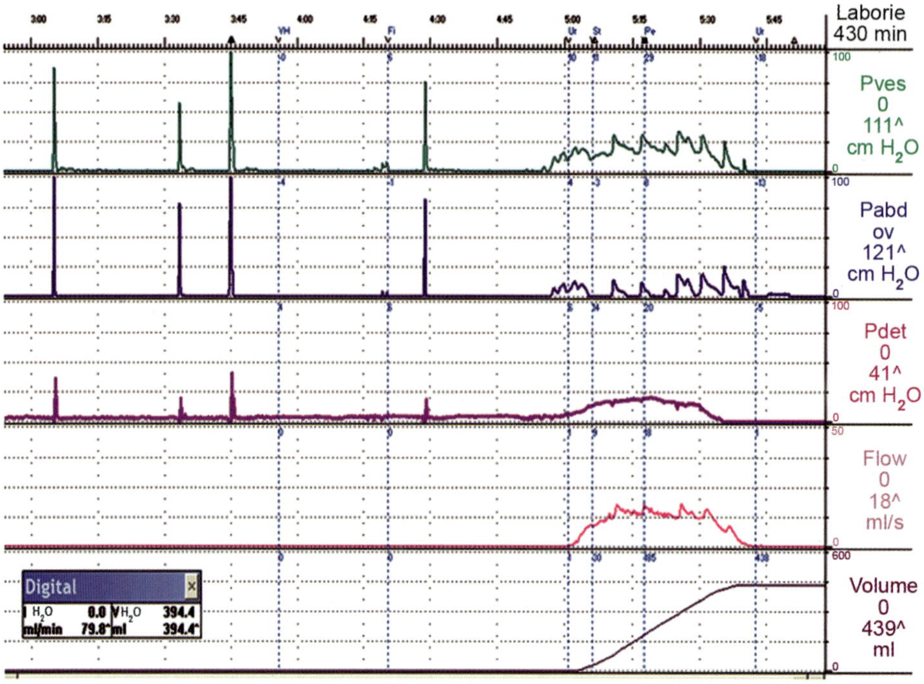

Fig. 3.8: Cystogram belonging to a patient with stress incontinence. The recording shows no unstable bladder contractions. *Courtesy: Specialist Hospital, Kochi*

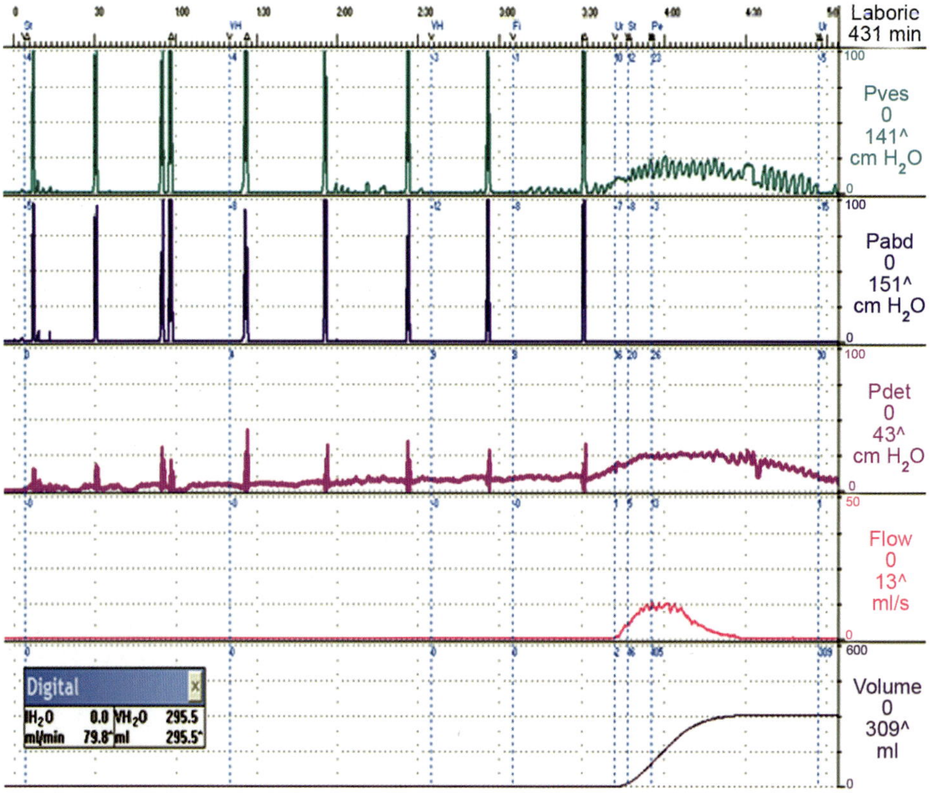

Fig. 3.9: Cystogram of a patient who presented with incontinence. Cystogram shows minimal detrusor pressure changes at rest but no urine leak. *Courtesy: Specialist Hospital, Kochi*

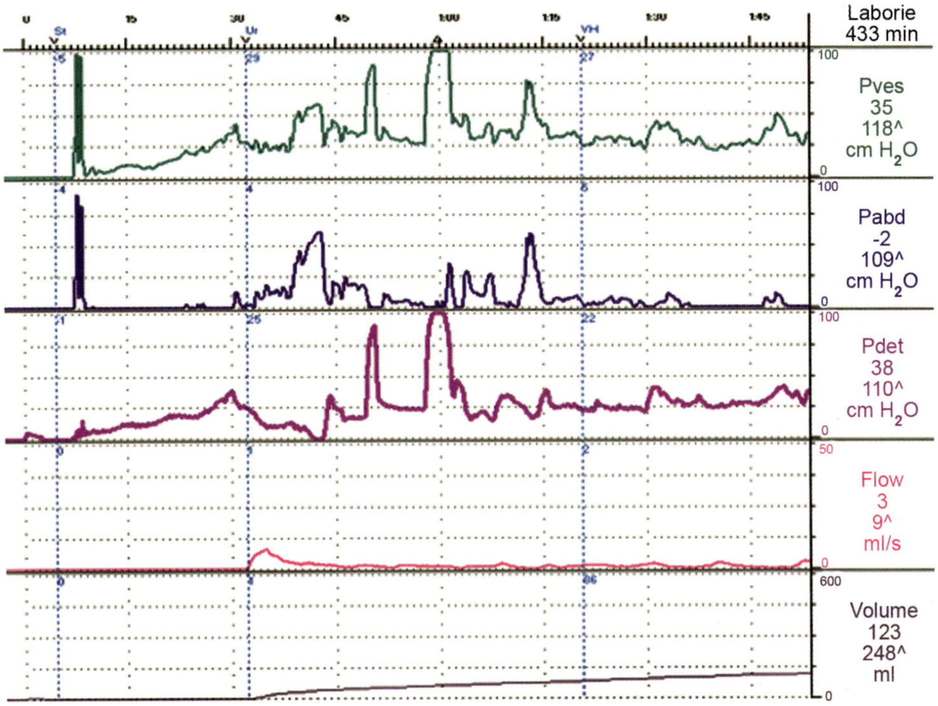

Fig. 3.10: Cystogram of a 21-year-old lady with nocturnal enuresis and severe urge incontinence. Detrusor contractions in the absence of increase in intra-abdominal pressure are seen. *Courtesy: Specialist Hospital, Kochi*

provoke detrusor contraction. The volume at which the woman feels the first desire to void and the maximum desire to void are noted. The detrusor pressure is noted at various quantities of filling and during coughing and running. After complete filling, the filling catheter is removed and the woman is asked to stand. She is then asked to cough and leakage is looked for. The occurrences of detrusor contraction on provocations as with sound of running water indicate detrusor over activity. The woman is then asked to void into a flow meter to measure urine flow rate, with the pressure lines *in situ*.

Normal Cystometry findings

1. Residual urine <50 ml
2. The first desire to void at about 200-250 ml of filling.
3. Bladder capacity—The volume at which the woman feels the strong desire to void. It should be more than 400 ml.
4. Normal detrusor pressure- Maximum detrusor pressure during filling <15 cm of H_2O. No detrusor pressure rise on filling.
5. Absence of cystometric detrusor contractions.
6. No leakage on coughing.
7. Detrusor pressure rise during voiding <50 cm of water with a peak flow rate >15 ml/sec at a voided volume over 150 ml.

Abnormal Cystometry

Leakage of urine during rise in intra-abdominal pressure in the absence of rise in detrusor pressure indicates stress incontinence. The test cannot confirm stress incontinence as the urethral pressure is not recorded in cystometrogram. Bladder neck descent can be conclusively made out only by imaging during voiding lateral cystometrogram. Detrusor instability can be made out by the presence of spontaneous or provoked detrusor contractions while the woman is not voiding. Low compliance is diagnosed by detrusor pressure rise >15 cm of water, when the bladder is filled with 500 ml of fluid and is maintained at that level even after filling is stopped.

Ambulatory Cystometry

Since cystometry is done in the laboratory setting it is inconclusive in 15-25% of women. This is thought to be due to the test occurring in an artificial environment during a short period. The normal filling is at a much slower rate than done during cystometry. Normally it is urine that fills the bladder, rather than saline. Hence ambulatory cystometry is introduced in which the pressure changes in the bladder during normal filling are studied. In ambulatory monitoring, portable digital storage device is attached to the woman's body over several hours till the end of the procedure. The device records the pressures automatically while the bladder fills and empties normally. At the end of the procedure the patient is made to do provocation tests. The recordings over the whole duration of the test are evaluated.

Assessment of Urethral Function

Poor urethral function is evidenced by:

1. Low valsalva leak point pressure
2. Low maximal urethral closure pressure
3. Visualization of open bladder neck at cystoscopy

Urethral closure pressure is urethral pressure minus vesical pressure. The urethral pressure should be higher than the intravesical pressure for maintaining continence. Hence assessment of urethral pressure is important in incontinent women. The instrument used is expensive and the investigation is not usually done as a routine procedure. The test is indicated before a repeat procedure for incontinence. The device consists of 2 micro-transducers mounted on a 7 F catheter at a distance of 6 cm. The bladder is filled with about 250 ml of saline and the catheter is introduced into the bladder so that both the transducers are inside the bladder. The catheter is connected to a catheter withdrawal mechanism, which withdraws the catheter through the urethra, at a rate of 5 cm/minute. As the catheter is pulled along the urethra, the intravesical pressure and the intraurethral pressure are recorded. The recording generates a curve called urethral pressure profile. The intravesical pressure is subtracted from the maximal urethral pressure to get the maximum urethral closure pressure. The static urethral pressure is the pressure in the urethra at rest. Dynamic urethral pressure is the difference between the maximal urethral pressure and the intravesical pressure while the woman coughs. Women having stress urinary incontinence will have a lower urethral closure pressure than continent women. Women who have a lower static urethral pressure (<20 cm of water) can be expected to have a 50% failure rate with the conventional continence procedures like Burch colposuspension. They need a more obstructive urethral procedure as treatment. The pressure reading obtained depends upon several variables like the orientation of the transducer, the rate of withdrawal of catheter, the position of the patient etc. The test has not gained popularity due to the lack of specificity and sensitivity.

Video Cystogram

This is the most advanced form of urodynamics. It is not a routine investigation, but is indicated in refractory stress incontinence when an initial surgery has failed.

If videography is added to cystourethrography a dynamic assessment of sphincteric integrity can be made. The intra vesical pressure at which leakage is recorded radiographically is the leak point pressure. A leak point pressure <60 cm of water denote intrinsic sphincter deficiency. The lesser the leak point pressure more severe will be the incontinence. The pressure is measured by keeping catheters placed in the bladder, rectum or vagina. It gives a measurement of the urethral resistance to increase in the intra abdominal pressure. The intravesical pressure at which leakage is identified during video urodynamic study can also be made out. The usefulness of the test is not yet established.

Cystourethroscopy

Cystoscopy is not routinely advised for all patients with lower urinary tract symptoms. But in the presence of persistence of bladder symptoms, associated hematuria or repeated surgical failure cystourethroscopy should be done to exclude bladder calculus, bladder tumor, urethral diverticulum and scarring of urethra and bladder neck. Visualization of an open bladder neck denotes poor urethral function.

3.9.5 Management

Conservative Management

Even though stress incontinence is a distressing symptom, it is not a life threatening condition. The etiology of the condition differs in different individuals. Success rate and complications of the surgical procedures vary. No one method is proved to be ideal for treating stress incontinence. Conservative treatment should be resorted to before surgical treatment. The woman who is suspected to have GSI, who has normal voiding diary and normal residual urine in ultrasound does not need urodynamic study before resorting to nonsurgical treatment.

Lifestyle modification: Women, who take more fluid than needed, should be advised to reduce fluid intake. Weight reduction has also been found to be effective in controlling urinary incontinence. Women with BMI>30 should be advised to lose weight.

Pelvic floor muscle strengthening program: The precise mechanism by which urethral tone, bladder neck and urethral mobility and the tone of the pelvic floor interacts to maintain continence remains unclear. However, it is clear that the tone of the levator ani muscle complex provides support for the urethra, vagina and rectum. The reflex contraction of levator ani in response to sudden increase in intra abdominal pressure while coughing or sneezing prevents development of stress incontinence. Hence it is prudent to rehabilitate the levator ani muscle,[9] to improve the continence mechanism.

Pelvic floor muscle exercise comprises contraction of pelvic floor muscles which can be performed as at least 8 contractions 3 times a day. If this is found to be beneficial it should be continued. There is good evidence that supervised pelvic floor muscle training for at least 3 months duration is a safe and effective initial treatment option for stress incontinence as well as mixed incontinence.

It was Arnold Kegel who first investigated the role of pelvic floor muscle strengthening exercise in the treatment of SUI. He developed a pneumatic bio-feedback device called the perineometer. A supervised pelvic floor muscle exercise is more rewarding than simply advising the patient to do the exercise. The introduction of a bio-feedback helps the patient to judge the progress. Supervision and feedback will make a drastic difference in the success rate of pelvic muscle rehabilitation.

Perineometry can be used as a bio-feedback, but it need not be routine. Perineometer is a cylindrical vaginal device which is kept in the vagina and the pressure generated while the pelvic floor muscles are contracted is recorded. It can be used for detecting improvement while performing pelvic floor exercises.

Weighted vaginal cones are available in a set of 3 or 5. They are of the same size but increasing weight. The cone is inserted in to the vagina to stimulate contraction of pelvic floor muscle. When cones of increasing weights are used subsequently the pelvic muscles get strengthened by the contractions induced in an effort to prevent the cone from falling.

Pelvic muscle exercises should be advised as an initial line of management for all women having GSI unless the incontinence is very severe. Most patients with mild incontinence will improve with exercise. Women with severe incontinence may not benefit from pelvic floor exercise. The exercise program has the advantage of involving the patient in her own care. Pelvic floor exercise simultaneously takes care of pelvic relaxation altogether which might prevent pelvic organ prolapse as well. In fact it can be incorporated as a routine program for the maintenance of women's health. All women should be advised pelvic floor exercise as a routine after delivery. Innovations in pelvic muscle rehabilitation, in the form of electrical stimulation of the muscle have been developed in an effort to improve the results.

One of the latest innovations in pelvic floor rehabilitation is pulsed magnetic technology to promote muscle strength of the pelvic floor. The therapy can be given while the patient sits on a chair. No intravaginal device is required and hence patient tolerance is better. The utility of this method of treatment is being evaluated.

Drug Treatment

The tone of the urethra and bladder neck is maintained by sympathetic system especially the α-adrenergic receptors. Hence drugs which increase the α-adrenergic activity will improve urethral tone and hence GSI. The drugs which are commonly used include imipramine (10-25 mg t.i.d.), ephedrine (15-30 mg t.i.d.) and phenyl-propanolamine (50-75 mg b.i.d). But these drugs being α-adrenergic will increase the vascular tone and hence cause hypertension especially in postmenopausal women. In this context it is worth remembering that women who are on α-blockers can have incontinence as an adverse effect. Drug treatment should not be offered as first line treatment for women with stress incontinence because of these side-effects.

Duloxetine (40 mg/day) is a selective serotonin and norepinephrine reuptake inhibitor (SNRI). The efficacy and safety of duloxetine[10] was evaluated in a randomized trial. It was found to decrease the episodes of incontinence and improve symptoms in a dose dependent manner. At a dose of 40 mg/day there was a decrease in frequency of incontinence in 59% of women treated. It can be offered to women who are not willing or are unfit for surgery. Nausea, dryness of mouth, headache and dizziness were reported as side effects. Duloxetine can be effectively combined with pelvic floor strengthening exercises.

Hormone Replacement Therapy

It was thought that estrogen administration could be beneficial in treating urinary incontinence in postmenopausal women. Contrary to this contention, it was proved in a large randomized trial (The WHI study) that both estrogen alone and estrogen and progesterone combination increased the incidence of stress urinary incontinence in postmenopausal[11] women.

Surgical Treatment of Stress Urinary Incontinence

When the conservative therapy fails surgery should be considered.

Selection of Patients for Surgical Treatment

The very fact that there are over 200 surgical procedures described for correcting the condition reveals that no one method is ideal. Surgical treatment should be planned only when conservative treatment by pelvic floor strengthening exercise fails. Before resorting to surgical procedures urodynamic study (cystometry) should be done to exclude voiding difficulty and detrusor overactivity. The presence of associated voiding difficulty or detrusor overactivity can change the surgical decision. The woman who has detrusor overactivity can be informed prior to surgery that the detrusor overactivity might worsen after surgery, so also the voiding difficulty. The first attempt of surgery is the best attempt for the patient.

The operations which are usually resorted to, fall under 2 main categories. The two main etiologies—urethral hypermobility and intrinsic sphincter deficiency determines this division. However it should be kept in mind that there can be a combination of the two in different proportions.

1. Procedures to correct incontinence caused by urethral hypermobility.
   a. Anterior colporrhaphy with Kelley 's bladder neck plication
   b. Abdominal bladder neck suspension procedures
      i. Retropubic bladder neck suspension / cystourethropexy
         - Marshall-Marchetti-Krantz procedure
         - Burch colposuspension
      ii. Paravaginal repair
      iii. Needle suspension procedures
         - Pereyera procedure
         - Modifications
2. Procedures to treat intrinsic sphincter deficiency
   a. Sling operations
      i. Organic materials- Autologous and heterologous
      ii. Synthetic materials- TVT and TVT-O
   b. Periurethral injections
      i. Teflon
      ii. Collagen
      iii. Fat
   c. Artificial urinary sphincter

1. Anterior Vaginal Repair

It consists of approximating pubo-vesico-cervical fascia in the midline to form a buttress for the bladder. The buttressing sutures placed in the region of the bladder neck reform the posterior urethrovesical angle and elevate the upper urethra. Randomized trials including anterior colporrhaphy and colposuspension reports a continence rate of 63% for anterior colporrhaphy, but at 1 year follow-up it fell to 36%. Due to the poor long-term results it is thought to be inferior to colposuspension procedures. Abdominal retropubic colposuspension procedure and Tension-free Vaginal Tape (TVT) are the procedures of choice at present.[12]

2. Retropubic Bladder Neck Suspension

Marshall-Marchetti-Krantz bladder neck suspension: Bladder neck suspension was originally described by Dr. Marshall, Marchetti and Krantz of the Cornell University Medical Centre. In bladder neck suspension surgeries, bladder neck and upper urethra are suspended with sutures placed on either side of bladder neck in the vaginal wall and anchored to the periosteum of pubic symphysis approaching through the retropubic space. This elevates the bladder neck and upper urethra and reforms the posterior urethrovesical angle. Because of the serious complication of periosteitis, this method is not commonly resorted to at present.

Burch colposuspension (Fig. 3.11): The procedure was described by John Burch Nashville[13] in 1961. In Burch colposuspension, bladder neck is anchored to the reflected part of the inguinal ligament (ileopectineal ligament). The bladder neck is approached transabdominally through the cave of Retzius. A Cherney incision is made 1 fingerbreadth above the pubic symphysis. For better exposure of the cave of Retzius, the rectus muscle is cut from its insertion on both sides. The peritoneal cavity need not be entered if hysterectomy is not otherwise required. The entire surgery is done in the retropubic space. The cave of Retzius is entered and the bladder and urethra are separated from the pubic symphysis. The bleeding points are coagulated. Bladder neck is identified by the bulb of the Foley catheter introduced before the procedure. As the assistant pushes the lateral vaginal fornix from below, sutures are taken from either side of the upper end of urethra, urethrovesical junction

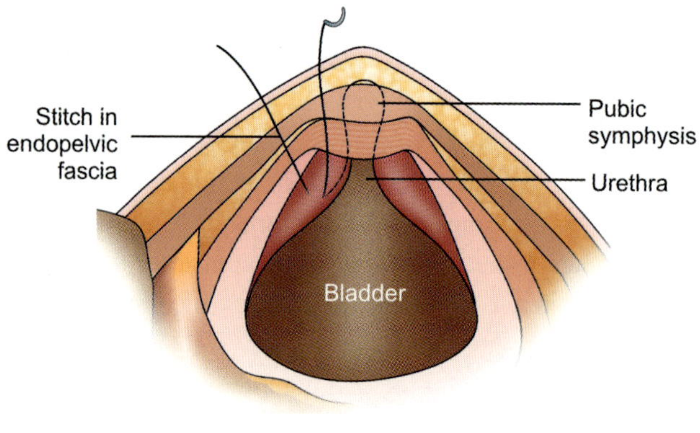

Fig. 3.11: Diagrammatic representation of Burch colposuspension. The suture is seen in the vaginal adventitia lateral to the urethrovesical junction. (Redrawn from TeLinde's operative gynecology 9th edition)

and lower end of bladder, through the endopelvic fascia over the vaginal wall but it should not cut through the vaginal mucosa. The sutures should not inadvertently pass through the urethra or bladder. The ileopectineal ligament is identified by tracing the inguinal ligament and the superior pubic rami. Laterally the obturator foramen and the obturator neurovascular bundle can be seen. Care should be taken not to injure the external iliac vein and artery which can be identified lateral to the femoral canal. The surgeon is likely to encounter considerable venous oozing from this area. The veins should be avoided while taking the sutures. Permanent (Prolene) or delayed absorbable (polydioxenone or PDS) sutures should be used. The procedure corrects cystocoele also. The detached muscles are approximated and the subcutaneous tissue and skin are closed. It is better to insert a retropubic drain if there is significant oozing from the cave of Retzius. As postoperative urinary obstruction is likely to occur, the patient should be on continuous bladder drainage for a few days. Regular complete bladder emptying should be ensured after removing the catheter. Suprapubic catheterization is an option, the advantage of which is that after the period of continuous catheterization is over, the suprapubic catheter can be clamped and the patient instructed to void so that the post void residual urine can be calculated. This avoids frequent introduction of transurethral catheter to measure post void residual urine. If the sutures are tight post operative voiding difficulty and later enterocele formation can follow.

Burch colposuspension is the most effective surgical procedure for stress incontinence. A Cochrane review has reported immediate success rate of 85-90% and a 5 year success rate of 70% following the procedure. Newer minimal access procedures like tension free vaginal tape look promising, but their long-term performance is not known. Laparoscopic colposuspension[14] entails speedier recovery but its relative safety and effectiveness is not known yet.

Complications of the Procedure Include

a. Voiding difficulty—might occur in 10.3% of women after colposuspension.
b. Detrusor overactivity—can occur de novo after the procedure. It is reported to occur in 8-27% of women.
c. Enterocele: Since the anterior vaginal wall is pulled up in colposuspension, the posterior vaginal wall is likely to prolapse. This has been reported to occur in 13.6% of women after surgery. If colposuspension is done along with hysterectomy, inserting an internal McCall's suture will prevent occurrence of enterocele.

3. Paravaginal Repair

This is based on the assumption that hypermobility of the bladder neck that results in descent of urethra and incontinence is because of the detachment of the endopelvic fascia from its normal attachment to arcus tendineus. In paravaginal[15] repair, endopelvic fascia is reattached to the arcus tendineus fascia bilaterally. The approach is the same as for Burch colposuspension. After reaching the cave of Retzius, the arcus tendineus is identified as a thin white band along the pelvic side wall over the obturator internus muscle from the pubic symphysis to the ischial spine. Care should be taken not to injure the obturator neurovascular bundle which runs above the level of the arcus tendineus over the pelvic side wall. This procedure is effective, durable and causes less voiding difficulty compared to Burch colposuspension. The cure rates are reported as 72% which is much lower than that of Burch colposuspension.

4. Endoscopic Retropubic Bladder Neck Suspension

With advance in endoscopy, Burch like procedure is done using the laparoscope. The retropubic space is entered with a laparoscope and the endopelvic fascia and the bladder neck are anchored to the Cooper's ligament. The endoscopic procedure is advised only for those who have not had previous surgeries. Women, who have had previous surgery for incontinence, will have significant scarring in the cave of Retzius, which makes endoscopic procedures difficult. This procedure should be done only by skilled endoscopic surgeons. Evidence from a Cochrane review on the subject is that laparoscopic colposuspension is as good as open colposuspension at two years postsurgery. The newer vaginal sling procedures (TVT and TOT) appear to offer even greater benefits and better objective outcomes. However, the long term successes of endoscopic procedures as well as the newer vaginal sling procedure are unknown.[16]

5. Needle Suspension Procedure

The procedure was first described by Armand Pereyra in 1959. In needle suspension procedure, the bladder neck is suspended using a suture which is introduced by a combined vaginal and abdominal approach using a long needle. A small suprapubic incision is made about two finger breadth above the pubic symphysis. The subcutaneous fat is separated to the level of the anterior rectus sheath. A long needle threaded with suture is passed through this incision blindly, through the cave of Retzius into the vagina. The vagina is incised in the midline at the region of the bladder neck and urethra.

The bladder neck is identified and dissection is carried on either side of the bladder upwards. During the dissection care is taken to dissect close to the pubic bone so that the bladder is not injured. The needle should exit through the vaginal incision at the level of the bladder neck. The bladder neck region is suspended with the help of suture to the abdominal fascia. Bladder injury should be excluded by cystoscopy at the end of the procedure. The vaginal and abdominal incisions are closed.

A Cochrane review of 8 trials including 327 women found that needle suspension procedures were more likely to fail than open retropubic procedures and the complication rates were also found to be high for needle suspension. Because of the high failure and complication rates, the procedure is not resorted to at present.

6. Sling Procedures

In sling procedures, the midurethra is elevated using either natural fascia or artificial materials and anchored to the anterior abdominal wall. Slings provide both urethral support and partial urethral compression. The procedure is effective in women who have bladder neck descent or sphincteric deficiency or both. It can be recommended to women who have previous suspension surgery failure. Sling procedures were in use since several years. Several different synthetic materials have been used as slings like nylon, marlex, mersilene, gore-TeX or homologous fascia lata, gracilis muscle, round ligament or rectus sheath.

Tension-free vaginal tape (TVT)

TVT is a minimally invasive surgical procedure for the treatment of stress incontinence. It was Ulmsten who first described slingplasty for the treatment of GSI in 1996. This is modified as the present TVT procedure. The procedure involves introduction of a knitted polypropelene mesh transabdominally to support the mid-urethra. After introduction the mesh will be interpenetrated by fibroblasts causing scar tissue which will hold the mesh in place for a long period without the need for inserting sutures. The procedure is done under conscious sedation so that intraoperatively the tightness of the sling can be checked. The device consists of a long prolene mesh (11 mm x 40 cm) with two 5 mm trochars at both ends. The skin, subcutaneous fat and the deep tissue behind the space of Retzius are infiltrated with local anaesthesia. Two small incisions are made suprapubically on either side of midline about 2.5 cm apart. If the incisions are more lateral there is risk of injury to the inferior epigastric vessels. Another incision about 1.5 cm is made in the vaginal wall over the mid-urethra. An 18 F Foley catheter is introduced into the bladder. The urethra is identified and the trocar is introduced by the side of the urethra blindly through the cave of Retzius to emerge through the abdominal incision. An identical procedure is repeated on the other side. Both the ends of the tape are pulled through the abdominal incision so that the mid-urethra is supported by the tape. The tightness of the tape is adjusted by asking the patient to cough. The tape is made tight so that no urine escapes while coughing. The redundant abdominal end of the tape is cut away along with the trochar so that the ends rest in the fatty tissue. The three incisions are then closed. Cystoscopy should be performed after insertion of each trochar in order to exclude bladder perforation. Since the trochar is inserted blindly, there can be serious complications like hemorrhage, hematoma formation or laceration of the iliac or inferior epigastric vessels if the trochar goes laterally. Rarely inadvertent intraperitoneal entry can cause bowel perforation. Hence the procedure should be performed by surgeons familiar with the relevant anatomy. The procedure can be performed quickly within 20-30 minutes. A long-term sequel is mesh erosion. If the mesh is tight during insertion, patient can have voiding difficulties. Rarely, voiding difficulty might require intermittent catheterization. Hence, these women should be taught intermittent clean self-catheterization. In the event of such a complication, removal of the tape is mandatory. The most commonly reported complication is bladder perforation.

The procedure is reported to carry 86% complete cure and a further 11% significant improvement at 3 years follow-up. The short term follow up of TVT and Burch colposuspension show similar continence rates16. But the long term follow up of TVT is still awaited. Even though the tape is expensive, the short hospital stay needed for the procedure makes it cost effective.

Transobturator sling procedure (TVT-O*)*

To reduce complications associated with retropubic vaginal tape, a modification in the form of transobturator sling procedure is developed. Here, the transobturator tape is introduced with the help of two specially designed needles through a vaginal incision to emerge lateral to the ischio-pubic rami. The procedure starts with a 2-3 cm incision in the anterior vaginal wall, 1 cm proximal to the external urethral meatus. After separating the endopelvic fascia from the vagina by sharp dissection, a finger is inserted through the vagina, in such a direction as to reach the under surface of the inferior ramus of the pubis. Another incision is made in the groin at about the level of insertion of the adductor longus tendon. In the outside-in procedure, the TOT trochar is passed directly posteriorly through the adductor muscles, the obturaror externus, obturator membrane and the obturator internus muscle. There will be a feeling of loss of resistance as the needle emerges from the obturator muscles. The direction of the trochar tip is turned medially till it comes in contact with the vaginal finger. The TOT tape is attached to the trochar and is then brought out through the groin incision. The same procedure is repeated on the opposite side and the other end of the tape is brought back out through the opposite groin. The tape thus forms a hammock mesh placed under the mid-urethra. The incisions are closed. Cystoscopy can be performed at the end of the procedure to exclude injury to bladder or urethra.

TVT-O is also not free of complications. It passes about 2-4 cm from the obturator nerve and vessels. Consequently, injury to the obturator nerve and vessels is a serious complication of the procedure. Even though initial studies reported improvement in about 80%, long term results are awaited.

7. Periurethral Injections

Women developing recurrence after colposuspension or sling procedures, who are identified as having intrinsic sphincter deficiency, can be given a trial of periurethral injections. The objective of the injection is to improve urethral coaptation at the level of the bladder neck. Bulking agents like gluteraldehyde cross-linked collagen, Teflon, fat, silicon etc are injected into the periurethral tissue around the bladder neck and proximal urethra or else transurethrally. Periurethral route is preferred because it avoids the leakage of collagen through the urethral puncture site. The success rate reported is 48%. Those who have detrusor overactivity are more likely to fail, and hence should be excluded from the procedure. The disadvantage of the procedure is the high long-term failure due to degradation of the injected material.

8. Artificial Sphincters

When all the other surgical procedures fail and the patient has severe intrinsic sphincter deficiency, placement of artificial sphincter is an option. The device is a small inflatable cuff that is implanted around the bladder neck and the proximal urethra. It is connected to a pump which is implanted within one of the labia majora and a reservoir which is placed in the abdomen beneath the fascia. The patient can deflate or inflate the cuff by squeezing the pump. When the pump is squeezed the fluid from the pump is emptied into the reservoir and the patient can void. After voiding, the cuff gets automatically reinflated. Thus the patient can void as and when she desires. As may happen with any other artificial implant, erosion or infection may occur. Cure rate of 80% and improvement rate of 90% have been reported.

3.10 MANAGEMENT OF MIXED INCONTINENCE

Many women may have both detrusor instability and GSI. There is a chance of exacerbation of detrusor overactivity when surgery for correcting urethral descent is done for women with mixed incontinence. But in some women, detrusor instability disappears after surgery. Rarely, detrusor instability not documented prior to surgery can develop postoperatively. Patient should be counseled for persistence or worsening of detrusor instability before being taken up for surgical procedures. It seems wise to give an initial trial of behavioral therapy or pharmacotherapy for detrusor instability before surgery.

3.11 MANAGEMENT OF RECURRENT INCONTINENCE

Women who present with recurrence of symptoms after initial surgery should be evaluated for the cause. It could be due to the associated detrusor instability which was overlooked or a failure of the procedure. These patients should be thoroughly evaluated with cystometry and cystourethroscopy. Cystometry identifies detrusor instability and cystourethroscopy identifies intrinsic problems of bladder and urethra. Those who have a scarred low pressure urethra should be advised sling operation. TVT is the treatment of choice. If severe sphincter deficiency is identified, periurethral bulking agents can be used. When all the methods fail, the last option is an artificial sphincter implantation.

3.12 DETRUSOR OVERACTIVITY

Detrusor overactivity is characterized by involuntary detrusor contractions during the filling phase of the bladder, which may be spontaneous or provoked. This is associated with symptoms of urgency. When the bladder pressure exceeds the urethral pressure, urge incontinence ensues. Detrusor overactivity can be further classified as neurogenic, non-neurogenic or idiopathic.

3.12.1 Types of Detrusor Overactivity

Neurogenic Detrusor Overactivity

When detrusor overactivity is associated with neurologic disorders, it is called neurogenic detrusor overactivity. It is also known as detrusor hyperreflexia. Lesions in the brain, spinal cord or peripheral nerves can affect micturition. The neural centre which coordinates voiding function is located in the pons, the pontine micturition center. When there is a lesion above the pons, the micturition reflex is intact and there is a co-ordinated relaxation of the sphincter during detrusor contraction. Patient may only lose the ability to either initiate or prevent micturition. The causes include stroke, Parkinson's disease, brain tumor, head injury and multiple sclerosis. Patients may have urgency, urge incontinence, or detrusor areflexia with overflow incontinence. The exact neurological pathways for suprapontine lesions are not yet described.

When the neural pathways connecting the pontine micturition center to the sacral micturition center is affected, detrusor overactivity and loss of coordinated sphincter relaxation result. This is called detrusor sphincter dyssynergia (DSD). Poor coordination of micturition reflex also causes weak, poorly sustained detrusor contractions. The lesions include spinal cord injury, spinal cord tumors, multiple sclerosis, myelodysplasia and transverse myelitis.

Sacral and peripheral neurologic lesions have varying effects depending on the extent of lesion. Sacral lesions are caused by disc prolapse, multiple sclerosis, and sacral cord tumors. Complete parasympathetic lesions cause areflexic bladder with retention. Sympathetic lesion causes loss of sphincteric function and nonfunctioning proximal urethra. Somatic neurologic lesions affect pudendal afferent and efferent nerves. This can cause loss of perineal and perianal sensations and impaired ability to contract urethral and anal sphincters voluntarily. Causes of peripheral nerve affection include extensive pelvic surgeries like abdomino-pelvic resection and radical hysterectomy, and diabetic neuropathy.

Non-neurogenic Detrusor Overactivity

The common non-neurological disease that causes unstable bladder contraction is cystitis. Bladder tumor, foreign bodies in the bladder, and bladder outlet obstruction can also result in unstable bladder. The causes of outlet obstruction in women include pelvic organ prolapse, urethral stricture, meatal stenosis, urethral diverticulum and primary bladder neck stenosis.

Idiopathic Detrusor Overactivity (detrusor instability)

Involuntary detrusor contraction in the absence of known neurologic or non-neurologic diseases is termed idiopathic detrusor overactivity.

3.12.2 Clinical Features

Women having detrusor overactivity can present with symptoms like urgency, urge incontinence, stress incontinence, nocturia etc. Urgency need not always be associated with incontinence. The diagnosis can only be made by urodynamic study with which detrusor contractions are made out.

3.12.3 Management (Table 3.3)

The aim of treatment is to reduce the severity of urgency or at least increase the warning time. Management is mainly conservative which includes bladder training and drug therapy.

Bladder training: Bladder training for a minimum of 6 weeks should be offered as first line treatment for women diagnosed to have urge incontinence or mixed incontinence. Bladder training includes gradual increase in duration between voids (habit retraining). The patient should be instructed to void every 1 ½ hrs during the day, gradually the interval can be increased by ½ an hour. Fluid intake should be just adequate. The woman should be instructed to keep a fluid chart. The patient has to be highly motivated for the success of treatment.

Drug treatment: If bladder training is not found to be effective oxybutynin should be offered as the first line drug treatment. Women, who cannot tolerate oxybutynin, should be offered tolterodine, trospium, solifenacin or transdermal or intravesical oxybutynin. The major side effect of oxybutynin is dry mouth. Tolterodine is a muscarinic receptor antagonist which has a relative selectivity for bladder receptors. Several randomized trials have reported significant reduction in incontinence with the administration of tolterodine. An extended release once daily preparation is presently available (UROTEL XL™). Trospium is also a muscarinic receptor antagonist. The incidence of dry mouth is less compared to oxybutynin. Solifenacin, a potent M3 receptor antagonist is given in a dose of 5 mg or 10 mg once daily. Darifenacin, a highly selective M3 receptor blocker is also found to be effective. Dry mouth is the major adverse effect of both solifenacin and darifenacin. Imipramine, a tricyclic antidepressant with anticholinergic properties is found to be beneficial in patients with nocturia.

Table 3.3: Management of detrusor overactivity

Behavioral Therapy	Bladder training
Drug Therapy	Drugs inhibiting bladder contraction
	a. Anticholinergic
	Tolterodine
	Trospium
	Solifenacin
	Darifenacin
	b. Antimuscarininc and muscle relaxants
	Oxybutynin
	Dropiverine
	Flavoxate
	c. Antidepressants
	Imipramine
	Amytryptilline
	Drugs reducing urine production
	DDAVP (Synthetic vasopressin)
	Intra vesical therapy
	Capsaicin
Neuromodulation	Sacral nerve stimulation
Surgical treatment	Clam cystoplasty
	Urinary diversion

Desmopressin, because of its antidiuretic effect can be used as a treatment for nocturia. Presently it is available as a nasal spray. But it should be used with care since it can cause hypernatremia especially in the elderly.

Intravesical therapy: Patients with neurogenic detrusor overactivity secondary to multiple sclerosis are found to benefit from intravesical capsaicin dissolved in 30% alcohol. The effect can last for about 6 months.

Botulinum toxin, which causes inhibition of calcium mediated release of acetylcholine at the presynaptic neuromuscular junction, can be made use of in the treatment of neurogenic detrusor overactivity. The use of the drug as direct injection into the detrusor under cystoscopic guidance is being studied in trials.

Neuromodulation: Drug treatment may not be tolerated by most women. Sacral nerve stimulation is recommended for such patients. The sacral nerves give parasympathetic and sympathetic innervations to the bladder. They also give somatic supply. Stimulation of these nerves is found to improve symptoms in patients with idiopathic as well as neurogenic detrusor overactivity. Up to 2/3rd of women respond to percutaneous sacral nerve stimulation. They will achieve either continence or have substantial improvement. Those who show improvement with cutaneous nerve stimulation can be offered permanent implant which is inserted under general anaesthesia. Studies have reported a 50% reduction in incontinence episodes. Even though the permanent implant is an expensive and invasive procedure, it is a choice for women with severe detrusor overactivity who do not respond to medical therapy. Older urge-incontinent patients have improvement with sacral neuromodulation but cure rates may be lower among younger population.[17]

Surgical treatment: Surgical treatment is the last resort for women with severe detrusor overactivity who do not respond to bladder training, drugs or nerve stimulation.

a. *Clam cystoplasty:* In Clam cystoplasty the bladder is bisected and a pouch of ileum is sutured to the bladder. This increases the bladder capacity and decreases the intra vesical pressure. The procedure is associated with urinary infection and several complications relating to the ileal graft. Hence this is not an accepted procedure.
b. *Urinary diversion:* In severe detrusor overactivity, where all the other measures fail, the only alternative is to divert urine to the ileal conduit.

3.13 CONCLUSION

Genuine stress incontinence and detrusor overactivity incontinence are the two common types of incontinence seen in women. Urinary infection should be excluded in all women with lower urinary tract symptoms. Genuine Stress Incontinence has several etiological factors including lack of urethral support, intrinsic sphincter deficiency and inadequate urethral pressure or it can be a combination of these in varying proportions. The diagnosis of GSI can be arrived from the history in a large percentage of women, but rarely, relying on the history alone can lead to misdiagnosis as there is overlap of symptoms of GSI and detrusor overactivity. Ideally subtraction cystometry should be done to exclude detrusor overactivity before proceeding for surgical management of GSI. Initially pelvic floor strengthening exercise should be advised for all women except when the incontinence is very severe. Based on available evidence, the initial surgery for women with bladder neck descent is either Burch colposuspension or TVT. Even though the results of Burch colposuspension and TVT are reported to be the same, long term follow up results after surgery are available only for Burch colposuspension. The surgery should be done by experienced surgeons familiar with the anatomy of the region. Before a repeat procedure, advanced urodynamic studies should be done to exclude associated conditions. Those who have decreased bladder neck mobility and scarring can be offered TVT as a repeat procedure. If still no relief is attained, periurethral bulking agents can provide short term positive results. The ultimate management is implantation of an artificial urethral sphincter. Detrusor overactivity is diagnosed by cystometric study. The treatment for detrusor overactivity is mainly medical. Antimuscarinic agents are the main stay of therapy. Though they are effective, side effects like dry mouth, constipation and blurred vision limit their use. Surgery should be thought of only as a last resort. Since no single treatment modality is fully effective, management should be highly individualized.

REFERENCES

1. Abrams P, Cardozo L, Fall M, et al. The standardisation of terminology of lower urinary tract function: report from the Standardisation Sub-committee of the International Continence Society. Neurourol Urodyn 2002;21:167-78.
2. Anders Foldspang, Seren Mommsen. The international continence society (ICS) incontinence definition: Is the social and hygienic aspect appropriate for etiologic research. J Clin Epi 1997;50(9):1055-60.
3. DeLancey, John O. L. Structural Support of the Urethra as It Relates to Stress Urinary Incontinence: The Hammock Hypothesis. Am J Obstet Gynecol 1994;170:1713-23.
4. Abrams P. Blaivas JG. Stanton SL et al 1988 The standardization of terminology of lower tract function. Scandinavian Journal of Urology and Nephrology 114(suppl):5.
5. James MJ, Jackson S, Shepard A, Abrams P Pure stress leakage symptomatology: is it safe to discount detrusor instability? British Journal of Obstetrics and Gynaecology 1999;101:371-74.
6. Resnick NM, Yalla SV. Management of urinary incontinence. The pathophysiology of urinary incontinence among institutionalized elderly persons. N Engl J Med 1989;320:1-7.
7. Walters MD, Diaz K. Q-tip test: a study of continent and incontinent women. Obstet Gynecol 1987;70:208-211.
8. Artibani W, Andersen JT, Gajewski JB, et al. Imaging and other investigations.Plymouth, UK: Plymbridge Distributors Ltd, 2002.
9. Hay-Smith EJC, Bo K, Berghmans LCM, et al. Pelvic floor muscle training for urinary incontinence in women. Cochrane Database Syst Rev 2001;CD001407.
10. PA Norton et al, Duloxetine versus placebo in the treatment of stress urinary incontinence. AMJ Obstet Gynaecol 2002;187:40-48.
11. Hentrix SL,Cochrane BB, Nygaard IE, et-al. Effects of estrogen with and without progestin on urinary incontinence. Jama 2005;293:935-48.
12. : Bergman A, Elia G. Three surgical procedures for Genuine Stress Incontinence: Five year follow up of a prospective randomized study. AMJ Obstet Gynaecol 1995;173:66-71.
13. Burch J. Urethrovaginal fixation to Cooper's ligament for correction of stress incontinence, cystocele and prolapse. Am J Obstet Gynecol 1961;81:281-90.
14. Lapitan MCM, Cody JD, Grant A. Open retropubic colposuspension for urinary incontinence in women. Cochrane Database of Systematic Reviews 2009, Issue 2. Art. No.: CD002912. DOI: 10.1002/14651858. CD002912. pub3.
15. Shull D.L, Vaden W.F. A six-year experience with paravaginal repair for Stress Urinary Incontinence. AMJ Obstet Gynaecol 1989;161:43-240.
16. Dean NM, Ellis G, Wilson PD, Herbison GP. Laparoscopic colposuspension for urinary incontinence in women. Cochrane Database of Systematic Reviews 2006, Issue 3. Art. No.: CD002239. DOI: 10.1002/14651858.CD002239.
17. Amundsen, Cindy L, Webster, George D. Sacral neuromodulation in an older, urge-incontinent population. Transactions of the Twenty-Eighth Scientific Meeting of the Society of Gynecological Surgeons. Am J Obstet Gynecol 2002;187(6):1462-65.

4 Primary Amenorrhea

B Presannakumari

4.1 INTRODUCTION

Arriving at a diagnosis of primary amenorrhea is considered a complex exercise but it can be sorted out and managed in most of the situations by the gynecologist. A few may need to be referred to the endocrinologist for diagnosis.

4.2 DEFINITION

Any patient fulfilling the following criteria should be evaluated as having the clinical problem of primary amenorrhea. Since the age of menarche has decreased over the past few decades, the definition of primary amenorrhea has undergone a modification.

1. No menstrual period by age 13 in the absence of growth or development of secondary sexual characteristics.
2. No menstrual period by age 15 regardless of the presence of normal growth and development including secondary sexual characteristics.

Even though the definition is as above, the evaluation of a patient should not be deferred until 15 years of age in all the situations. If the girl has cyclic lower abdominal pain, she should be evaluated even if she is less than 15 years for cryptomenorrhea which is a possibility. The incidence of primary amenorrhea is reported as less than 1%. The commonest condition presenting as primary amenorrhea is Turner syndrome. Turner syndrome, if diagnosed early can have the benefit of stature correction with the administration of growth hormone.

Another common condition presenting as primary amenorrhea is abnormality of the mullerian tract. We very often see mullerian anomalies with a functioning uterus and the patient will have cryptomenorrhea. Delay in treatment will result in damage to the internal genitalia and increased incidence of endometriosis. These patients usually present early because of cyclical lower abdominal pain and urinary retention.

5α-reductase deficient individuals will be brought up as girls and will have virilizing puberty. If the parents prefer to bring them up as females, it is better to interfere early. Hence, whenever the parents bring a child for not attaining menarche, an effort should be made to categorize with the necessary diagnostic investigations. At the same time, unnecessary expensive and invasive diagnostic investigations should be avoided.

4.3 NORMAL SEX DIFFERENTIATION

Certain conditions presenting as primary amenorrhea are due to abnormal sex differentiation. Hence it is worth going into the basics of sex determination.

4.3.1 Male Development

With advances in cytogenetics and molecular genetics, the molecular basis of sex determination is better understood.[1] Using cloning and DNA sequencing techniques the gene determining testicular development is identified as the SRY (sex determining region of Y) gene. Another gene, known as the SOX-9 gene also is involved in testicular differentiation. Under the influence of these genes the totipotent gonad develops into the testis. The fetal testis elaborates mullerian inhibiting factor (MIF) and testosterone.

MIF from the fetal testis causes regression of mullerian ducts and hence uterus, tubes and vagina will not develop in a male fetus. Testosterone secreted by the fetal testis stimulates the development epididymis, vas deferens and the seminal vesicles from the wolffian duct. The external genitalia develops under the influence of dihydrotestosterone, which is formed from testosterone by the enzyme 5 α reductase. This is the reason for the absence of virilization of the external genitalia in complete androgen insensitivity (AIS) as well as in 5 α reductase insufficiency which will be discussed later. Male internal genitalia develop in 5 α reductase deficient individual because testosterone action is normal; whereas male internal genitalia will be absent in AIS individuals.

4.3.2 Female Development

Female development is the neutral norm. So far only one gene is identified as responsible for ovarian development- the DAX-1 gene. In the mouse model, it has been found that DAX-1 expression continues during ovarian development but stops in the testis after SRY expression. The wolffian structures regress due to lack of testosterone stimulation. Reminders of the wolffian duct can persist in the form of hydatid of Morgagni or as Gartner's duct cysts.

Normal female and male sex determination, differentiation and development are elaborated diagrammatically in Figures 4.1 and 4.2.

4.4 PUBERTY

It is pertinent to understand the physiology and timing of normal puberty and its abnormalities, before proceeding to primary amenorrhea.

Puberty is the period of life during which the capacity for reproduction is achieved and is characterized by the development of secondary sexual characteristics along with growth spurt. On an average, this period spans about 3-4 years. Maturation of secondary sexual characteristics includes that of breasts, external genitalia, pubic and axillary hair. These physical changes are brought about by complex physiological events culminating in menarche, the first menstruation. Adolescence is a longer period which spans longer than puberty and it involves the social and psychological adaptations to the hormonal changes of uberty.

4.4.1 Timing of Puberty

The age of onset of puberty is not uniform among all ethnic groups. This variation from the usual need not always be

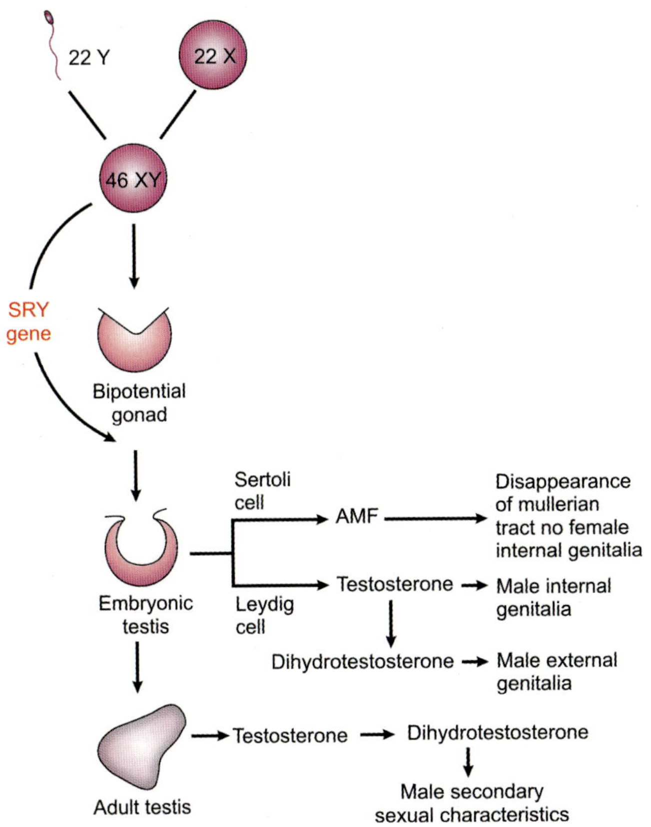

Fig. 4.1: Diagrammatic representation of normal male sex differentiation. (AMF: Anti-mullerian factor)

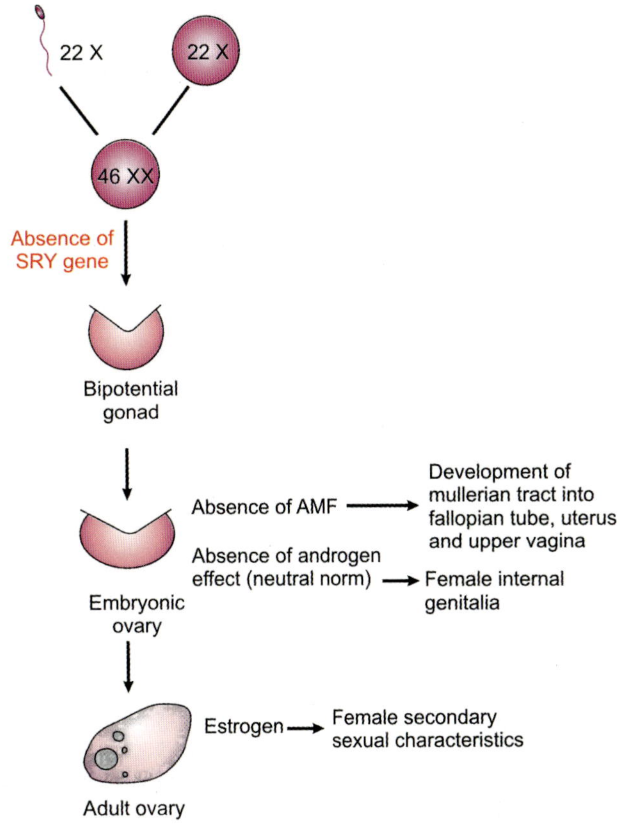

Fig. 4.2: Diagrammatic representation of normal female sex differentiation. (AMF: Anti-mullerian factor)

taken as a clinical disorder but can be attributed to the differences in the maturational program of GnRH secretion.

Studies by Tanner and Davis established the average age of pubertal development in North American girls as breast budding at 10.7 years with an SD of 1 year and the average age of menarche as 12.7 years with an SD of 1.3 years.[2]

Precocious puberty is defined as breast budding occurring less than 2.5 SD's from the mean or younger than 8 years.

Delayed puberty is defined as absence of secondary sexual characteristics by an age that is 2–2.5 SD beyond the mean for the population (approximately 13 years in girls and 14 years in boys).

Recent data derived from cross sectional studies show a trend towards earlier onset of puberty among girls[3]. It was found that 6.7% of White and 27. 2% of Afro American girls had evidence of breast and pubic hair development before the age of 8 years. Hence, following traditional definitions would result in a high proportion of girls being diagnosed and evaluated for precocious puberty.

In 1999, the Drug and Therapeutic and Executive Committees of the Lawson Wilkins Pediatric Endocrine Society (LWPES) published new recommendations for the definition of precocious puberty. The cut off for precocious puberty should be decreased to 7 years in White girls and to 6 years in Afro American girls.[4] Since these recommendations are based on cross sectional studies, additional well defined prospective studies are required before redefining the age limit of precocious puberty.

4.4.2 Events of Puberty

Puberty is characterized by a sequence of predictable events. The normal sequence of pubertal events are:

1. **Adrenarche:** Adrenarche is the activation of adrenal cortex leading to the production of adrenal androgens.
2. **Gonadarche:** Gonadarche is the activation of gonads brought about by the secretion of FSH and LH by the pituitary.
3. **Pubarche:** Pubarche is the appearance of pubic hair.
4. **Thelarche:** Thelarche is the appearance of breast tissue.
5. **Menarche:** Menarche is the onset of first menstrual period.

The onset and progression of pubertal changes are variable. The sequence of changes in secondary sexual characteristics has been categorized into several stages. The widely utilized staging system is the one published by

Marshall and Turner and is commonly referred to as Tanner staging.

4.4.3 Tanner Staging (Tables 4.1 and 4.2)

As per Tanner staging, breast development and pubic hair development are rated on a 5 point scale, which is given in tables below.

4.4.4 Physiology of Puberty

The occurrence of various events of puberty requires an intact hypothalamopituitary gonadal axis (HPG axis). In addition to this, an intact hypothalamopituitary adrenal axis is also important for normal pubertal development.

Gonadarche

The HPG axis is active during fetal life and continues in infancy. After infancy, it enters a quiescent phase known as the *'juvenile pause'*. The onset of various events of puberty is brought about by the activation of the quiescent HPG axis leading to the pulsatile secretion of GnRH, which occurs before the physical signs of puberty appear.

The hypothalamus starts secreting GnRH in a pulsatile manner, first at night and later, throughout the day. In response to GnRH from the hypothalamus, pituitary releases gonadotropins, LH and FSH. Initially, the LH peaks occur exclusively during sleep under the influence of the nocturnal pulsatile GnRH release. Later, the LH peak amplitude increases around 10 fold and the FSH amplitude doubles. During pubertal progression of breast development from Tanner stage 2 to 3, further increase in LH pulse amplitude occurs and this will be greatest during sleep.

As breast development advances to Tanner stage 4, LH pulses become diurnal and reach the adult pattern. As puberty progresses, the diurnal pattern of gonadotropin secretion changes and pulsatile gonadotropin secretion with high peaks occur throughout the day. Under the influence of FSH, the estradiol levels increase and become detectable throughout the day. After about a year of consistently high estradiol levels, menarche occurs and at this time, breast development reaches Tanner stage 4. There is a difference in gonadotropin peak levels in girls and boys in that peak level of gonadotropins are reached in early morning in boys and in mid morning in girls.

Table 4.1: Tanner staging of breast development

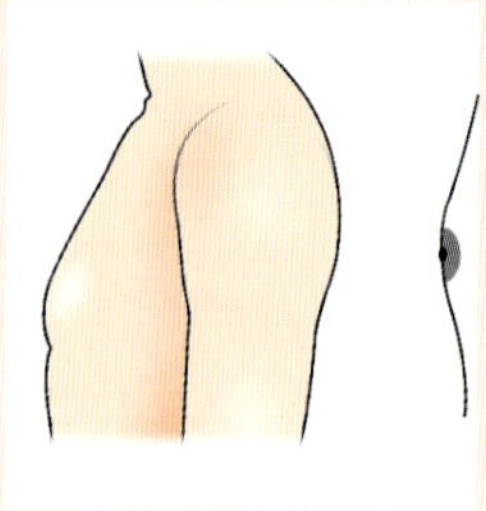	I: Preadolescent
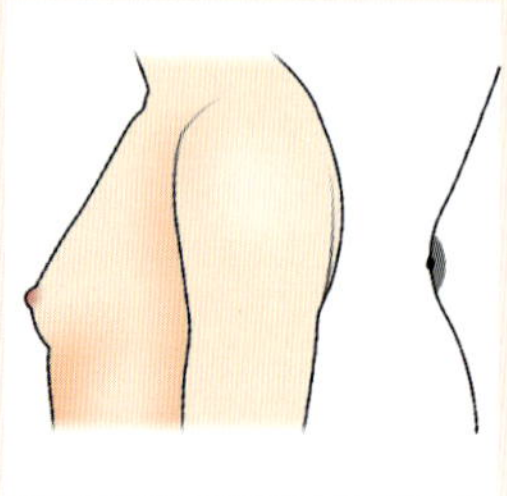	II: Breast budding
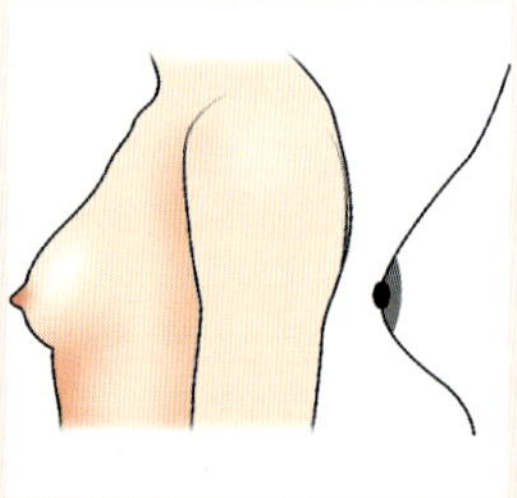	III: Continued enlargement
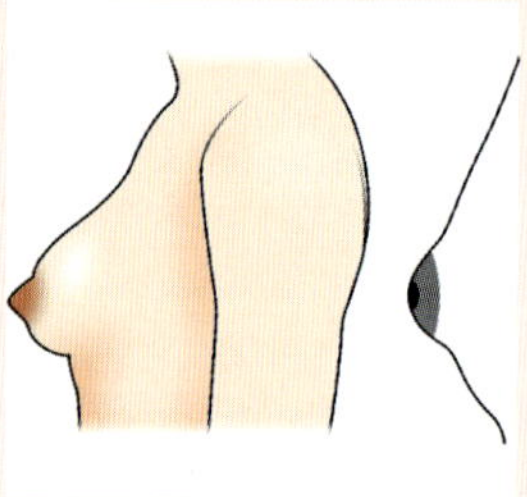	IV: Areola and papilla from secondary mound
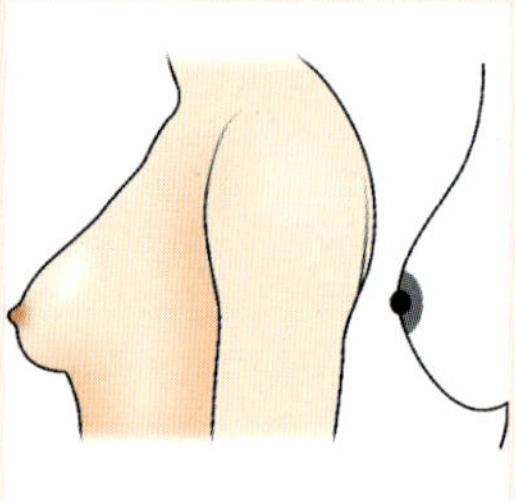	V: Mature breasts

Adrenarche

Adrenarche also plays an important role in the development of the physical changes of puberty. The maturation of zona reticularis of the adrenal gland results in increased production of adrenal androgens. It is under the influence of the adrenal androgens DHEA, DHEAS and androstenedione that the pubic hair, axillary hair, body odor and acne develop.

Like gonadarche, adrenarche is also a gradually progressive maturation process. Adrenarche precedes gonadarche by 1- 2 years in boys and girls. However, the

Table 4.2: Tanner staging of pubic hair development

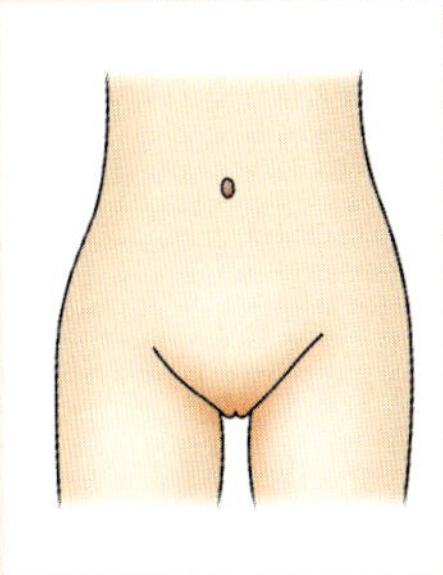	I: No pubic hair
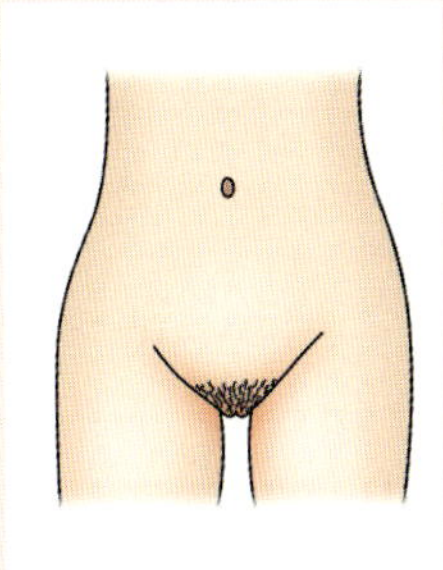	II: Sparse long pigmented hair chiefly along labia majora
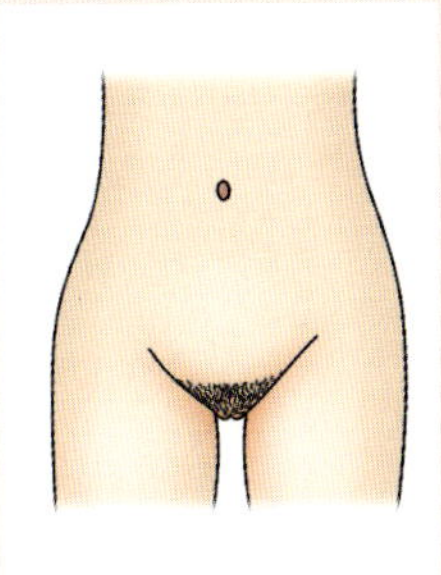	III: Dark course curled hair sparsely spread over mons also
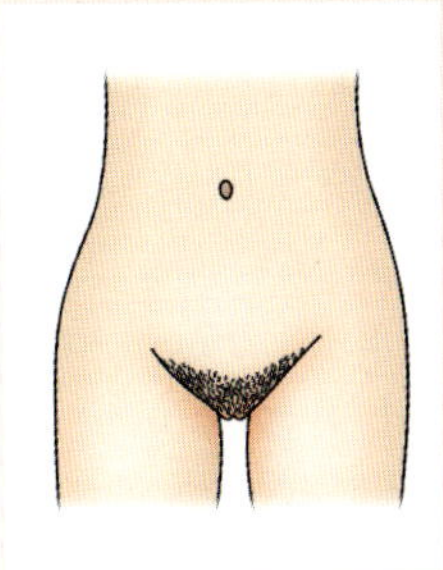	IV: Adult type hair, abundant but limited to mons
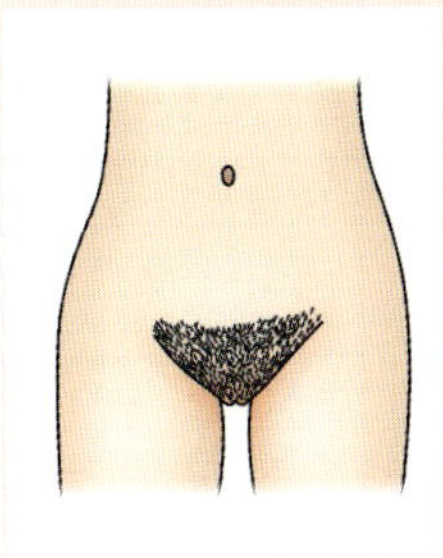	V: Adult type spread in quantity and distribution

Source: Marshall WA, Tanner JM. Variations in pattern of pubertal changes in girls. Arch DisChild 969; 44(235):291–303.

timing of clinical expressions can vary. Adrenarche may overlap with gonadarche but they are both separate processes regulated independently.

4.4.5 Chronological Sequence of Pubertal Changes (Fig. 4.3 and Table 4.3)

On an average, the sequence of events of puberty starts with growth spurt which will be followed by breast development, pubic and axillary hair development and ends with menarche. The duration of these events usually spans for a period of 4.5 years with a range of 1.5-6 years.[5]

4.4.6 Regulation of Pubertal Timing

The timing of puberty differs in different ethnic groups. The most important factor determining pubertal timing is genetic. (Fig. 4.4) Environmental influence has a significant role in modifying the genetic factors. Geographic location, exposure to light, general health and nutrition and psychological factors are all found to influence the initiation and the rate of progression of puberty. Children living close to the equator,

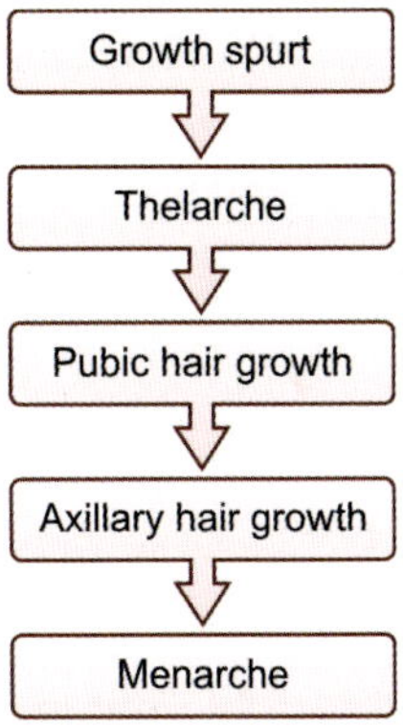

Fig. 4.3: Chronological sequence of pubertal changes

Table 4.3: Relationship between pubertal events and endocrine system

Estrogen secretion	Breast development
Testosterone secretion	External genitalia in males
FSH secretion	Stimulates sertoli cells/follicular cells
Adrenal androgen secretion	Pubic/axillary hair development
Sex steroids, thyroxine and GH secretion	Growth
Pulsatile LH secretion as a result of pulsatile GnRH	Ovulatory menstrual cycle

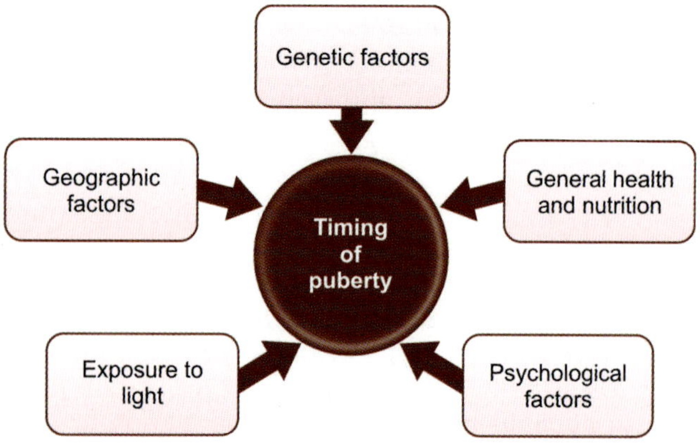

Fig. 4.4: Factors affecting timing of puberty

those living at lower altitudes, those who belong to the urban areas and are obese are found to have earlier onset of puberty than those living at higher altitudes and with lower weight. There is good correlation between the timing of menarche among mothers and daughters as well as among sisters. The recent trend towards an earlier onset of puberty can presumably be due to improved nutrition.

Genetic Factors

The identification of genes responsible for hypogonadotrophic hypogonadism has provided an insight into the possible genetic basis of GnRH neuronal development. The understanding that the defect in leptin/leptin-receptors results in hypogonadotropic hypogonadism led to the speculation that leptin could be a trigger for the onset of puberty.[6,7]

Mutation in several genes that are critical in the hypothalamopituitary development has been identified in individuals with hypothalamic hypogonadotropic hypogonadism. These include DAX 1, steroidogenic factor 1 (SF-1), HESX-1, LHX3 and PROP-1.

Mutations in GPR 54 also have been identified in hypogonadotropic hypogonadism. However, the exact role of these genes identified in these disorders in regulating the onset of puberty is not definite. It is probable that less severe genetic variations due to gene polymorphism could be the reason for the variation in pubertal timing seen in the general population.

4.4.7 Neuroendocrine Regulation of Pubertal Onset (Fig. 4.5)

The exact factors responsible for the dampening of the HPG axis after infancy (the juvenile pause) and its re-emergence before puberty are not well established. GABA neurons appear to play a prominent role in regulating the *'juvenile pause'*.[8]

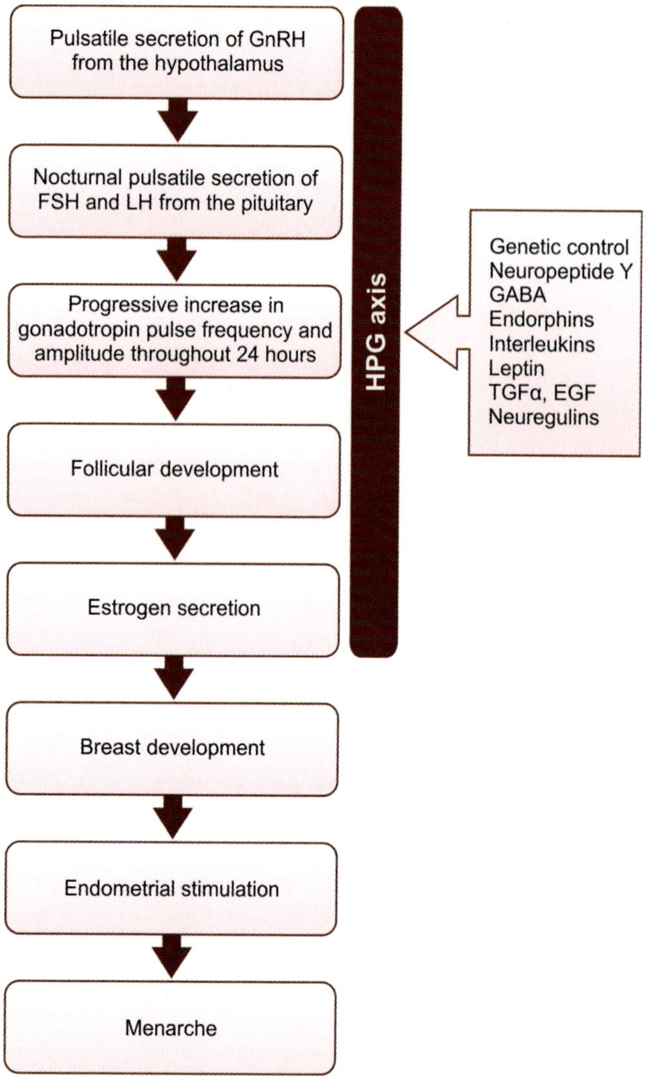

Fig. 4.5: Neuroendocrine regulation of puberty

Studies in monkeys have shown that neuropeptide Y mRNA expression in the hypothalamus of juvenile monkeys is higher than in neonatal monkeys. Hence, neuropeptide Y may be a factor that governs *'juvenile pause'*. Endogenous opioids and melatonin may also be contributing to the *'juvenile pause'*.

The important excitatory neurotransmitter is glutamate. Leptins, nor epinephrine, dopamine, TNF α, kisspeptins, neuregulins and galanin like peptides are also considered stimulators of GnRH secretion.

Relation of Obesity to Pubertal Timing

The increased adiposity may be a contributing factor for the shift towards earlier puberty. Higher BMI scores were observed among pubertal girls compared to age matched prepubertal girls.[9,10] The National Heart Lung and Blood Institute Growth and Health Study found that girls who had earlier onset of menarche had greater BMI scores than girls with normal or late menarche.[11]

However in the same study, it was found that in obese boys, pubertal development was less sensitive to nutritional status. Since menarche occurs earlier in obese girls, it was hypothesized that leptin, which correlates with BMI, may have a permissive role in signaling the onset of puberty by its action on the HPG axis.

Influence of Environment on Puberty

Some interesting observations have emerged from recent studies on the environmental influence on the timing of puberty. Possible association between girls exposed to cosmetics/hair care products containing estrogen like chemicals and the earlier occurrence of puberty has been postulated, based on studies in animals. Polychlorinated biphenyls, organochlorine pesticides and phthalates can bind with estrogen receptors and alter GnRH gene expression.[12] Foods containing soy products may also influence the HPG axis maturation due to the presence of phytoestrogens.

4.4.8 Disorders Pubertal Development

Premature Pubertal Development

Premature pubertal development can be isolated or generalized.

Classification

1. Premature thelarche
   a. Isolated premature thelarche
      i. Classical form
      ii. Non-classical form
   b. Slowly progressive precocious puberty
2. Isolated premature menarche
3. Premature adrenarche
4. Precocious puberty
   a. Gonadotropin dependent/Central
      i. Idiopathic
      ii. Secondary: Suprasellar tumors-Hypothalamic hamartoma, astrocytoma, optic glioma, pineal tumor, arachnoid cyst, cranial irradiation
   b. Gonadotropin independent
      i. McCune-Albright Syndrome
      ii. Primary hypothyroidism
      iii. Ovarian /adrenal tumors

Incomplete Precocious Puberty

Precocious puberty can be incomplete with isolated thelarche or pubarche. Isolated premature thelarche is characterized by breast development which occurs usually under the age of 2 years in the absence of other signs of puberty. Growth and bone age of these children will be normal and the condition is self limiting. The non-classical form affecting older girls is characterized by associated menstrual bleeding. The condition is not found to have any long term effect on puberty and fertility. Hence treatment is not required.

However, it should be kept in mind that early thelarche may be part of the HPG axis maturation and can progress to central precocious puberty.

Premature adrenarche is precocious development of pubic or axillary hair or both before 8 years of age without other signs of puberty. The condition is due to premature androgen secretion from zona reticularis. Skin changes, acne and adult type perspiration can also be associated. Due to the production of androgens, these children will be taller than normal girls and will have advanced bone age. Their plasma levels of DHEA and androstenedione will be in the range that is seen among older pubertal children. Premature pubarche associated with obesity and acanthosis may be a fore runner of metabolic syndrome. Premature adrenarche can also be due to pathological disorders like late onset CAH or androgen secreting ovarian tumors.

HPG axis activation can be incomplete resulting in unsustained and intermittent but slowly progressing sexual maturation. The etiology of the condition is unknown but genetic basis involving mutations in Gs-α have been identified in girls with fluctuating pubertal development.

Isolated premature menarche is characterized by repeated vaginal bleeding without other signs of pubertal development. The exact reason for this is unknown. It could be due to the activation of HPG axis resulting in FSH secretion and estradiol levels sufficient to stimulate the endometrium, but not sufficient enough to produce breast development. However local lesions in the genital tract should be considered and excluded in such a clinical situation. No treatment is required as the condition is self limiting and will not have any long term sequelae.

4.4.9 Precocious Puberty

Precocious puberty is defined as the development of secondary sexual characteristics before the age of 8 years in girls and 9 years in boys.

Centrally Mediated Precocious Puberty (CPP)

Centrally mediated precocious puberty results from the activation of the HPG axis. The biological events usually follow the same pattern of normal pubertal development. Rarely, girls with centrally mediated precocious puberty can present with isolated development of pubic hair or menses. In girls, centrally mediated precocious puberty is often idiopathic while in boys, idiopathic precocious puberty is rare and there will usually be an underlying pathology. Girls who develop precocious puberty will have significant bone age advancement (usually >2 S.D's for the age). Growth spurt and development of secondary sexual characteristics will be present. These girls will have high LH and estradiol levels. Ovarian and uterine measurements also will be advanced for age.

Since early production of sex steroids causes advanced epithelial maturation and closure, these girls will have compromised adult height. Hence, short stature is one of the hazards of precocious puberty. Early pubertal development and menarche causing psychosocial stress is another important issue.

Etiology of centrally mediated precocious puberty

About 85% of centrally mediated precocious puberty is idiopathic. However, lesions in the brain can influence GnRH pulse release and cause centrally mediated precocious puberty. Central nervous system tumors like astrocytomas, hamartomas, adenomas and gliomas, CNS infections, head injury and iatrogenic causes like radiation, chemotherapy can all cause CPP.

Peripherally Mediated Precocious Puberty (PPP)

Peripherally mediated precocious puberty is due to the production of sex steroids either from an ovarian or adrenal tumor. There will not be any activation of the HPG axis. However, in some cases, secondary activation of HPG axis can occur.

Diagnostic Work-up (Flow Charts 4.1 and 4.2)

A detailed history regarding the preceding growth spurt, symptoms related to any CNS or ovarian tumors, drug intake, surgeries, radiation as well as onset and sequence of pubertal progression should be taken as the first step towards proper evaluation of precocious puberty. Measurement of LH and estradiol levels and ultrasound measurement of volume of uterus and ovaries will give a clue to the etiology of precocious puberty. Those who have virilization should have measurement of DHEA and DHEAS to make out the source of androgen.

Imaging of the brain should be done if the clinical situation warrants. Gonadotropin response to GnRH stimulation is the gold standard in diagnosing central precocious puberty. Demonstration of bone age is important as it will be advanced in central precocious puberty but will be appropriate for age in peripherally mediated precocious puberty.

In isolated premature thelarche and premature adrenarche, gonadotropin levels will be in the prepubertal range. The testosterone and estradiol levels will not be significantly increased. Children with premature adrenarche usually will have DHEA and DHEAS levels in the pubertal range. Children with androgen secreting ovarian tumors may have raised testosterone levels.

Management

Management of central precocious puberty

Children who are diagnosed to have central precocious puberty should be treated to attain the adult height as well as to minimize the psychosocial stress associated with precocious puberty.

GnRH agonist administration is the treatment of choice as these agents downregulate the pituitary and limit pubertal progression. For this purpose, the preferred treatment modality is depot injection on a 3 monthly basis. GnRH agonists can cause a transient flare up of gonadotropin levels resulting in a transient advancement of secondary sexual characteristics but, pituitary down regulation will soon follow.

There can be concerns about GnRH agonist treatment adversely affecting bone mineral density. However, the peak bone mineral density attainment is thought to occur during the time when the girl completes puberty. There is no consensus as to when GnRH agonist therapy has to be discontinued. The optimum outcome of GnRH therapy is achieved in children whose treatment is started sufficiently early.

Management of peripherally mediated precocious puberty

Since peripherally mediated precocious puberty is secondary to pathological conditions like ovarian or

Flow Chart 4.1: Diagnostic work-up for individuals who have precocious puberty

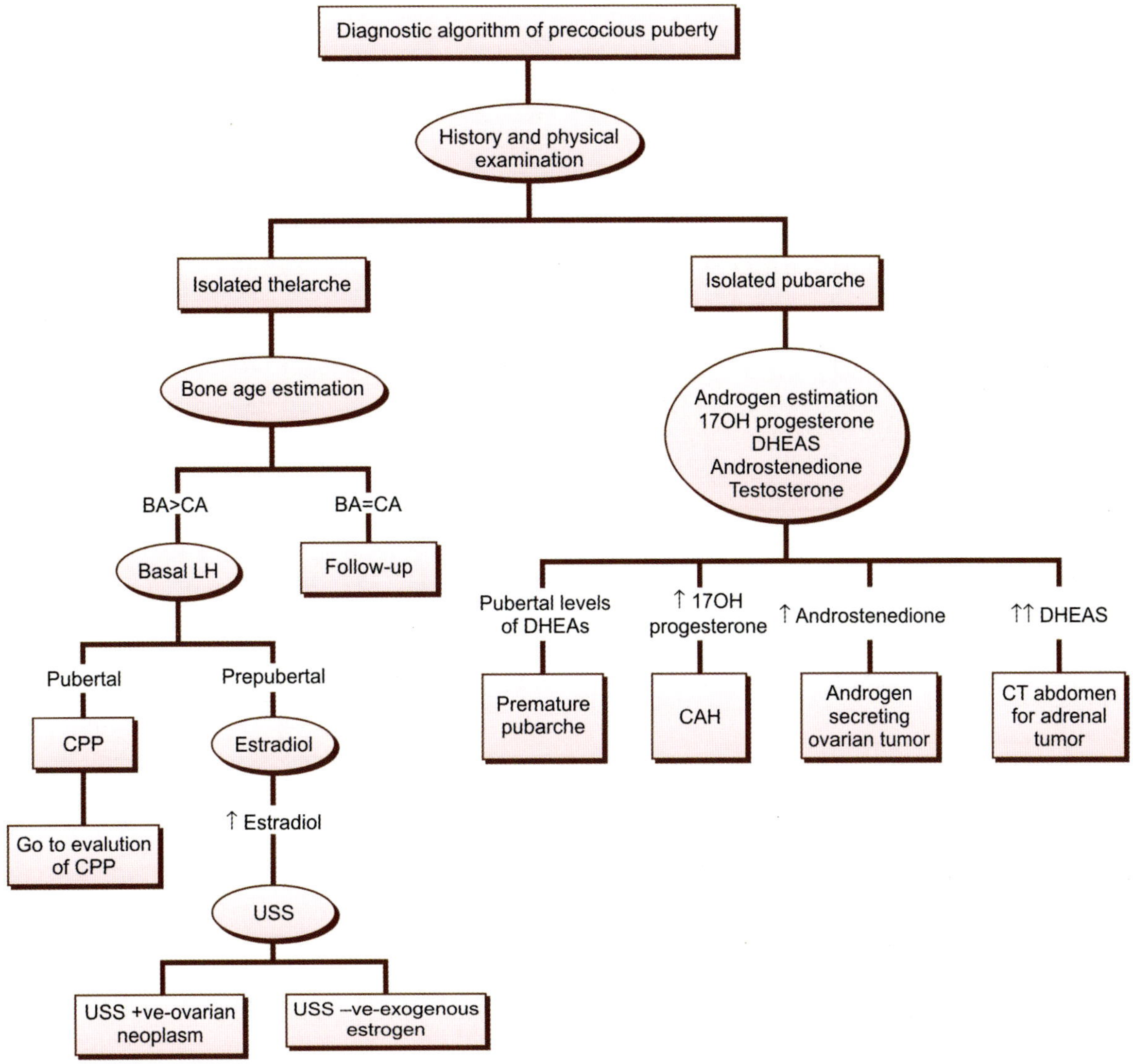

adrenal tumors, treatment of the underlying disorder gives the cure.

Premature pubarche and thelarche can be limited by giving androgen receptor inhibitors like spironolactone, ketoconazole and estrogen receptor inhibitors like tamoxifen or aromatase inhibitors like anastrozole respectively.

4.4.10 Delayed Puberty

Delayed puberty is defined as the absence of secondary sexual characteristics by an age that is 2–2.5 SD beyond the mean for the population (approximately 13 years in girls and 14 years in boys).

The commonest cause is constitutional delay but permanent hypogonadotropic hypogonadism should be considered as constitutional delay is a retrospective diagnosis.

Individuals with constitutional delay eventually will undergo spontaneous pubertal development. Often, there will be a positive family history. Trend of acquisition of delayed puberty among families suggest an autosomal dominant inheritance with variable penetrance.

Adult height will be less in children with constitutional delay. The differentiation between constitutional delay and permanent hypogonadotrophic hypogonadism is a challenge to the clinician. The definitive diagnosis of constitutional delay can be made only when the girl attains spontaneous puberty. But, individuals with constitutional delay will have

Flow Chart 4.2: Diagnostic algorithm for premature menarche

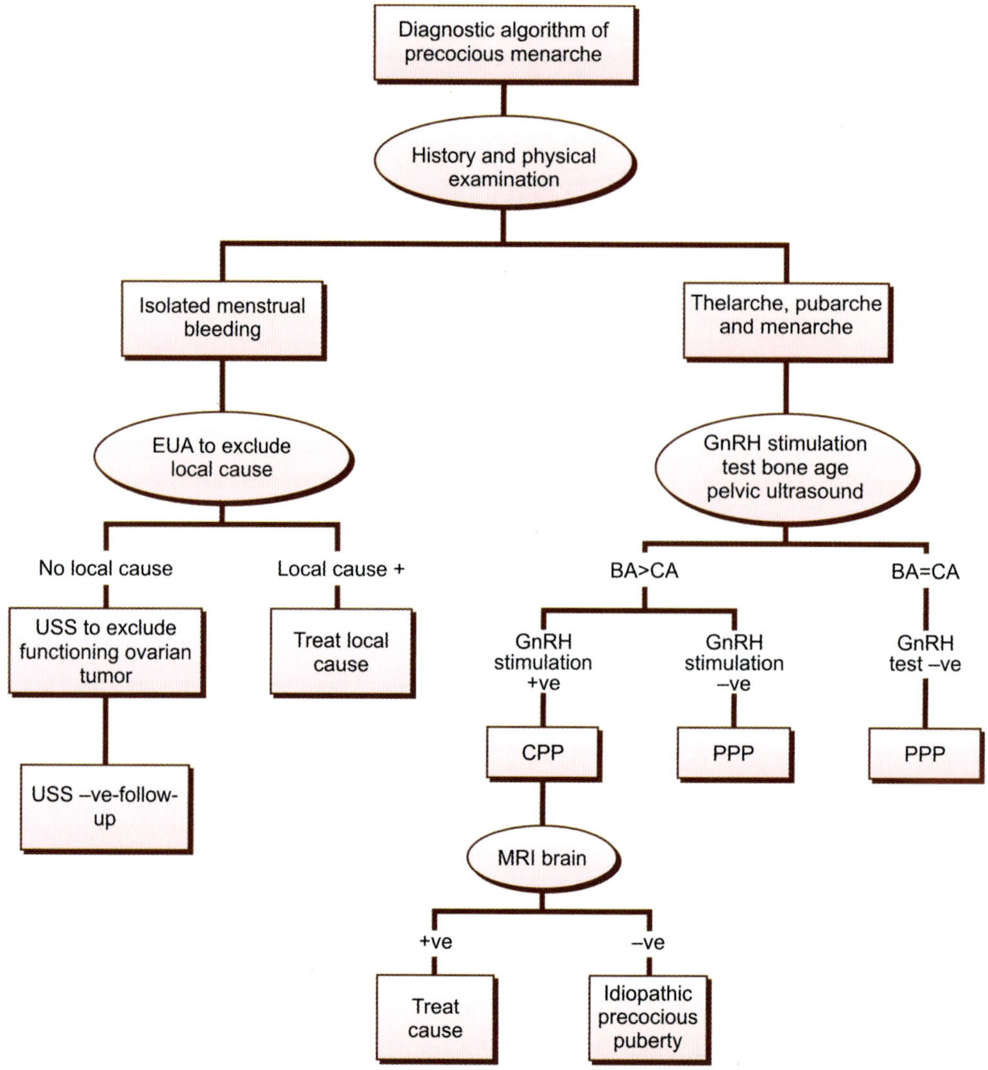

delayed bone age. But, this delay is not more than 1 year of chronological age.

4.5 BASIC PRINCIPLES OF MENSTRUATION

For normal menstruation, there should be a mature hypothalamo-pituitary-ovarian axis and a normal outflow tract from the uterus to the vaginal introitus. The endocrine control of menstruation is a delicate orchestra involving hormones and autocrine and paracrine factors produced by the hypothalamus, pituitary and ovary. The hypothalamus is influenced not only by the feedback effect from pituitary and ovary, but also by signals from higher centers in the CNS through neurotransmitters like dopamine, norepinephrine, endorphins, serotonin and melatonin. The hypothalamus controls the pituitary through the production of GnRH (Fig. 6.2). GnRH is released in pulses and reaches the anterior pituitary through the hypothalamo-hypophyseal portal system. Under the influence of GnRH, pituitary releases FSH and LH in a pulsatile manner. The pulse frequency and amplitude varies in the different phases of the menstrual cycle. The pulsatile release of these two gonadotropins FSH and LH regulate the ovarian cycle. The cyclical release of ovarian hormones in turn causes cyclical changes in the endometrium resulting in menstruation. Even if the HPO axis is normal, an individual may be amenorrheic because of a congenital or acquired problem with the uterovaginal canal.

Absence of menstruation can be due to faults in any one of the previously mentioned sites. An etiological classification can be derived based on the defects in the following 4 compartments

- Compartment I- Disorders of the outflow tract (uterus and vagina) (Table 4.4)
- Compartment II- Disorders of the ovary
- Compartment III- Disorders of the anterior pituitary
- Compartment IV- Disorders of the CNS

4.6 COMPARTMENT I

4.6.1 Mullerian Anomalies

Anomalies of mullerian tract are a spectrum of disorders ranging from complete absence of uterovaginal canal to an imperforate hymen with a bulging hematocolpos.

Mayer- Rokintansky- Kustner- Hauser (MRKH) Syndrome

Complete absence of the uterovaginal canal is one of the common causes of primary amenorrhea, second only to ovarian dysgenesis. Reported to be occurring in approximately 1 in every 5000 female births, these patients have absence of uterus, vagina and fallopian tubes. Rarely in the place of uterus, there may be a rudimentary bicornuate cord. Because ovarian development is completely different from the mullerian development, the ovaries are completely normal in structure and function. Needless to say, their external genitalia will be of normal female type and will be appropriate for age. The individuals will have absolutely normal female phenotypic appearance.

The exact etiology of the condition is not known. Occurrence is usually sporadic. The possibility of a genetic basis as the etiology of the disease is being investigated. A mutation has been identified in the gene responsible for galactose-1- phosphate -uridyl transferase in individuals with mullerian agenesis and their mothers. Increased intrauterine exposure to galactose may be the reason for mullerian agenesis in this group.[7]

Table 4.4: Disorders of the outflow tract

Congenital	a. MRKH syndrome
	b. Mullerian anomalies
	i. Transverse septa
	ii. Partially non canalized vagina
	Hematocolpos
	Hematometra
Acquired	a. Asherman's syndrome
	i. Tuberculous
	ii. Non-tuberculous

Since one third of these patients will also have associated renal anomalies, their urinary tract should also be evaluated. 12% or more of them can have associated skeletal anomalies like absent digits or syndacty and rarely cardiac anomalies.

Diagnosis is based on the normal female phenotypic appearance, normal female karyotype-46, XX and the demonstration of non canalized vagina and absent uterus.

If imaging of the uterus by ultrasound is ambiguous, MRI is the investigation of choice. Invasive investigations like diagnostic laparoscopy need not be done. These patients can have their own children by retrieving their ova for in-vitro fertilization and growing the embryo in a surrogate mother. For coital function, vaginoplasty may be done a few months before marriage with split skin grafts or amniotic membrane. Care should be taken not to injure the urinary tract or the rectum. An alternative to vaginoplasty is progressive dilatation with vaginal dilators (Frank).[13,14]

Other Mullerian Anomalies

There can be a spectrum of various types of agenesis of the vagina with a functioning uterus. The mildest form of mullerian tract abnormality is imperforate hymen presenting with cryptomenorrhea. The condition can be diagnosed by the bulging bluish hymen which can be tackled by a cruciate incision. Vaginal examination and even pressing the abdomen should not be done as it may suck the micro organisms from the outside and cause infection. Patient should be given a sterile pad and allowed to walk about for drainage of the hematocolpos. If the cervix is atretic and the uterus is functioning, there is no alternative but hysterectomy, even though reconstruction of cervix is occasionally reported. With a normal functioning uterus and cervix, there can be various types of transverse vaginal septa

MRKH syndrome

- Normal female phenotype with well-developed breast, pubic and axillary hair
- Absent uterus and vagina
- Normal ovaries
- Associated renal/skeletal anomalies
- Karyotype: 46, XX

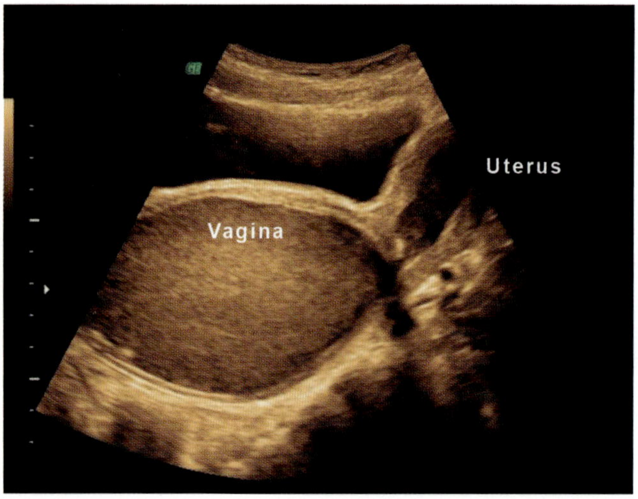

Fig. 4.6: Transabdominal scan showing hematocolpos as a consequence of non-canalized lower 1/3rd of vagina

and partially non canalized vagina. Because of the functioning uterus and the cervix, the patient will be menstruating and the menstrual blood will get collected in the patent part of the vagina. These girls may present early as soon as they reach puberty with cyclical abdominal pain or urinary retention. This hematocolpos can present as a cystic mass in the hypogastrium, sometimes mistaken for an ovarian cyst (Fig. 4.6). The problem can be diagnosed by rectal examination when the hematocolpos can be felt anteriorly.

When the hematocolpos is due to partially non-canalized vagina, the surgical correction should be done via the vaginal route by an experienced team because if the initial correction is not proper, the vagina will get closed and during a repeat procedure the chance of injuring the rectum and bladder is high. Simple drainage by approaching transvaginally without making an effort to keep the vagina patent or draining the hematocolpos by a needle is despicable, because of the problems which can occur during a repeat procedure, as already mentioned. After careful dissection in the plane between the urethra and bladder anteriorly, and the rectum and anal canal posteriorly the hematocolpos can be reached. If the raw area is a smaller portion, like the lower 1/3rd of vagina or a transverse septum it can be corrected by vaginal advancement. Because of the hematocolpos, the vagina will be greatly dilated and there will be sufficient redundant vagina for a successful vaginal advancement. If the raw area is extensive like the lower 2/3rd of vagina or middle third of vagina, vaginal advancement may not be feasible. In this situation, patency of the vagina should be maintained by keeping a mould with a graft for the epithelization of the neo-vagina.[15] The graft can be a split skin graft or amniotic membrane.

One rare cause for amenorrhea in a patient with well developed secondary sexual characteristics, uterus and vagina is pelvic tuberculosis occurring in childhood. It usually presents later in life as oligomenorrhea, dysmenorrhea, miscarriages, etc. Tuberculosis should be suspected if ultrasound shows calcification in the endometrium. Diagnosis can be confirmed with endometrial aspiration and culture of the material obtained. Treatment with anti-tuberculous drugs will be effective in checking the infection but future fertility prospects are not very favorable. Uterine schistosomiasis is the other rare condition which can produce amenorrhea due to end organ failure. This situation can also be confirmed by examination of the uterine curettings.

4.6.2 Androgen Insensitivity Syndrome (AIS)

Even though classified under compartment I, AIS is due to the defect in the intracellular receptor for androgen in an individual who has testis and male karyotype. Since MIF is produced by the testis, the uterus and upper vagina will be absent. The lower vagina will be present since it is developed from the urogenital sinus. Androgen action depends on receptors. Hence defective receptors will fail to express androgens and the external genitalia will be of female type, but infantile.

Due to unopposed action of estrogen produced from the testis, these individuals will have breast development up to Tanner III with no axillary or pubic hair due to the androgen insensitivity. Their gonads will be in the abdomen or anywhere in the inguinal canal or even in the labium majus, as testicular descent depends upon androgen action. Some individuals will give a history of inguinal hernia repair in childhood which is actually the partially descended testis which might have been mistakenly removed. Defective androgen action and deficiency of estrogens lead to delayed epiphyseal closure. These individuals have long arms and legs and will attain

Androgen insensitivity syndrome (AIS)

- Female appearance
- Breast development- *Tanner* stage III
- Absent axillary and pubic hair
- Shallow blind ending vagina
- Absent uterus
- Karyotype: 46,XY
- Gonadectomy for preventing development of gonadoblastoma

Table 4.5: Differences between mullerian agenesis and androgen insensitivity syndrome

Mullerian agenesis	*Complete androgen insensitivity syndrome*
Normally developed breasts	Breast development -Tanner stage III
Normal pubic and axillary hair	Axillary and pubic hair absent
Normal vulva, non-canalized vagina	Shallow blind ending vagina
Absent uterus	Absent uterus
Karyotype 46, XX	Karyotype XY

normal or above normal height. Their androgen levels will be normal and hence 17-keto steroid level will also be normal. As there is no androgen action due to defective receptors, they cannot be converted to a phenotypic male by giving exogenous androgens. They can only be reared as females.

Their gonads are prone to develop malignancies after puberty in 22%. Hence the gonads should be removed after attaining puberty or breast development. Though their testis harbors immature spermatozoa, mature sperms are not produced.[16]

Androgen insensitivity can be incomplete. These individuals present at birth with ambiguous genitalia or at puberty with virilization. They will have enlarged clitoris, axillary and pubic hair development along with some amount of breast development.

The differences between mullerian agenesis and complete androgen insensitivity syndrome is provided in Table 4.5.

4.7 COMPARTMENT II

4.7.1 Gonadal Dysgenesis

Individuals with absent ovarian function and quantitative alteration of sex chromosomes are classified as gonadal dysgenesis.

Turner syndrome

- Short stature,
- Normal intelligence,
- Web neck, cubitus valgus, low hairline, shield chest.
- Congenital cardiac defects
- Renal anomalies
- Skeletal defects
- Autoimmune thyroiditis
- Diabetes insipidus

Turner Syndrome

The commonest gonadal dysgenesis encountered is Turner syndrome, which is the commonest cause of primary amenorrhea also.

The karyotypes can be:

- Turner syndrome -45, X.

Mosaic Turner Syndrome

- 45, X/46, XX
- 45, X/46, XX/47, XXX
- 45, X/46, XY

X chromosome deletions

- 46, XXpdel 21-22
- 46, XXqdel 13-26

The commonest karyotype is 45, X. This is the only monosomy which survives to adult life. Only one X chromosome is enough for the initial differentiation of the female fetal gonad, but a second X chromosome is necessary for the follicular development and maturation. Hence the fetus with 45, X karyotype will have follicles in the early intrauterine life. But nearly all the follicles will become atretic by the time the fetus is born. But a mosaic Turner will have a few follicles and may attain puberty and can even give birth to children. They will undergo premature menopause.[17]

The typical phenotype of Turner syndrome is characteristic. They will have webbed neck (Fig. 4.7), short stature, shield chest, cubitus valgus, low hair line, congenital cardiac defects, renal anomalies, skeletal anomalies, normal intelligence, autoimmune thyroiditis and diabetes mellitus.

Individuals with structural abnormalities of X chromosome like Xp deletion, also presents with primary amenorrhea and features similar to Turner syndrome. But individuals having Xq deletion will not have features of Turner syndrome, even though they will also be amenorrheic. They can be of normal stature and eunuchoid in appearance.

4.7.2 Pure Gonadal Dysgenesis

Phenotypic females with streak gonads and no chromosomal abnormalities are classified as pure gonadal dysgenesis. Because of several unrelated etiologies, the gonads may not develop in an otherwise normal individual. This results in a female phenotype irrespective of the genotype, i.e. whether 46,XX or 46,XY. All these individuals will be phenotypically females as female development is the neutral norm. They will have high gonadotropin levels. The etiology can be viral infection, metabolic abnormalities or genetic mutations. Individuals

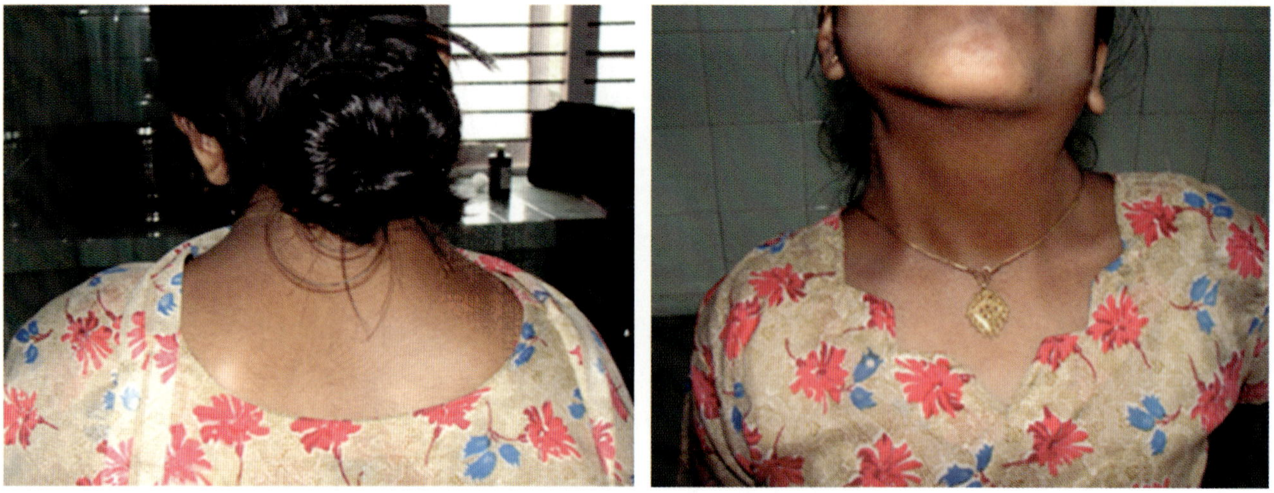

Fig. 4.7: Webbed neck typical of Turner syndrome

with XY karyotype should have their gonads removed. They will have sexual infantilism, primary amenorrhea, tall or normal stature and will have phenotypically female characteristics irrespective of karyotype. A few individuals may have a reduced ovarian function so that they have some development of secondary sexual characteristics and a few menstrual cycles.

46,XY pure gonadal dysgenesis is otherwise called Swyer syndrome.

Swyer Syndrome

Swyer syndrome is a 46,XY female with sexual infantilism. The gonads do not develop in these individuals due to mutations in the SRY gene of Y chromosome.

Other mutations of the Y chromosome are also reported to result in a dysgenetic male gonad. These are SOX9, DAX1 and SF1. The genetic abnormalities will result in defective gonadal development. Because of the absence of anti-mullerian hormone, the mullerian duct will persist and the patient will have a rudimentary uterus and vagina. This is one of the differences between androgen insensitivity and Sweyer syndrome. Since these individuals are at risk for gonadoblastomas, their gonads should be extirpated.

Gonadal dysgenesis in individuals with 46,XX is due to the presence of small fragments of Y chromosome in their genome. This cannot be diagnosed by conventional karyotyping. It can only be diagnosed by doing PCR with Y chromosome probe.[18,19] Hence all individuals with gonadal dysgenesis and karyotype 46,XX should be screened with Y specific DNA probe.

Features of Swyer syndrome

- Mutations of the SRY gene on the Y chromosome
- Eunuchoid features
- Phenotypic female
- Secondary sexual characters not developed
- Infantile uterus and vagina
- Karyotype 46,XY

Streak gonads (should be removed as there is a 30% chance for malignancy)

4.7.3 Mixed Gonadal Dysgenesis

Patients with streak gonad on one side and malformed testes on the other side are classified as mixed gonadal dysgenesis. They will have ambiguous genitalia. Mutations of SRY gene is identified as one of the etiology of the condition.

4.7.4 Resistant Ovary Syndrome

This rare disorder, otherwise called Savage syndrome is characterized by normal female karyotype and female phenotype. The ovaries will have follicles but ovulation will not occur. The exact etiology is unknown but it is postulated that it could be due to abnormal FSH receptors in the ovary. They will have high gonadotropin levels. Autoimmune premature ovarian failure presenting as primary amenorrhea can also have the same clinical features. Ovarian biopsy differentiates the two conditions as there is no lymphocyte infiltration in the former. Since there is not much difference in the management, ovarian biopsy is not mandatory.

4.7.5 Enzyme Deficiencies

17 α-hydroxylase and 17, 20 desmolase Deficiency

These can present as hypogonadism, as sex steroids are not produced in the absence of 17α-hydroxylase. The karyotype can be 46,XY or 46,XX. Uterus is absent in individuals with 46,XY. Since 17 α-hydroxylase is necessary for synthesis of cortisol, its production will also be reduced. There will be an excess production of mineralocorticoid resulting in Na^+ retention, K^+ loss and hypertension.

Aromatase Deficiency

In this condition androgen cannot be converted to estrogens due to the deficiency of aromatase enzyme. This disorder is an autosomal recessive abnormality caused by mutations of CYP 19 gene.[20] Female child will be virilized with ambiguous genitalia. At puberty virilization will worsen and the individuals will not attain menarche. Gonadotropins will be high and androgen and estrogen level would be low.

4.7.6 Premature Ovarian Failure

If ovarian failure occurs before attaining menarche, patients can present as primary amenorrhea.

Etiologies

1. Chromosomal anomalies like 45,X/46,XX or 47,XXY or 46,XX delXp or Fragile X premutation
2. Autoimmune disorders
3. Galactosemia
4. Destruction of follicles due to infections like mumps
5. Radiation exposure

(Since almost all of these individuals present as secondary amenorrhea, a detailed description on this is included in the Chapter 5, Secondary amenorrhea)

4.8 COMPARTMENT III

Pituitary causes of amenorrhea can be congenital or acquired. It is very rare for pituitary tumors to present as primary amenorrhea. The pituitary disorders can be enlisted into:

- Congenital isolated gonadotropin deficiency
- HPO dysfunction—PCOD
- Late onset congenital adrenal hyperplasia
- Pituitary adenomas

4.8.1 Congenital Disorders of the Anterior Pituitary

Hypopituitarism

Congenital pan-hypopituitarism will present early in childhood. They will have amenorrhea because of lack of gonadotropins. One such syndrome is Laurence-Moon-Bardet-Biedl syndrome characterized by sexual infantilism, obesity, mental retardation and several morphologic anomalies.

Isolated FSH Deficiency

Isolated gonadotropin deficiency has been reported to produce primary amenorrhea. These individuals have very low FSH levels and high LH levels. Hence if an individual with amenorrhea has low FSH levels, LH should also be estimated. These individuals can be treated with exogenous FSH.

4.8.2 Acquired Causes

Pituitary tumors can produce amenorrhea due to prolactin secreting adenomas or non prolactin secreting lesions like craniopharyngioma, meningioma, glioma, chordoma and metastatic lesions. Craniopharyngiomas compress the optic chiasma and produce visual symptoms. They cause amenorrhea by compressing the pituitary stalk. Non neoplastic intracranial lesions of the sella, like tuberculosis, cysts, sarcoidosis and fat deposits can cause pituitary compression leading to hypogonadotropic amenorrhea. Nearby lesions like internal carotid artery aneurysm and obstruction of the aqueduct of Sylvius can also cause amenorrhea. Prolactin secreting tumors can rarely occur in childhood and can cause primary amenorrhea.[21] They can be identified by high prolactin levels (usually >100 ng/dl).

4.9 COMPARTMENT IV

4.9.1 Congenital-Kallmann Syndrome

Kallmann syndrome is due to deficient secretion of GnRH. There will be associated anosmia or hyposmia. As the condition runs in families there will be positive family history. The karyotype will be 46,XX. Since their gonads are responsive to gonadotropins, ovulation can be induced with exogenous gonadotropins.

4.9.2 Acquired Causes

Anorexia Nervosa

Anorexia nervosa usually presents as secondary amenorrhea. The presentation can vary from a short period of amenorrhea to a state of severe malnourishment with life threatening problems. The etiology is psychological and could be due to personal, familial or cultural factors. Primary amenorrhea can also be caused due to anorexia nervosa. The normal weight gain at puberty may be misinterpreted as excessive and the girl may develop anorexia. Teenagers presenting as primary amenorrhea with normal female phenotype and subnormal secondary sexual characters should be investigated for anorexia nervosa if they have the following features:

- Weight loss of 25% or weighing 15% below the requirement for the age and height.[22]
- Special food habits—denial or unusual hoarding or handling of food and self induced vomiting.
- Excessive growth of lanugo hair.
- Constipation.
- Low blood pressure
- Diabetes insipidus

Extreme Exercise, Stress and Obesity

Extreme exercise, stress and obesity are causes for secondary amenorrhea. Hence, they are detailed in the chapter on Secondary Amenorrhea.

Other Hormonal Factors

Excessive secretion of GH, TSH, ACTH and prolactin causes feedback inhibition of GnRH pulses and can lead to amenorrhea. This is the reason behind amenorrhea in patients with acromegaly, Cushings syndrome and thyroid disorders.

Constitutional Delay

Constituitional delay as a cause of primary amenorrhea is a retrospective diagnosis. These individuals will have delayed maturation of the HPO axis. Their bone age will also be delayed.The delay is not more than one year of chronological age. It is difficult to differentiate these individuals from those having hypothalamopituitary failure. However girls with constitutional delay will be shorter than those who have hypothalamopituitary failure. Follow-up is needed to confirm the diagnosis.

4.10 DIAGNOSTIC WORK-UP AND MANAGEMENT

When a girl is brought with primary amenorrhea, a diagnosis can be arrived at with the aid of:

- History
- Physical examination
- Imaging studies
- Hormonal evaluation
- Karyotyping

An invasive diagnostic procedure like laparoscopy is not required and should not be done simply for diagnostic purpose. After physical examination, the investigations can be channeled. There can be three main groups of patients based on physical examination:

1. individuals without secondary sexual characteristics
2. individuals with female type secondary sexual characteristics
3. individuals with virilising puberty

4.10.1 Primary Amenorrhea with Sexual Infantilism (Fig. 4.8)

These individuals can be short or tall. Detailed management work-up for each are discussed below

Short Individuals without Secondary Sexual Characteristics and Primary Amenorrhea

If the patient is short, stigmata of Turner syndrome should be looked for. Individuals with Turner syndrome will have typical features as described earlier. Karyotype should be done for confirmation. Karyotype is 45, X. Due to gonadal failure, they will have very high levels of gonadotropins.The other karyotypes of individuals with features of Turner syndrome are:

45, X/46, XX
45, X/46, XX/47, XXX
45, X/46, XY
46, XXpdel 21-22

The deletion can be missed in conventional karyotyping.

Turner syndrome individuals need hormonal replacement for development of secondary sexual characteristics as well as for cardiovascular and skeletal protection. They can be started on low dose of estrogens (0.3 mg conjugated equine estrogens). Later on, estrogen dose can be increased and progestagens added. If the individual is very short, growth hormone administration

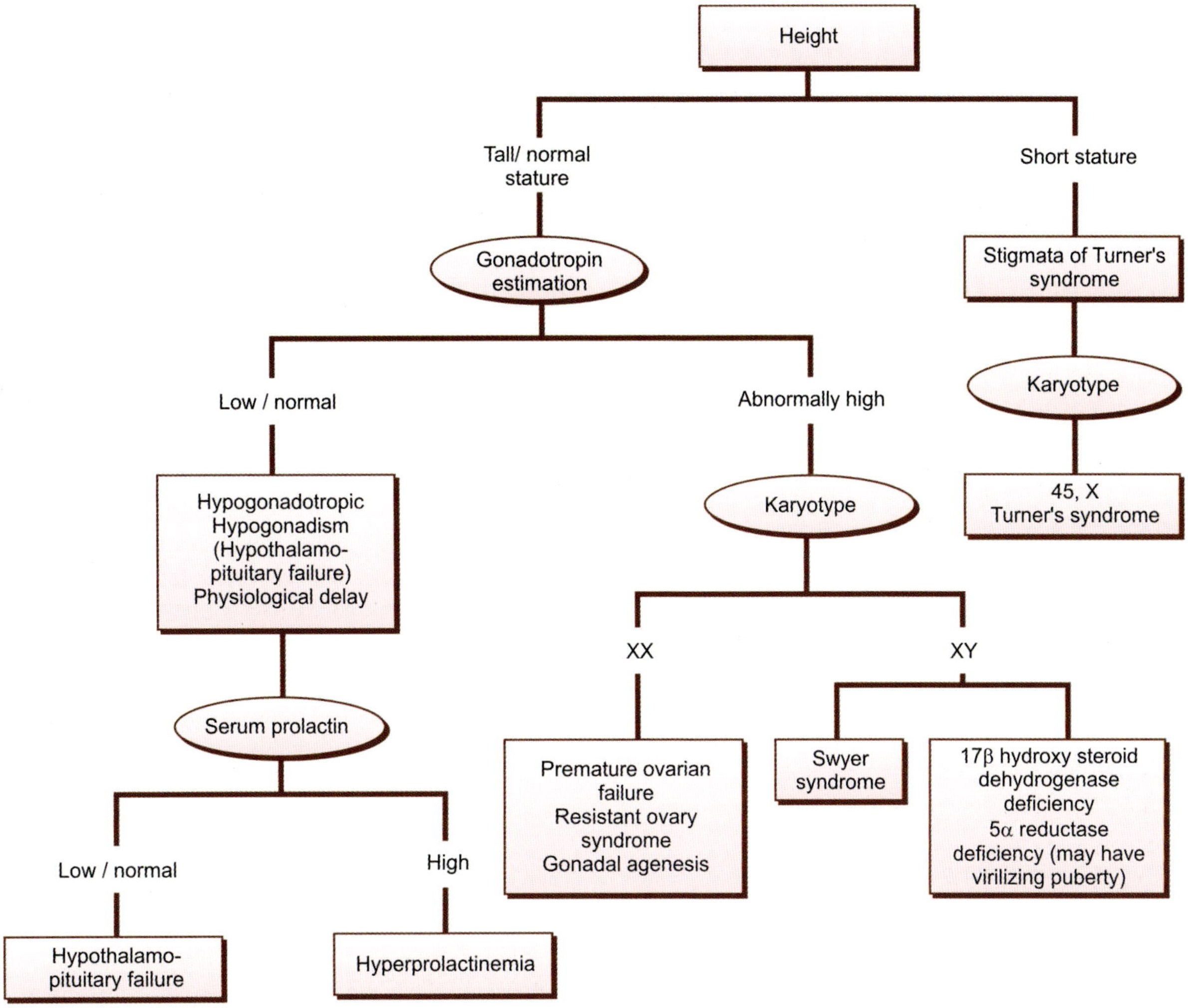

Fig. 4.8: Diagnostic work-up of patients with primary amenorrhea and sexual infantilism

can be considered for attaining height. Mosaic Turner with Y chromosome should have their gonads removed to prevent gonadal malignancies developing in later life. These individuals need not necessarily have features of virilization.

Individuals with Turner syndrome should be investigated for co-morbidities like cardiovascular and other endocrine disorders. About 30% of them will have coarctation of the aorta. Turner syndrome individuals are capable of becoming surrogate mothers with donated ovum and ART. They have a risk of aortic dissection during pregnancy, which should be discussed with the couple.

The mosaic Turner usually presents as secondary amenorrhea. They may not be as short as 45,X individuals.

Individuals having Xq deletion (46, XXqdel 13-26) will also have primary amenorrhea, but will not have features of Turner syndrome. They will have normal stature.

Tall/normal Statured Individuals without Secondary Sexual Characteristics and Primary Amenorrhea

The tall/normal statured girls with primary amenorrhea and absent secondary sexual characteristics may be having either primary or secondary gonadal failure. Their tall nature is due to the delayed epiphyseal union as a consequence of absence of sex steroids. Serum FSH estimation can give the clue as to whether it is primary or secondary gonadal failure.

Hypergonadotropic (Table 4.6)

It is needless to say that patients with primary gonadal failure will have elevated gonadotropin levels. *All individuals with high FSH levels should undergo karyotyping to find out Y chromosome fragment, even if these individuals do not show features of virilization. Individuals with Y chromosome fragment should have their gonads removed* due to the high risk for developing gonadoblastomas.

Indications for karyotyping

- Hypogonadism and high FSH to exclude Y chromosome
- Normal puberty and absent uterus-to confirm MRKH syndrome
- Virilizing puberty to exclude partial androgen insensitivity syndrome, 5a reductase deficiency and mixed gonadal dysgenesis.

Table 4.6: Causes of gonadotropin level >35 IU/ml

Congenital
- Turner syndrome
- Pure gonadal dysgenesis
  - XX gonadal dysgenesis
  - XY gonadal dysgenesis or Swyer syndrome
- Enzyme deficiencies
  - 17α hydroxylase deficiency in XX individuals
  - Galactosemia

Acquired gonadal failure
- Infections like mumps
- Radiation and chemotherapy

This subgroup mainly includes:

A. Genetic

- Pure gonadal dysgenesis
- Swyer syndrome
- Other mutations of the Y chromosome

Gonadal dysgenesis in individuals with 46,XX is due to the presence of small fragments of Y chromosome in their genome. This cannot be diagnosed by conventional karyotyping. It can only be diagnosed by doing PCR with particular target DNA. It is important to search for these fragments of Y chromosome[1] since they are at high risk for development of gonadoblastomas.

Other Genetic Causes of Ovarian Failure

Deletion of a portion of X chromosome can lead to ovarian failure. One such deletion identified is Xq del 13-26.These individuals usually present as secondary amenorrhea.

Individuals with fragile X pre-mutations will also develop premature ovarian failure but they usually present as secondary amenorrhea.[23]

B. Enzyme Deficiencies

17α hydroxylase deficiency and 17, 20 desmolase deficiency

Individuals with 17 alpha hydroxylase deficiency and 46,XX as well as 46,XY karyotype will present with primary amenorrhea. They will be having high FSH levels. Since 17 hydroxylation is not required for mineralocorticoid production, they will have high levels of minerlocorticoids, which in turn makes them hypertensive. Sex steroids are not produced either in the adrenals or in the ovary. Hence such individuals with 46, XY will not have virilization and will be sexually infantile.

C. Acquired

Apart from the above mentioned causes, irradiation of the ovaries and chemotherapy with alkylating agents can lead to primary amenorrhea resulting from ovarian failure.

Hypogonadotropic Hypogonadism

If the FSH levels are low, the patient may have a defective pituitary or hypothalamus. Delay in the pulsatile release of GnRH is the commonest reported cause. Puberty usually occurs at a later age. Diagnosis is established by estimating bone age in X-Ray (left wrist), which will also be delayed. Confirmation is done by GnRH challenge. GnRH agonist is given at a dose of 100 micrograms subcutaneously, after a week's treatment with ethinyl oestradiol 0.01mg daily. It will increase the level of gonadotropins in individuals with constitutional delay but not in individuals with pituitary failure.

Absence of the olfactory sense in a girl presenting with primary amenorrhea, sexual infantilism and low FSH leads to a diagnosis of Kallman Syndrome.

Isolated FSH deficiency also is reported to cause hypogonadotropic primary amenorrhea. Since their LH levels are high, LH estimation should also be done when a girl is found to have primary amenorrhea and low FSH. These individuals may respond to exogenous FSH.

Hypogonadotropic patients with primary amenorrhea should have their CNS evaluated with CT or MRI to exclude prolactinomas or other space occupying lesions that interfere with the hypothalamo-hypophyseal portal system.

Treatment

Aims of treatment include:

- Treating the primary cause for amenorrhea,
- Substituting hormones for the development of secondary sexual characteristics and preventing the adverse effects of estrogen deprivation especially osteoporosis.

Treatment of the Primary Cause of Amenorrhea

Hyperprolactinemia is treated with bromocriptine. It should be started at a low dose of 2.5 mg and then increased to a maximum of 7.5 mg. Patients should be warned about the side-effects of bromocriptine which mainly include gastric irritation and hypotension. Craniopharyngiomas and other tumours need surgical interference. Isolated FSH deficiency can be treated with FSH administration when pregnancy is desired.

Treatment of Hypothalamic Amenorrhea

These patients need long term GnRH treatment. But the problem is the long term use of GnRH pump. Hence hormone replacement with estrogen and progestogens can be started from childhood and GnRH treatment resorted to when pregnancy is desired.

Management of Individuals with Y Chromosome in their Genome

Individuals with Y chromosome or even SRY gene translocated to the X chromosome are at risk of development of gonadal tumors. Individuals with XX karyotype and hirsutism may be having SRY gene translocated onto X chromosome. These individuals should have gonadectomy even if the gonad is streak. SRY gene can be identified by PCR.

Hormone Replacement

For the development of secondary sexual characteristics, these girls should be treated with low dose unopposed estrogens initially. Treatment can be started with either 0.3 mg conjugated equine estrogens or 0.5 mg estradiol daily. After about 6 months to 1 year, the dose can be stepped up to 0.625 mg conjugated equine estrogens or 1 mg oestradiol. 5 mg of medroxyprogesterone acetate or an equivalent progestin can be added for the first 14 days of each month. With this treatment, the individuals usually will have development of secondary sexual characteristics. Bone mineral density will also be taken care of. The individual will be having regular withdrawal bleeds. The low dose of estrogens administered will promote bone growth and development and at the same time will not cause premature closure of epiphyses. Hence full height potential is achieved.

For individuals with Turner syndrome who are characteristically short, treatment with recombinant growth hormone can be considered. With 2 years of GH treatment, an average gain in height of 5-6 cm can be achieved.[24]

Orthotropic ovarian transplantation[25] has been successfully reported in individuals with Turner syndrome.

> Individuals with all forms of gonadal failure need cyclical estrogen progestin therapy for initiation and maintenance of secondary sexual characters as well as to prevent osteoporosis

4.10.2 Amenorrhea with Secondary Sexual Characteristics (Fig. 4.9)

Individuals with Female Type Secondary Sexual Characteristics

If a girl has well developed secondary sexual characteristics, with Tanner stage 4 or more breast development, axillary and pubic hair development, she will be probably having mullerian anomaly. If she has a functioning uterus and a partially non developed vagina or transverse vaginal septum or imperforate hymen, she will present early due to the symptoms of hematocolpos. The exact nature of the anomaly can be diagnosed by abdominal examination, examination of the vulva and rectal examination. An imperforate hymen will present as a bluish bulge in the vulva.

Breast development up to Tanner stage 3, with absent axillary and pubic hair and blind ending vagina is the typical phenotypic feature of androgen insensitivity syndrome. Rectal examination can make out the absence of the uterus. Imaging studies can confirm absent uterus and can locate the gonads. If the gonads are in the abdomen, it can be made out by ultrasound. If it is somewhere in the inguinal canal, CT or MRI may be needed for locating the gonads. Karyotyping is necessary for confirming the diagnosis. Gonadectomy should be deferred till puberty so that the small amount of estrogen elaborated by the testis (unopposed by androgen) will result in breast development. Since the end organ is defective, these individuals cannot be reared as males by administering exogenous androgens. However, in partial androgen insensitivity syndrome, the management depends upon the gender identity preferred by the patient and the parents. They should undergo gonadectomy at the earliest to avoid further virilization provided their choice is to be reared up as females. Individuals who prefer male gender identity may be treated with testosterone or dihydrotestosterone after orchipexy. Dihydroteststerone is preferred because it cannot be aromatized to oestrogen in the periphery. Osteoporosis and psychological sequelae are the reported complications.

The vexing problem after diagnosis is about disclosing the genetic sex to the parents as well as to the individual. After proper counseling, it is better to disclose the genetic sex and give the reasons for continuing the gender identity as either male female depending up on the situation.

Individuals with Virilization (Fig. 4.10)

5α-reductase deficiency

If the individual who is reared as a girl has virilising puberty and absent breast development, the likely diagnosis

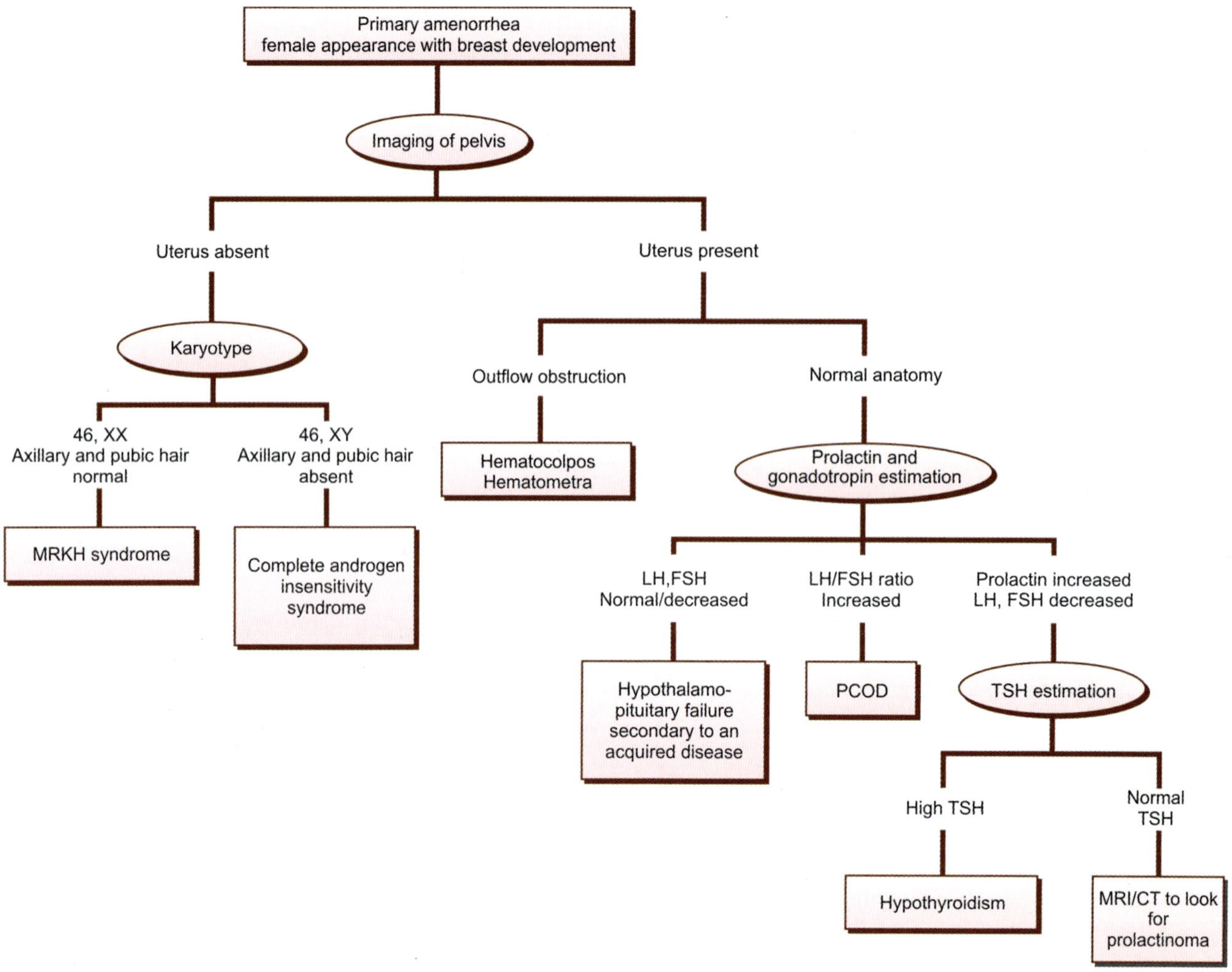

Fig. 4.9: Diagnostic work-up of individuals with primary amenorrhea and female appearance with breast development

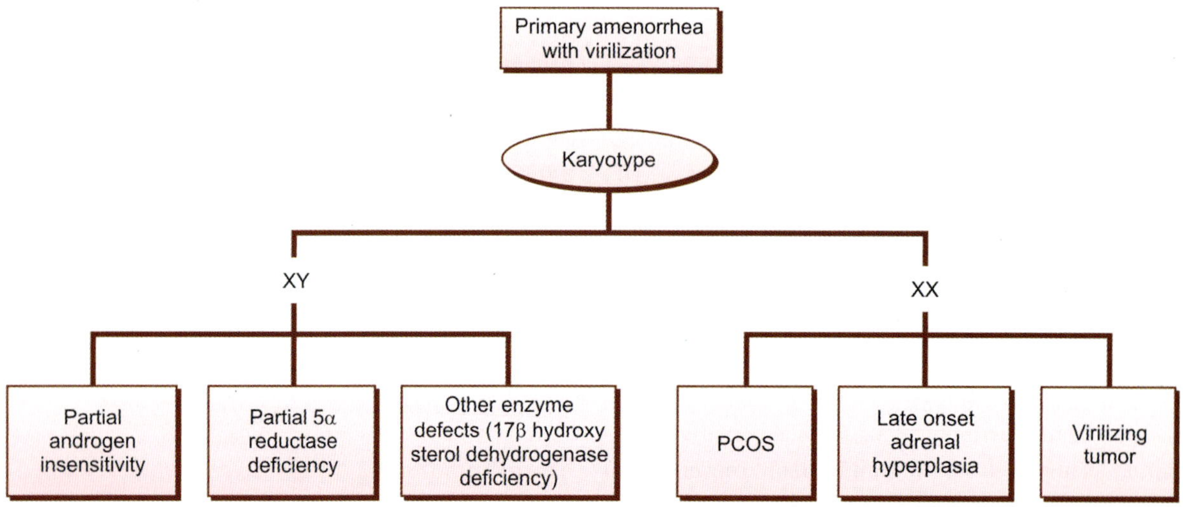

Fig. 4.10: Etiology of individuals with primary amenorrhea and virilization

is 5α-reductase deficiency. Their genitalia will be abnormal at birth with fusion of labioscrotal folds and urogenital opening or separate urethral and vaginal openings. At puberty, virilization occurs. These individuals resemble partial androgen insensitivity syndrome. Karyotype will be 46,XY. They will have internal duct system since its development depends upon testosterone production. But dihydrotestosterone dependant structures like prostate and external genitalia development will be affected. Dihydrotestosterone level is found to be decreased but testosterone levels will be normal. Hence, the levels of FSH and LH will be normal. The management depends upon the choice of the individual and the parents. Because the individual is reared as a girl till puberty, the parents may prefer to rear the child as a girl. Orchidectomy should be done to prevent further virilization and also development of gonadoblastoma. These individuals can also be reared as males by giving exogenous dihydrotestosterone but orchidectomy is indicated to prevent gonadoblastoma if the gonad is in the abdomen. If orchipexy is possible, it may be done.

Adolescent type 21 hydroxylase deficiency

21 hydroxylase deficiency usually presents at birth. But, the late onset type (attenuated or acquired) usually present at puberty with hirsutism, amenorrhea or irregular menstruation. It is prudent to think of this possibility in a girl who presents with amenorrhea and hirsutism. The disorder is inherited as autosomal recessive trait. The gene is identified as CYP21B located on chromosome 6. A variety of mutations have been identified and most patients are compound heterozygotes. The diagnosis is based on the elevated levels of 17 hydroxyprogesterone. Since 17 hydroxyprogesterone may be marginally elevated in patients with polycystic ovarian disease, ACTH stimulation test will help in distinguishing between the two. There will be a dramatic increase in 17 hydroxyprogesterone level, 60 minutes after ACTH administration in patients with 21 hydroxylase deficiency. The condition can be treated with 3.5-5 mg/m^2 of prednisone.

Polycystic Ovarian Syndrome

Rarely, patients with PCOS can present as primary amenorrhea. They have normal stature and breast development but show obesity, hirsutism and can have clitoromegaly. Ovaries will be polycystic. As mentioned above, they rarely have elevated 17 hydroxyprogesterone levels. Treatment is required to prevent endometrial hyperplasia as well as to normalize their lipid profile. If the lipid profile is abnormal with low HDL and high LDL, protection against cardiovascular diseases is necessary.

Even if contraception is not needed, these girls should be treated with low dose combination oral contraceptive pills. For those who are worried about hirsutism, a combination OCP containing drosperinone may be preferred. Endometrial hyperplasia prevention can be achieved by administering medroxy progesterone acetate 10 mg daily for at least 10 days a month so that they will have regular withdrawal bleeding. (Detailed discussion of PCOS is provided in Chapter 9, PCOS)

4.11 CONCLUSION

The cause of primary amenorrhea can be sorted out in most of the situations by careful history and physical examination. The important aspects of the physical examination include examination for secondary sexual characteristics and anatomic abnormalities. Early diagnosis of conditions like Turner syndrome is important since early interference in the form of GH administration is essential in achieving stature correction. A girl who has normally developed secondary sexual characteristics and amenorrhea, may be having mullerian agenesis. Invasive investigation like laparoscopy is not necessary for diagnosis in most of the situations and should not be resorted to unnecessarily. The diagnosis of mullerian agenesis can be confirmed by imaging. They can be advised vaginoplasty before marriage. When the secondary sexual characteristics are absent, estimation of FSH levels should be performed to differentiate between hypergonadotropic and hypogonadotropic hypogonadism. All individuals with high FSH, irrespective of presence or absence of virilization should be karyotyped to look for Y-chromosome component. Individuals with Y-chromosome should have gonadectomy done for preventing the development of gonadoblastoma. By correct evaluation and proper management women having primary amenorrhea can attain menstruation and even fertility. Even when menstruation and fertility cannot be achieved, the girl can be helped to lead a healthy life by medicines and appropriate surgical interference.

4.12 CLINICAL SCENARIOS

Case Scenario 1

29 yr old Mrs.R presented with primary infertility. She was married for 4 years. She did not attain spontaneous menarche and gave history of regular withdrawal bleeding after taking OCP which was prescribed by a local physician.

There was no relevant family history. She was short statured with a height of 145 cm. Her breast, axillary and pubic hair showed Tanner stageIII. Local examination revealed female type infantile external genitalia. Rectal examination revealed uterus to be smaller.

What are the possible diagnoses?

Regular withdrawal bleeding with OC pills indicates that she has a patent uterovaginal canal. At the age of 29 her breast and pubic hair development is only up to tanner stage III which is subnormal indicating that she is not exposed to endogenous estrogen. Since she gives history of hormone intake, the present breast development can be assumed to be due to the same. In short, she is a 29 year old short statured lady with primary amenorrhea, sexual infantilism, female type genitalia and patent uterovaginal canal. The possibility is hypogonadism

What investigation will sort out whether she has ovarian failure or pituitary-hypothalamic failure?

Gonadotropin level. Hormonal profile was done and her FSH was estimated to be 62 IU/l and LH 46 IU/L.

What do you infer?

Her hypogonadism is due to primary ovarian failure. Hypothalamus and pituitary are normal.

What else should you look for?

Since she is short statured with sexual infantilism, the stigmata of Turner syndrome have to be looked for.

Her neck showed webbing and she had cubitus valgus. Ultrasound showed uterus measuring 6 × 3 × 3 cm.

What particular investigation will clinch the diagnosis?

Karyotyping

What will you expect?

45,X

The karyotype came as 46,XX.

Since physical features were suggestive of Turner syndrome the karyotype was repeated. The result was 46,XX/45,X. She was a mosaic turner.

If the karyotype is confirmed as 46,XX, what is the possibility?

Xp deletion can also present with primary amenorrhea. They can also have features of Turner syndrome. On conventional methods their karyotype will be reported as 46,XX.

How will you diagnose the deletion?

FISH or PCR using the appropriate probe

Case Scenario 2 (Figs 4.11 and 4.12)

Miss V, 17 yr old college student presented with primary amenorrhea. Her family history did not reveal anything relevant. On examination she was of normal built. Her height was 156 cm and she weighed 55 kg. She was a normal looking adolescent, with breasts, axillary and pubic hair of Tanner stage 4. Examination of external genitalia revealed normal vulva except for absence of vaginal orifice. On rectal examination, the uterus was not felt.

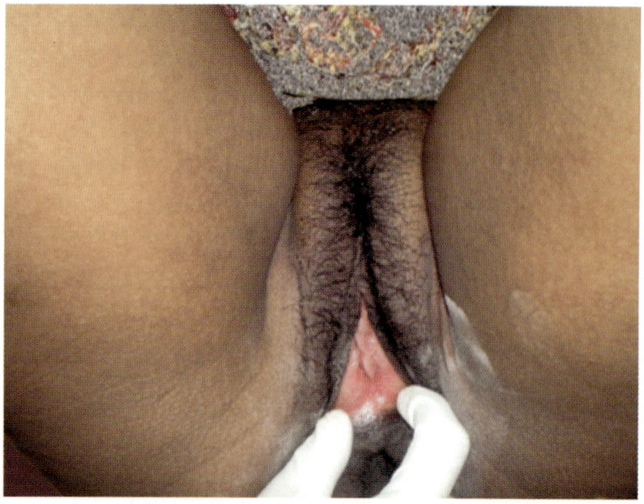

Fig. 4.11: External genitalia showing non-canalized vagina (situation 2)

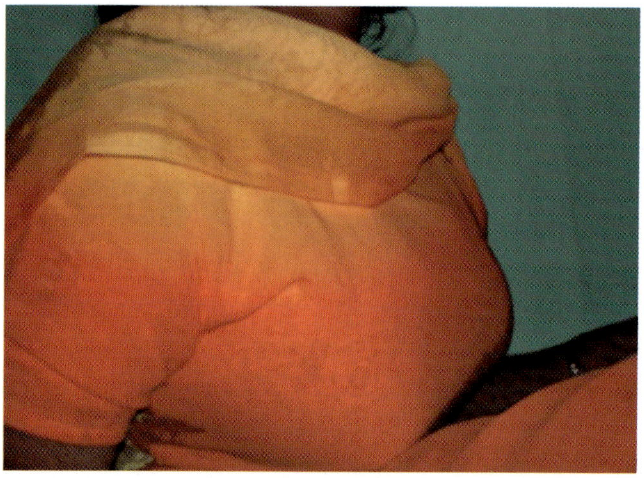

Fig. 4.12: Figure showing normal breast development (situation 2)

What could be the probable diagnosis?

The two conditions presenting with primary amenorrhea, breast development and absent uterus are mullerian agenesis and testicular feminization syndrome. In testicular feminization syndrome, axillary and pubic hair will be absent and a short vagina which is developed from the urogenital sinus will be present. Hence the diagnosis is mullerian agenesis due to the normal female appearance with well developed axillary and pubic hair and breast development appropriate for age with absent uterus.

How will you confirm the clinical examination finding?
Ultrasound examination to visualize the ovaries and confirm absence of the uterus and exclude cryptomenorrhea. However girls with cryptomenorrhea will present early with monthly pain abdomen and examination will reveal a mass in the hypogastrium or a mass on rectal examination. Since the girl is 17 years of age with secondary sexual characters appropriate for age, cryptomenorrhea is unlikely.

Should you do karyotyping of this girl?
Karyotyping need not be done as there is no suspicion about the diagnosis. If the clinical picture is not typical because of the presence of incompletely developed breast and pubic as well as axillary hair, incomplete testicular feminization is a possibility, karyotyping should be done.

What else should be done to complete the investigation?
Exclude renal and skeletal anomalies which can be associated with mullerian anomaly.

What management will you advise?
Vaginoplasty about 6 months before marriage

Karyotype of 46, XX confirmed the diagnosis. She was advised vaginoplasty about 6 months before marriage.

Case Scenario 3

30 yr old Mrs. V presented with dyspareunia. She claimed to be having infrequent menstruation. She gave a history of surgery in the right inguinal region in childhood. On examination, she was tall with height-170 cm and weight 65 kg. Her breast was of Tanner stage 3. Her axillary and pubic hairs were absent. Her vulva appeared infantile and she had a shallow vagina, which ended blindly. On rectal examination, the uterus was not felt.

What is the most probable diagnosis?
Considering the absence of pubic and axillary hair, breast development of Tanner stage 3, blind ending vagina and absent uterus, the most probable diagnosis is androgen insensitivity syndrome (AIS).

What investigation will confirm the diagnosis?
Karyotyping

What will you expect?
46,XY

What might have been the surgery done in the inguinal region?
One or both of the gonads of individuals with AIS can be anywhere between the abdomen and the labium majus, which can be mistaken for hernia and might have been removed.

What management protocol will you advise for this patient?
The other gonad has to be located. It is likely to be in the abdomen and has to be removed to prevent development of gonadoblastoma.

What postoperative management will you advise?
After gonadectomy there is a high risk for osteoporosis. Hence, she should be advised to take estrogen preparation continuously. Since uterus is not present there is no need to add progesterone. With estrogen, breast development also will occur and her vaginal dryness with the resultant dyspareunia will be relieved.

Can she be converted to a male?
Not possible even if gonads had not been removed. Because of defective receptor, exogenous as well as endogenous androgen will not act.

Case Scenario 4

16 yr old Miss R was referred as primary amenorrhea. Her height was 154 cm and she weighed 65 kg. She had hirsutism with a score of 8, breasts tanner stage 4, pubic and axillary hair normal, vulva normal, hymen intact and no clitoromegaly. Rectal examination showed normal sized uterus.

What are the probable diagnoses?
This 16 year old girl is having virilizing puberty and amenorrhea. Hence, the diagnoses are partial AIS, 5α-reductase deficiency, adult onset adrenal hyperplasia, PCOS and androgen secreting ovarian tumor.

How will you make a differential diagnosis between all these conditions?
Trans-abdominal ultrasound

Her ultrasound examination revealed uterus measuring 4.1 × 3.5 × 3.1 cm, endometrium 6 mm, both ovaries polycystic. No adnexal mass. Since the uterus is present, partial AIS and 5α reductase deficiency were excluded. Since there is no adnexal mass androgen secreting tumor is unlikely. However, since androgen secreting tumors can be very small, they can be missed at ultrasound.

How will you differentiate between CAH and PCOD?
Estimation of 17 hydroxyprogesterone should be done. It will be elevated in CAH and the diagnosis should be confirmed by ACTH stimulation test which will be abnormal in CAH.

Provisional diagnosis of PCOD was made and she was advised micronised progesterones for 10 days a month for withdrawal bleeding. She reported 2 weeks later with withdrawal bleeding, which indicates that her HPO axis is normal. She was advised to take medroxy progesterone acetate from 1st to 10th of each month. Progesterone treatment will prevent endometrial hyperplasia and endometrial cancer developing in these women. This regime was preferred because she did not have a severe degree of hirsutism. If hirsutism and acne were of concern for her, a combination oral contraceptive pill containing anti-androgen cyproterone acetate would have been preferred.

Case Scenario 5

One lady bystander of a patient in the post-natal ward appeared like a man in feminine attire. At night, the other patients and relatives alerted the security staff about this particular person, as only women were allowed at night in the female ward. She was a 28 yr old individual dressed in purdah. The duty medical officer came to clear the situation. The lady revealed that she had not attained menarche. She attended the outpatient clinic for evaluation the next day. She was a tall thin individual with no obvious breast development. Her height was 181 cm. Her breast was Tanner stage 1. She had no axillary hair, but had sparse pubic hair. Her vulva was infantile. Vagina was patent, but narrow. A probe could be passed into the vagina. Since speculum could not be passed the presence of cervix or uterus could not be made out. Ultrasound revealed a hypoplastic uterus.

What are the most probable diagnoses?

She is an individual with hypogonadism- gonadal or hypothalamopituitary.

How will you make out whether the condition is gonadal failure or hypothalamopituitary failure?

Estimation of FSH level is the investigation which will sort out the situation. Patients with gonadal failure will have gonadotropins in the menopausal range which distinguishes them from hypothalamo-pituitary failure whose FSH levels are extremely low.

Her FSH was found to be 55 IU/L and LH was 40 IU/L.

What is the next step in investigation?

Karyotype. The reason is that patients with 46, XX as well as 46,XY and individuals with fragments of Y chromosome in their genotype can present with gonadal dysgenesis and hypogonadism. Even the streak gonad of individuals with Y chromosome should be removed to prevent development of gonadoblastoma. The karyotype came as 46, XY. A diagnosis of Swyer Syndrome was thus confirmed.

Is it possible that the karyotype be 46,XX in such a clinical situation?

Yes, XX pure gonadal dysgenesis can be caused by small Y chromosome fragments in their genome. This can be identified only by PCR using Y sequence and not by conventional karyotyping. Gonadectomy for prevention of malignancy is advised for such individuals also.

What management will you advise?

She should be advised laparotomy for removal of the dysgenetic gonads and hormones to prevent development of osteoporosis in later life.

Case Scenario 6

19 yr old Miss P was brought with complaints of amenorrhea for 6 months. There was no relevant past medical or surgical history. On questioning, it was made out that the so called periods were actually withdrawal bleeding after hormone therapy. She was tall, breasts of tanner stage 3, axillary and pubic hair scanty, vulva female type but infantile. USS revealed small uterus 2.7 × 1.7 × 1.1 cm, ovaries were not convincingly identified.

Diagnosis of hypogonadism was made. Her gonadotropin levels were estimated and found to be elevated (FSH: 59.4 mIU/ML, LH: 22.2MIU/ml, prolactin: 12 ng/ml, estradiol 41 pg). In view of her high gonadotropin levels, karyotyping was advised. Karyotype came as 46,XX. Hence the diagnosis was pure gonadal agenesis. She should have been ideally put on ethinyl oestradiol for 6 months and then progestogens added. Since this girl already had combination OCPs, she was advised to continue OCPs for further breast development and for prevention of steoporosis which these type of individuals are prone for.

Case Scenario 7 (Figs 4.13A to E)

A 14 yr old girl was brought with recently developing hirsutism and primary amenorrhea. On examination, she was found to have a normal stature with a height of 157 cm, no breast development, had hirsutism with a score of 8, clitoromegaly and labial fusion. Imaging showed absent uterus and gonads in the inguinal canal.

What are the probable diagnoses?

5α reductase deficiency, partial androgen insensitivity, intersex and CAH

What is the essential investigation which should be done?

Karyotyping

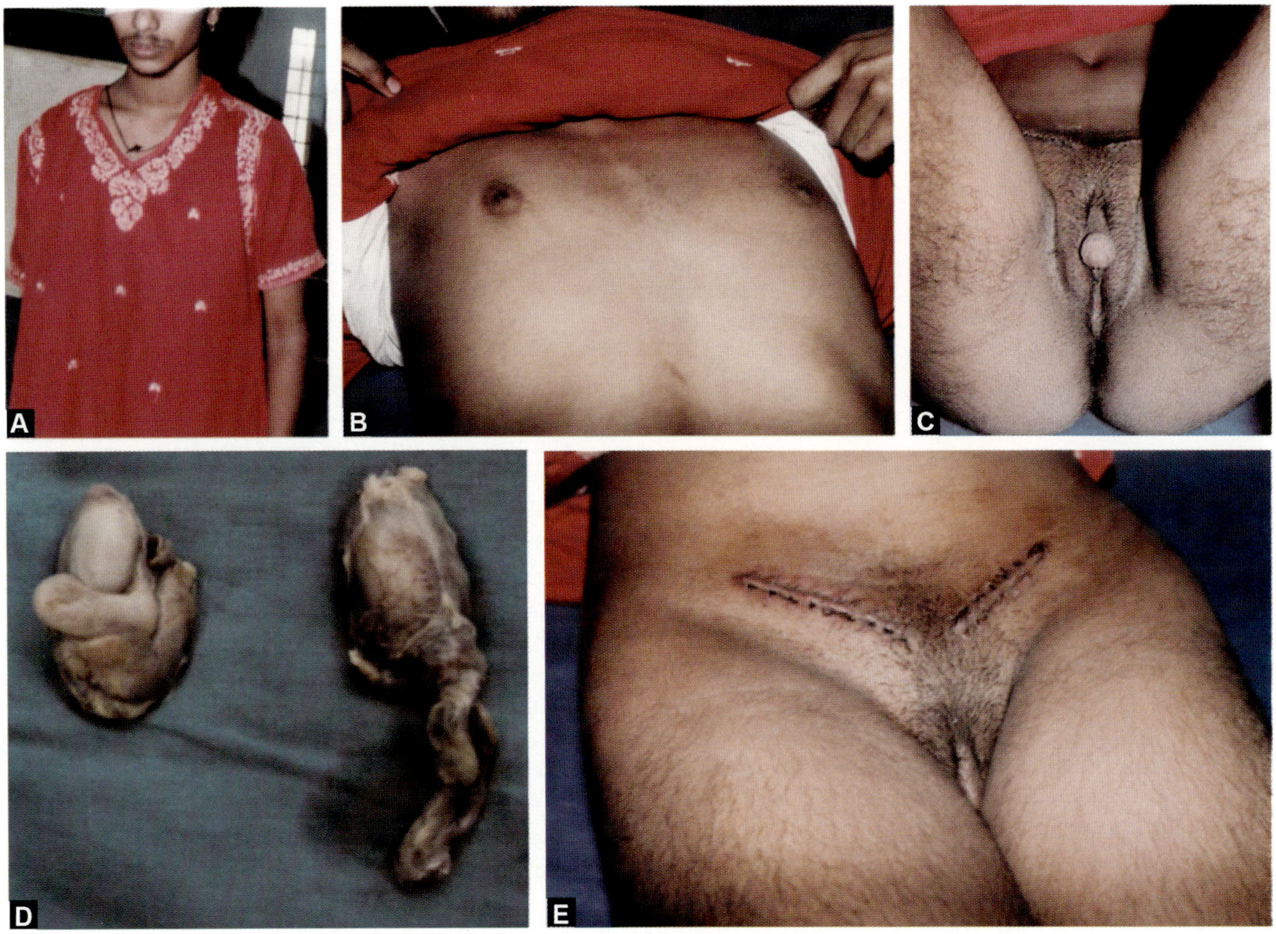

Figs 4.13A to E: Features of girl with 5α reductase deficiency (A). Breast development Tanner Stage I (B). External genitalia showing clitoromegaly (C). Extirpated gonads (D). Gonadectomy incisions in the inguinal region (E)

The karyotype was 46,XY. Should you estimate 17-OH progesterone?

The karyotype of 46,XY excludes possibility of this being an individual (female) having CAH and virilization and hence 17 OH progesterone need not be estimated.

What is the next step in management?

Counseling the parents. Whether to rear as female or convert to male should be decided by the parents and the patient.

What should be done if the decision is to rear as male?

Orchiopexy and plastic surgery for external genitalia

The parents opted to rear the individual as a girl only. The need for gonadectomy (30% risk of gonadoblastoma) was discussed with the parents. She was taken for gonadectomy, had bilateral gonadectomy done and was discharged from the hospital with advice to undergo electrolysis for her facial hair and estrogen-progesterone supplementation for development of breasts and bone protection. She was also advised to come for review if she has problems with sexual intercourse.

REFERENCES

1. Pailhoux E, Jaubert F, et al. Molecular genetics of sex determination. Semin Reprod Med 2002;20:157-67.
2. Marshall WA, Tanner JM. Variations in pattern of pubertal changes in girls. Arch Dis Child 1969;44(235):291-303.
3. Herman-Giddens ME, Slora EJ, Wasserman RC, et al. Secondary sexual characteristics and menses in young girls seen in office practice: a study from the Pediatric Research in Office Settings network. Pediatrics 1997;99(4):505-12.
4. Kaplowitz PB, Oberfield SE. Re-examination of the age limit for defining when puberty is precocious in girls in the United States: implications for evaluation and treatment. Drug and Therapeutics and Executive Committees of the Lawson Wilkins Pediatric Endocrine Society. Pediatrics 1999;104:936-41.
5. Marshall WA, Tanner JM. Variations in pattern of pubertal changes in girls. Arch DisChild 969;44(235):291-303.
6. Strobel A, Issad T, Camoin L, et al. A leptin missense mutation associated with hypogonadism and morbid obesity. Nat Genet 1998;18:213-5.

7. Farooqi IS, Wangensteen T, Collins S, et al. Clinical and molecular genetic spectrum of congenital deficiency of the leptin receptor. N Engl J Med 2007;356:237-47.
8. Mitsushima D, Hei DL, Terasawa E. Aminobutyric acid is an inhibitory neurotransmitter restricting the release of luteinizing hormone-releasing hormone before the onset of puberty. Proc Natl Acad Sci USA 1994;91(1):395-9.
9. Kaplowitz PB, Slora EJ, Wasserman RC, et al. Earlier onset of puberty in girls: relation to increased body mass index and race. Pediatrics 2001;108(2):347-53.
10. Parent AS, Teilmann G, Juul A, et al. The Timing of normal puberty and the age limits of sexual precocity: variations around the world, secular trends, and changes after migration. Endocr Rev 2003;24(5):668-93.
11. Biro FM, McMahon RP, Striegel-Moore R, et al. Impact of timing of pubertal maturation on growth in black and white female adolescents: the National Heart, Lung, and Blood Institute Growth and Health Study. J Pediatr 2001;138(5): 636-43.
12. Gore AC. Environmental toxicant effects on neuroendocrine function. Endocrine 2001;14(2):235-46.
13. Cramer DW, Goldstein DP, Fraer C, et al. Vaginal agenesis (Mayer–Rokitansky–Kuster–Hauser syndrome) associated with the N314D mutation of galactose–1–phosphateuridyl transferase (GALT). Mol Hum Reprod 1996;2:145-8.
14. Frank RT. The formation of an artificial vagina without operation. Am J Obstet Gynecol 1938;35:1053-5.
15. Roberts CP, Haber MJ, Rock JA. Vaginal creation for mullerian agenesis. Am J Obstet Gynecol 2001;185:1349-52.
16. Wisniewski AB, Migeon CJ, Meyer-Bahlburg HF, et al. "Complete androgen insensitivity syndrome: long-term medical, surgical, and psychosexual outcome". The Journal of Clinical Endocrinology and Metabolism 2000;85(8): 2664-9.
17. T Morgan. Turner syndrome: diagnosis and management. Am Fam Physician. 2007;76:405-10.
18. Fechner, Patricia Y. Partial gonadal dysgenesis in a patient with a marker Y chromosome. American Journal of Medical Genetics 1992;42(6).
19. Osipova GR, Karmanov ME, Kozlova SI, et al. PCR detection of Y specific sequences with Ullrich-Turner Syndrome: Clinical implications and limitations. AMJ Med Genet 1998; 76:283-87.
20. Ghosh D, Griswold J, Erman M, Pangborn W (January 2009). "Structural basis for androgen specificity and oestrogen synthesis in human aromatase". Nature 457 (7226): 219-23.
21. Koenig MP, Suppinger K, Leichti B. Hypoprolactinemia as a cause of delayed puberty: successful treatment with bromocriptine. J Clin Endocrinol Metab 1977;45:825-8.
22. Leah M Kalm Richard D. Semba, "They Starved So That Others Be Better Fed: Remembering Ancel Keys and the Minnesota Experiment," Journal of Nutrition, Vol. 135, June 2005;1347-52.
23. Uzielli ML, Guarducci S, Lapi E, et al. Premature ovarian failure (POF)and Fragile X premutation female:from POF to Fragile X carrier identification,from Fragile X carrier diagnosis to POF association data. AMJ Med Genet 1999;84: 300-303
24. Hintz RI, Attie KM, Baptista J, Roche A Effect of growth hormone treatment on adult height of children with idiopathic short stature.Genentech Collaborative Group. New Engl J Med 1999;18:502
25. Mhatre P, Mhatre J, Mahotra R. Ovarian Transplant a new frontier. Transplant Proc 2005;37(2):1396-8.

5 Secondary Amenorrhea

B Presannakumari

5.1 INTRODUCTION

Even though the etiology of primary amenorrhea and secondary amenorrhea overlap to a great extent, it is prudent to discuss secondary amenorrhea separately. Conditions like testicular feminization syndrome or MRKH exclusively present as primary amenorrhea. Certain conditions present either as primary or secondary amenorrhea. The typical examples are mosaic turner syndrome and HPO dysfunction .The acquired diseases of genital tract like Asherman syndrome, autoimmune premature ovarian failure and tumors of the pituitary or hypothalamus usually present as secondary amenorrhea. When these acquired disorders occur in a girl before puberty, she can present as primary amenorrhea. This chapter describes a protocol for arriving at the organ system responsible for causing amenorrhea. Once the diagnosis is arrived at, management can be planned.

5.2 DEFINITION

Secondary amenorrhea is defined as the absence of menstruation for a length of time equivalent to a total of at least 3 of the previous cycle intervals or 6 months in a woman who has had at least a few spontaneous periods.

5.3 ETIOLOGY

The cause of secondary amenorrhea can fit into any of the following compartments

- Compartment I : disorders of the outflow tract
- Compartment II : disorders of the ovary
- Compartment III: disorders of the anterior pituitary
- Compartment IV: disorders of the hypothalamus

5.3.1 Compartment I: Disorders of the Outflow Tract

The commonest condition causing secondary amenorrhea due to outflow tract abnormality is Asherman's syndrome. The condition is characterized by intrauterine adhesions. The adhesions follow vigorous curettage of the uterine cavity after abortion or delivery. Intrauterine adhesions can also occur in tuberculosis or schistosomiasis of the endometrium.

5.3.2 Compartment II: Disorders of the Ovary

1. Autoimmune ovarian failure
2. Chromosomal/genetic
   a. Mosaic Turner syndrome (45,X /46,XX or 45, X/46,XY), rarely Turner syndrome
   b. 47,XXX (triple X) or 48,XXXX
   c. Deletion of portions of X chromosome –Xq13-26, Xp11
   d. Autosomal dominant familial ovarian failure
   e. Fragile X carrier
   f. Galactosemia
3. Iatrogenic
   a. Radiation
   b. Chemotherapy
   c. Surgical removal
   d. Infections (pelvic tuberculosis, mumps)
4. Idiopathic

5.3.3 Compartment III: Disorders of the Anterior Pituitary

1. Prolactinomas
2. Other hormone secreting tumors of the pituitary
3. Non-functioning tumors
4. Pituitary necrosis—Sheehan's syndrome

5.3.4 Compartment IV: Disorders of the Hypothalamus

1. Dermoid cyst
2. Tuberculous granuloma
3. Hypothalamic dysfunction
   a. Anorexia nervosa
   b. Emotional stress
   c. Extreme exercise
   d. Chronic illness

Premature Ovarian Failure

Premature ovarian failure (POF) is ovarian failure occurring before the age of 40 and is characterized by amenorrhea, estrogen deficiency and elevated gonadotropin levels. It is seen in 1% of women. This may be due to decreased follicular reserve or accelerated atresia of follicles. The condition may occur due to a variety of causes as enlisted above. Advances in molecular biology and genetics have sorted out many of the etiologies leading to premature ovarian failure. But still, only in 1/3rd of women the cause may be clearly identified. Chromosomal and genetic causes are the common condi-tions which are identifiable. The common chromosomal causes for premature ovarian failure are mosaic Turner (45,X /46,XX or 45,X/46,XY), triple X (47,XXX),48,XXXX and structural abnormalities of X chromosome.

Genetic causes of premature ovarian failure are fragile X pre-mutation, galactosemia and autosomal dominant premature ovarian failure.[10] About 22% of fragile X pre-mutation carriers will have premature ovarian failure.[11,12,16] The condition can be suspected from the family history of male members being affected with fragile X syndrome exhibiting the typical phenotype.

Galactosemia is due to mutation in galactose-1-phosphate uridyl transferase gene. Gonadal failure occurs due to the accumulated galactose interfering with the migration of germ cells from the yolk sac to the urogenital ridge in fetal life.

Autoimmune Premature Ovarian Failure

This is one of the commonest causes of premature ovarian failure. All women with secondary amenorrhea having normal phenotypic appearance should be suspected to have autoimmune ovarian failure. These women are likely to develop autoimmune failure of other endocrine glands as well.[5,6] Detection of ovarian antibodies is not conclusive in diagnosing the disease. They should be tested periodically to look for failure of other endocrine organs as well. The following tests should be done to screen for other endocrine disorders

1. Serum calcium and phosphorous
2. Fasting blood sugar
3. Morning cortisol level
4. Free T3, T4 and TSH
5. Thyroid antibodies
6. Complete blood count and ESR
7. ANA and rheumatoid factor
8. Albumin globulin ratio

The usual endocrine abnormality associated with premature ovarian failure is hypothyroidism. Since ovarian failure usually precedes adrenal failure, it is worth estimating the cortisol levels periodically. If the cortisol level is normal, testing for ACTH is not necessary.

Rare conditions associated with POF are myasthenia gravis, idiopathic thrombocytopenic purpura, rheumatoid arthritis, vitiligo and autoimmune hemolytic anemia.

Radiation and Drugs

Radiation administered as a part of treatment for malignancy can lead to premature ovarian failure. Because of the improved survival of malignancy patients treated with radiotherapy and chemotherapy, an increase in the number of women with premature ovarian failure is encountered. Abdomino-pelvic irradiation will destroy ovarian follicles thus causing premature ovarian failure. High dose cranial irradiation can also lead indirectly to POF due to the adverse effect on pituitary. Chemotherapeutic agents especially alkylating agents cause ovarian failure due to destruction of follicles.

Hyperprolactinemia

Approximately 15-20% of women have hyperprolactinemia as the cause of secondary amenorrhea. Normally prolactin secretion is regulated by inhibition from the hypothalamus through dopamine. This inhibition is not subjected to negative feedback by peripheral hormones. Prolactin secretion is stimulated by peripheral estrogen. Hyperprolactinemia causes amenorrhea by inhibiting GnRH pulse release. Causes of hyperprolactinemia are listed in Table 5.1. Pathological hyperprolactinemia may be induced by drugs like phenothiazines, butyrophenones, cimetidine, reserpine and α-methyl dopa.

Only one half of women who present with hyperprolactinemia have galactorrhea and only half of the women who report with galactorrhea have hyperprolactinemia.[13-15] Serum prolactin levels should be estimated for all patients presenting with secondary amenorrhea irrespective of the presence of galactorrhea. About 3-5% of the patients would be having hypothyroidism as a cause for hyperprolactinemia. Hence, TSH should be estimated when prolactin levels are high.

Table 5.1: Pharmacological agents associated with hyperprolactinemia

Agents
Phenothiazines
Perphenazine
Chlorpromazine
Thioridazine
Trifluoperazine
Prochlorperazine
Butyrophenones
Haloperidol
Pimozide
Benzamides
Metoclopramide
Clebopride
Cimetidine
Rauwolfia alkaloids
Reserpine
Methyldopa

Amenorrhea Associated with Extreme Exercise and Stress

A decrease in the body fat may be the underlying pathology in excessive exercise. A minimum of 17% body fat[1,2] is required for the initiation of menses and 22% for its maintenance.

Rather than percentage of body fat, inappropriate calorie intake is recently thought to be the cause for amenorrhea in individuals who exercise extremely.[7,8] Leptin has been proposed as a mediator between adipose tissue and gonads. A threshold level of leptin is necessary for normal reproductive function. A low intake of calories results in low insulin levels which is sensed by the adipose tissue resulting in low leptin levels. The low leptin levels in combination with associated stress induced high cortisol levels and low T3 levels result in inhibition of GnRH pulse release. An athlete's menstrual dysfunction is thus due to a combination of inadequate nutrition, associated with eating disorders and the psychological stress of competition. They are at high risk for osteoporosis.

Stress

Stress can cause increase in the endogenous opioids, ACTH, prolactin, adrenal androgens, cortisol or melatonin. This in turn affects GnRH pulse release from the hypothalamus leading to amenorrhea.

Obesity

Obesity causes menstrual irregularities rather than amenorrhea. Obese women will elaborate estrone by the peripheral conversion of androstenedione. Their sex hormone binding globulin levels are low and hence their free androgen levels are high. The free androgens will cause hirsutism. The increased free androgens and estrogens will alter the GnRH pulse release from the hypothalamus and cause menstrual irregularities and amenorrhea.

5.4 EVALUATION

fsAs in any other clinical situation a careful history gives important clues to the diagnosis. A history of how the amenorrhea started, whether it followed uterine curettage, whether it was a gradual decrease in the frequency of menses etc is important. If a woman has not regained menses after child birth a history of post partum collapse and lactation failure will lead to the suspicion of Sheehan's syndrome.

History of chronic intake of medications which can cause amenorrhea, like phenothiazines should be elicited. Endocrine disorders can rarely be the cause of secondary amenorrhea. The commonest endocrine disorder causing secondary amenorrhea is hypothyroidism. Women with hypothyroidism can present with galactorrhea also. Autoimmune premature ovarian failure can be associated with multiple endocrine dysfunction. Hence it is important to go into the history suggestive of other endocrine failure also. Rarely pituitary tumors can be the reason for secondary amenorrhea. These patients will give a history of symptoms suggestive of raised intracranial tension like headache and visual disturbances. Menopausal symptoms like hot flashes favor premature menopause rather than end organ failure. Symptoms like change in voice and hirsutism point to the development of an androgen secreting tumor. Emotional stress, recent weight gain or weight loss, extreme exercise etc lead to the diagnosis of hypothalamic amenorrhea. Detailed medical and surgical history, irradiation of cranium or abdomen must be taken. As conditions like premature menopause run in families, family history of secondary amenorrhea must be enquired into.

5.4.1 Clinical Examination

Keeping the history in mind, a detailed clinical examination should be done. General examination should note the height, weight, features of hypothyroidism or features of Cushing's syndrome. Evidence of defeminisation and virilisation like breast atrophy, clitoromegaly, hirsutism, voice change, etc. points towards the presence of excess androgen. Expressible galactorrhea should be elicited even if the patient does not complain of galactorrhea. Fundoscopy and visual field testing should be done in women suspected to have an intracranial lesion. Pelvic examination should make out vaginal atrophy, size of uterus and presence of any adnexal mass.

5.4.2 Transvaginal Ultrasound (TVS)

TVS can give valuable information as to the status of the endometrium, presence of intrauterine adhesions, hematometra, adnexal pathology like androgen secreting tumor and pelvic inflammatory masses (tuberculosis). Nature of the ovaries, whether small and inactive or enlarged and polycystic can be made out by TVS.

5.5 MANAGEMENT (FIG. 5.1)

5.5.1 Investigations

If the history and clinical examination point towards a particular etiology, the investigation can be channeled. For example, if a woman presents with history of amenorrhea following uterine curettage or any other surgery on the uterus and ultrasound examination suggests intrauterine adhesion, the initial investigation can be hysteroscopy rather than estimation of hormone levels. If the woman has amenorrhea as well as galactorrhea, estimation of TSH and prolactin should be the initial investigation. A woman who has menopausal symptoms along with amenorrhea should have gonadotropin estimation at the outset.

Investigations for women with virilization and amenorrhea

Testosterone

DHEA

DHEAS

17-hydroxy progesterone

In most of the situations, there will not be any clue either in the history or clinical examination. It is prudent to proceed in a stepwise manner in such a circumstance. *The initial investigation should comprise estimation of TSH, prolactin, FSH and LH. The level of these 4 hormones will give the clue as to whether the amenorrhea is due to hypothyroidism, hyperprolactinemia, ovarian failure or pituitary failure.* Raised prolactin level can be either due to primary hypothyroidism or due to prolactinoma which can be sorted out by seeing the TSH. Patients with ovarian failure will have gonadotropins in the menopausal range. Patients with pituitary or hypothalamic failure have very low gonadotropins and patients with HPO dysfunction will have normal or slightly abnormal gonadotropin levels. Women with amenorrhea and virilization should have estimation of serum testosterone, DHEA and DHEAS to make out the source of androgen. 17-hydroxy progesterone also should be tested to exclude juvenile type congenital adrenal hyperplasia. Elevated DHEAS level will be seen in adrenal tumors. Cortisol level should be tested if the examination suggests Cushing's syndrome.

If the prolactin levels are above normal (20 ng/ml), imaging of the sella should be done to exclude prolactinomas and non functioning pituitary tumors. Non functioning pituitary tumors can compress the pituitary stalk and interfere with the dopamine pathway to the pituitary causing hyperprolactinemia. The prolactin levels in these patients may not be as high as in women having prolactin secreting pituitary tumors. The serum prolactin level will be >100 ng/ml in women with prolactinoma.

Most clinicians advise prolactin and TSH estimation initially. If these two hormones are normal, FSH estimation is advised to make out whether primary ovarian failure is the cause for the amenorrhea.

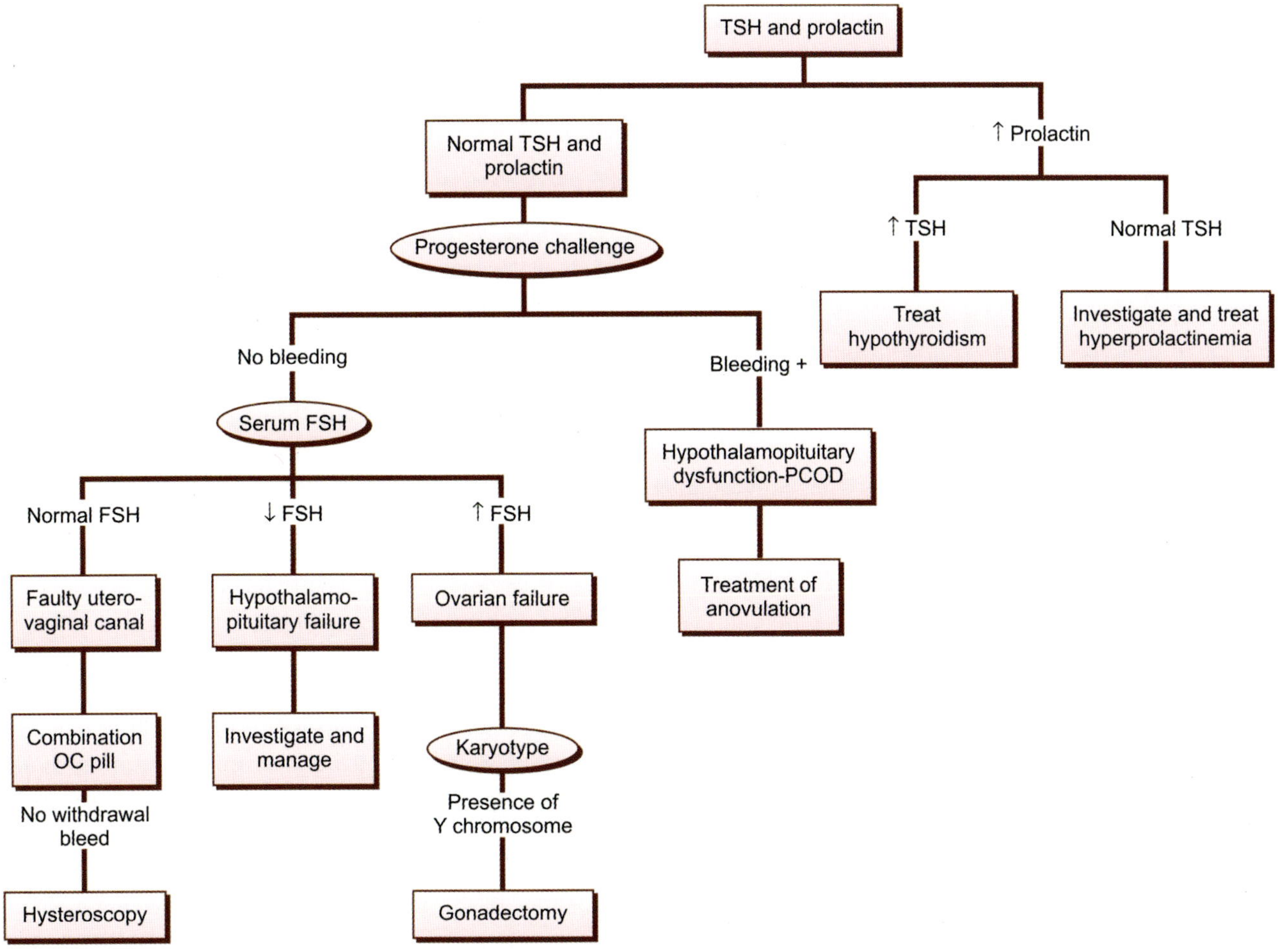

Fig. 5.1: Management algorithm for secondary amenorrhea (This chart applies to women without virilization. Those with virilization need estimation of androgen level)

Based on FSH levels, patients with secondary amenorrhea without virilization can be divided into

1. Patients with high FSH: gonadal failure
2. Patients with normal FSH: abnormalities of uterovaginal canal like Asherman's syndrome
3. Patients with very low FSH: hypothalamopituitary failure. These patients should have imaging of the brain to evaluate the sella turcica and the supra-sellar area to exclude pituitary or supra-sellar lesions, though hypothalamic amenorrhea due to emotional stress as well as other hypothalamic causes is commoner than tumors.

Progesterone Challenge Test

Level of endogenous estrogen and the patency of the outflow tract can be verified by progesterone challenge test. A progestagen without any estrogenic effect should be preferred. Oral micronized progesterone 300 mg/day for 5 days or medroxyprogesterone acetate 10 mg/day for 5 days can be advised. The woman who has some amount of endogenous estrogen and a normal outflow tract will have withdrawal bleed within 2 to 7 days of stopping the medication. Occasionally, women with high androgen levels as in PCOS may not have withdrawal bleeding. If withdrawal bleed occurs, it could be inferred that:

1. The woman has anovulation
2. Her HPO axis is intact
3. She has a patent uterovaginal canal

In an occasional patient, it can trigger ovulation and she might conceive. In the presence of uterovaginal canal defect or extreme hypoestrogenic state either due to ovarian failure or pituitary failure, progesterone withdrawal bleed will not occur. To differentiate between these two, combination of estrogen and progesterone should be given. One of the combination oral contraceptives can be advised. Those who do not bleed after stopping this combination should be evaluated for endometrial pathology like Asherman's syndrome by hysteroscopy.

5.5.2 Treatment

Women with no Withdrawal Bleed after Progesterone Challenge

These patients have blocked uterovaginal canal or a total absence of endogenous estrogen. Those who do not have endogenous estrogen may be having either ovarian failure or pituitary failure. Patients with ovarian failure will have very high levels of gonadotropins (FSH >20 IU/L, LH >40 IU/L). Those with pituitary failure will have very low levels of gonadotropins (FSH <5 IU/L). Women with outflow tract obstruction have gonadotropins in the normal range. They can be suspected in TVS by the 'broken IUD appearance' of the endometrium.

When there is no withdrawal bleed after progesterone challenge, a combination of estrogen and progesterone should be given. Patients without flow obstruction will not have withdrawal bleed. Confirmation of the diagnosis and treatment by adhesiolysis can be done by hysteroscopy. After lysis of adhesions through a hysteroscope, the uterine cavity can be kept patent by inserting an IUD. The patient can be given cyclical OCP for a few months.

Prolactin-secreting ectopic tumors are rarely encountered. Prolactin secretion can be associated with prolactin secreting bronchogenic carcinoma, renal carcinoma or teratoma of the ovary.

Patients with high gonadotropin level

The gonadotropin levels are very high in patients with ovarian failure. Before labeling a patient as ovarian failure, repeat estimation after one month interval should be done to exclude transient high levels. On rare occasions, gonadotropin secreting pituitary adenoma may be the reason. These women will have symptoms like headache and visual disturbances. They can be identified by the high level of α-subunit of the hormone. Hence if there is a clinical suspicion of pituitary tumor, the α-subunit of the gonadotropins should be estimated and brain imaging should be done.

Amenorrhea with high gonadotropin level-gonadal failure

- Pregnancy has to be ruled out
- Karyotype to be done if amenorrhea occurs < 30 yrs of age to exclude Y chromosome.
- Y chromosome fragment should be excluded even if karyotype is 46,XX by molecular testing.
- Gonadectomy should be advised if Y chromosome or fragment is present.
- Autoimmune gonadal failure should be thought of and other endocrine failure should be looked for.

The FSH levels will be elevated before attaining menopause and this is the case even in premature menopause. Occasionally patients with premature menopause will spontaneously ovulate and can conceive. *The chance of pregnancy should also be kept in mind when a patient has high FSH level.*

Karyotype should be done when the gonadotropin levels are high. Presence of Y chromosome warrants gonadectomy to prevent development of gonadoblastoma.[4] Patients with mosaic Turner syndrome may be short statured measuring <160 cms in height. Fragile X premutation should be suspected if there is a family history of fragile X syndrome. The genetic abnormality can be confirmed by PCR.

All other patients who are normal looking should be suspected to have auto immune ovarian failure.

Rarely patients with autoimmune premature ovarian failure will resume spontaneous ovulation and can conceive, but the chances are very rare. Hence the patient should be counseled appropriately. Patients with premature ovarian failure whose FSH is not higher than LH and serum estradiol more than 50 pg/ml may respond to ovulation induction. They may respond to gonadotropin but not to GnRH agonists. Women with resistant ovary syndrome can present with either primary or secondary amenorrhea. Their ovaries contain follicles which are resistant to gonadotropins. Mutations of the gonadotropin receptor gene are identified as the reason for the unresponsiveness of the ovarian follicles. Diagnosis by ovarian biopsy is not necessary as differentiating it from premature ovarian failure does not alter management.

The usual endocrine abnormality associated with POF is hypothyroidism. Since adrenal failure also can occur, it is worth estimating the cortisol level periodically. As long as the cortisol level is normal, testing for ACTH reserve is not necessary.

Patients with low gonadotropin levels

Patients with abnormally low levels of gonadotropins may have pituitary or hypothalamic cause for amenorrhea.[3] Brain imaging should be done to exclude pituitary or supra-sellar tumor. Pituitary tumors elaborating prolactin can be microadenomas or macroadenomas. Microadenomas are <10mm in diameter. Non-prolactin-secreting tumors can compress the pituitary stalk and interrupt the normal dopamine regulation of prolactin secretion. In this situation too, the prolactin levels will be elevated.

Women with hyperprolactinemia and high TSH will respond to treatment with thyroxine. Their prolactin level would normalize without dopamine agonist treatment.

> **Amenorrhea with low gonadotropin level**
> - Hyperprolactinemia to be excluded
> - Brain imaging to exclude intracranial lesion
> - History of obstetric shock- Sheehan's syndrome is a possibility
> - Normal imaging and normal prolactin is in favor of hypothalamic amenorrhea
> - Hormone replacement should be advised to protect skeletal and cardiovascular systems

Hyperprolactinemia patients with normal TSH should be treated with dopamine agonists like bromocriptine or cabergoline. The advantage of cabergoline is the once weekly dosage. Before starting treatment, patients should be properly counseled regarding side effects like hypotension especially while rising from bed. They should be advised to take the drug on full stomach before going to bed. Bromocriptine can be started at a low dose of 2.5 mg at bed time and can be increased to a maximum of 7.5 mg. Cabergoline can be started at a dose of 0.25 mg twice weekly and increased to a maximum of 3 mg a week. If indicated, the dosage can be increased to twice weekly.

A rare pituitary cause for secondary amenorrhea is postpartum pituitary necrosis—Sheehan's syndrome. The etiology is pituitary necrosis following post partum collapse. The vascularity of the pituitary gland is normally increased during pregnancy. Profound hypotension following delivery can result in hypoperfusion of the enlarged pituitary gland leading to necrosis and hypofunction. Lactation suppression would be the first to manifest. The patient will continue to be amenorrheic years after delivery due to the abnormally low gonadotropin levels. This will be followed by reduced TSH production and hypothyroidism and hypoadrenalism. Hormone supplementation is the treatment. If pregnancy is desired, ovulation induction can be achieved with gonadotropins.

Hypogonadotropic patients with normal prolactin levels and normal imaging studies are classified as hypothalamic amenorrhea, which is the result of functional suppression of the hypothalamus due to a stressful situation. This is diagnosed by excluding pituitary causes. The mechanism of amenorrhea in these patients is the altered GnRH pulse release from the hypothalamus. Amenorrhea of eating disorders like anorexia nervosa and bulimia nervosa as well as amenorrhea of athletes are also due to deranged hypothalamic function. The diagnosis can be suspected by excluding anorexia and weight loss from the history and physical examination. These patients will not have withdrawal bleed after the progesterone challenge due to the extreme hypoestrogenic state. Patients considered as having hypothalamic amenorrhea should be evaluated annually for development of a pituitary or supra-sellar lesion by prolactin assay and imaging of the brain. Amenorrhea associated with weight loss or psychological stress might recover spontaneously over several years. Women who have anorexia nervosa need psychological counseling by a professional. Amenorrhea associated with extreme exercise usually improves with gain in body weight but weight gain may not be practically possible in these patients as they will be unwilling to give up their routine exercise. If they continue to be amenorrheic, cyclical hormone therapy should be advised to protect from osteoporosis as well as adverse cardiovascular effects. They should be advised to reduce the amount of exercise to improve weight gain when pregnancy is planned. If regular menstrual cycles do not resume with gain in weight, ovulation induction should be advised.

Post-pill Amenorrhea

Amenorrhea occurring after discontinuation of oral contraceptive pill is termed post-pill amenorrhea. It was believed to be due to the persistent suppressive effect of the drug. However it is presently understood that there is no cause-effect relationship between hormone use and amenorrhea. Hence if a woman is amenorrheic 6 months after discontinuation of oral contraceptive or 12 months after the last injection of depot-provera, she should be investigated to identify the cause of amenorrhea.

Hormone Therapy

All hypoestrogenic patients should be supplemented with hormones to prevent the adverse effects of hypoestrogenism. Long-term hypoestrogenic state will lead to decreased bone density and cardiovascular disease. Exercise induced bone deposition cannot balance the effect of hypoestrogenism on the bones. Thus patients with gonadal failure as well as those with hypothalamic amenorrhea should be advised treatment with estrogen-progestin combination. An accepted schedule is to start with 0.625 mg conjugated estrogen or 1mg estradiol daily, along with 5mg medroxy progesterone acetate for 2 weeks every month. Bone density has to be periodically assessed and treatment modified accordingly. Withdrawal bleed usually occurs on the third day of stopping progestin. If irregular bleeding occurs in between, it signifies a resumption of endogenous hormone production. Hormone therapy should be stopped and the patient monitored for resumption of ovulation and menstruation. Dietary advice with calcium supplementation 1000-1500 mg/day should be encouraged. Since hypothalamic amenorrhea can revert spontaneously, it is better to prescribe one of the oral contraceptive preparations which would provide hormone replacement as well as contraception.

Patients with normal gonadotropin levels

The commonest condition leading to amenorrhea with normal gonadotropin levels is polycystic ovarian disease. These patients will usually have withdrawal bleeding after progesterone challenge. Occasionally there may not be withdrawal bleeding due to the decidualisation produced by the high androgen level. Here the management depends upon whether they pursue conception or not. Those who wish to conceive may be managed by ovulation induction.

Those who do not wish to conceive should have regular withdrawal bleeding which can be achieved with 10 mg MPA given for at least 10 days a month. This will protect against development of endometrial hyperplasia. They should be treated from adolescence to prevent the risk of developing endometrial hyperplasia and endometrial carcinoma. Women who need contraception also can be treated with combination oral contraceptive pill. Women with hirsutism or acne may be given pills containing either ethinyl estradiol and cyproterone acetate or ethinyl estradiol and drosperinone. The advantage of drosperinone is the absence of weight-gain due to the anti-mineralocorticoid activity.

Detailed management of PCOS is discussed in the Chapter 9: Polycystic ovarian syndrome.

5.6 CONCLUSION

Causes of secondary amenorrhea may be in the uterovaginal canal, ovary, pituitary or the hypothalamus. Most often history will give clue to the diagnostic category. A stepwise evaluation is to estimate TSH and prolactin initially. However, if the history and examination is suggestive of a particular compartment defect, investigation and management can be channeled appropriately. All patients with raised prolactin (even if less than 100 ng/ml) should have imaging of the brain. Supra-sellar tumors can compress the pituitary stalk and interfere with dopamine pathway causing hyperprolactinemia. Women with premature ovarian failure (especially before 30 years of age) and high gonadotropins should have karyotyping done to exclude presence of Y chromosome. Those with Y chromosome should have gonadectomy to prevent development of germ cell tumors. Autoimmune premature ovarian failure is one of the common causes of POF which can be associated with other endocrine gland failure. Hence hypothyroidism and hypoadrenalism should be watched for. Women having hypoestrogenism either due to ovarian failure or due to hypothalamo-pituitary failure should be supplemented with hormones to prevent osteoporosis and cardiovascular disease. Amenorrhea of anorexia nervosa and extreme exercise need lifestyle modification and counseling.

5.7 CLINICAL SCENARIOS

Scenario 1

32-year-old M/s B presented with amenorrhea of 10 months duration. Her periods were irregular for a few months before the amenorrhea. She had no other complaints. She is para 1 with a full-term normal delivery 8 years back. She did not give a history of radiation or chemotherapy for any indication. There is no history of uterine curettage. She has no symptoms of menopause. On examination, she did not have any gross abnormality. Her weight was noted to be 68 kg and height 5ft (BMI=30). There was no galactorrhea, even expressible. Pelvic examination: vagina showed evidence of hypoestrogenism. Uterus appeared normal in size and there was no adnexal mass. TVS: uterus normal size, endometrium thin, ovaries polycystic but no hyperthecosis, no corpus luteum or dominant follicle seen.

How will you proceed to arrive at the cause for her amenorrhea?

Hormonal profile which should include prolactin, TSH, FSH and LH.

What is the rationale of doing all 4 hormone tests?

The history as well as examination including TVS does not point towards any of the diagnostic probabilities. The hormonal profile will give the clue as to whether the defect is hyperprolactinemia, hypothyroidism, hypothalamo-pituitary failure or ovarian failure.

Hormonal profile: Serum prolactin: 13.3 ng/ml; TSH: 1.48 μIU/ml; LH: 0.85 mIU/ml; FSH: 1.08 mIU/ml. What is the possible diagnosis?

FSH and LH are very low. Prolactin and TSH are in the normal range excluding hyperprolactinemia and hypothyroidism. Hence hypothalamic amenorrhea is the probable diagnosis.

Why can't it be premature ovarian failure?

When there is ovarian failure, gonadotropin levels will be very high whereas in this patient, gonadotropin level is abnormally low

What is the next step in diagnosis?

Progestagen challenge is the next step.

Medroxy progesterone 10mg was given for 5 days. She did not have withdrawal bleeding.

What does it indicate?
It indicates that she does not have endogenous estrogen.

What other investigation should be done?
CT/MRI brain to exclude pituitary or supra-sellar lesion as the patient is having unusually low gonadotropin level

What drug treatment would you advise?
Combination OC pill

What is the rationale behind administration of OC pill?
To protect the bones and cardiovascular system as well as to provide contraception as this lady has a rare chance for resuming hypothalamo-pituitary function and ovulation

If she is pursuing conception, how will you proceed?
Ovulation can be induced with either GnRH or gonadotropins

How will you follow-up the patient?
She should have yearly prolactin estimation and brain imaging to exclude development of pituitary or hypothalamic lesion which can be missed in the early phase of the disease.

Scenario 2

M/s A, 27 year old married lady presented with complains of inability to conceive. She was married for 10 years. Her husband was working in the Middle East. They had stayed together for about 8 months. She did not give history of any coital problems. She revealed that she was not having spontaneous periods since 8 years. She attained menarche at the age of 12 years. She had regular monthly periods for about one year. Thereafter she had only withdrawal bleeding. She has one sister who also is having secondary amenorrhea and has one child born by IVF. She was advised to take COC pills by the local physician, which she has been continuing. She was diagnosed to have mitral regurgitation but was hemodynamically stable. She gave no history suggestive of raised intracranial tension.

On examination she was tall built and obese. Height was 167 cm, Weight 80 kg. She has no hirsutism or galactorrhoea. Her secondary sexual characters were normal. She had no features of Turner syndrome.

Pelvic examination
Vulva appeared normal. Vagina showed less rugosity. Cervix was unremarkable. Bimanual examination showed uterus to be smaller than normal. There was no adnexal mass. TVS showed a smaller than normal uterus and small ovaries.

What is the most probable diagnosis?
As she has withdrawal bleeding after taking COC pills she has no obstruction to the uterovaginal canal. Since withdrawal after taking progestagen alone has not been checked, integrity of the HPO axis cannot be taken as normal from the history.

How will you proceed to arrive at a diagnosis?
Since she has been continually on COCs, progestagen challenge has no role.

At this stage what are the probable diagnoses?
The diagnoses could be either ovarian failure or hypothalamo-pituitary failure.

What investigations will help you to arrive at a diagnosis?
Estimation of FSH, LH, Prolactin and TSH. Prolactin and TSH may be tested initially. If found normal, FSH testing may be resorted to.

Serum FSH level will be very high (above 35 IU/ml) in ovarian failure and will be very low in hypothalamo-pituitary failure.

Her serum FSH was 40 IU/ml, suggesting ovarian failure.

What could be the probable cause for ovarian failure in this lady?
Autoimmune ovarian failure, chromosomal causes like mosaic Turner syndrome, X deletions, genetic causes like Galactosemia, autosomal dominant premature ovarian failure and resistant ovary syndrome form the spectrum of probable causes.

What further test is mandatory?
Karyotype. Since she developed ovarian failure before 30 years of age, the reason could be chromosomal. If her karyotype shows Y chromosome or fragment of Y she needs gonadectomy for preventing the development of gonadoblastoma.

As her sister also had POF, the most probable cause is autosomal dominant POF.

How will you confirm the diagnosis?
If the gene probe is available it can be diagnosed. Since there is no specific advantage in diagnosing as far as the management is concerned, we need not pursue the same.

Does she need any other test?
Tests for autoimmune disease like ANA, RA factor, and anti dsDNA should be done. Even if they are negative, periodic testing for other endocrine abnormalities like hypothyroidism, hypoparathyroidism and hypoadrenalism should be done as we are not sure whether she has

autoimmune ovarian failure, even though she has an affected sister.

If she is desirous of having a child how will you help her?

She can conceive by ART using donated ovum.

Scenario 3

26 year old M/s b presented with amenorrhea of 10 months. She is a parous lady with one child aged 3 years. She had pregnancy termination (surgical) at 8 weeks amenorrhea 2 years ago and had copper IUD insertion. She had her IUD removed about a year ago, after which she had only one period. She has no galactorrhea, menopausal symptoms or symptoms suggestive of raised intracranial tension. There is no history of loss or gain of weight or any psychological stress.

What are the diagnostic possibilities?

Considering the fact that her amenorrhea started after IUD removal Ashermann's syndrome is a probability, even though she had one period after removing IUD.

What is the next step in management?

TVS should be done initially because it gives valuable information about the presence of intrauterine adhesion, the hormonal status by the appearance of endometrium and the ovaries.

Contrary to what was expected, the endometrium did not show any evidence of intrauterine adhesion, instead was very thin and atrophic. The ovaries also appeared inactive and the ovarian volume was 3.2 ml, less than expected in a woman of child bearing age.

What is the next step in investigation?

Since the picture is of ovarian failure, she needs estimation of Prolactin and TSH. If these are normal FSH level should be tested (However, Prolactin, TSH and FSH can be tested together so that the diagnosis can be arrived without delay). Her serum prolactin level was found to be 65ng/ml which is well above normal and TSH was 3.1 which are within normal limit. Hence it was concluded that her amenorrhea is due to hyperprolactinemia.

Should you advise imaging study of brain?

Ideally it should be done, as elevated prolactin level can be due to nonfunctioning tumors of the pituitary interfering with dopamine pathway. Imaging was not done as she could not afford expensive investigations. Since she did not have any symptom suggestive of intracranial lesion brain imaging was not insisted.

How will you treat?

She should be started on dopamine agonists. This lady was started on bromocriptine, 2.5 mg/day. She was given warning about gastric discomfort and hypotension, which can cause fainting attacks. She had episodes of vomiting which was treated at the local hospital with antiemetics and i/v fluids. After 2 and half months of starting bromocriptine, she reported again because she had severe vomiting.

On detailed questioning she revealed that she had one period about a month after starting medicine and continued to be amenorrheic afterwards and her vomiting was severe since one week.

How will you proceed?

TVS should be done to find out the response to treatment by assessing the endometrium and the ovaries.

TVS revealed an intrauterine gestational sac with a tiny embryo with cardiac pulsations!

She was 6 weeks pregnant. Hyperprolactinemia is one condition which promptly responds to treatment.

Scenario 4

Miss P, 23 yrs presented with amenorrhea of 8 years duration. She attained menarche at the age of 11 years and was having regular cycles till 14 years and later had hypomenorrhea before being amenorrheic from 15 years. She had straw colored vaginal discharge after becoming amenorrheic. She was being treated for the same for the past 4 years. She was given several times Norethisterone as well as combined OCPs but had no withdrawal bleeding. At the age of 20 years, she had laparotomy done for an ovarian cyst diagnosed by USS. Laparotomy findings revealed peritoneal adhesions and adhesions involving uterus, omentum and descending colon and a thin walled cyst in the right ovary with dark hemorrhagic fluid. Left ovary and tube could not be visualized due to adhesions. The biopsy report came as follows–Section shows a multiloculated cyst with a fibrous wall. Cyst is lined by flat and cuboidal cells. The cyst wall shows focal lymphocytic infiltration. The diagnosis was given as multiloculated serous cystadenoma ovary. She continued to remain amenorrheic after the surgery.

1. **What do you infer from this history?**
   Since she was not responding to several cycles of combined oral contraceptive pills, it should be an acquired defect of the uterovaginal canal.
2. **If she had come to you with secondary amenorrhea and without taking hormone tablets, what should have been your first step?**
   First step should have been checking for the integrity of HPO axis by testing for a progestagen withdrawal bleed.

3. **If she had no withdrawal bleeding after progestagen, what are the possibilities?**
   There are two possibilities –
   - It could be a state of extreme hypoestrogenism due to either primary or secondary ovarian failure.
   - It could be an acquired defect of the uterovaginal canal.

   Women who have hyperandrogenism, the commonest being PCOS, rarely may not bleed after progestagen withdrawal due to the changes in the endometrium caused by the hyperandrogenic state.

   This lady does not have any features of hyperandrogenism, hence that possibility is unlikely.
4. **How will you differentiate between ovarian failure and acquired UV canal defect?**
   If withdrawal bleeding occurs after giving combined OCPs, it excludes the possibility of UV canal defect. However, rarely, if the patient has ovarian failure of several years duration, she may need several cycles of OCP's before she responds with a withdrawal bleed. Since this lady had no withdrawal bleed after several cycles of OCPs, possibility of primary or secondary ovarian failure is unlikely.
   But, because she is unmarried, instead of directly evaluating the UV canal, a serum FSH and serum prolactin may be tested.
   Her S. FSH was 6.7 mIU/ml and S prolactin was 13.2 ng/ml which were both within normal limits.
5. **Is a Transabdominal scan indicated?**
   The commonest acquired UV canal defect presenting with secondary amenorrhea in an unmarried lady is tuberculosis. Asherman's syndrome as a result of curettage is a possibility but this lady gives no such history.

   Tuberculosis can lead to adnexal masses which are usually unilateral as well as encysted ascites; all of these can be made out by USS. Endometrial calcification is another finding which can be made out with an USS. Intrauterine adhesions may give a broken IUCD appearance in USS.

   This patient's USS was unremarkable; endometrial calcification or adhesions were not made out.
6. **What is the place of blood investigations like TC, DC, ESR and ADA (adenosine deaminase) estimation?**
   The routine blood investigations (TC, DC, ESR) may not be abnormal in pelvic tuberculosis, which we are suspecting. ADA estimation is more specific for pleural tuberculosis.
   But, in this lady, it was elevated to 57 IU/ml.
7. **How will you evaluate the UV canal of this lady?**
   Inspite of the fact that she is unmarried; a hysteroscopic evaluation is indicated for her. The hysteroscopy was done and the findings were as follows – Endometrium whitish, uterine cavity narrowed. Both the ostia were not visualized. Cervical biopsy and endometrial curettings were taken.
   Histopathology report: Chronic granulomatous inflammatory lesion involving the endometrium, picture consistent with tuberculous etiology.
   She was referred to state TB center for taking ATT.
8. **What is the prognosis for this patient?**
   She is currently taking ATT. She has gained 2 kg weight since then, but has not attained menstruation yet.

   Tuberculous endometritis carries worse prognosis than other types of chronic bacterial or viral endometritis in that even after treatment, there will usually be significant uterine scarring and very low pregnancy rates.
9. **Can she conceive with IVF?**
   Even with IVF, fertility rates are very low since she had tuberculosis of the endometrium (implantation rates are very low).

REFERENCES

1. Frisch R E, McArthur D A. Menstrual cycles; Fatness as a determinant of minimum weight for height necessary for the maintenance or onset. Science 1974;185:949-95.
2. Frisch RE. Body fat, menarche, and reproductive ability. Semin Reprod Endocrinol 1985;3:45-4
3. Vance ML. Hypopituitarism. N Engl J Med 1994;330:1651-1662.9.
4. Manuel M, Katayama KP, Jones HW Jr. The age of occurrence of gonadal tumors in intersex patients with a Y chromosome. Am J Obstet Gynecol 1976;124:293-300.
5. Mignot MH, Shoemaker J, Kleingel M, et al. Premature ovarian failure. I: the association with autoimmunity. Eur J Obstet Gynecol Reprod Biol 1989;30:59-66.
6. de Moraes–Ruehsen M, Blizzard RM, Garcia–Bunuel R, et al. Autoimmunity and ovarian failure. Am J Obstet Gynecol 1972;112:693-703.
7. Olson BR. Exercise induced amenorrhea. Am Fam Physician 1989;39:213-21.
8. Highet R. Athletic amenorrhea: an update on a etiology, complications and management. Sports Med 1989;7:87-108.
9. Speroff L, Glass RH, Kase NG. Clinical gynecologic endocrinology and infertility. 6th ed. Baltimore, MD: Williams & Wilkins, 1994.
10. Mattison DR, Evan MI, Schwimmer WB. Familial premature ovarian failure. Am J Hum Genet 1984;36:1341-48.

11. Allingham–Hawkins DJ, Babul–Hirgi R, Chitayat D, et al. Fragile X premutation is a significant risk factor for premature ovarian failure: the International Collaborative POF in Fragile X Study: preliminary data. Am J Med Genet 1999;83: 322-25.
12. Murray A. Premature ovarian failure and the FMR1 gene. Semin Reprod Med 2000;18:59-60.
13. Bohnet HG, Dahlen HG, Wuttke W, et al. Hyperprolactinemic anovulatory syndrome. J Clin Endocrinol Metab 1976; 42:132-43.
14. Franks S, Murray MA, Jequier AM, et al. Incidence and significance of hyperprolactinaemia in women with amenorrhea. Clin Endocrinol (Oxf) 1975;4:597-607.
15. Jacobs HS, Hull MG, Murray MA, et al. Therapy–orientated diagnosis of secondary amenorrhoea. Horm Res 1975;6: 268-87.
16. A Murrey, J Wete,S Gimley,G Convey, P Jacob. Studies of FRAXA and FRAXE in women with premature ovarian failure. J Med Genet 1995;35:637-40.

6 Abnormal Uterine Bleeding

B Presannakumari

6.1 INTRODUCTION

Abnormal uterine bleeding (AUB) is one of the commonest problems with which women present to the gynecology outpatient department. The problem can present in a wide variety of clinical types and can be due to multiple, unrelated etiologies.

The terms used to describe abnormal menses are:

- **Menorrhagia**–defined as regular cycles with increased amount or duration of menstrual bleeding.
- **Metrorrhagia**–irregular bleeding both in duration and amount and the patient may not be able to differentiate the normal periods from the abnormal flow. This type of bleeding occurs in anovulatory cycles.
- **Hypomenorrhea**–regular periods with decreased flow.
- **Oligomenorrhea**–defined as infrequent periods which are usually irregular.
- **Amenorrhea**–defined as absence of menstruation for more than 90 days in a woman with a regular 28–30 day cycle. In women with infrequent cycles, amenorrhea is the absence of menstruation for more than 3 cycle intervals.
- **Polymenorrhea**–defined as menstruation occurring at intervals less than 21 days.

6.2 MECHANISM OF NORMAL MENSTRUATION

It is important to learn the mechanism of normal menstruation to understand the pathology of abnormal uterine bleeding. Normal menstruation is dependent on a patent utero-vaginal canal and a normal hypothalamo-pituitary-ovarian (HPO) axis. Normal menstruation occurs at an interval of 21-35 days and the duration is 2-7 days. The average normal loss is about 30 ml/cycle. Variations from these are considered abnormal. If the flow exceeds 80 ml/cycle, it can cause anemia. During normal menstrual cycle, cyclical changes occur in the ovary which in turn result in cyclical changes in the endometrium. The ovary is under

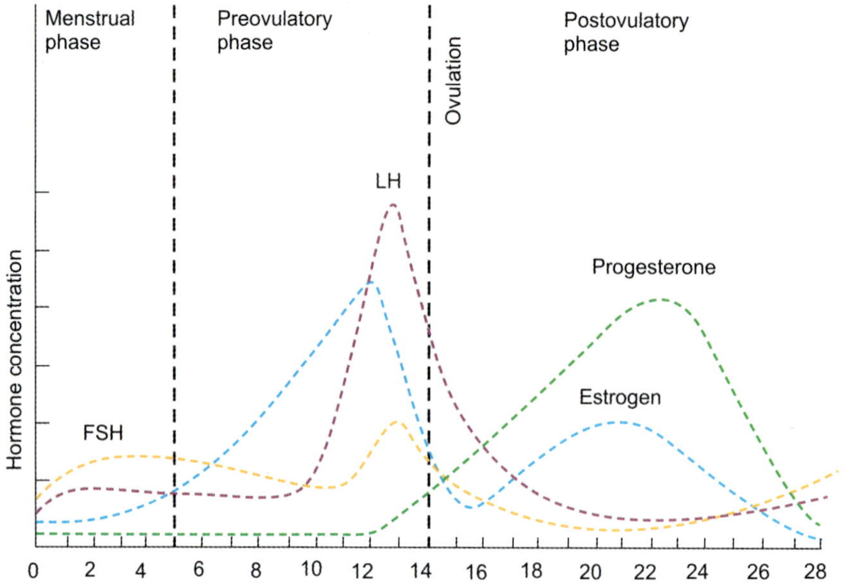

Fig. 6.1: Hormonal events of menstrual cycle

the influence of hypophysis through gonadotrophins which in turn is controlled by the hypothalamus. The hypothalamus is influenced by other centers in the brain. Abrupt changes in weight, either gain or loss, intake of drugs like anti-convulsants and anti-depressants and extreme exercise can influence the HPO axis and cause abnormal menstruation. The thyroid and adrenal glands also influence the menstrual cycle.

The menstrual cycle (Fig. 6.1) can be separated into two distinct phases – the follicular phase and the luteal phase. In the follicular phase, the follicle enlarges under the influence of LH and FSH secreted by the anterior pituitary. FSH and LH are secreted by the anterior pituitary under the influence of GnRH which is secreted in a pulsatile manner from the arcuate nucleus of the hypothalamus. The HPO axis (Fig. 6.2) is thus fine regulated by the hypothalamus and GnRH is the hormone which regulates the cyclicity of menses. Disturbances in the pulsatile release of GnRH affect this cyclicity. The pituitary production of gonadotropins is under the influence of GnRH produced by the hypothalamus and the feedback influence of the ovarian steroids, estrogen and progesterone.

As the follicle matures, it secretes estrogen. The follicle that has the highest sensitivity to FSH secretes the highest level of estrogen and becomes the dominant follicle. The estrogen produced by the dominant follicle inhibits the secretion of FSH by the pituitary through negative feedback. Estrogen also has positive feedback on the pituitary to secrete LH. Inhibin A and B, produced by the ovary causes negative feedback on the pituitary which decreases the production of FSH. Activin produced by the ovary increases the sensitivity of the follicle to FSH and promotes the growth of the follicle.

As the estradiol level peaks at about the 12th-14th day of the cycle, LH surge is triggered resulting in ovulation. LH surge occurs 24–36 hours prior to ovulation.

During the follicular phase, the endometrial stroma, glands and blood vessels proliferate under the influence of estrogen. Vascular endothelial growth factor is involved in the angiogenesis of the endometrium. The thickness of the endometrium increases. In ultrasound, the endometrium is described as trilaminar, the three lines constituted by the central cavity line and the two endometrial-myometrial interfaces.

Progesterone production starts 24 hours before ovulation. After ovulation, the corpus luteum will produce progesterone which peaks by the 21st day of the cycle. This increased level of estrogen and progesterone exerts negative feedback on the pituitary and the hypothalamus causing a decrease in the production of FSH and LH, the levels of which gradually fall. The corpus luteum has a life span of 14 days after which it involutes, resulting in sudden fall of progesterone and estrogen. As the progesterone level falls, the inhibition on FSH and LH is removed and the hypothalamus starts secreting GnRH in a pulsatile manner.

During the secretory phase, the endometrial changes are characterized by the presence of secretions. The earliest morphological evidence of ovulation is the presence of secretory vacuoles which can be seen initially in the subnuclear region. The stroma will become more edematous and the glands, tortuous. Later the secretions migrate by

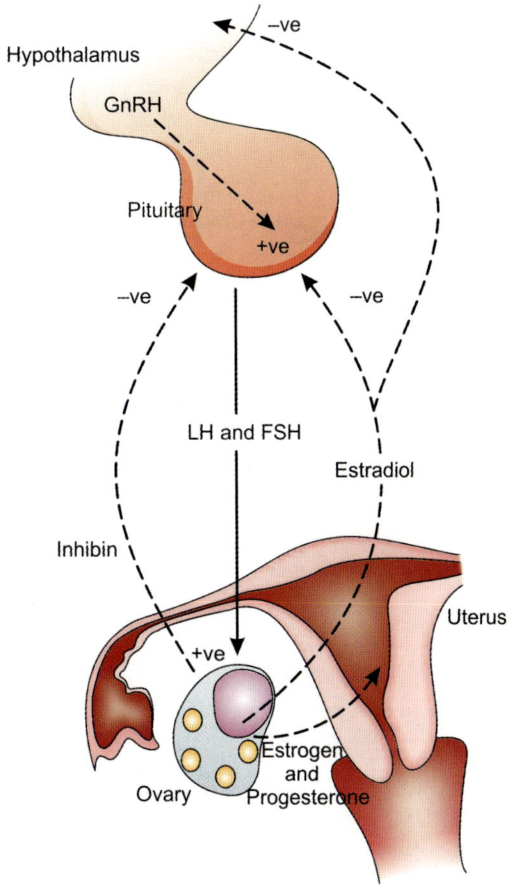

Fig. 6.2: Diagrammatic representation of hypothalamo-pituitary-ovarian axis

the side of the nucleus into the lumen of the glands. The spiral arterioles will become more coiled. The endometrial thickness increases and in ultrasound scan, the trilaminar pattern would be lost.

Towards the end of the secretory phase, progesterone withdrawal causes destabilization of lysosomal membranes causing release of phospholipase A2 which results in synthesis of arachidonic acid from phospholipids of the cell wall. This further leads to activation of the cyclooxygenase cascade leading to prostaglandin production. This results in episodic constriction and relaxation of endometrial spiral arterioles leading to endometrial ischemia and shedding of endometrium. There will be local release of cytokines, tumor necrosis factor α (TNF α) and other signaling molecules. The degradation of extra cellular matrix is thought to be due to activation of pro-inflammatory cytokines and release of endometrial matrix metalloproteinases. These molecules cause degradation of extracellular matrix, causing breakdown of endometrium. The functional layer of the endometrium is shed and expelled along with blood and tissue fluid resulting in the menstrual flow.

As the corpus luteum degenerates, the negative feedback on the pituitary is lost and FSH production starts at the beginning of menstruation. Estrogen production gradually increases, leading to proliferative changes in the endometrium which starts by the third day of menses usually leading to cessation of flow by the seventh day. Local growth hormones are also involved in the repair and regeneration of the endometrium.

6.3 MECHANISM OF ABNORMAL BLEEDING IN OVULATORY CYCLES

The abnormal bleeding appears to be due to defective vasoconstriction and hemostasis. An increase in the total prostaglandin release and disproportionate rise in PGE_2 and PGI_2 has been demonstrated. The myometrium of these women synthesize more PGI_2 from precursors in the endometrium. Increased endometrial tissue plasminogen activator content and increased local fibrinolytic activity were also demonstrated. Increased enzymatic activity of lysosomes may contribute to abnormalities in tissue breakdown and remodeling.

Genetic predisposition also has been explained. A gene called 'endometrial bleeding associated factor' located on chromosome 1 has recently been demonstrated in women with normal menstruation and the expression is found to be stronger in women with abnormal menstruation.

6.4 MECHANISM OF ABNORMAL BLEEDING IN ANOVULATORY CYCLES

In anovulatory cycles, the endometrium is exposed to unopposed estrogen action which will lead to endometrial proliferation and hyperplasia. The exact mechanism of anovulatory bleeding is unknown. Large tortuous vessels are formed due to prolonged stimulation by estrogens, as estrogen stimulates vascular endothelial growth factor (VEGF) expression. Vessel wall fragility will also be increased. The blood vessels will become large tortuous and thin walled with increased fragility. Due to the deficiency of progesterone there can be abnormalities in the steroid receptors as well as local prostaglandins which are involved in normal hemostasis of menstruation. Absence of progesterone leads to imbalance in the prostaglandin production causing more prostaglandin E than prostaglandin F. After some time, the endometrium outgrows its blood supply and sheds irregularly causing prolonged bleeding. Increased nitric oxide production as a result of estrogenic stimulation also contributes to increase in bleeding. Deficiency in the production of PGF_2 due to progesterone deficiency leads to reduced vascular tone and increased bleeding.

Inter-menstrual bleeding

Inter-menstrual bleeding is due to surface lesion of the genital tract. HPO axis would be normal. The patient will be able to differentiate the normal menses from the abnormal flow. The usual causes are cervical polyp, erosions, carcinoma cervix or submucous fibroid. Rarely, infections and benign and malignant lesions of the vulva and vagina can also cause intermenstrual bleeding.

6.5 BREAKTHROUGH BLEEDING

In women taking continuous progestagens, the low estrogen level causes erratic breakdown of endometrium. Disturbed angiogenesis, increased spontaneous tissue breakdown and defective repair contribute to breakthrough bleeding in long term progestagen users. This is also the reason for abnormal bleeding among HRT users.

6.6 CAUSES OF MENORRHAGIA

Menorrhagia is defined as menstrual bleeding of more than seven days duration or more than 80 ml per menstrual cycle. Only 40% of women who complain of excessive blood loss will have it confirmed by objective methods. The blood loss assessed by the number of sanitary pads or tampons need not be accurate. It was Halberg et al who first demonstrated by objective method, measuring hemoglobin extracted from sanitary pads using alkali hematin technique that the normal blood loss ranges between 15 and 50 ml, the average being 35 ml. The upper limit for the diagnosis of menorrhagia was set at 80 ml because about 2/3rd of women who lose more than 80 ml of blood will have iron deficiency anemia. Even though alkali hematin method gives the accurate estimate of blood loss, it is not clinically feasible.

Abnormal uterine bleeding can be with or without an organic cause. Dysfunctional uterine bleeding (DUB) is abnormal uterine bleeding without pelvic pathology. Hence DUB is a diagnosis of exclusion. With the widespread use of transvaginal ultrasound (TVS), the number of patients classified as having DUB has come down significantly.

AUB can be due to:
1. Pelvic pathology
2. Systemic diseases
3. Iatrogenic causes
4. DUB
5. Pregnancy complications

6.6.1 Pelvic Pathology

Women presenting with regular cycles and abnormal bleeding may have some pelvic or systemic pathology. Most common cause for AUB is local pelvic pathology which can be any of the following
- Myomas
- Adenomyosis
- Endometrial or cervical polyp
- Pelvic inflammatory disease (PID)
- Malignant and premalignant conditions

Myoma

Myomas are a common cause for abnormal uterine bleeding in the child bearing age group. Submucous and intramural myomas cause menorrhagia. Submucous myoma projecting into the cavity and myomatous polyp coming out through the cervical canal can also present as metrorrhagia. The mechanism of heavy bleeding due to myomas has been postulated to be due to abnormal release of regulatory molecules with angiogenic activity such as vascular endothelial growth factor, fibroblast growth factor and transforming growth factor β.

Adenomyosis

It is one of the causes for menorrhagia in women during the fifth decade. Establishing a diagnosis of adenomyosis is

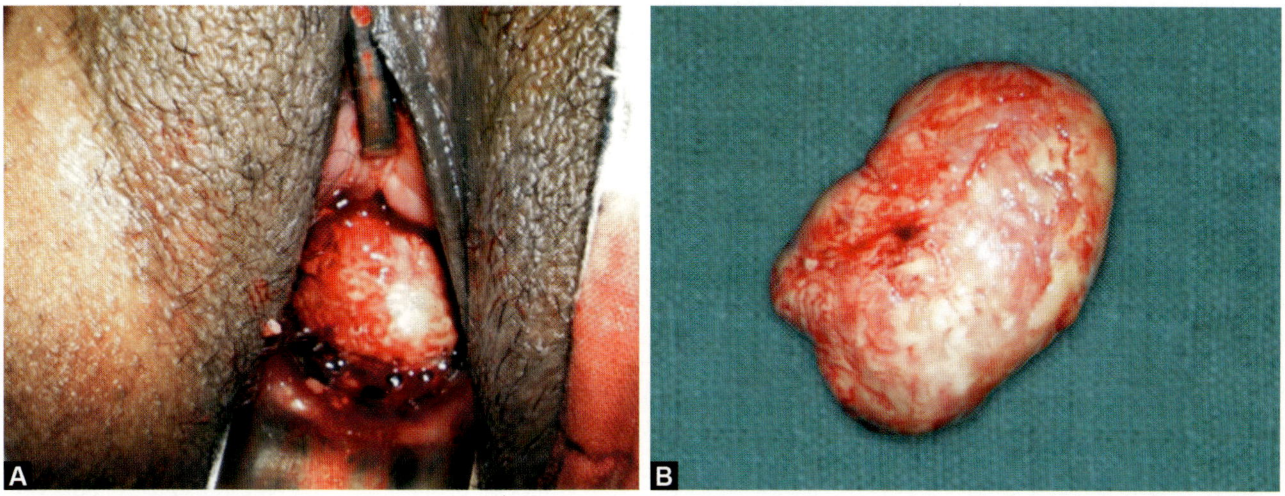

Figs 6.3A and B: Fibroid polyp projecting out through the external os. Patient presented with irregular vaginal bleeding, TVS delineated a single fibroid polyp with thin pedicle. The polyp was removed by avulsion. The removed specimen is shown on the right

difficult because it can be diffuse, nodular or multifocal. It cannot be diagnosed by hysterosalpingogram or hysteroscopy. With the evolution of sonography, adenomyosis can be predicted with reasonable accuracy. Usually adenomyosis produces typical appearance in ultrasound. Rarely adenomyosis can be focal producing fairly circumscribed lesions in the anterior or posterior wall. In these circumstances, MRI may be necessary to distinguish it from fibroid.

Endometrial or Cervical Polyp (Figs 6.3 to 6.8)

Women with mucous polyp or fibroid polyp can present with metrorrhagia or menorrhagia. Submucous fibroid sometimes protrudes out of the uterine cavity as fibroid polyp and may be seen in the vagina. Rarely large polyps may even present outside the vulva. Fibroid polyps can also arise from the cervix itself and can attain huge size.

Pelvic Inflammatory Disease (PID)

Patients with chronic PID can also present with menorrhagia because of the associated pelvic congestion. Patients with acute PID can present with an episode of abnormal uterine bleeding.

Malignant and Premalignant Conditions

Patients with malignant and premalignant conditions can also present with AUB. Endometrial hyperplasia which is usually seen in patients with chronic anovulation associated with PCOD presents with periods of amenorrhea followed by profuse bleeding.

Premenopausal women who have endometrial malignancy can present with irregular bleeding or menorrhagia

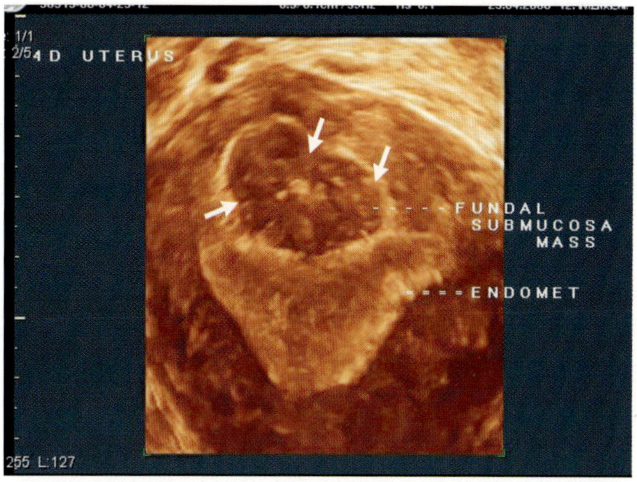

Fig. 6.4: Submucous myoma delineated with 4D ultrasound

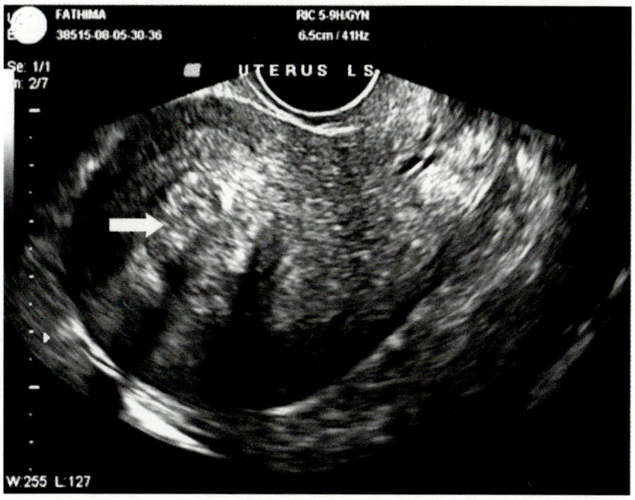

Fig. 6.5: Submucous myoma in a 32-year-old lady who presented with progressively increasing menorrhagia. On clinical examination the size of the uterus did not appear to be enlarged

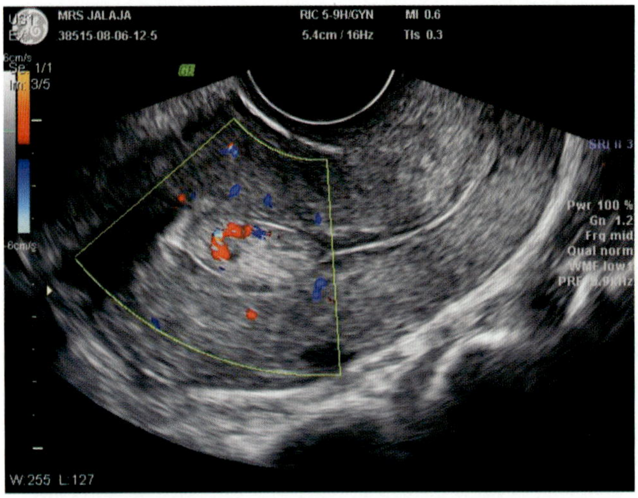

Fig. 6.6: Fibroid polyp showing vascularity (the pedicle sign) which distinguishes it from blood clot in the uterine cavity

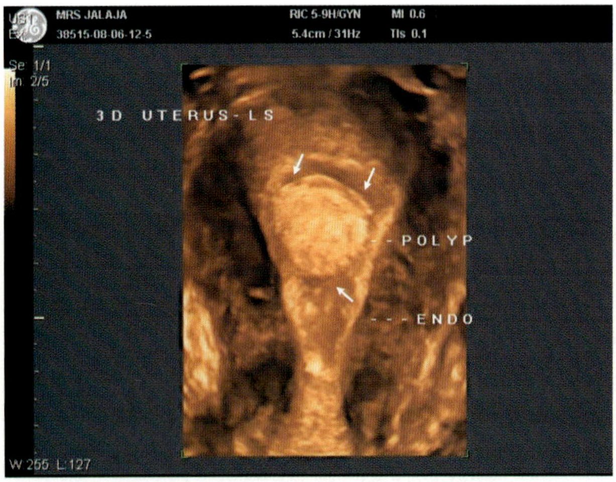

Fig. 6.7: 4D ultrasound delineating fibroid polyp of the same patient as in Figure 6.5

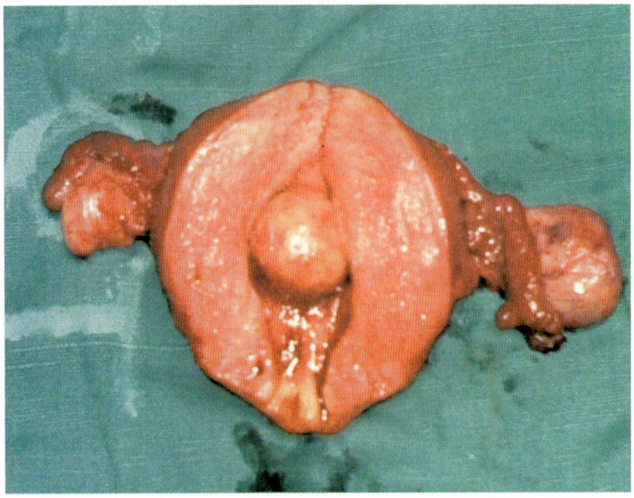

Fig. 6.8: Cut section of the uterus showing Type I submucous myoma. This myoma could have been removed hysteroscopically

(40% present with menorrhagia). Cervical cancer and local non cancerous lesions of cervix like polyp or cervicitis usually present with inter menstrual or post coital bleeding. Malignancies and other lesions of the vagina as a cause of bleeding is very rare.

6.6.2 Systemic Disease

Systemic diseases contribute to menorrhagia in only a small percentage of women. Inherited abnormalities like Von Willebrand disease, platelet function defects and other rare inherited defects of coagulation usually present during adolescence as profuse or prolonged bleeding.

Acquired causes like immune thrombocytopenia or leukemia can occur at any age and present as acute onset of menorrhagia. Hence, it is important to exclude these conditions in patients who present with recent onset of severe menorrhagia. Sometimes, acute menorrhagia will lead to the diagnosis of leukemia or an acquired bleeding disorder.

Endocrine abnormalities like thyroid disorders can present with menorrhagia. Hypothyroidism usually causes anovulation and hence anovulatory bleeding. If a woman's menorrhagia is unexplained, thyroid disorder should be looked for.

6.6.3 Iatrogenic or Drug Induced

In some situations, AUB could be iatrogenic due to the use of hormonal contraceptives or intra uterine devices or other medications like anticoagulants, antidepressants and tranquilizers.

6.6.4 Dysfunctional Uterine Bleeding (DUB)

When all the above situations are excluded, the diagnosis of DUB can be made. DUB is defined as excessive bleeding (excessively heavy, prolonged or frequent) of uterine origin which is not due to any demonstrable pelvic disease, complications of pregnancy or systemic disease. DUB accounts for 50% of menorrhagia. In the rest of the patients menorrhagia may be due to some local pathology. Even if bimanual examination does not reveal pelvic pathology, transvaginal ultrasound scan (TVUS) is helpful in revealing pathologies like small submucous fibroids, endometrial polyp or adenomyosis.

Anovulatory bleeding is due to a disturbance in the hypothalamo-pituitary ovarian axis. It usually presents as irregular bleeding following varying periods of amenorrhea. Chronic anovulation occurs in polycystic ovarian disease (PCOD). Anovulatory cycles are frequent at the extremes of reproductive life, but intermittent cycles may also be ovulatory, thus causing irregular menses.

6.7 ABNORMAL UTERINE BLEEDING IN ADOLESCENT AGE GROUP

The etiology, pathology, investigations and management of AUB varies in the three different age groups of women–adolescent, child bearing and perimenopausal, even though there is some overlap. It is important to have knowledge about the etiology in the different age groups, so that a logical diagnostic workup can be evolved, to arrive at a diagnosis and plan treatment.

Abnormal uterine bleeding in this age group is usually due to the immature HPO axis but rarely may be part of a generalized bleeding disorder like Von Willebrand disease or thrombocytopenia. The HPO axis continues to mature after puberty. In the first few years after menarche, FSH, LH, estrogen and progesterone are all below the normal adult levels. Within five years after menarche, their levels gradually reach that of adults. The anovulatory irregular cycles will become regular and ovulatory, one to two years after menarche. Anovulatory DUB is the usual cause of AUB in adolescents and these girls will have irregular menses. Generalized bleeding disorders contribute to 20% of adolescent AUB and present as menorrhagia or as irregular bleeding. These patients on detailed questioning will usually give a history of bleeding from wound sites and gums.

6.7.1 Evaluation and Management of Adolescent AUB

Medical History

The patient should be asked specifically about recent weight gain or weight loss, eating and exercise habits, and about any psychosocial stress. Any history suggestive of bleeding disorder like bleeding from gums should also be elicited. Family history of bleeding disorder can give the clue. Patients should also be enquired about history suggestive of hyperandrogenism.

Examination

The important points to be noted in the general examination are height, weight and BMI. Features of virilization like acne, hirsutism, clitoromegaly and presence of acanthosis nigricans should be looked for. Thyroid enlargement should also be noted. Pointers of serious bleeding disorders like petechiae and bruises should not be overlooked.

If the patient has severe bleeding not responding to treatment and is not sexually active, a one finger vaginal examination should be done to rule out rare local causes like foreign body or tumors like sarcoma botryoides or clear cell carcinoma of the vagina. Acute onset of profuse fresh bleeding may be due to a vaginal laceration as a result of sexual assault. Pregnancy associated conditions should also be kept in mind.

Investigations

The basic investigation is a complete blood count to assess the severity of bleeding and also to know the adequacy of platelets. A laboratory diagnosis of iron deficiency anemia is definitely an objective evidence of menorrhagia. Hence, any patient who presents with excessive blood loss should have their hemoglobin estimated to know the basal level of hemoglobin so that response to treatment can be assessed. It also gives an idea about the severity of blood loss. Patients with severe bleeding should be tested for coagulation disorders. PT and APTT are not sensitive enough to diagnose inherited disorders of coagulation. One of the common inherited disorders of coagulation is von Willebrand disease. Hence von Willi brand's panel should be tested. It includes vWF antigen assay, Factor VIII level and Ristocetin co-factor assay. Patients with severe bleeding and normal von Willebrand panel should be referred for further tests of coagulation. Thyroid function tests need be done if there is a clinical suspicion of thyroid dysfunction. Pregnancy test or imaging studies should be done as the clinical situation warrants.

Treatment

The most common cause for bleeding in this age group is anovulation due to immaturity of the hypothalamo-pituitary-ovarian axis. After excluding generalized bleeding disorders, the parents should be counseled. If the bleeding is not very profuse as to produce anemia, the initial treatment can be a combination of anti-prostaglandin and anti-fibrinolytic agents.Simultaneously, hematinics can be given and a nutritious diet should be advised.

In a few patients, the bleeding can continue for several days and produce severe anemia. In such a situation, hormonal therapy is warranted. Even though the bleeding is usually anovulatory, endogenous estrogen will also be deficient. Hence, they have insufficient endometrium on which progesterone can exert its action. These patients need a combination of estrogen and progesterone.

Patients with heavy bleeding and severe anemia need a higher dose of hormones. They can be started on combination oral contraceptive (COC) pills 4 times daily which can be gradually tapered to once daily in a span of 2 to 3 weeks. Since high dose estrogen can cause nausea and vomiting, an anti-emetic should also be prescribed. Afterwards, COC may be given once daily cyclically for 3 to 6 months. The patient should be followed up after stopping hormones for recurrence of symptoms.

Hospitalization

If hemoglobin is <8 gm% or if the patient has orthostasis, hospitalization is necessary. Even if the Hb is >8 gm%, if the patient has severe bleeding she should be admitted. Anemia should be corrected by blood transfusion. When bleeding is acute and heavy, high dose estrogen may be deemed necessary i.e. conjugated equine estrogen (CEE) 25mg (high dose) every 4th hourly may be given until bleeding stops.[1]

This estrogen acts at the capillary level to reduce hemorrhage. 24 hrs after the bleeding ceases, hormonal treatment can be continued as a COC pill which can be given for 21 days and stopped for withdrawal bleed. COC pill should be started at a high dose of 4 tablets a day and later tapered to one tablet a day. If the girl is anemic, instead of stopping after a period of 21 days it can be continued for a period of 2-3 months without interruption, but not more than that as prolonged use can lead to breakthrough bleeding. The cyclical combination COC pill can be continued for 3-6 months. If the bleeding is not profuse, a lower dose of oral estrogen, like 1.25 mg of conjugated estrogen can be given 4 hourly. When bleeding stops, it can be tapered to a single daily dose for 7-10 days. Later, after 10 days, progestagen like medroxyprogesterone acetate 10 mg/day can be added for another 10 days and both estrogen and progesterone can be withdrawn together. Estrogen alone should not be withdrawn, as it might lead to profuse bleeding. This can be followed by cyclical COC pills. In situations where estrogens are contraindicated, progestagen like medroxyprogesterone acetate can be administered. A high dose of 10 mg four times daily should be started and tapered to 10 mg daily. It can be maintained with the progestin only pill. Simultaneously anemia should be corrected by administering oral iron.

Inherited Abnormalities of Hemostasis

Approximately 20% of adolescents with menorrhagia have an underlying systemic disorder. In more than 50% of these women, the underlying cause may be a coagulopathy such as thrombocytopenia, von Willebrand disease or rarely leukemia. The first manifestation of a bleeding disorder could be as abnormal bleeding when the girl attains menarche.

Von Willebrand Disease (vWD)

Von Willebrand disease is the commonest inherited disorder of coagulation characterized by decreased or defective production of von Willebrand protein. Von Willebrand protein is a plasma protein which circulates in plasma with factor VIII, forming a complex with it and protects it from proteolytic enzymes. It is involved in platelet function and also serves as a stabilizing agent for coagulation. Thus it acts as a bridge between platelets and damaged endothelium. The disease is highly complex in pathology. There are three types of vWD. Type I and type III are characterized by a quantitative abnormality while type II is a qualitative abnormality. Type I is the most common (70%). Type III is a severe deficiency of von Willebrand protein. When an adolescent girl is brought with heavy menstrual bleeding, taking a proper medical history is very important. History of bleeding from nose or gum, bleeding from minor injuries, joint or muscle bleeding or history of gastrointestinal bleeding should arouse the suspicion of the presence of an inherited bleeding disorder.

Investigation: Routine coagulation tests like PT or aPTT are not helpful in diagnosing vWD. Women who do not respond to treatment and have normal coagulation profile should have specialized coagulation tests done like factor VIII assays, von Willebrand test and platelet function tests. These tests are available only in specialized laboratories which is the reason why most of the patients with von Willebrand disease are not usually diagnosed. Testing for von Willebrand disease is by von Willebrand panel which includes von Willebrand factor antigen assay, Ristocetin co-factor activity and factor VIII coagulant activity. All three tests should be done initially. Ristocetin co-factor activity is used to assess the risk of bleeding. There is considerable variability between laboratories and between the different days of the menstrual cycle when the tests are done. It is recommended to do the tests during the first four days of the menstrual cycle. When the test results happen to be normal for a patient with a high index of clinical suspicion, it should be repeated.

Treatment: Desmopressin is the treatment of choice in the presence of severe bleeding. If the patient does not respond to Desmopressin, von Willebrand factor concentrate should be administered.

Thrombocytopenia

Thrombocytopenia, due to immune or non-immune reasons or as a result of bone marrow failure can lead to menorrhagia or irregular bleeding in adolescent as well as adult women. Bleeding manifestations are determined by the etiology and severity of thrombocytopenia. Unlike platelet function abnormalities, thrombocytopenia is easily diagnosed. Since a complete blood count is routinely done for all adolescents with abnormal bleeding, the condition will be promptly diagnosed.

Thrombasthenia

These are a group of platelet function defects which can present as heavy menstrual bleeding. They are diagnosed by platelet function tests when other tests are inconclusive. Rare types of platelet function abnormalities include Glanzmann thrombasthenia and Bernard-Soulier syndrome.

Other Inherited Abnormalities of Hemostasis

Women who are carriers of hemophilia will have decreased levels of factor VIII or IX. They may also be at risk of bleeding. Dysfibrinogenemia, hypofibrinogenemia, prothrombin deficiency, deficiency of factors V, VII, X, XI or XIII can also present with menorrhagia.

6.7.2 Adolescent PCOS

It is not rare for PCOS to present in the adolescent age group. Typically these patients have obesity, hirsutism and oligomenorrhea. Sometimes they may have profuse bleeding following amenorrhea. These patients should be definitely treated from adolescence, to decrease the high level of LH and to prevent the endometrial hyperplasia from unopposed estrogen. The cycles can be regularized by administering medroxy progesterone 10 mg/day from day1 to day10 of every month to ensure patient compliance. After six months, treatment can be withheld, to find whether the cycles have regularized. If the cycles are still irregular, it is better to continue the same treatment. Patients having hirsutism and acne might need a combination of Drosperinone and Ethinyl Estradiol or a combination of Cyproterone and Ethinyl estradiol. The advantage of Drosperinone is decreased weight gain due to its anti mineralocorticoid action. The theoretical disadvantage of giving combination OCP for these young girls is premature epiphyseal fusion, affecting adult height.

If the patient is not responding to treatment, pelvic imaging should be done. Rarely, they can have submucus fibroids or malignancies like sarcoma botryoides. Imaging study can be a transabdominal ultrasound. In the event of inconclusive ultrasound examination, MRI should be resorted to. If there is endometrial calcification, an endometrial study to rule out tuberculosis should be performed.

6.8 AUB IN REPRODUCTIVE AGE GROUP

Abnormal bleeding in the reproductive age group can be due to the following conditions (Table 6.1):

Table 6.1: Causes of AUB in reproductive age group

1.	Pregnancy related conditions
2.	Pelvic pathology
3.	Dysfunctional uterine bleeding
4.	Endocrine disorders
5.	Systemic diseases
6.	Inherited or acquired disorders of coagulation
7.	Iatrogenic and drug related

6.8.1 Causes of AUB in Reproductive Age Group

Pregnancy Related Conditions

Recent onset of abnormal bleeding in the reproductive age group should arouse the suspicion of pregnancy related conditions. Threatened miscarriage, incomplete miscarriage, molar pregnancy and ectopic pregnancy can be suspected from a careful history. A pregnancy test should be done if there is a clinical suspicion. Whenever clinical examination is doubtful, transvaginal ultrasound will help to differentiate between the different pregnancy conditions.

Pelvic Pathology

Fibroid

The commonest uterine pathology causing abnormal bleeding is fibroid. Submucous and intramural fibroid are the ones that cause menorrhagia. Submucous fibroids cause dysmenorrhea which can be very severe. Submucous fibroids and fibroid polyps may cause intermenstrual bleeding also because of the local infection and trauma over the polyp.

Adenomyosis

Adenomyosis causes dysmenorrhea and menorrhagia which usually occurs in the fourth decade of the woman's life. Adenomyosis is typically seen in multiparous women, but rarely it can occur in nulliparous women also, associated with endometriosis. Bimanual examination will usually show a uniformly enlarged uterus which will be firmer and harder than fibroid. The uterine size will not be more than 10-12 weeks pregnancy. Diagnosis is by TVS. The usual appearance of adenomyosis in TVS is pine leaf pattern (Fig. 6.9). The appearance can also be like multiple small hypo echoic areas distributed throughout the myometrium. The diffuse adenomyosis can involve either the anterior or posterior wall, more frequently the posterior wall. Characteristically the disease is asymmetrical. If in doubt MRI is more predictive than Ultrasound. Adenomyosis can also be focal. Focal adenomyosis (adenomyoma) should be differentiated from fibroid. Fibroid will have a pseudo capsule formed by the

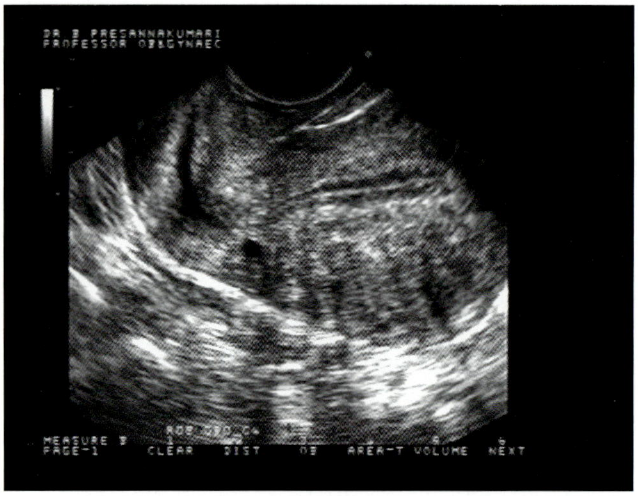

Fig. 6.9: TVS showing adenomyosis of the posterior wall of the uterus

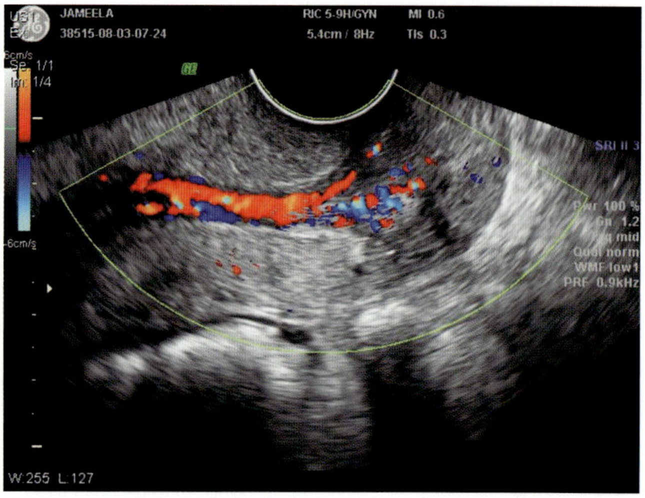

Fig. 6.10: Fibroid polyp seen protruding through the cervical canal showing feeding vessel. Polyps will always have feeding vessels which can be identified by Doppler

surrounding compressed myometrium where as adenomyoma will not have a definite capsule. Hence, it is difficult to enucleate an adenomyoma. If hysterectomy is not the option of treatment, it is important to differentiate between adenomyoma and fibroid. Menorrhagia due to adenomyosis is difficult to treat medically compared to that caused by dysfunctional uterine bleeding.

Polyp

Polyps are more common in the perimenopausal age group but can be seen in younger women as well. Patients with polyp will usually present with menorrhagia but can also present with irregular bleeding. They can be mistaken for hyperplastic endometrium in TVS (Fig. 6.10). Sono hysterography will help to differentiate between thickened endometrium and polyp.

When patients present with irregular bleeding, it could be due to polyps in the endometrial cavity or a pregnancy condition like incomplete miscarriage with retained products. Clots in the endometrial cavity can also appear as an echogenic mass on TVS. All these can be differentiated from each other by Doppler study. A feeding vessel can be identified in polyp whereas no vessels will be seen in retained products (incomplete miscarriage) or blood clot.

Endometrial hyperplasia and cancer

Women at risk of endometrial cancer in the child bearing age group are those who have chronic anovulation. They will have infrequent periods and menorrhagia. Since 40% of women having endometrial carcinoma will present with menorrhagia, endometrial[2,3] sampling is indicated in such women if the endometrial thickness is more than 11 mm.

Dysfunctional Uterine Bleeding (DUB)

Definition

The definition of DUB by Fraser and Sengurtekin is- excessive bleeding (excessively heavy, prolonged or frequent) of uterine origin which is not due to demonstrable pelvic disease, complications of pregnancy or systemic disease. This definition is endorsed by the European Society for Human Reproduction and Embryology. With the widespread use of TVUS, women classified as having DUB are much less than that was thought earlier. DUB accounts for 50% of menorrhagia. Causes like small submucus fibroids or adenomyosis which were not evident in clinical examination can now be delineated by TVUS. Previously these women were classified as having DUB. Dysfunctional uterine bleeding[4] can occur in ovulatory as well as anovulatory cycles. 80% of DUB are ovulatory.

Ovulatory DUB

In ovulatory cycles, menorrhagia occurs due to altered local vasoconstriction. Vasoconstriction is the normal mechanism of control of bleeding during menses. A number of endometrial products can alter the degree of vasoconstriction and cause abnormal bleeding. It has been found that the total endometrial prostaglandin content is proportional to the amount of blood loss. An increase in PGE 2 and PG I 2 receptors as well as a disproportionate increase in PGE2 have been demonstrated in the endometrium of patients with ovulatory DUB.

Anovulatory DUB

In anovulatory DUB there is a disturbance in the hypo- thalamopituitary-ovarian axis. Anovulatory bleeding usually occurs following menarche or in the perimenopausal age group. The condition can be chronic also as in PCOS. In anovulatory bleeding there will be varying periods of amenorrhea followed by irregular vaginal bleeding. This type of bleeding can occur sporadically at any time among women in the childbearing age group. Occasional anovulatory cycles can occur at any time in the reproductive age group. The typical history will be a period of amenorrhea for a few months followed by irregular vaginal bleeding. The follicle matures and produces estrogen but the LH surge will not occur. As a consequence the follicle does not rupture but continues to produce estrogen. Under the influence of estrogen, endometrium undergoes hyperplasia. Later on, the endometrium will irregularly shed causing irregular bleeding. This condition used to be known as Metropathia Hemorrhagica.

Hematological Disorders

Menorrhagia due to congenital disorders of coagulation will date back to menarche. Acquired abnormalities of hemostasis can also be the cause for menorrhagia. Commonest acquired cause is thrombocytopenia. It is important to keep this in mind when women complain of abrupt onset of severe menorrhagia. Clinical examination should include looking for petechial spots (Fig. 6.11), hepatosplenomegaly, lymphadenopathy etc because rarely menorrhagia may be the first symptom of thrombocytopenia or leukemia.

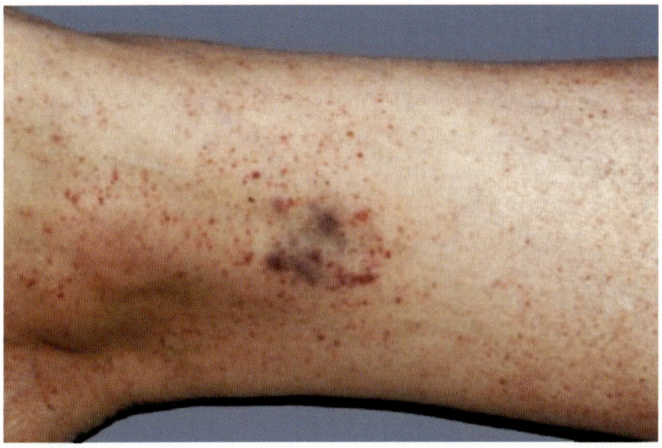

Fig. 6.11: Petechial spots in a lady who presented with severe menorrhagia of 2 months duration and severe headache. Since the platelet count was only 10000, she was admitted and treated with platelet transfusion and immunoglobulin, but she died following intracranial hemorrhage

Endocrine Disorders

The commonest endocrine disorder which causes abnormal bleeding is hypothyroidism. Anovulation associated with hypothyroidism is the etiological factor. Thyroid function should be tested in women who give a history suggestive of, or have clinical evidence of thyroid disorder. Treatment of the thyroid disorder will usually cure the abnormal bleeding. Hyperthyroidism also can lead to abnormal bleeding. Women with hyperprolactinemia may experience irregular anovulatory periods and amenorrhea.

Systemic Disease

Systemic diseases like chronic liver disease can cause menorrhagia due to deficiency of clotting factors.

AV Malformations

A very rare cause for menorrhagia is acquired AV fistula following procedures like curettage. The usual presentation is profuse bleeding after a procedure like uterine curettage. Clinical examination and B-mode ultrasound will be unremarkable. Doppler examination will clinch the diagnosis. Uterine artery embolization may be resorted to if the uterus is to be conserved.

Iatrogenic and Drug Related

Women on anticoagulant therapy for artificial heart valves or other conditions can present with severe menorrhagia. Treatment is problematic since most of the medicines used to treat menorrhagia are contraindicated in such women because anti-coagulation is their requirement and the drugs given for menorrhagia are pro-coagulants. Post-IUCD-insertion menorrhagia is a usual occurrence in the first few cycles. This can be managed by antifibrinolytic agents and antiprostaglandins. After a few cycles, menorrhagia usually abates.

6.8.2 Management of AUB in the Reproductive Age Group

Approach to the Patient

A proper history including past medical and surgical history of the patient who presents with abnormal bleeding will lead the clinician to diagnostic possibilities. Information regarding use of drugs (anticoagulants, hormones) and coagulation disorders (history of easy bruising, bleeding gums, increased bleeding during any previous surgery) should be elicited. A detailed menstrual history should give a clue as to whether the abnormal bleeding is a pregnancy related condition. A sudden change from a regular menses to irregular bleeding suggests pregnancy related conditions. An acute onset of severe menorrhagia may be due to acquired coagulation defects like thrombocytopenia or even leukemia. Regular menses with irregular intermenstrual bleeding suggests local pathologies like submucus fibroid, fibroid polyp, malignant or premalignant lesions of the cervix or vagina. Regular menses with symptoms of ovulation like mid menstrual pain and discharge per vaginum and premenstrual symptoms suggests ovulatory bleeding. Anovulatory bleeding is usually irregular without a definite pattern. It could be prolonged spotting or severe hemorrhage but characteristically painless. When women complain of menorrhagia, a careful history of how it affects her normal life should be elicited. A history of passing clots definitely gives a clue that bleeding is more than normal and at the same time suggesting that the coagulation cascade is normal.

Examination

The general condition of the patient depends on the amount of bleeding. Rarely the bleeding can be severe enough to compromise the general condition of the patient in which case, establishing hemodynamic stability should be given the first priority. Looking for anemia gives a clue as to the severity of menorrhagia. A meticulous complete general examination should be done to exclude generalized disease.

Investigations

A complete blood count (CBC) should be done for all women with menorrhagia. A basal level of PCV is imperative to assess the severity of menorrhagia and repeated assessment is important in gauging the response to treatment. Even though thrombocytopenia and leukemia are very rare causes of menorrhagia, these should not be overlooked. Thyroid function should be tested if there is clinical suspicion of a thyroid disorder or when there are no other causes of menorrhagia. If the history is suggestive of a bleeding disorder, tests for bleeding disorders especially von Willebrand panel should be done. ACOG recommends testing for von Willebrand's panel in adult women with severe menorrhagia and in women undergoing hysterectomy for the sole reason of menorrhagia. If the history is suggestive of a pregnancy condition, a urine pregnancy test should also be done.

Endometrial evaluation of women with menorrhagia

Transvaginal ultrasound (TVS) should be done for all women presenting with menorrhagia. TVS helps detect submucous myoma, adenomyosis, endometrial polyp, endometriosis, endometrial hyperplasia and endometrial cancer which cannot be diagnosed by pelvic examination. The sensitivity of diagnosing endometrial cancer is 91-96%. In young women presenting with cyclical menorrhagia, ultrasound evaluation may be deferred. Otherwise

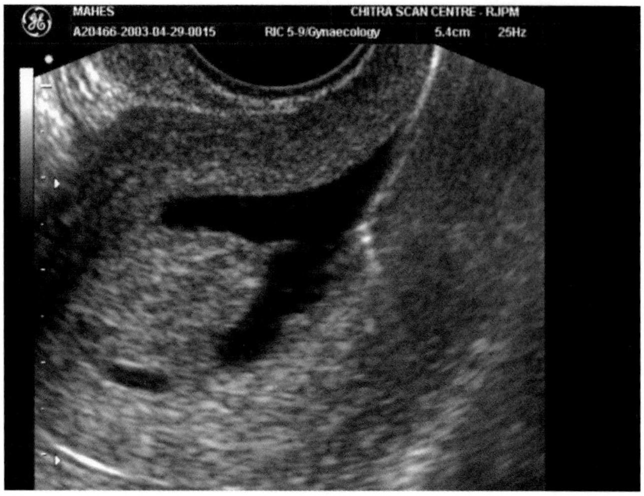

Fig. 6.12: Saline hysterosonography showing clearly depicted endometrial polyp

endometrium should be evaluated. Women with anovulatory cycles are prone for endometrial hyperplasia and malignancy at an younger age. Histopathological evaluation of the endometrium is mandatory for such women.

The simplest way to get a sample of the endometrium is by endometrial biopsy. It can be done as an office procedure using Pipelle endometrial aspirator.

Saline sonohysterogram (Fig. 6.12): A thick endometrial shadow in TVS may be hyperplastic endometrium or a polyp. The two can be differentiated by saline sonohysterogram. A few cc of saline infused into the endometrial cavity through a no. 8 Foley catheter will delineate the polyp by the presence of surrounding fluid.

Hysteroscopy: Hysteroscopy has an important role in the evaluation and management of AUB. Polyps and submucus fibroids suspected by ultrasound can be confirmed by hysteroscopy. Hysteroscopy is highly accurate in diagnosing frank cancer. The role of hysteroscopy lies in confirming endometrial lesions suspected in TVS and also in directing the biopsy site. Operative hysteroscopy has a definite role in endometrial resection and in the management of submucous fibroids. Cochrane database analyzed the accuracy of the above three diagnostic procedures in women with AUB. It appeared that all three procedures help in predicting the presence of anatomic lesions and have good negative[5] predictive value.

Endometrial biopsy: A thick endometrium made out by TVS needs biopsy. Endometrial sampling helps to diagnose the type of endometrium and also to exclude hyperplasia and malignancy. The traditional way of managing abnormal uterine bleeding used to be dilatation and curettage. The accuracy of blind curettage is at present considered inferior to sampling the endometrium using aspiration methods

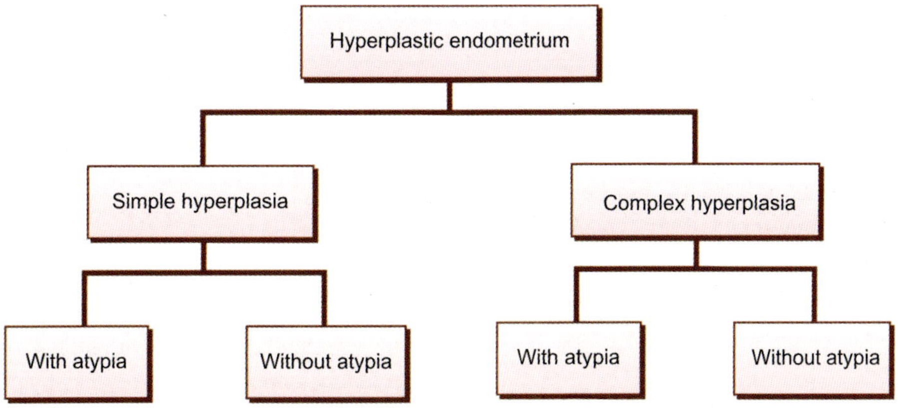

Fig. 6.13: Classification of hyperplastic endometrium

which use negative pressure, like the Pipelle. However, a patient who has bleeding following a period of amenorrhea will definitely benefit from a thorough curettage, if the endometrium remains thick even after several days of bleeding. Women presenting with abnormal bleeding in the postpartum or post abortive period may have chronic endometritis which can be diagnosed by examination of the curetting. Hyperplastic endometrium can be classified based on the pathological types (Fig. 6.13). The incidence of hyperplasia progressing to malignancy in the four categories is listed in Table 6.2.

Table 6.2: The chance of hyperplasia progressing to malignancy

Simple hyperplasia without atypia	1%
Simple hyperplasia with atypia	8%
Complex hyperplasia without atypia	3%
Complex hyperplasia with atypia	29%

Source: Kurman RJ, Kaminski PF, Norris HJ. The behavior of endometrial hyperplasia: a long term study of untreated hyperplasia in 170 patients. Cancer 1985;56:403-12

After investigations, most women with abnormal bleeding can be diagnosed as having some underlying anatomic cause. After excluding all the anatomic causes a diagnosis of Dysfunctional Uterine Bleeding (DUB) can be reached. Women presenting with varying periods of amenorrhea followed by bleeding will most probably be having anovulatory DUB. Irregular vaginal bleeding can occur due to causes other than anovulation like fibroid polyp, endometrial hyperplasia, endometrial carcinoma, malignancies of the cervix and vagina, pregnancy conditions and coagulopathies.

Medical management

The aim of treatment is to decrease the amount of bleeding as well as to achieve predictable withdrawal bleeding. Management should be based on the following:

- The underlying cause for the bleeding
- The severity of bleeding
- The need for contraception
- The woman's choice, her health status, affordability as well as the facilities available

Heavy menstrual bleeding used to be a major indication for hysterectomy. But with the introduction of medical treatment including medicated intrauterine devices, as well as minimally invasive procedures like endometrial ablation and uterine artery embolisation, the number of hysterectomies for the sole indication of heavy menstrual bleeding is gradually coming down.

Compliance to treatment protocol is of utmost importance in achieving the optimum success. Hence it is important to counsel the woman and her family about the significance of following treatment protocol as well as about other treatment options available if the initial treatment fails, to accomplish the desired effect.

Management of Anovulatory DUB

Irregular bleeding especially following amenorrhea will be usually anovulatory. Rarely regular menses can also be anovulatory. Endometrial sampling differentiates between proliferative, hyperplastic and secretory endometrium. Irregular menses poses great anxiety to women. Management depends upon the severity of bleeding and the need for child bearing. The aim of treatment of anovulatory bleeding is to arrest the acute bleeding episode as well as to decrease the risk of endometrial hyperplasia and cancer, if the woman has chronic anovulation. *Patients should be counseled about the need for regular treatment. Irregular medication can cause more erratic bleeding.*

Progestagens: Since progesterone deficiency is the fundamental defect in anovulatory bleeding, the first line management can be progestagens. When the woman presents with bleeding, 19-nor testosterone derivatives should be preferred for hemostasis. Norethisterone 5mg thrice daily can be started. It will take minimum 48 hours for the bleeding to stop. If bleeding persists, the dose can be increased to 10mg thrice daily. This can be continued for a minimum of 15 days and then withdrawn. On the fifth day of withdrawal bleed, the woman can be started on a safer progestagen like Medroxyprogesterone. A minimum of three cycle treatment should be advised. If the endometrium shows complex hyperplasia, long term cyclical progestagen treatment of about 9 months should be advised and the endometrium re-evaluated after treatment to check whether the hyperplasia has reversed. Women with chronic anovulation can be managed by progestagen given in the second half of menstrual cycle so that they will have regular withdrawal bleeding, which will prevent development of endometrial hyperplasia and endometrial cancer.

Role of antifibrinolytics: Since the pathology is progesterone deficiency, treatment with antifibrinolytics may not be effective. However it can be given along with progestagens to decrease the amount of blood loss in the initial phase.

Combination oral contraceptive pill: Women having anovulatory bleeding can also be treated with a combination of estrogen and progestagen in the form of combined oral contraceptive pill, especially if contraception also is needed. The transdermal contraceptive patch or the vaginal contraceptive rings are the other choices. Based on a Cochrane review no randomized trials have compared the effectiveness of progestagens vs. progestagen estrogen combination in the management of anovulatory bleeding[6].

If the woman wishes to conceive, ovulation induction can be undertaken.

Levonorgestrel intrauterine system (LNG IUS): The levonorgestrel intrauterine system which delivers 20 μg of Levonorgestrel in the endometrium is superior to oral progestagens in treating both ovulatory as well as anovulatory DUB. It obviates the systemic side effects of oral progestagens. Inserting the device into the uterine cavity is a onetime office procedure and patient satisfaction is much more than oral progestagen therapy. Irregular bleeding can occur in the initial few months after insertion. About 86% of women will have their menstrual flow reduced within 3 months of insertion and 80 % of women become amenorrheic within one year of insertion. The LNG-IUS can be advised for women who want to preserve their fertility because of the reversibility after removal of the device. The lifespan of the device is 5 years.

Management of (Ovulatory Bleeding) Menorrhagia

Women with regular cycles and heavy bleeding may be having some pathologic cause for the heavy bleeding. It may be due to submucus myomas, adenomyosis or chronic pelvic inflammatory disease. All these can be diagnosed by TVS and if necessary hysteroscopy can be resorted to. After excluding pelvic pathology, the abnormal bleeding is classified as dysfunctional uterine bleeding (DUB). The first line treatment of women with ovulatory DUB can be tranexamic acid combined with mefenamic acid. Tranexamic acid reduces menstrual blood loss by 50% and mefenamic acid reduces menstrual cramps as well as bleeding. Patients who do not respond to these drugs need hormonal therapy. It can be combined oral contraceptive (COC) pill if there are no contraindications for its use. COC is especially preferred if the woman wants contraception also. Ethamsylate does not significantly reduce menstrual blood loss. Another choice of treatment is LNG-IUS. A Cochrane review reported that LNG-IUS is more effective in relieving menorrhagia than 21 day treatment with progestagens. For the woman who cannot tolerate oral medication LNG-IUS should be preferred because of its lack of systemic effects.

Other Medical Methods

Danazol: Danazol act on the pituitary and suppress gonadotropin production thereby preventing ovulation and ovarian steroidogenesis. Consequently endometrium will undergo atrophy resulting in hypomenorrhea or amenorrhea. It is very effective in controlling both ovulatory and anovulatory bleeding, but the associated androgenic side effects deter its use in the treatment of DUB.

GnRH analogs: GnRH antagonists as well as agonists in high doses given monthly will suppress the pituitary and cause amenorrhea. The disadvantage is the extreme hypoestrogenic state which can be caused due to its prolonged use. Hence long term treatment is not feasible, but if the patient is severely anemic, GnRH can be tried for a few months during which time the patient's anemia can be corrected and the other treatment modality can be planned.

Surgical treatment

Surgery should be offered to women who do not respond to medical therapy and those who cannot tolerate medical therapy especially if she has completed her family.

The traditional treatment for menorrhagia was dilatation and curettage and hysterectomy if no relief. Over the past few decades this has changed from hysterectomy to medical treatment followed by intrauterine devices and minimally invasive surgical procedures. The minimally invasive surgical treatment includes uterine artery embolisation and the different methods of endometrial ablation. Women with submucous fibroids can be managed by hysteroscopic resection of myoma.

Minimally Invasive Surgical Procedures for DUB

These procedures involve destruction of the endometrium leaving the uterus intact.

Different types of energy sources are used to destroy the endometrium. The entire endometrium up to the upper endocervical canal is destroyed. Deep endocervical canal destruction can result in stenosis and hematometra and hence should be avoided. The desired after effect is amenorrhea. Even though amenorrhea may not be achieved always, there will be a reduction in blood loss resulting in eumenorrhea. Endometrial ablation is found to be 90% effective in reducing bleeding or causing amenorrhea. Hence patients should be counseled appropriately. Compared to hysterectomy, duration of hospital stay, recovery time and hospital expenses are much less.

Endometrial ablation using hysteroscope: The first generation methods involved the use of hysteroscope.

Resectoscopic Endometrial Ablation (REA)

This technique of destroying the endometrium instead of performing hysterectomy started in the early 1980s. The procedure actually evolved from trans-urethral resection of the prostate.

Women who have ovulatory DUB are the ones who will benefit from endometrial ablation. But those whose menorrhagia is due to bleeding disorders like von Willibrands disease and those on anticoagulants may also benefit from ablation done as an adjunctive procedure. Ablation can be tried in patients with small fibroids (less than 3 cm) and adenomyosis. The reported rate of amenorrhea following endometrial resection is 35% but satisfaction rates after 1 year of follow up has been reported to be 90%.

Women who have anovulatory bleeding are not good candidates for endometrial ablation. They should be treated with progestagens. The benefit of treating anovulatory bleeding medically, in women who have completed child bearing was addressed in the M/S trial. Women were more satisfied with surgical therapy than medical therapy. However, because of the less cost and risk of medical therapy compared to surgical therapy it should be offered to women before advising surgery.

Women with polycystic ovaries should be treated medically from the time of diagnosis. Since they are at high risk for endometrial hyperplasia and endometrial cancer they should not be treated with endometrial ablation as endometrial assessment after ablation is not possible.

Diagnostic hysteroscopy and endometrial biopsy should be done prior to the procedure to exclude endometrial pathology. Women found to have submucous fibroids or endometrial polyps can be treated by hysteroscopic resection.

Procedure: For endometrial resection, the surgeon needs the following:

- A non- electrolyte distension medium like glycine, dextran , sorbitol or mannitol.
- Hysteroscope with a resectoscope which has provision for fluid inflow, optics, channel for instruments and fluid outflow.
- A power source which can be LASER or electrocautery

The uterine cavity is distended with a non-electrolyte solution. By using a wire loop electrode the endometrium is shaved off in small strips measuring 7mm wide and 3-4mm deep. The resectoscope has a second fluid channel for the egress of fluid and debris produced by the resection. The procedure is called TCRE or Trans Cervical Resection of the Endometrium.[7]

Laser ablation of the endometrium: Under hysteroscopic guidance, endometrium is destroyed using Nd: YAG laser. Goldrath et al developed laser ablation of the endometrium in 1979.Nd Yag laser is used to effect coagulation of the endometrium to a depth of 6 mm. Even though success rates obtained were as high as 83%, laser failed to be widely used as the equipment was very costly and the learning curve was very high.

Roller ball endometrial ablation: Resection of the endometrium using wire loop electrode needs a lot of experience and skill. To overcome this difficulty an easier procedure of roller ball ablation was introduced. Using a 3 mm ball electrode the entire endometrium is ablated with mono polar current. The distension medium used is the same as that for endometrial resection. Preoperative endometrial thinning is mandatory before roller ball ablation. The procedure is quicker and safer than endometrial resection, as it is less likely to perforate the uterus. The roller ball is good for ablating the cornual region. In the presence of endometrial polyps or submucus fibroids, endometrial resection should be preferred. Both can be used in a combined procedure. The cornual region and fundus can be ablated with ball electrode and the rest can be resected with a wire loop.

Medical preparation of the endometrium: Use of GnRH analogue or Danazol[8] prior to ablation causes significant thinning of the endometrium resulting in technical ease of the procedure as well as improved success rate.

A Cochrane review clearly demonstrated the advantage in terms of ease of the procedure, shorter surgical time, higher rate of post surgical amenorrhea and lower rate of post surgical dysmenorrhea following pre-operative thinning of the endometrium using either GnRH or Danazol for a period of four weeks.

Complications of endometrial ablation: The two important serious complications of EA procedures are:

1. Distension medium related complications
2. Injury to viscera following perforation of the uterus during the procedure

Distension of the uterine cavity is mandatory for hysteroscopically directed procedures. When monopolar current is used, electrolyte solution like normal saline cannot be used for distending the uterine cavity because of the danger of transmitting electricity into neighboring structures. The usual distention medium used is a non electrolyte solution like 3% sorbitol, 1.5% glycine, 5% mannitol or a mixture of sorbitol and mannitol. Excepting mannitol, all other solutions which are hypo-osmolar, if absorbed signi-ficantly into the circulation can cause dilutional hypo-natremia, hypoosmolality and brain edema. Premenopausal women are more prone for brain edema due to the inhibitory effect of estrogen and progesterone on the sodium pump. The development of hysteroscopic bipolar electro surgical system which can be operated in electrolyte rich fluid medium like normal saline has obviated the complication of hyponatremia, but fluid overload can occur even when normal saline is used as distention medium. Pre-operative use of GnRH reduces the incidence of fluid overload. Automated systems which measure fluid deficit will give an idea about the amount of intravasated fluid. If the deficit exceeds 750 to 1500 ml, serum electrolytes should be monitored and frusemide should be given intravenously. When the serum sodium falls to 125 mEq/L or the deficit exceeds 1500 to 2000 ml, the procedure should be stopped.

Long term sequels of ablation are development of hematometra and pelvic pain. If the woman develops endometrial hyperplasia or carcinoma, there can be delay in diagnosis due to inadequate sampling of the endometrium. Women who are below 45 years of age as well as those who have adenomyosis should be expected to have high failure rate following the procedure.

Thirty to forty percent of women who had EA had to undergo a repeat procedure in a four year follow up study. Resource utilization is less for EA procedures. Even though the initial hospital expense for EA is less than hysterectomy, the need for a repeat procedure in the follow up period of four years will nearly equalize the expense of both.

Non-resectoscopic Endometrial Ablation (NREA) - Second generation EA

EA using resectoscope has several disadvantages. The equipment is costly, the surgeon needs training and the use of distention medium carries with it problems which are already mentioned. To overcome these difficulties several methods of endometrial destruction without using resectoscope were developed. These devices are kept in the uterine cavity and the endometrium is destroyed using different types of energy sources. These techniques need less training, have fewer complication rates and can be performed in a shorter time. Even though chance of uterine perforation is less, it has been reported with these techniques also. Success rates reported are not inferior to resectoscopic methods. Following are the various non resectoscopic endometrial ablation methods.

Thermal balloon ablation: The procedure involves keeping a balloon in the endometrial cavity and distending the balloon with pre heated fluid. The fluid temperature is electronically controlled and maintained by a controlling unit. The earliest of such device is the Thermachoice system. The system comprises of a disposable balloon catheter of size 5.5 mm outer diameter, with a heating element inside. A connecting cable connects it to an electrically operated controller unit. . The balloon pressure, the fluid temperature and treatment duration can be set in the controller unit. 5% Dextrose is injected into the balloon. The temperature of dextrose is controlled by the controlling unit. The balloon temperature is maintained at 87°C at a pressure of 160-180 mm of mercury. The duration of treatment is eight minutes. Preoperative treatment with GnRH analogue or preoperative curettage improves the result of treatment. The procedure can be performed under local infiltration anesthesia or short general anesthesia. Compared to EA, complications like electrolyte imbalance and perforation of the uterus are almost nil in thermal ablation group.

Another device using thermal balloon is Caveterm Plus. The balloon in this device is made of flexible silicone.

Because of the flexibility, the balloon will approximate better to the endometrium. A pump maintains continuous flow of glycine to the balloon at a temperature of 75°C for a period of 15 minutes.

There have been randomized trials comparing endometrial ablation with thermal balloon ablation. Clinical outcome and patient satisfaction rates were similar for the two methods. Women with heavy menstrual bleeding due to submucous myomas were also found to benefit from thermal balloon ablation. A randomized trial involving 93 subjects compared thermal ablation with radio frequency endometrial ablation in women with type 2 myomas less than 50% diameter within the uterine cavity and up to 3 cm in size. Clinical outcome was similar in the 2 groups.

Microwave endometrial ablation: In this procedure endometrium is destroyed with microwave energy at a fixed frequency of 9.2 G Hz at an operating power of 42 W. This combination of power and frequency destroys the endometrium to a depth of 5-6 mm. One important complication of the procedure is perforation of the uterus with either the probe or the microwave energy which can lead on to inadvertent injury to the bowel. Amenorrhea rate of 53% and satisfaction rates of 87% has been reported.

Endometrial laser intrauterine thermo therapy procedure (ELITT): Generalized endometrial destruction is produced with a device consisting of multiple laser fibers. This was developed by Donez et al and Johns et al. Nd: YAG laser or diode laser is used for the procedure. The endometrium is destroyed to a depth of 6mm in 5 minutes.

Cryotherapy: In cryotherapy endometrium is destroyed using very low temperature (–90°C.)The device comprises of a probe of 4.5 mm outer diameter, which is passed in to the uterine cavity and a controller unit. When activated, a freeze zone 1.5 mm deep is produced. In 10 minutes the endometrium is destroyed. Clinical outcome is almost similar to RFEA (84.6% Vs 88%).

Thermal destruction with preheated fluid: Since thermal balloon cannot uniformly destroy the endometrium in women with distorted uterine cavity, devices which can destroy the endometrium with free fluid were dis-covered. One such device is Hydrothermablater (HTA). Free fluid is instilled into the uterine cavity under hysteroscopic guidance via a narrow disposable sheath of 2.7 to 3 mm diameter introduced through the operating channel of hysteroscope. The fluid inflow is controlled by a controller unit which can be attached to the sheath. The cervix is dilated and the telescope with a sheath is introduced into the uterine cavity. Fluid at 90 degree is instilled into the uterine cavity under a controlled pressure of less than 40 cm of water for a period of 3 minutes. For another 1 minute the fluid is allowed to cool and is then collected back through a closed system attached to the cervix.

Radiofrequency endometrial ablation (RFEA): This device uses radiofrequency energy for automated endometrial ablation. A single use 7.2 mm diameter probe is used to deliver bipolar current .The probe is attached to a microprocessor based control unit . The device available in the market is Novasure. No mechanical or medical thinning of the uterine cavity is required. The procedures can be carried out under local anesthesia with sedation .The probe is inserted into the uterine cavity after cervical dilatation. After insertion, the electrode is allowed to touch the endometrium by retracting the outer sheath. The electrode is activated for 80 to 90 seconds. The depth of desiccation is controlled automatically. Uterine cavity measuring up to 10 cm can be treated with this device .The 1 year satisfaction rates were recorded as 92.8.

Photodynamic therapy: With the help of a photosensitizer, the endometrium is destroyed by light of an appropriate wave length. 5 Aminolevulinic acid is the photosensitizer used.

Advantages of Endometrial Ablation (EA) over Hysterectomy

A Cochrane systematic review compared the randomized trials involving oral medical therapy, LNG-IUS, endometrial ablation and hysterectomy .Oral therapy can be persisted long term in a minority of women. LNG-IUS can be inserted in an office visit whereas REA or NREA need theatre setting. For women who have contraindication for medical treatment or who refuse medical treatment, endometrial ablation is the option, provided fertility preservation is not needed. For women who wish to preserve fertility, LNG-IUS should be preferred. The duration of surgery,hospital stay and recovery time were shorter for endometrial ablation than hysterectomy. Patient satisfaction rates were as high as 95% following hysterectomy compared to endometrial ablation.[9]

Hysterectomy

Heavy menstrual bleeding used to be a major cause for hysterectomy. But with the introduction of medical treatment including medicated intrauterine devices as well as minimally invasive procedures like endometrial ablation and uterine artery embolisation, the number of hysterectomies for the sole indication of heavy menstrual bleeding is gradually coming down.

For women who do not respond to medical or minimally invasive therapy, those who cannot tolerate medical therapy and those who have recurrence of symptoms following minimally invasive therapies, hysterectomy is the option.

6.9 AUB IN PERIMENOPAUSAL AGE GROUP

6.9.1 Etiology

Menstrual cycles become shortened and anovulatory as women approach menopause. Progesterone deficiency occurs in anovulatory cycles. Even in ovulatory cycles the estradiol levels will be less in premenopausal women. Malignant and premalignant lesions of the genital tract should be kept in mind in perimenopausal women. The causes can be DUB or benign or malignant lesions of the vulva, vagina, cervix, endometrium or ovary. About 20-25% of cancer of the endometrium occurs in premenopausal women. A rare cause is malignancy of the fallopian tube. The benign lesions can be endometritis, atrophic endometrium,uterine polyp or endometrial hyperplasia. Even though tuberculous endometritis commonly occurs in the child bearing age group, it rarely occurs in the postmenopausal age group and may present with postmenopausal bleeding. Uterine polyps can be fibroid polyps or endometrial polyps due to inflammation, hyperplasia or malignancy. Rare malignant tumors like mixed mullerian tumor can present as uterine polyps, which typically will be arising from the fundal region of the uterus . Women on HRT can have bleeding resulting from missed pills, medication interaction,or malabsorption.

History should elicit the regularity of period, period of amenorrhoea, amount of blood loss , presence of postcoital bleeding, bleeding while straining for stool, associated vaginal discharge etc. History of hormone intake should be elicited.

6.9.2 Examination

A complete general examination should be done to look for anemia and to exclude systemic and endocrine disorders which can cause abnormal bleeding. Abdominal examination should be done to look for masses. The vulva, vagina and the cervix should be examined carefully for any lesions. It should be kept in mind that bleeding from urethral caruncle, hemorrhoids etc can be mistaken for vaginal bleeding. Careful bimanual examination should be done to make out the consistency of the cervix, cervical enlargement, uterine enlargement and adnexal masses. Functioning ovarian tumors can be very small but cause irregular bleeding due to the associated endometrial hyperplasia or even malignancy.

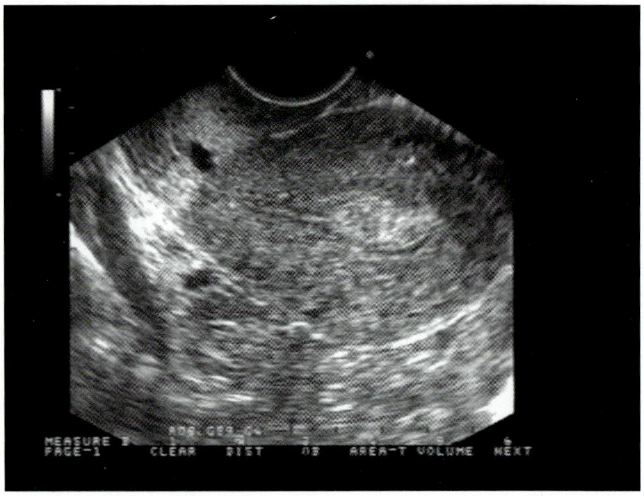

Fig. 6.14: Endometrial polyp in a 55-year-old lady who presented with postmenopausal bleeding

6.9.3 Investigations

Cervical smear should be examined if not done recently. The routine cervical smear should also include smear from endocervical canal with endocervical brush, so that endocervical malignancy and premalignant lesions are not missed. Transvaginal ultrasound should be done to evaluate the endometrium, endocervix, myometrium and adnexa.

TVS (Fig. 6.14)

In the absence of obvious lesions in the vulva, vagina and the cervix, pathology should be looked for in the endocervix, endometrium and adnexa. A detailed evaluation of the cervix, endometrium, myometrium and the adnexa should be done by transvaginal ultrasound. Depending upon the sonography findings an abnormal endometrium should be sampled. Women taking Tamoxifen should have endometrial evaluation by hysteroscopy if they happen to have abnormal bleeding. These women should have periodic endometrial evaluation by TVS even if asymptomatic and a higher cutoff of 9 mm should be taken as indication for biopsy. Suspected endometrial polyp can be delineated by sonohysterogram. However, hysteroscopy should be preferred, as both diagnosis as well as treatment can be done by hysteroscopy.

Endometrial Sampling

All perimenopausal or postmenopausal women who have abnormal bleeding should have endometrial sampling. However, if TVS shows the endometrial thickness to be < 4mm, with no irregularity and normal sub-endometrial halo, sampling may be deferred as chances of endometrial malignancy in such instances are negligible. But repeat episode of bleeding warrants endometrial sampling. The risk of recurrent bleeding is more in the presence of malignancy and less if the cause of bleeding is due to atrophic changes in the endometrium.

If endometrial thickness is > 4 mm, endometrium has to be sampled; the type of sampling (hysteroscopic or blind biopsy) is determined by the nature of the lesion (focal or diffuse) which has to be made out by saline infusion sonography.

Dilatation and curettage is not the preferred method of sampling the endometrium, especially in this age group, for fear of missing malignancy. Curettage prior to hysterectomy showed that endometrial lesions were missed in 10% of the patients. Sampling devices like Pipelle or the Vabra aspirator, which use negative pressure permits aspiration of tissue into the device, should be preferred over blind curettage. Complication rates are much less with the use of these methods. A comparison between Pipelle endometrial aspiration and curettage among postmenopausal women showed that, specimen adequate for histological diagnosis were obtained in 84.1% by Pipelle, whereas by curettage specimen was adequate in only 45%. Curettage as well as vacuum aspiration can miss focal lesions.

Hysteroscopy is better at diagnosing polyps, other benign lesions as well as malignancy. All suspicious areas should be biopsied during hysteroscopy. Mere visualization is unreliable for diagnosing malignancy. Hysteroscopy is associated with complications like perforation of the uterus, hemorrhage as well as anesthetic complications but these are much less in experienced hands.

6.9.4 Treatment

Management of malignant and premalignant lesions of the genital tract is discussed in the corresponding chapters.

Hysteroscopic removal is preferred for the management of endometrial polyps due to the less recurrence risk compared to removal using forceps. All polyps should be subjected to histopathological evaluation. If the pathological examination shows hyperplasia with atypia, hysterectomy should be advised to prevent malignancy.

Treatment of Anovulatory Bleeding

When no cause is found the bleeding may be anovulatory. If the woman has no contraindication for estrogen therapy, low dose estrogen containing COC pills can be prescribed. The woman on cyclic HRT who has irregular bleeding can be managed by increasing the dose of progesterone. If the bleeding is in the middle of the cycle, the estrogen dose can be increased. Most women on HRT will have irregular bleeding in the first 3-4 months and later the bleeding will abate. For those whose bleeding continues, HRT should be stopped and the woman should be re-evaluated. Women who have proliferative endometrium without atypia can be managed by either giving medroxyprogesterone 10 mg daily for 10 days a month or by cyclical medroxyprogesterone. The levonorgestrel IUS is effective in treating patients who have hyperplasia. Atypical hyperplasia warrants hysterectomy.

Those who continue to have recurrent bleeding should be advised hysterectomy even if no pathology is identified.

6.10 CONCLUSION

- Assessment of the severity of menorrhagia should be based on how much the symptoms affect the daily activities of the woman rather than the actual volume of bleeding.
- The basic investigations should include a blood count which is used to assess the severity of loss and also to form a basis for evaluation of the effectiveness of treatment.
- Disorders of coagulation should be suspected in girls presenting with abnormal bleeding in adolescence.
- Transvaginal scan should be done for all adult women who have abnormal bleeding to exclude uterine pathologies like polyps or submucus myomas.
- For women with cyclical bleeding a trial of antiprostaglandins and antifibrinolytic agents should be tried as initial treatment.
- Adolescent girls presenting with infrequent periods should be treated with progestagens for at least 10 days a month to reduce the long term sequels of chronic anovulation.
- Judicious use of TVS has reduced the need of invasive endometrial sampling procedures.
- The decision of invasive endometrial sampling must be taken liberally in the perimenopausal age group, whereas it must be done only rarely in adolescent age group either as a diagnostic or therapeutic modality.
- For acyclical and irregular bleeding, progesterone is the treatment of choice. Levonorgestrel intrauterine system has the maximum patient acceptance.
- Minimally invasive surgical techniques should be resorted to after proper patient counseling.
- Malignancy should be excluded in perimenopausal women who presents with AUB.
- Hysterectomy solely for menorrhagia should only be done as the last resort.

REFERENCES

1. DEvora GR,Owens KaselI'. Use of Premarin in the treatment of dysfunctional uterine bleeding- a double blind randomized control study. Obstet Gynaecol 1982;59:288.
2. Farquhar C, Ekeroma A, Furness S, et al. A systematic review of transvaginal ultrasonography sonohysterography and hysteroscopy for the investigation of abnormal uterine bleeding in premenopausal women, Acta Obstet Gynecol Scand 2003;82:493-504.
3. Haynes etal. Patterns of menstrual blood loss in menorrhagia. Research and Clinical Forums 1979;1:73-78.
4. Mark Livingstone and IanS Fraser Human reproduction update 2002;8(1):60-67.
5. van Dongen H, de Kroon CD, Jacobi CE, Trimbos JB, Jansen FW. Diagnostic hysteroscopy in abnormal uterine bleeding: a systematic review and meta-analysis. BJOG: an International Journal of Obstetrics and Gynaecology 2007;114(6):664-75.
6. Cochrane Database of Systematic Reviews 2007, Issue 4. Art. No.: CD001895. DOI: 10.1002/14651858. CD001895. pub2.
7. Decherney A, Polan ML. Hysterocopic management of intrauterine lesions and intracatable uterine bleeding. Obstet Gynaec 1983;61:392-39.
8. FraserIS, Healy DL, Torode H, SongJY, MAmers P, WildeF. Depot goserelin and danazol pretreatment before rollerball endometrial ablation for menorrhagia. Obstet Gynaecol 1996; 87:544-550
9. Lethaby A, Shepherd S,Cooke I, Faquhar C. Endometrial resection and ablation versus hysterectomy for heavy menstrual bleeding. Cochrane Database of Systematic reviews 1999, issue2. Art No: CD000329.DoI:10.1002/ 14651858.C000329.
10. Carlson et al. Transvaginal USS of the endometrium in women with PMB, Am J obstet Gynecol 1995;172:1 488-95.
11. Guido RS, et al. Pipelle endometrial sampling. Sensitivity in the detection of endometrial cancer. J Reprod Med 1995; 40:553-5.

7 Male Factor Infertility

K Jayakrishnan

7.1 INTRODUCTION

A gynecologist is often the first person to evaluate an infertile couple and is often expected to assess the male partner too. An understanding of the male reproductive function, its assessment and treatment modalities is expected of every practicing gynaecologist.

The male partner may contribute to 30-40 % cases of infertility and he may be solely responsible in 20 % of cases.[1] Introduction of micromanipulation techniques in the last decade has revolutionized the way male infertility is treated.[2]

This chapter aims to brush up the readers understanding of the anatomy and physiology of the male reproductive system and the methods of evaluating it. This will be followed by a discussion on the treatment modalities.

7.2 PHYSIOLOGY

The male reproductive organs (Fig. 7.1) are influenced by hormones secreted in the hypothalamus and the pituitary. Gonadotropin releasing hormone (GnRH) is released from the medial basal hypothalamus in a pulsatile pattern approximately every 70-90 minutes. The half-life of GnRH is 2-5 minutes. GnRH release is inhibited by testosterone and inhibin. Its secretion is also decreased by corticotropin-releasing hormone (CRH) and opiates. This is clinically evident at times of illness and stress, when there is a decreased production of gonadotropins.

Follicle stimulating hormone (FSH) and luteinizing hormone (LH) are glycopeptides secreted by the gonadotrops in the anterior pituitary in response to GnRH secretion. LH acts on the interstitial cells of Leydig to increase steroidogenesis (synthesis and secretion of testosterone and other androgens). LH release is controlled by the feedback of steroids from the testicle. FSH participates in protein synthesis and the initiation of spermatogenesis at the level of the seminiferous tubules in conjunction with testosterone. It stimulates the Sertoli cells to secrete inhibin. FSH release is controlled by the feedback of inhibin from the testicle. Androgens at physiological levels do not suppress FSH secretion. LH and FSH also control their own release by negative feedback to the hypothalamus. FSH binds to Leydig cells and increases the number of LH receptors on the cells.

Spermatogenesis (Fig. 7.2) occurs in the testes at the seminiferous tubules, which form most of the testis. Sertoli cells, which rest on the basement membrane of the seminiferous tubules, serve mainly to support, nourish and

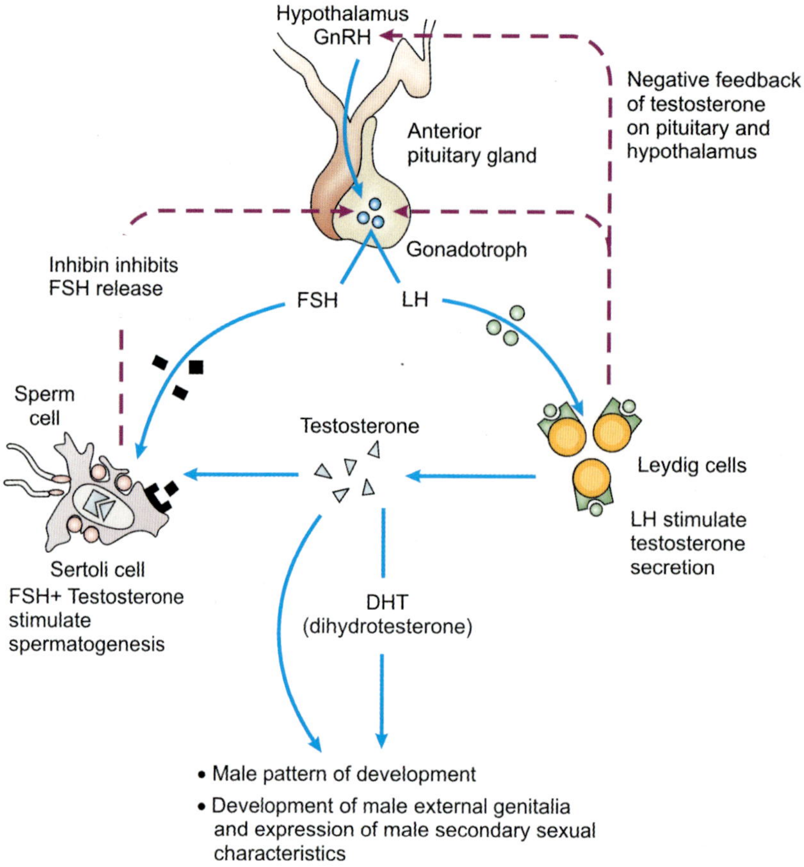

Fig. 7.1: Hormonal control of spermatogenesis and androgen production from the testis

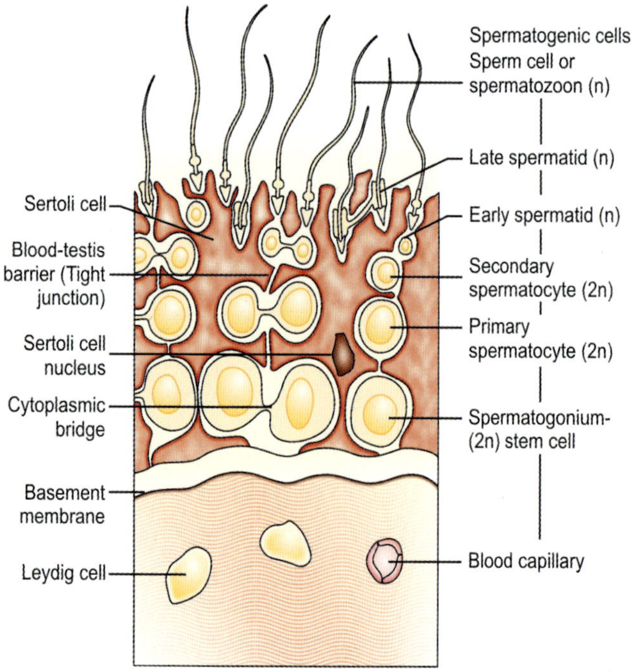

Fig. 7.2: Seminiferous tubules showing stages of sperm production

protect the developing germ cells. Spermatogonia undergo mitotic division to form the primary spermatocytes. They undergo meiotic division to form secondary spermatocytes. These secondary spermatocytes mature to become spermatids and undergo spermiogenesis to become spermatozoa. This involves casting excess cytoplasm away as a residual body, the formation of the acrosome and flagella, and the migration of cytoplasmic organelles to their final cellular location. These sperms travel to the epididymis before appearing in the ejaculate. Here they mature and acquire the capacity to fertilise. Sperms take around two to three weeks to traverse the epididymis. Sperms are stored near the tail portion and in the vas deferens until they are ejaculated. The whole process takes around 72-74 days. Semen is composed of secretions from the prostate, the vas deferens, the seminal vesicles, bulbourethral glands and the peri-urethral glands. The seminal vesicles contribute prostaglandins and fructose and are responsible for two-thirds of the volume of the ejaculate. The prostate contributes acid phosphatase, zinc and citric acid. Qualitative fructose is useful for verifying the presence of the vas deferens.

7.3 SEMEN AND ITS ANALYSIS

Semen is collected by masturbation after a period of abstinence of 2-3 days. A longer period of abstinence may show a lower sperm count. Semen should be collected in a wide mouthed, dry and clean container and should be brought to the laboratory within one hour of collection. Till then it should be kept at a temperature close to the body temperature. For those uncomfortable with collecting semen by masturbation, it should be collected in a non-toxic sheath. Condoms should not be used. The WHO reference values for semen analysis are described in Table 7.1.[3] [IV]

Semen consists of spermatozoa and seminal plasma from the accessory glands. Before being able to fertilize the ovum, liquefaction of semen, capacitation of sperm and the acrosome reaction must occur. Semen normally liquefies in 20 to 30 minutes. Semen might be abnormally viscid and may take a longer time for liquefaction. Analysis may be performed after repeatedly pushing the semen through a No 19 needle. If the post coital test is negative, such abnormal semen might be implicated as a cause for infertility and intrauterine insemination might be helpful.

Before going into further parameters of a semen analysis, it must be understood that the WHO criteria are described as 'reference' values rather than 'normal' values. Variations in reports might be seen between samples from the same person, in the same sample when analyzed by two different persons and even when analyzed by the same person at two different occasions. Automated methods have not been able to correct this problem. Though computer-aided semen analysis (CASA) produces good qualitative data, it is a labor-intensive procedure that includes a high initial cost and is plagued with inaccuracies when sperm concentrations are very high or very low. Hence it is important to understand that a better picture might be obtained only by repeated testing. Semen analysis is usually performed after an interval of two to four weeks, even though the optimal time for checking a second sample is at least three months after the initial study [III]. Another important aspect is that a person who has semen parameters below the 'normal' values might not be infertile and fertile men do occasionally have values in the 'abnormal' range. Individual tests evaluate only one aspect of a quality necessary for fertility and do not imply the ability or inability to achieve conception. Table 7.2 summarizes causes of abnormal semen parameters.

Assessment of sperm morphology may vary from one laboratory to another. Most andrology laboratories follow the "strict" or the Tygerberg criteria[4] which has been mentioned in the latest WHO recommendations.[3] Though it classifies even minor abnormalities as 'abnormal sperms', it has a better co-relation with fertilization and pregnancy rates at IVF and other ART procedures. Results were more reproducible when the strict criteria were adopted. When the routine criteria are followed, 30% or more sperms should be of normal morphology.

Table 7.1: Semen analysis: Normal reference values (WHO, 2000)

Parameter	Value
Volume	$\geq$ 2.0 ml
Liquefaction time	Within 60 minutes
pH	$\geq$ 7.2
Sperm concentration	$\geq$ 20 million/mL
Total sperm number	$\geq$ 40 million/ejaculate
Percent motility	$\geq$ 50% (grade A and B) or $\geq$ 25% grade A (within 60 minutes of ejaculation)
Normal morphology	15% or 30%
Vitality	75% or more live sperms
White blood cells	< 1 million/mL

Grade A: rapid progressive motility
Grade B: slow or sluggish progressive motility
30%; or 15% if based on strict morphological criteria

7.4 SPERM FUNCTION TESTS

Many tests have been used to study sperm function as semen analysis gives an idea about the sperm quality only. Most tests try to assess a particular function of the sperm. These tests are more of academic interest and are not commonly performed even at specialized infertility centers; as most of them are cumbersome, do not provide a clear prognosis, may not be standardized and sometimes not very specific [IV]. The more important sperm function tests are elaborated in Table 7.3.

Intrauterine insemination is currently used for the treatment of infertility in unexplained as well as those due to immunological causes. Empirical treatment with corticosteroids is therefore not recommended now. Considering the above facts, testing for immunological causes of infertility itself is controversial.

7.5 HISTORY TAKING AND EXAMINATION

A careful history might be useful in pointing out the cause for infertility. The duration of infertility and details regarding prior workup and treatment should be asked for. Enquiries regarding previous medical and surgical problems,

Table 7.2: Abnormalities in semen parameters

Parameter	Causes	Comments
Reduced semen volume	Short period of abstinence Spillage of sample Retrograde ejaculation Absence of the vas deferens or seminal vesicles Ductal obstruction Hypogonadotropism	Post-ejaculation urine microscopy Trans-rectal USG Hormonal evaluation
Increased semen volume	Prolonged abstinence Accessory gland inflammation Contamination with urine	Semen culture Antibiotics
Semen that does not coagulate	Ejaculatory duct obstruction Absence of seminal vesicles	Trans-rectal USG Semen fructose
Reduced sperm concentration (oligospermia)	Idiopathic (most common) Accessory gland infection Chemotherapy Cryptorchidism	Physical examination for varicocele Anti-sperm antibody evaluation Hormonal analysis Trans-rectal USG
Decreased motility (asthenospermia)	Drugs Endocrine Environmental toxins	Toxins include pesticides, lead, carbon disulfide
Increased morphologically abnormal sperms (teratospermia)	Epididymal causes Increased scrotal temperature Occupational Radiation Smoking Systemic illnesses Varicocele	Drugs which may affect semen parameters include spironolactone, cyproterone, ketoconazole, cimetidine, tetracycline, nitrofurantoin, sulfasalazine, colchicine, methadone, methotrexate, phenytoin, thioridazine and calcium channel blockers
Azoospermia	Obstructive azoopermia • Congenital bilateral absence of vas deferens (CBAVD) • Vasectomy • Infective causes Non obstructive azoospermia • Klinefelter's syndrome • Young syndrome • Cryptorchidism • Chemotherapy • Radiation	Examination Serum FSH levels Semen fructose Karyotyping Sperm centrifuged to verify azoospermia Post-ejaculation urine (retrograde ejaculation) Hormonal evaluation Testicular biopsy (testicular failure) Trans-rectal USG (ejaculatory duct obstruction) CBAVD – evaluate for cystic fibrosis mutations and renal tract abnormality
Increased in WBCs	Prostatitis May be mistaken for immature sperm cells	Increased round cells may reflect poor prognosis of fertilization

chemotherapy, radiation, use of therapeutic and recreational drugs, smoking and alcohol intake should be made. Ask for any history of trauma or surgery to the testes and testicular involvement during mumps. It is also important to enquire about the sexual habits of the couple. The frequency of sexual intercourse and problems related to erection and ejaculation should be specifically asked or they are likely to be missed.

Following a general and systemic examination, local examination of the genitals should be performed. Look for

Table 7.3: Sperm function tests

Test	Description
Sperm penetration assay or Zona free hamster oocyte test (SPA)	Tests the ability of sperm to penetrate the egg. Patients with a poor SPA should proceed directly to ICSI.
Human zona binding assay	Tests zona penetrating or zona binding ability of human sperm.
Hypo-osmotic swelling test	Assessment of functional disturbance of the tail membrane to differentiate between viable but immotile sperm and dead sperm. Used clinically to select viable (but nonmotile) sperm for ICSI.
Capacitation assay	To evaluate the ability of sperm to undergo capacitation, Sperm that do not undergo capacitation portend a poor response to IVF, and ICSI should be considered.
Acrosome reaction	Tests the ability of the sperm to undergo the acrosome reaction when exposed to inducing substances. Results correlate with IVF success; abnormal test require ICSI.
Postcoital test	Effect of cervical mucus on sperm viability and function
Test for sperm antibodies	Immunobead test Mixed agglutination test (SpermMar)

anatomical abnormalities of the penis; presence, size, and consistency of the testicles and palpate the epididymis, vas deferens and the spermatic cord. To check for the presence of a varicocele, the patient should perform a Valsalva manoeuvre in the sitting and standing positions in a warm room. Grade 1 varicocele is defined as one palpable only with Valsalva, while grade 2 is palpable at standing, and grade 3 is visible at rest.

7.6 TREATMENT

Encourage patients to stop smoking cigarettes [IIb] and to limit environmental exposure to harmful substances and/or conditions. Stress relief therapy and consultation of other appropriate psychological and social professionals may be advised. Broad management protocols are outlined first while management of specific conditions is elaborated later.

7.6.1 Medical Management

Treatment of disorders diagnosed during evaluation should be undertaken. This would include correction of endocrine disorders like hyperprolactinemia, thyroid disorders, etc. Infections should be treated with antibiotics [Ib]. Counseling and medications like sildenafil may be required for patients with erectile dysfunction [Ia]. Retrograde ejaculation may be treated with imipramine or alpha-sympathomimetics, such as pseudoephedrine. If medical treatment of retrograde ejaculation fails, the use of penile electrovibration stimulation and sperm recovery from the urine can be considered.

A variety of empirical treatments have been used in an attempt to improve semen characteristics and fertility. The use of such medications for improving semen parameters is controversial. Clomiphene citrate which increases serum levels of FSH, LH and testosterone may improve the total sperm count but has not yet been proven to increase pregnancy rates when compared with those who receive no treatment.[5][Ia]. The use of androgens like mesterolone and testosterone undecanoate has no difference when compared to placebo in the treatment of patients with oligoasthenospermia[6,7] [Ia]. Human chorionic gonadotropin has been used in a dose of 2500 IU twice weekly for 6 – 8 weeks in men with hypogonadism[8] [II] and those with isolated Leydig cell dysfunction.[9] Its use in normogonadotropic oligozoospermia though is not effective[10] [Ib]. Antioxidants like vitamin C and E, selenium and glutathione have shown some promise in improving semen parameters but further studies are required[11-13] [Ib]. Other commonly prescribed drugs like L carnitine, co enzyme Q derivatives, N acetyl cysteine and arginine may have shown improvement in semen parameters in some studies but good evidence regarding improvement in pregnancy rates is lacking.

7.6.2 Surgical Management

Surgical correction of penile deformities is sometimes required. The most common surgical procedure is that for correcting a varicocele. A varicocele is an abnormal tortuosity and dilatation of the veins of the pampiniform plexus within the spermatic cord. It is more commonly seen in the left side, because of the insertion of the vein into the renal vein in contrast to the right side where it drains into the inferior vena cava. Varicoceles are seen in 20-40 % of infertile males and in 10-15 % of fertile men! Rise in testicular temperature, reflux of toxic metabolites from the renal vein and germ cell hypoxia have been attributed as a cause of infertility in patients with varicocele. Surgical correction by open or laparoscopic route is possible. Whether surgery results in higher fertility is controversial. Studies showing improvement in fertility[14,15] and no differences abound[16-21] Though evidence based on clinical trials lacks support for varicocelectomy [Ia], most clinicians will recommend surgical correction if varicoceles are diagnosed by examination[22] Surgical correction of varicocele diagnosed purely by scrotal ultrasound probably would not improve fertility.

Men who desire to have children after vasectomy may be offered microsurgical vasovasostomy or vasoepididymostomy. Success rates for couples with female partner aged 40 or older was lower than for those with the female partner aged 39 or younger (14% vs. 56%).[23] Patients with a known or suspected obstruction of the ejaculatory ducts may be eligible for a transurethral resection of the ejaculatory ducts (TURED) [III]. Recovery and cryopreservation of spermatozoa for use in assisted reproduction should be considered during surgical reconstruction to avoid a second surgical procedure at a later date.

7.6.3 Intrauterine Insemination

This involves placement of processed semen into the uterine cavity. Intrauterine insemination (IUI) allows the sperm to be placed past the inhospitable cervical mucus and increases the chance of natural fertilization. IUI involves placement of 0.3 to 0.5 ml of semen which is processed by various techniques using a very thin flexible catheter via the transcervical route into the uterine cavity. IUI is indicated in male factor infertility, in those with anti-sperm antibodies, infertility due to cervical factors and in cases of unexplained infertility. Placement of unprocessed semen into the uterine cavity is not practiced as prostaglandins and proteins in semen can cause uterine cramping and occasionally allergic reactions.

Processing of semen aims to obtain a sperm population of uniform morphology and good motility, devoid of dead sperm, miscellaneous cellular elements and seminal plasma which is re-suspended in a medium. The commonly used methods are described. In conventional washing, semen is washed and centrifuged in commercial media, the supernatant discarded and the pellet overlaid with media again. This process may be repeated 2-3 times. After the final wash, the pellet is re-suspended in media and used for IUI. Such a technique is used with near normal samples. Alternatively in the swim up technique, following sperm preparation by the conventional method, the tube is incubated and sperms 'swim-up' from the pellet to the overlaying media, which is then used for insemination. Such inseminates have lesser levels of contamination from dead sperms and cellular debris. The gradient method involves centrifugation through a dense liquid phase (density gradient). Commercially available gradient media are overlaid with semen and subjected to centrifugation. Motile sperm cells migrate to the bottom of the tube, which are used for IUI after further washing. The swim up and gradient density techniques have better results than the conventional method, the gradient density technique being used when the sperm concentration is lower and the number of dead and abnormal cells are high.

IUI is usually combined with superovulation of the female partner [Ib]. Follicular monitoring with transvaginal sonography is followed by an ovulation trigger with hCG. Some centers time IUI after a natural LH surge identified by a urinary LH kit.

Protocols regarding timing and number of IUIs performed vary. When a single IUI is performed, it may be performed 36 hours following the administration of hCG. Those centers which advocate two IUIs usually space them at least 12 hours apart, between 24 and 48 hours after the administration of hCG. Both protocols have their advocates, with studies showing either no difference in pregnancy rates[24, 25] or a significant increase.[26] The Cochrane review states that double intrauterine insemination showed no significant benefit over single intrauterine insemination in the treatment of sub-fertile couples with husband semen [Ia].[27]

Success rates per cycle in different studies vary from 8 to 30 %. Variables which determine success rates depend on semen parameters (total number of sperms per inseminate and morphology), method of preparation, age and presence of uterine, tubal or ovarian pathology in the female partner and the use of medications for superovulation.[28-30] IUI is more successful in unexplained infertility than in pure male factor infertility. A couple may be offered 3-6 cycles of super-ovulation with IUI before moving to assisted reproductive technologies. Generally, IUIs are performed if the total inseminate contains more than 1 million sperms. If this is not achieved, an early recourse to ICSI should be made.

7.6.4 Donor Insemination

Therapeutic donor insemination (TDI) is useful in patients with azoospermia or severe oligospermia, when ICSI is not possible or desired. This may be in cases of non-obstructive azoospermia; when there is a possibility of a disease being transmitted from the male partner (inherited, sexually transmitted) or due to financial reasons.

Donor semen available from sperm banks should be collected from healthy young donors after screening by history and appropriate laboratory test for transmittable diseases (HIV, hepatitis B, hepatitis C, syphilis, gonorrhea, chlamydia, and cytomegalovirus) [IV]. Semen thus obtained is cryopreserved. Tests which may become positive after an incubation period should be repeated and only then semen should be made available for TDI (e.g. HIV, which should be tested after 6 months). A freeze and thaw cycle results in sperms which are of an inferior quality compared to a fresh sample [Ib]. Success rates up to 30 % per cycle have been reported. TDI may be performed for 6 to 12 months [III]. If conception does not occur, the female partner should be assessed.

7.6.5 Assisted Reproductive Technologies (ART)

ART involves fertilization of the human oocyte by human sperm in vitro. In in-vitro fertilization (IVF), oocytes are obtained following controlled ovarian hyperstimulation followed by ultrasound guided transvaginal aspiration. Semen is washed in a way similar to that before an IUI and 50,000 to 100,000 capacitated sperms are placed in culture with a single oocyte. Fertilization is assessed after 16 to 20 hours and embryos are transferred in to the uterine cavity between days 2 to 5.

IVF was very useful in cases of male factor infertility, but what really revolutionized treatment in severe male factor infertility was intracytoplasmic sperm injection (ICSI). This involves micromanipulation techniques to inject a viable sperm into the ooplasm of the egg. After cumulus and corona cell removal (denudation), oocytes are used for microinjection. ICSI is carried out on metaphase II oocytes. Motile sperms are selected and immobilised under an inverted microscope equipped with micromanipulators and microinjectors. The microinjectors are used to either fix or release the oocyte with the holding pipette, or to aspirate and inject a spermatozoon with the injection pipette. The oocyte is held in position by means of minimal suction by the holding pipette. The oocyte is manipulated so that the polar body is located at the six o' clock position, which avoids damage to the spindle. The oolemma is ruptured using the injection needle and the sperm is released into the oocyte. ICSI is also useful in azoospermia when sperm can be retrieved from the testes or the epididymis. Sperms can be collected from the epididymis by microsurgical epididymal sperm aspiration (MESA) or percutaneous epididymal sperm aspiration (PESA). The latter might be a less invasive procedure, but the number of sperms obtained is less and pregnancy rates slightly lower [III]. Testicular sperm is obtained by open microsurgical testicular sperm extraction (TESE) or testicular sperm aspiration (TESA). Both open procedures might provide for more quantity of sperms which can be cryopreserved for future use. Fresh and frozen–thawed spermatozoa appear to have comparable fertilization and ongoing pregnancy rates when used for ICSI. Fertilisation and pregnancy rates in pure male factor infertility depend on the etiology. The rates are lower in patients with testicular when compared to post-testicular causes.

An area of concern has been about the possibility of congenital malformation in children conceived following ART. Current evidence showed higher risk of major malformations in IVF and ICSI children compared to spontaneously conceived children, but there were no significant differences in the risk when IVF and ICSI were compared.

7.7 AZOOSPERMIA AND ITS MANAGEMENT

Absence of sperm in the ejaculate is seen in 1% of all men.[31] Azoospermia has been traditionally classified into 'obstructive' and 'non-obstructive'. Because of overlapping and confusion with respect to certain etiologies, azoospermia is currently divided into causes due to deficient hormonal stimulation of the testis, testicular dysfunction, and seminal ducts obstruction or dysfunction -pre-testicular, testicular, and post-testicular causes respectively (Table 7.4).[32]

Management of azoospermia depends on the cause. In pre-testicular azoospermia, low levels of gonadotropins (LH and FSH) and testosterone are seen. Treatment involves pulsatile GnRH therapy or sequential therapy with hCG (1,000-2,500 IU twice a week) followed by hMG (150 IU three times weekly) after serum testosterone and estradiol levels are back in the normal range. In testicular azoospermia,

Table 7.4: Causes of azoospermia

Type	*Causes*
Pre-testicular	• Hypogonadotropic hypogonadism • Congenital (Kallmann's syndrome, Noonan syndrome) • Acquired (trauma, tumor) • Idiopathic.
Testicular	• Congenital (Klinefelter's syndrome, Y-deletion) • Acquired (radiotherapy, chemotherapy, torsion, mumps, orchitis) • Developmental (testicular maldescent)
Post-testicular	• Ductal obstruction • Dysfunction (retrograde ejaculation)

LH and FSH levels are elevated and serum levels of testosterone are low. Testicular biopsy and karyotyping is indicated. Testicular azoospermia can be treated if spermatozoa are obtained from the testes for ICSI. ICSI is also indicated in post-testicular azoospermia. Exceptions include patients who have undergone vasectomy who can initially opt for a reversal surgical procedure; and in retrograde ejaculation, where sperms obtained from urine can be used for IUI or ART depending on the yield.

Truly azoospermic patients should be evaluated for ejaculatory duct obstruction by TRUS (Transrectal ultrasound). TRUS is indicated in patients with azoospermia or severe oligospermia to rule out a complete or partial ejaculatory duct obstruction. TRUS is also useful to evaluate the presence of seminal vesicles. Those patients with ejaculatory duct obstruction are candidates for transurethral resection of the ejaculatory ducts

REFERENCES

1. Thonneau P, Marchand S, Tallec A, Ferial ML, Ducot B, Lansac J, Lopes P, Tabaste JM, Spira A. Incidence and main causes of infertility in a resident population (1,850,000) of three French regions (1988-1989). Hum Reprod 1991;6:811-6.
2. Palermo G, Joris H, Devroey P, Van Steirteghem AC. Pregnancies after intracytoplasmic injection of single spermatozoon into an oocyte. Lancet 1992;340:17-18.
3. World Health Organization. WHO Laboratory Manual for the Examination of Human Semen and Sperm Cervical Mucus Interaction. Cambridge: Cambridge University Press; 2000.
4. Kruger TF, Menkveld R, Stander FS, Lombard CJ, Van der Merwe JP, van Zyl JA, Smith K. Sperm morphologic features as a prognostic factor in in vitro fertilization. Fertil Steril 1986;46:1118-23.
5. World Health Organization. A double–blind trial of clomiphene citrate for the treatment of idiopathic male infertility. Int J Androl 1992;7:1067-72.
6. Gerris J, Comhaire F, Hellemans P, Peeters K, Schoonjans F. Placebo-controlled trial of high-dose Mesterolone treatment of idiopathic male infertility Fertil Steril 1991;55:603-7.
7. Mesterolone and idiopathic male infertility: a double-blind study. World Health Organization Task Force on the Diagnosis and Treatment of Infertility. Int J Androl 1989;12:254-64.
8. European Metrodin HP Study Group Efficacy and safety of highly purified urinary follicle-stimulating hormone with human chorionic gonadotropin for treating men with isolated hypogonadotropic hypogonadism Fertil Steril 1998; 70:256-62.
9. Yamamoto M, Hibi H, Katsuno S, Miyake K. Human chorionic gonadotropin adjuvant therapy for patients with Leydig cell dysfunction after varicocelectomy. Arch Androl 1995;35:49-55.
10. Schill WB, Jungst D, Unterburger P, Braun S. Combined hMG/hCG treatment in subfertile men with idiopathic normogonadotrophic oligozoospermia. Int J Androl 1982;5:467-77.
11. Scott R, MacPherson A, Yates RW, Hussain B, Dixon J. The effect of oral selenium supplementation on human sperm motility. Br J Urol 1998;82:76-80.
12. Suleiman SA, Ali ME, Zaki ZM, el-Malik EM, Nasr MA. Lipid peroxidation and human sperm motility: protective role of vitamin E. J Androl 1996;17:530-7.
13. Lenzi A, Culasso F, Gandini L, Lombardo F, Dondero F. Placebo-controlled, double-blind, cross-over trial of glutathione therapy in male infertility. Hum Reprod 1993;8:1657-62.
14. Madgar I, Weissenberg R, Lunenfeld B, Karasik A, Goldwasser B. Controlled trial of high spermatic vein ligation for varicocele in infertile men. Fertil Steril 1995;63:120-24.
15. Matthews GJ, Matthews ED, Goldstein M, Induction of spermatogenesis and achievement of pregnancy after microsurgical varicocelectomy in men with azoospermia and severe oligoasthenospermia. Fertil Steril 1998;70:71.
16. Baker HWG, Burger HG, de Kretser DM, Hudson B, Rennie GC, Straffon WGE, Testicular vein ligation and fertility in men with varicoceles, Br Med J 1985;291:1678-80.
17. Kamischke A, Nieschlag E. Analysis of medical treatment of male infertility. Hum Reprod 1999;14(suppl 1): 1-23.
18. Nilsson S, Edvinsson A, Nilsson B. Improvement of semen and pregnancy rate after ligation and division of the internal spermatic vein: fact or fiction? Br J Urol 1979;51:591-96.
19. Breznik R, Vlaisavljevic V, Borko E. Treatment of varicocele and male infertility. Arch Androl 1993;30:157-60.
20. Yamamoto M, Hibi H, Hirata Y, Miyake K, Ishigaki T. Effects of varicocelectomy on sperm parameters and pregnancy rate in patients with subclinical varicocele: a randomized prospective controlled study. J Urol 1996;155:1636-38.
21. Nieschlag E, Hertle L, Fischedick A, Abshagen K, Behre HM. Update on treatment of varicocele: counseling as effective as occlusion of the vena spermatica. Hum Reprod 1998;13:2147-50.
22. Agarwal A, Deepinder F, Cocuzza M, Agarwal R, Short R, Sabanegh E, Marmar J. Efficacy of Varicocelectomy in Improving Semen Parameters: New Meta-analytical Approach. Urology 2007;70:532-8.
23. Gerrard ER Jr, Sandlow JI, Oster RA, Burns JR, Box LC, Kolettis PN. Effect of female partner age on pregnancy rates after vasectomy reversal. Fertil Steril 2007;87:1340-4.

24. Ransom MX, Blotner MB, Bohrer M, Corsan G, Kemmann E. Does increasing frequency of intrauterine insemination improve pregnancy rates significantly during superovulation cycles? Fertil Steril 1994;61:303-7.
25. Alborzi S, Motazedian S, Parsanezhad ME, Jannati S. Comparison of the effectiveness of single intrauterine insemination (IUI) versus double IUI per cycle in infertile patients. Fertil Steril 2003;80:595-9.
26. Ragni G, Maggioni P, Guermandi E, Testa A, Baroni E, Colombo M, Crosignani PG. Efficacy of double intrauterine insemination in controlled ovarian hyperstimulation cycles. Fertil Steril 1999;72:619-22.
27. Cantineau AEP, Heineman MJ, Cohlen BJ. Single versus double intrauterine insemination (IUI) in stimulated cycles for subfertile couples. Cochrane Database of Systematic Reviews 2003, Issue 1. Art. No.: CD003854. DOI: 10.1002/14651858.CD003854.
28. Sunde A, Kahn J, Molne K. Intrauterine insemination: A European collaborative report. Hum Reprod 1988;3(Suppl 2):69-73.
29. Guzick DS, Carson SA, Coutifaris C, Overstreet JW, Factor-Litvak P, Steinkampf MP, Hill JA, Mastroianni L, Jr., Buster JE, Nakajimi ST, Vogel DL, Canfield RE, for the National Cooperative Reproductive Medicine Network. Efficacy of superovulation and intrauterine insemination in the treatment of infertility. New Engl J Med 1999;340:177-83.
30. Botchan A, Hauser R, Gamzu R, Yogev L, Paz G, Yavetz H. Results of 6139 artificial insemination cycles with donor spermatozoa. Hum Reprod 2001;16:2298-2304.
31. Willott GM. Frequency of azoospermia. Forensic Sci Int 1982;20:9-10. 32.Sharif K. Reclassification of azoospermia: the time has come? Hum Reprod 2000;15:237-38.

LEVELS OF EVIDENCE

Ia Systematic review and meta-analysis of randomized controlled trials Ib At least one randomized controlled trial IIa At least one well-designed controlled study without randomization IIb At least one other type of well-designed quasi-experimental study III Well-designed non-experimental descriptive studies, such as comparative studies, correlation studies or case studies IV Expert committee reports or opinions and/or clinical experience of respected authorities.

INFORMATION RESOURCES

1. Indian Council of Medical Research, National Academy of Medical Sciences (India). National guidelines for accreditation, supervision and regulation of ART clinics in India. New Delhi: Ministry of health and family welfare, government of India; 2005. [Guidelines for ART clinics in India]
2. www.icmr.nic.in/art/Chapter_4.pdf [consent forms for IUI/TDI and IVF]

8 Female Factor Infertility

B Presannakumari

8.1 INTRODUCTION

The prevalence of infertility is estimated to range from 13.3 to 15%. Even though the prevalence has not increased over the past few decades, the demand for infertility care is on the rise owing to changing lifestyles. Deliberate delay in child bearing also contributes in part to this increase.

Population data suggests that among the couples experiencing infertility, half will subsequently conceive without treatment. About 50% of those who do not conceive will be having primary inability to conceive and the rest will be having secondary infertility. The chance of spontaneous conception is influenced by duration of infertility, previous pregnancies and the cause of infertility.

8.2 DEFINITIONS

Infertility is defined as inability to conceive after one year of unprotected intercourse. Infertility can be classified as primary infertility where no pregnancy has ever occurred or secondary infertility where a pregnancy has occurred in the past, not necessarily resulting in a live birth. *Fecundability* is the probability of becoming pregnant within a single menstrual cycle and fecundity is the probability of achieving live birth within a single menstrual cycle. The normal conception expected is 84% in 12 months and 92% in 24 months.[1]

Adapted from Templeton et al Management of infertility for the MRCOG and beyond. The past few decades have seen tremendous advances in the diagnostic modalities and the management of the different factors contributing to infertility. Presently, treatment of infertility is rewarding. The success rate following treatment of anovulatory infertility has seen great improvement with advances in ultrasonography and ovulation inducing drugs. With advances in endoscopic surgery, the diagnosis and success rate of treatment for infertility due to endometriosis and

Table 8.1: Diagnostic categories of infertility

Factors	Primary (%)	Secondary (%)
Anovulation	20	15
Male factor	25	20
Tubal	15	40
Endometriosis	10	5
Unexplained	30	20

pelvic inflammatory disease (PID) too are much better than before. With the evolution of hysteroscopic surgery, endometrial pathologies like uterine septa, submucus fibroids, polyps and intrauterine adhesions also can be treated with high success rate. The final answer to the treatment of male infertility has evolved in the form of intracytoplasmic sperm injection (ICSI). The abnormal cervical factor and the damaged fallopian tubes are bypassed by ART procedures.

The important factors contributing to infertility (Table 8.1) include male factor, ovulatory disorders, tubal damage including blocks as well as peri-tubal adhesions which may be due to pelvic inflammatory disease or endometriosis, uterine factors like fibroids, uterine anomalies, infections like tuberculosis, coital problems, cervical factors and immunological factors. In spite of all investigations, infertility remains unexplained in 10-30% of couples. Even though the etiologies of primary and secondary infertility are the same, their proportion varies. Usually a single factor is identified but different causes can coexist like male factor along with anovulation or male factor along with endometriosis or two different female factors.

8.3 APPROACH TO A COUPLE WITH INFERTILITY (FIG. 8.1)

8.3.1 History

The couple seeking treatment for infertility will be emotionally distressed and most of them might have had previous work up and treatment. They should be approached with concern and both partners should be evaluated together. A very careful history about medical, surgical and gynecological aspects forms the basis of the evaluation. History about outcome of previous conceptions, history suggestive of pelvic inflammatory disease, intrauterine manipulations, pelvic surgery, etc. should be elicited. A detailed menstrual history will give a clue as to whether the cycles are ovulatory or not. Regular cycles with mid menstrual pain, discharge and premenstrual symptoms are pointers to an ovulatory cycle. History of severe dysmenorrhea which begins a few days prior to the periods and gets aggravated as the period progresses is the most common symptom of endometriosis. Both partners should be interrogated individually and together regarding coital problems. The male partner should be asked about previous history of developmental defects, genital trauma, past genital surgery, infections like mumps and also about chronic medications. Occupational history of both partners especially the male partner should be elicited. An enquiry into the history suggestive of systemic diseases which can contribute to infertility, like endocrine disorders, collagen vascular diseases, etc. should be made. Family history of premature ovarian failure, hereditary disorders etc. have a bearing on pre-conceptional counseling. It is of utmost importance to win the confidence of the couple through patient hearing and an empathetic but pleasant approach.

8.3.2 Examination

A proper history will give a clue to the cause of infertility in most of the situations. Irregular and infrequent periods suggest anovulation. Endometriosis should be suspected in a woman who has severe dysmenorrhea. Pelvic adhesions should be anticipated in a woman who had previous abdominal or pelvic surgery like appendicectomy. These points in the history should be kept in mind while examining the patient.

General examination (Table 8.2) of the female partner gives important clues especially in ovulatory dysfunction.

Table 8.2: Clinical examination

General examination
- Height, weight, BMI
- Thyroid-enlargement
- Breast-Tanner stage, galactorrhea
- Hyperandrogenism-hirsutism, frontal baldness, acne

Abdominal examination
- Abdominal mass
- Hirsutism

Gynecological examination
- Pubic hair
- Vulva clitoromegaly
- Speculum examination—Mullerian anomalies of vagina and cervix

Vaginal infections

Cervicitis
- Bluish nodules (endometriosis)
- Bimanual examination—size and mobility of uterus, nodules in the pouch of Douglas, adnexal masses

The typical polycystic ovary syndrome patient will be obese, hirsute, and may or may not have galactorrhoea. If she has secondary amenorrhea and/or galactorrhea, features of Cushing's syndrome, pituitary disorders, and of other endocrine dysfunctions should be looked for. The normality of the secondary sexual characters should be determined, for rarely one may encounter a 'woman' presenting with infertility who is actually having androgen insensitivity syndrome! The vulva, vagina and cervix should be examined for signs of infection, congenital anomalies, evidence of endometriosis like bluish nodules etc. A careful bimanual examination should be performed to elicit tenderness of the uterus and adnexal structures, enlargement or displacements of the uterus and nodules or masses in the fornices. *TVS cannot replace bimanual examination.*

8.3.3 Investigations

Even though investigations for infertility are usually started after the couple had unprotected intercourse for one year, *the couple should be evaluated whenever they feel like having a fertility problem.* Targeted investigations should be done when the history and clinical examination point toward the existence of a problem. For example if the female partner complains of severe dysmenorrhoea and dyspareunia and has clinical features of pelvic disease like endometriosis or PID, investigations should be planned early. For the couple who has no significant abnormality made out from the history and physical examination, explaining the normal pattern of conception, advice about fertile period and lifestyle modification would be enough.

Indications for Laparoscopy as Initial Investigation

- History and clinical examination suggestive of endometriosis
- History and examination suggestive of PID
- History of pelvic/abdominal surgery eg. appendicectomy

Based on the history and clinical examination, the investigations can be channeled. All investigations for infertility cannot be done at the same period of the menstrual cycle. Tubal patency should be tested in the immediate post-menstrual period. Follicular tracking for ovulation detection should be started on the ninth day. Semen analysis is done

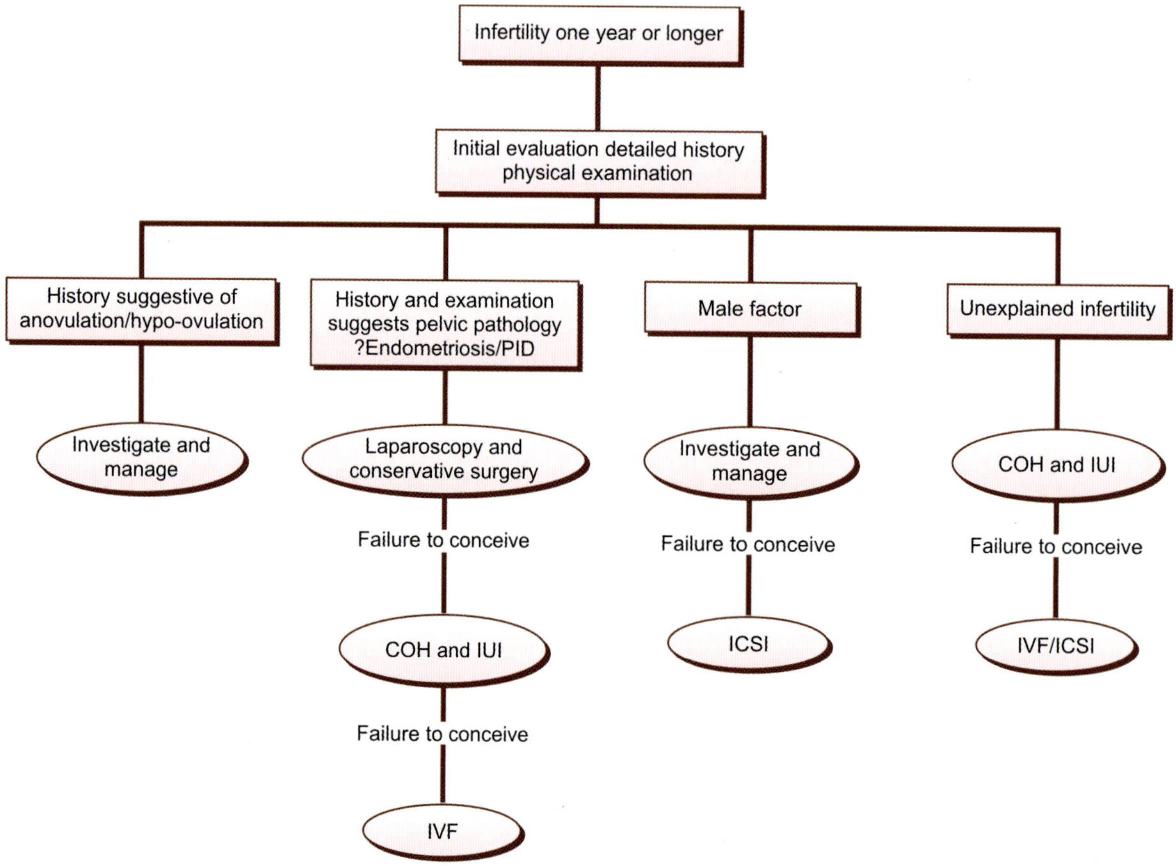

Fig. 8.1: Management algorithm of infertility

after three days of abstinence which can conveniently be done at the time the female partner is having her periods. Hence *an individualized evaluation plan should be formulated for each couple and the same explained to them in detail.* The evaluation should be completed within a period of two to three menstrual cycles. All couples may not need all the investigations. The most rewarding and least invasive tests should be performed initially. Further evaluation should be channeled according to the etiology suspected at initial evaluation.

There will be pointers in the history and clinical examination as to the cause of infertility. A lady with history and examination suggestive of polycystic ovarian disease can have tests for ovulation and hormonal assay and started on ovulogens deferring HSG or laparoscopy. The chance for a woman with polycystic disease presenting with primary infertility, having concurrent tubal factor is extremely rare. But if she does not conceive after many cycles of successful ovulation, tubal patency then needs to be checked. On the contrary, if the history and findings suggest a disease like endometriosis, laparoscopy can be done as a primary investigation.

Indications for Early Testing for Tubal Patency

- Secondary infertility
- Previous ectopic
- Previous septic abortion
- History of tubal surgery
- History suggestive of PID or endometriosis

The initial investigation to be performed is semen analysis. Abnormal semen is the cause of infertility in 35% of infertile couples. If the semen analysis report is abnormal, the male partner has to be examined and investigated as has been detailed in the chapter on male infertility. When the semen analysis is normal, the investigations should be pointed towards the female partner. Documentation of ovulation is one of the preliminary tests for the female partner.

Post-coital Test (PCT)

Just before ovulation estrogen levels peak. As a result the cervical glands produce copious thin watery secretions which most women appreciate in the pre-ovulatory phase. The PCT is performed around the time of LH surge which can be made out either by noting the mature follicle using ultrasound or by testing for LH peak by LH test. Between 2-8 hours after coitus mucus is collected from the os. There is no added advantage in collecting the mucus from different levels of the cervical canal as sperm distribution after intercourse is uniform in the mucus. As the mucus is being collected in a syringe, Spinn-Barkeit is assessed. Spinn-Barkeit is the threadability of cervical mucus.

Normally the mucus can be threaded to 8-10 cm or more. Poor mucus can be a barrier to sperm penetration. The mucus is examined for the number of motile sperms – sperms with progressive forward motility. Normally there should be 5-20 motile sperms per high power field. The approximate sperm count will be 20 million/ml if there are 20 sperms per high power field in the test. If the test is positive it defines that the mucus is normal, the sperms are normal in number and motility and there is no coital problem.

Poor test results can be due to incorrect timing which can be excluded in the subsequent cycle by proper training of the couple. If it is abnormal when done in the proper time, it could be due to poor mucus, immunological causes or abnormal semen. Abnormalities in the semen can be made out by semen analysis. Poor mucus can be treated by conjugated estrogens 0.625 mg orally daily for 10 days from the 7th to the 17th day of the cycle. The post coital test is not widely used at present and irrespective of whether the test is negative or positive, controlled ovarian hyper stimulation and IUI can be proceeded with. The success rate of IUI in women with negative PCT is better than in women with a positive PCT. IUI can be tried for three to four (a maximum of six) cycles. Further persistence with IUI is not reasonable. The couple should be advised IVF without wasting time as *age is the most important factor affecting success in IVF cycles.*

Documentation of Ovulation

Ovulation disorders account for 30-40% cases of female infertility. Ovulation disorders can be easily diagnosed and treated with a very high success rate.

Women with regular cycles, premenstrual symptoms and dysmenorrhea can be thought to have normal ovarian cycles while those with infrequent and irregular cycles can be assumed to have anovulation. As ovulation is an absolute prerequisite for conception it must be documented in all women complaining of infertility.

Methods of Detecting Ovulation

Basal body temperature (BBT) charting

Following ovulation, due to the thermogenic effect of progesterone there would be a temperature rise of 0.58°F over the basal range of 97-98.8°F. This gives a bi-phasic temperature chart. The rise will last for 10 days through the luteal phase. The temperature should be recorded as first thing in the morning before the woman rises from bed, eats drinks or smokes. Use of a BBT thermometer is preferred due to its precision in the temperature range. Though inexpensive, this method is not fool-proof because even in ovulatory cycles, temperature recordings usually do not show the typical bi-phasic pattern and even when the charting is monophasic, it can be an ovulatory cycle. Hence, considering the practical difficulties associated with the emotional trauma to the patient and the poor compliance of women with the procedure as evidenced by clinical experience, this method of laboriously charting the basal body temperature should be abandoned in favor of more patient-friendly tests like the ultrasonogram and serum progesterone estimation.

Mid-luteal Progesterone

Serum progesterone estimation on Day 21-23 can be used to confirm ovulation in women with normal ovulatory cycles. The level of progesterone in ovulatory cycles varies from 3-10 ng/ml. The normal mid-luteal level is 6.5 ng/ml. However, patients with irregular and infrequent cycles need repeated weekly estimations till she attains her next period and the progesterone levels are interpreted retrospectively. RCOG recommends this method as the test for ovulation detection.

Ultrasound Monitoring (Table 8.3)

With the advent of ultrasound, ovulation is detected by serial transvaginal scanning beginning from day-9. Follicular size reaches an average of 21-23 mm before it ruptures and becomes the corpus luteum. Ovulation might occur even when the follicle diameter is 17 mm. At times it may reach up to 29 mm before it ruptures. In the routine evaluation of infertile women with regular cycles, mid-luteal progesterone estimation is more convenient than serial ultrasonogram. However in women undergoing ovulation induction, ultrasound should be preferred as the number of developing follicles should be ascertained and hyperstimulation and higher order-multiple pregnancy avoided. Ovulation detection by transvaginal scan has so many advantages. The uterus and endometrium can be evaluated; luteal phase insufficiency can be predicted by noting the thickness, homogenesity and blood flow of the endometrium. The ovaries can be evaluated for PCOS and premature ovarian failure can be suspected by the appearance of the ovaries. Associated pelvic pathology like endometriosis, PID etc. can also be suspected on ultrasonogram.

Endometrial Biopsy

Endometrial biopsy used to be the method of diagnosing ovulation as well as luteal phase defects. With the advent of ultrasound and serum progesterone estimation this is no longer performed routinely as it is an invasive procedure and carries the risk of infection.

Luteal Phase Defect (LPD)

LPD has been defined as a lag of two days in the histology of the endometrium compared to the day of menses. About 3-4% of infertility is believed to be due to LPD. It can occur in isolated cycles among normal women. Only if it occurs repeatedly can it be attributed to cause infertility. It is identified in 5% of women with recurrent miscarriage. There is controversy as to what are the criteria to diagnose this condition. LPD is the result of decreased hormone production by the corpus luteum. The root cause of LPD is decreased FSH production leading to abnormal LH secretion and inadequate progesterone production. Hyperprolactinemia and hypothyroidism can lead to inadequate FSH production and LPD. Mid-luteal progesterone estimation and endometrial biopsy has been used to diagnose LPD. As the basic defect is insufficient FSH production, treatment with gonadotropins and clomiphene citrate are reasonable options.

Table 8.3: Ultrasonogram vs mid-luteal progesterone estimation in detecting ovulation

Ultrasonogram	*Mid-luteal progesterone estimation*
• Number of follicles can be ascertained. Hence, USS is a must during ovulation induction • Endometrial evaluation and assessment of other pelvic pathologies possible • Noninvasive	• Useful mainly in patients with regular cycles. Need multiple weekly tests and retrospective interpretation in patients who have irregular cycles. • Number of follicles cannot be determined • Hence not useful in ovulation induction • Other pelvic pathologies cannot be assessed • Diagnosis of ovulation is retrospective • Hence not useful in timing coitus or artificial insemination • Less expensive

Tests to assess ovarian reserve

Tests used to assess ovarian reserve are:

1. Day-3 FSH in the serum
2. Serum Inhibin B level
3. Serum MIS (Mullerian Inhibiting Substance)
4. Clomiphene citrate challenge test
5. Ultrasound measurement of antral follicle count and mean ovarian volume measurement.

1. **Day 3 FSH:** Before the rise in FSH levels to menopausal range there will be a rise in the basal FSH at day-3 as an initial event which could give a clue as to whether the woman is reaching the end of ovarian reserve. Basal FSH estimation gives a better prediction of success with IVF, than the age of the woman. Women with day-3 FSH levels >15 IU/L is 3.9 times more likely to have an unsuccessful IVF, the specificity being 96% and positive predictive value being 26%.
2. **Serum inhibin B:** Inhibin is normally secreted by the granulosa cells of pre-antral follicles. Inhibin B levels usually rise during the transition from luteal to follicular phase. This increase depends on the number of follicles recruited during the cycle. In one study it was found that patients with Serum Inhibin B levels <400 pg/ml had significantly less number of follicles than others.
3. **Mullerian inhibiting substance (MIS):** MIS is produced by granulosa cells as well as by the antral and pre-antral follicles. MIS levels decline with age and becomes undetectable after menopause. As ovarian reserve decreases serum MIS concentration decreases. Hence serum MIS can also be used as a measure of ovarian reserve.
4. **Clomiphene citrate challenge test (CCCT):** It is worthwhile to screen all women who are 30 years and above, women of any age with unexplained infertility and poor responders to ovulation induction with CCCT and day-3 estradiol. 100 mg clomiphene citrate is given for 5 days from day-5 to day-9. Serum FSH and estradiol are measured on day-3 and day-9. The test need to be done only for women with day-3 FSH value >10-15 IU/L or estradiol level >65 pg/ml. An increase in FSH to 15 IU/L or more can be assumed to be associated with failure to achieve pregnancy. It is important to remember that values of FSH can vary between different laboratories. In women with poor ovarian reserve there is a high incidence of an exaggerated response. This exaggerated response is a better predictor of ovarian reserve than basal FSH.

   In women over 40 years, even a normal test does not ensure adequate ovarian reserve. An abnormal test can definitely be taken as a reason for considering ovum donation. Although an abnormal test indicates poor prognosis it should not be taken as an absolute inability to achieve pregnancy.
5. **Antral follicle count:** Antral follicle count and anti-mullerian hormone estimation were found to be the most significant predictors of poor response to ovarian stimulation during ART.[2]

8.4 OVULATORY DISORDERS

Anovulation or infrequent ovulation is seen in about 25% of the couples presenting with infertility. Women who are found to be anovulatory should be evaluated for pointing out the reason for anovulation. WHO has classified anovulation into three types:

1. **WHO type I** – hypothalamopituitary failure (discussed in Chapter 5: Secondary amenorrhea). Gonadotropins are in the normal or near normal range.
2. **WHO type II** – hypothalamopituitary dysfunction
3. **WHO type III** – ovarian failure (discussed in Chapter 5: Secondary amenorrhea)

Differences can be made out by estimation of serum FSH, LH, TSH and prolactin. FSH and LH levels will be very low/undetectable or even in the normal range in hypothalamopituitary failure and normal/raised in hypothalamopituitary dysfunction. Patients with primary ovarian failure have very high levels of FSH and LH. Since there is a likelihood of an abnormal Y-chromosome component in these women, karyotyping becomes mandatory.

Other causes of defective ovulation include congenital adrenal hyperplasia, adrenal tumors and androgen producing ovarian tumors. Hirsutism and obesity are present in most women with PCOS. But women with juvenile type of congenital adrenal hyperplasia, androgen secreting ovarian tumors and adrenal tumors, will present with hirsutism and features of virilization, especially so with androgen producing ovarian tumours.

Polycystic Ovarian Syndrome (PCOS) *(For details refer Chapter 9: PCOS)*

PCOS is the most common cause of anovulation /oligo-ovulation. Clinical features can vary in different individuals and also in the same individual over time. Large proportion of women will be obese with hirsutism and oligomenorrhea or amenorrhea. A small group of women with PCOS will be lean.

Revised Rotterdam ESHRE/ASRM 2003 diagnostic criteria for PCOS is provided in Table 8.4.

Table 8.4: Revised Rotterdam ESHRE/ASRM 2003 diagnostic criteria for PCOS

Diagnosis of PCOS includes two out of three features listed below:

1. Oligo and/or anovulation
2. Clinical (hirsutism, acne, and rarely androgenic alopecia) and/or biochemical (increased free androgen, increased free androgen index, or elevated DHEAS) evidence of hyperandrogenism
3. Polycystic ovaries Exclusion of other etiologies (congenital adrenal hyperplasia, androgen secreting tumors and Cushing's syndrome)

Reference: Rotterdam ESHRE/ASRM sponsored PCOS consensus workshop group. Revised 2003 consensus on diagnostic criteria and long term health risks related to polycystic ovary syndrome. Human reprod 2004;19 (1):41-7

Ultrasound Criteria of Polycystic Ovaries

Presence of ≥ 12 follicles in each ovary measuring 2-9 mm in diameter and increased ovarian volume more than 10 ml is diagnostic of PCO. The distribution of follicles can be of two types, either a peripheral distribution giving a pearl necklace pattern or a uniform distribution in the ovarian stroma. Even if one ovary satisfies the criteria it is considered as PCO. Ovarian volume >10 ml is considered significant but multiple cysts can be seen in ovaries with normal volume also. Women with clinical features of PCOS can have ovaries with increased volume without the polycystic appearance. In the presence of a dominant follicle or corpus luteum it is difficult to assess the polycystic nature of the ovaries. Also in women who are on COC the polycystic nature of the ovaries can change.

Management of PCOS (Fig. 8.2)

The first line intervention in all obese PCOS women before starting drug treatment is weight reduction. Weight loss reduces insulin resistance and consequently hyperinsulinemia and hyperandrogenism. A weight loss of even 5% might result in spontaneous ovulation and pregnancy. The effectiveness of ovulation inducing drugs also will be increased by weight reduction.

Clomiphene Citrate (CC)

CC binds to estrogen receptors in the hypothalamus inhibiting ovarian hypothalamic feedback loop leading to increased GnRH pulse release from the hypothalamus. As a result, gonadotropin secretion from the pituitary is increased leading to folliculogenesis and ovulation. The anti-estrogenic effect of clomiphene on the endometrium and the cervix is a disadvantage which may be the reason for the disparity in ovulation and pregnancy rates in CC induced cycles. 80-85% of the treated women will ovulate but only 40% has been found to conceive. CC binds to estrogen receptors for an extended period of about 2 months. Hence, it is better to stop induction with CC after 3 consecutive induction cycles. If a further course is needed Clomiphene can be restarted after a 2-month off-period for a maximum of three more cycles.

Adverse effects: Visual abnormalities, nausea, vasomotor flashes etc are encountered rarely. Multiple pregnancy rates reported is 5-8% among which twin pregnancies are the most frequently encountered. Further higher order pregnancies are extremely rare. Very rarely even ovarian hyperstimulation syndrome (OHSS) can occur.

Dosage: CC is started at a dose of 50 mg/day starting from day 2 to day 6 of a spontaneous period or withdrawal bleed. For a woman who has infrequent periods or amenorrhea, the drug should be started after inducing withdrawal bleed. Ovulation should be monitored by ultrasound from day 9. A baseline ultrasound should be undertaken on day 3 to assess whether there is a functional cyst persisting from the previous cycle which can interfere with the interpretation of follicular development. After day 9, TVS should be repeated on alternate days. If the woman is found to be ovulating at this dose of CC, the same dose can be persisted with for a minimum of three cycles. For non-responders, the dose can be increased in increments of 50 mg to a total of 150 mg/day.

Documentation of ovulation can also be done using a home urine LH kit. LH surge is detected by this kit and serum progesterone may be estimated one week after the surge. Its disadvantage over ultrasound monitoring is the inability to detect the number of follicles and the endometrial response. Advice should be given to the couple to have sexual intercourse around the time of ovulation. In the presence of a dominant follicle if no LH surge is detected, HCG 5000 IU or GnRH 250 microgram can be administered to trigger ovulation. If even after 6 ovulatory cycles conception has not occurred it is not advisable to continue CC as maximum conception with CC induced cycles will occur in six months time.

Insulin Sensitizers

Insulin resistance can be assessed by testing fasting glucose insulin ratio. If it is <4.5 it is a marker of insulin resistance and insulin sensitizers would be useful in such women.

Insulin resistance is usually seen in obese women with hirsutism and PCOS. It is also reported in thin women with PCOS. Insulin sensitizers like metformin and rosiglitazone have been studied in several randomized control trials. Metformin reduces insulin resistance and promotes glucose utilization by muscle and adipose tissue. The drug also reduces intestinal absorption of glucose and significantly decreases hepatic glucose output. It reduces hyperinsulinemia, basal and stimulated LH levels, free testosterone levels and PAI-1 levels in obese PCOS patients. It is cleared by the kidney. The combination of metformin and CC is more effective in inducing ovulation than using CC alone. In a randomised trial of CC, CC and metformin, and metformin alone in 626 patients, live birth rate was 22.5% in CC group, 26% in CC and metformin group and 7.2% in the metformin alone group. Multiple pregnancies were 6% in CC group, 0% in metformin group and 3.1% in the CC and metformin group.[3] Metformin is found to be beneficial not only in obese women but also in normal weight women with anovulatory infertility.[4]

Adverse effects: Metformin can cause minor side effects like nausea, vomiting, bloating sensation etc. Fatal lactic acidosis has been reported to occur in patients with underlying renal compromise. Hence liver and renal function tests should be done before starting on metformin.

Dosage schedule: Metformin should be started at a dose 500 mg OD after breakfast in the first week. The dose is increased to 500 mg BD from the second week and 500 mg TDS from the third week onwards, to be continued at this dose. For working women, 1000 mg BD is a convenient dosage.

If metformin alone is given, a few months may elapse before ovulation occurs. Hence follicle tracking is not feasible. Serum progesterone estimation may be done weekly and the results interpreted retrospectively once the woman attains her periods. If CC is combined with metformin, it is advisable to add CC once the full dose of metformin is reached. If ovulation does not occur, dose of CC can be increased to 150 mg/day.

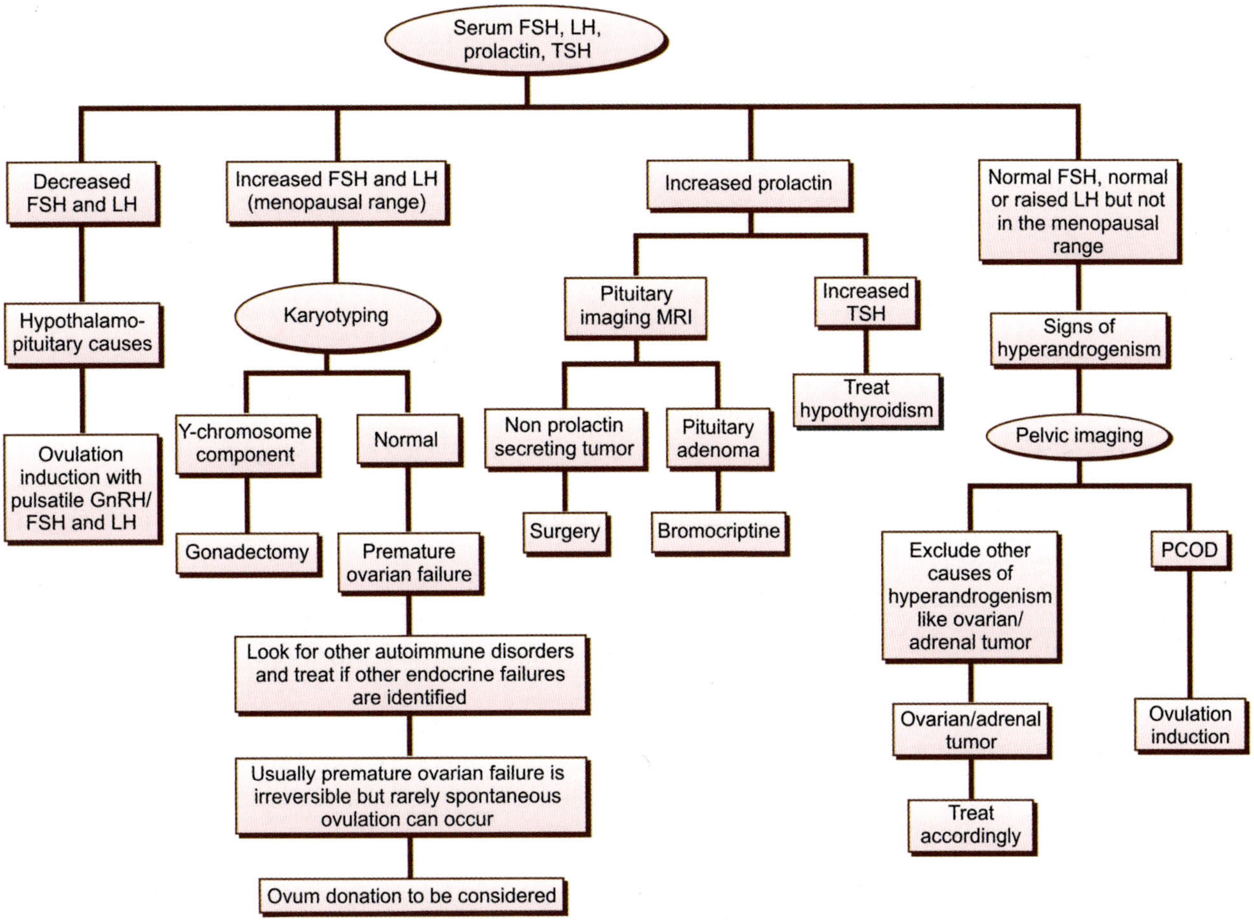

Fig. 8.2: Management algorithm of anovulatory infertility

Even though these earlier reports on the efficacy of metformin were encouraging, recent trials have shown that metformin alone is inferior to the metformin-CC combination in treating infertility associated with PCOS.[5]

Metformin continuation in pregnancy: Metformin being a category B drug and not a known teratogen, PCOS patients who conceive while on metformin treatment may be advised to persist with the drug especially in the wake of studies which show a decreased incidence of gestational diabetes mellitus as well as abortions in such women.

Rosiglitazone, a thiozolidinedione has been found to be effective[6] for inducing ovulation in obese clomiphene resistant patients with PCOS. Pregnancy rate can be increased by combining rosiglitazone with CC.

Letrozole

Letrozole inhibits aromatase enzyme which converts androgen to estrogen. The reduced estrogen causes enhanced GnRH pulsatility and increases FSH production. This results in enhanced follicular development. The half life of letrozole is very short- 45 hours. Hence it is quickly and completely removed from the body and has much less adverse effect on the endometrium and the cervix. When used along with gonadotropins it reduces the amount of gonadotropin required, thus reducing cost of therapy without compromising pregnancy rate. Several studies have shown that Letrozole and Letrozole-FSH combination had the highest pregnancy rate and lowest multiple pregnancy rate. The conception rate in each cycle was found to be 25%.

Dosage: The dose is 2.5 mg /day starting from day 2 or 3 for 5 days. The dose can be increased to 7 mg/day. It can also be given as a single dose.

Adverse effects: Adverse effects of letrozole include headache, hot flashes and breast tenderness. Pregnancies following letrozole are not reported to carry increased risk of abortion or congenital anomalies. If the woman does not conceive after 3-6 cycles she should be investigated for other causes for infertility. Trials are ongoing on ovulation induction with Anastrozole,[7] another aromatase inhibitor.

If the woman is not conceiving there are two options:
- Ovarian drilling and
- Induction of ovulation with gonadotropins

Laparoscopic Ovarian Drilling (LOD)

In olden days surgical management for PCOS was in the form of wedge resection of the ovaries. It was effective in achieving regular ovulation and menstruation by reducing the androgen output from the ovaries. Due to the occurrence of peri-tubal ovarian adhesions as well as loss of considerable amount of ovarian tissue following the procedure, it went into disrepute. With the advent of laparoscopic surgery alternative procedure of laparoscopic ovarian drilling came into practice. The procedure involves puncturing the follicular cysts which reduces the androgen secreting tissue from the ovary. Androgen withdrawal causes reduction of estrone which is produced by conversion of androgen. The fall in estrone results in decreased negative feedback on the pituitary production of FSH. The resulting increase in FSH production results in normal follicular growth and ovulation. Thus the HPO axis is normalized. Laparoscopic puncture also appears to decrease the spontaneous abortion rates in PCOS patients. Prior ovarian drilling favourably affects pregnancy rates in IVF cycles. Drilling can be done with laser or electrocautery. Drilling with electrocautery is the most commonly adopted method. After inserting the primary trocar and telescope, the pelvis is inspected systematically. The ovary is immobilised by catching hold of the ovarian ligament using an atraumatic grasper. An insulated puncture needle is inserted and the cysts are punctured using a cutting current of 100 W and then coagulated with coagulation current of 40 W for 2 seconds.[8] Regarding the number of punctures, recommendations vary, but up to even 15 punctures is reasonable. The procedure is then repeated on the opposite ovary. At the end of the drilling, the ovaries should be washed with normal saline to decrease the temperature of the ovaries as heat can destroy the ovarian follicles. It is questionable as to whether there is a chance of premature ovarian failure following the procedure. Peritubal and periovarian adhesions can follow laparoscopic puncture as well. When second look laparoscopy was done one year after LOD, it was found that four among fifteen women had adhesions.[9] After the procedure 73% ovulated spontaneously, 24% with CC while 1.8% required gonadotropins.

Treatment with Gonadotropins

Induction with gonadotropins avoids the risks associated with laparoscopy. However it has the disadvantages of being costlier than laparoscopy and of causing ovarian hyperstimulation and multiple pregnancies. Before initiating treatment the patient should be counseled about the risks involved.

Hypogonadotropic Hypogonadism (WHO type I)

Pituitary/hypothalamic disorders can cause very low levels of gonadotropins and hence will present with amenorrhea.

Congenital disorders like Kallmann's syndrome due to GnRH deficiency presents with primary amenorrhea. These individuals will have associated anosmia. Among the acquired causes of hypogonadotropic hypogonadism is Sheehan's syndrome due to pituitary necrosis caused by obstetric shock. In this situation the woman presents with lactation failure and amenorrhea after delivery. She may also have features of other endocrine gland failure. The diagnosis is made from history and hormonal estimation. Another acquired cause of hypogonadotropic amenorrhea is weight loss or excessive exercise causing hypothalamic amenorrhea. Rare causes are space occupying pituitary lesions. Clinical examination including visual field testing and imaging the pituitary fossa will clinch the diagnosis.

Management

Management of hypogonadotropic hypogonadism is ovulation induction with gonadotropins which is discussed in detail later in this chapter.

Hyperprolactinemia

Raised levels of prolactin interfere with GnRH secretion resulting in low levels of gonadotropins causing oligomenorrhea and amenorrhea. Hyperprolactinemia can be the result of prolactin secreting pituitary adenomas or tumors of the pituitary stalk obstructing dopamine from reaching the pituitary. Primary hypothyroidism can cause hyperprolactinemia due to the raised levels of TSH interfering with GnRH release. Chronic intake of drugs such as metoclopramide, phenothiazines, reserpine and methyldopa can cause dopamine depletion and hyperprolactinemia. (Management is discussed in Chapter 5: Secondary amenorrhea).

Hypergonadotropic Hypogonadism (WHO Type III)

Very high levels of gonadotropins indicate ovarian failure. Ovarian failure can be primary or secondary. The common cause of primary ovarian failure is Turner syndrome or gonadal dysgenesis. Turner syndrome patients will have the characteristic stigmata like short stature, webbed neck, shield chest and cubitus valgus. Patients with mosaic Turner and other acquired diseases causing premature ovarian failure, present with secondary amenorrhea and infertility.

Management

Karyotyping is indicated for all women presenting with premature ovarian failure and high gonadotropins to exclude Y chromosome component as the presence of a Y chromosome warrants gonadectomy, even if it is a streak gonad, to prevent future development of germ cell tumors in these gonads.

Surrogacy: With advances in ART procedures individuals who have premature ovarian failure can accept ovum from another normal individual to become surrogate mothers. Individuals who have Turner syndrome are likely to have coarctation of aorta, they are prone for aortic dissection during pregnancy and labor. Hence cardiovascular evaluation and counseling should be done before venturing to surrogacy in these women. As endogenous hormones are lacking, they need hormonal substitution with estrogen and progesterone simulating normal cycles. Their endometrial response should be tested in a mock cycle with exogenous hormones before the ART cycle.

8.5 UTERINE AND CERVICAL FACTORS OF INFERTILITY (TABLE 8.5)

Uterine factors are rare causes of infertility. They are usually responsible for recurrent pregnancy loss (RPL) rather than inability to conceive. 20% of infertility is attributed to uterine and cervical factors.

Uterine Factors

The uterine factors identified as causing 15% of infertility include the following.

Leiomyoma

When leiomyomas are diagnosed in infertile patients it may not always be the sole cause for infertility. Submucous myomas, myomatous polyps and large myomas which distort the uterine cavity can be considered to cause infertility. Distortion of the uterine cavity, altered contractility, abnormal placentation and imbalance in prostaglandin

Table 8.5: Uterine and tubal factors causing infertility

Uterine factors	*Tubal factors*
Submucous fibroids	Pelvic inflammatory disease
Intrauterine adhesions	• *Chlamydial*
Mullerian anomalies	• *Gonococcal*
In utero exposure to	• *Tuberculosis*
Diethyl stilbestrol	Endometriosis
Endometrial polyps	Previous pelvic surgeries
	Pelvic and abdominal infections
	Salpingitis isthmica nodosa
	Cornual fibroids

production are the factors suspected as causes for infertility. Before advising myomectomy sufficient time should be given for conception. Myomectomy can be performed by laparotomy or laparoscopy. Pregnancy rates reported following the procedure are the same for both. Earlier reports of laparoscopic myomectomy showed increased scar rupture during pregnancy and labor, but later ones does not show such high incidence of rupture due to improvements in laparoscopic suturing. Submucous myomas even if small can cause infertility. They will function as a foreign body in the uterine cavity. It can be removed by hysteroscopic resection.

Intrauterine Adhesions

Adhesions can occur following thorough curettage of the uterine cavity after abortion, postpartum hemorrhage, etc. Severe adhesions can also occur following tuberculosis or schistosomiasis of the genital tract. Tuberculous adhesions are highly refractory to treatment and chances of conception are meagre even with IVF.

Release of adhesions through hysteroscopy is the treatment of choice and carries good success rate, if it occurred as a sequel of curettage. Adhesions can be cut hysteroscopically. An IUCD should be inserted to prevent further adhesions. Post operative treatment with conjugated estrogen at a dose of 2.5-5 mg/day for about 4-8 weeks will help regenerate the endometrium. Success rates reported are as high as 80% after the procedure provided the adhesions are mild to moderate. Severe adhesions[10] are difficult to treat and carry very poor success rates.

Mullerian Anomalies

Among mullerian anomalies, septate uterus causes reproductive failure, obstetric complications and infertility. Uterus didelphys rarely causes reproductive failure and infertility. A rare mullerian anomaly which can be attributed to infertility is transverse vaginal septum. A perforated transverse vaginal septum can cause infertility even though menstruation occurs normally. This condition can be diagnosed by speculum examination. Other mullerian anomalies should be excluded by imaging and the septum excised by a simple procedure. Vertical vaginal septum need not cause infertility, but may be associated with fusion anomalies of the uterus.

Septate and bicornuate uterus can be differentiated by ultrasound, especially 4D ultrasound. Women with septate uterus should have septal resection done if she has repeated abortion or if she presents with infertility. Septal resection significantly decreases the risk of repeated abortion. Hysteroscopic septoplasty is the surgical treatment of choice. The septum is cut with cautery from below upwards till both the ostia are seen in a single field. Laparoscopic guidance is preferable during the procedure. 25% of mullerian anomalies are associated with cervical incompetence and hence it should be anticipated in all women with mullerian anomalies.

In utero Exposure to Diethylstilbestrol (DES): T Shaped Uterus

In utero exposure to DES can cause various types of uterine anomalies. The T shaped uterus is one among them. This can be diagnosed by ultrasound and HSG. Surgical correction by lateral metroplasty is not reported to improve fertility significantly and hence not advised.

Endometrial Polyp

Endometrial polyps can also cause infertility and miscarriage. Diagnosis can be suspected at TVS. Confirmation of diagnosis and management can be done hysteroscopically.

8.6 TUBAL AND PERITONEAL FACTORS

Forty percent of secondary and 15-20% of primary infertility can be attributed to tubal factors. Tubal damage results as sequelae of pelvic inflammatory disease, tubal surgery or endometriosis. Abnormal tubal function does not always imply tubal block but it could mean loss of integrity of the endosalpinx which is necessary for the normal function of the tube. Pelvic surgery can result in peri-tubal and peri-ovarian adhesions which can interfere with motility of the tube.

Pelvic Inflammatory Disease (PID)

A single episode of PID carries up to 10% risk of future infertility due to tubal damage. *Chlamydia* has been identified as the most common microorganism causing PID, to the extent of 50%. Factors associated with high incidence of chlamydia infection include multiple sexual partners, alcohol addiction, cigarette smoking and poor socioeconomic status. Chlamydia usually inhabits the gland crypts of the endocervix. Instrumentation of the uterine cavity takes the organism to the fallopian tubes and hence unnecessary uterine instrumentation should be avoided, especially in women who have not completed childbearing.

After infection the organism multiplies intracellularly and releases elementary bodies by rupturing the cell it has invaded, causing cellular damage. The infection however is usually silent so that treatment is often delayed and at times not started at all resulting in extensive tissue destruction and sequelae of PID. The damage produced to the fallopian tube is permanent and consequently infertility and ectopic pregnancy can result. Tissue damage produced by Chlamydia also favors secondary infection with aerobic and anaerobic bacteria. In the past few decades awareness about chlamydial infection has led to treatment of PID with drugs that cover Chlamydia trachomatis also, like *Doxycycline* or *Azithromycin*.

Gonococcus is the other organism that causes tubal damage. However gonococcal infection presents with systemic symptoms and the organism can easily be identified by simple Gram staining of fluid collected from the cul-de-sac. Infection causes severe damage to the endosalpinx. This damaged environment favours growth of aerobic and anaerobic organisms as well.

Comparatively higher incidence of *Mycoplasma hominis* and *Ureaplasma urealyticum* is found in the cervical mucus and semen of infertile couples. Treatment with doxycycline decreases the presence of this organism in the mucus and semen. Whether treatment improves pregnancy rate has not been established.

Tuberculosis (TB) of the genital tract is common in Asia, Middle-east and Latin America, but rare in the United States. Genital tuberculosis is usually secondary to pulmonary TB. Fallopian tubes are the usual site of genital tuberculosis. About half of these patients develop endometrial TB also. The usual organism producing pelvic TB is *Mycobacterium tuberculosis* or *M.bovis*. There are two types of pelvic TB—the wet type where there is ascites and the entire peritoneum is studded with miliary tubercles and the dry type with extensive adhesions and possible tubo-ovarian abscess formation which is usually unilateral. Women with pelvic TB can present with pelvic pain, infertility and menstrual irregularities, mainly amenorrhea. Treatment does not usually restore fertility and post-treatment conception rate is only 5%. Hence conservative surgery for preserving fertility is not advised, unless the disease is very minimal.

Other causes of tubal block

Endometriosis: Usually endometriosis does not produce tubal block, but due to the distortion in anatomy, the tubal function may be impaired. Rarely, it may lead to cornual block.

Fibroids: Fibroids in the cornual region can cause distortion of the intramural portion of the tube and obstruction. Tubal patency may be regained after myomectomy.

Previous pelvic surgery: Previous tubal surgeries like salpingotomy for ectopic, ovarian cystectomy, wedge resection of the ovaries, myomectomy, etc. carry risk of tubal block or peritubal adhesions and interference with tubal motility.

Infections in the abdomen and pelvis: Inflamed or ruptured appendix can cause severe pelvic adhesions.

Salpingitis isthmica nodosa: It is a nodular thickening of the isthmic region of the fallopian tube. The etiology is unknown but the most recent concept is that it is a congenital abnormality.

Assessment of the Fallopian Tube

Assessment of the fallopian tube includes determination of the patency as well as assessment of the internal and external appearance of the tubes. The tubal mucosa and tubal motility are important factors necessary for the transport of gametes and fertilized ovum. Hence assessment of patency alone may not be sufficient. Damage of the endosalpinx can also result in tubal block. Restoration of the block will not restore fertility if the endosalpinx is damaged along with the block. Hence tubal factor assessment should include establishment of tubal patency as well as visualization of the endosalpinx.

Hysterosalpingogram (HSG)

Hysterosalpingography gives important information about the uterine cavity and the fallopian tube. It is complimentary to laparoscopy and not a substitute for it. In this investigation, the uterine cavity and fallopian tubes are delineated by injecting radiopaque dye transcervically into the uterine cavity. Either a *Leech Wilkinson cannula* or a *number 8 Foley* can be used to inject dye into the cavity. The dye can be water soluble or oil based. The advantage of oil based dye is that obstruction of the tube by mucus plug can get relieved by it. A Cochrane review has noted significant increase in fertility rates after tubal flushing with oil based media.[11] The iodine in the dye may exert a bacteriostatic effect also. However, anaphylactic reactions tend to be more and there is also a chance for formation of oil granuloma. Sometimes venous or lymphatic intravasation may occur and uterus and fallopian tubes may not be delineated.

Procedure: Patient should be administered an analgesic and antispasmodic before the procedure. To prevent chlamydial infection prophylactic *doxycycline 100 mg BD* should be started two days before the procedure and continued for 5 days. The patient should be kept in the dorsal position and under aseptic precautions either a Leech-Wilkinson cannula or a No.8 Foley catheter is introduced into the uterine cavity and the bulb inflated. Usually three films are taken. The first picture is taken before the dye is injected to verify the position of the cannula. 3-6 ml of the dye is injected and the second picture is taken which delineates the uterine cavity and the tubes. The third picture is taken after the dye has escaped into the peritoneal cavity.

Timing: HSG should be done in the immediate postmenstrual period. If performed in the luteal phase there is a high incidence of false negative result due to the thick endometrium occluding the internal ostia. The procedure may disturb the implanted ovum if conception has occurred in that particular cycle.

Contraindication: Acute PID is an absolute contraindication for this procedure. Performing HSG in the presence of PID can cause serious flare up of infection. In the case of a doubt of pelvic infection, ESR should be assessed. If the ESR is abnormal, the patient should be treated with a course of antibiotic and the decision for HSG should be taken on reassessment after one month. A better option would be to proceed with laparoscopy. If there is evidence of PID at laparoscopy, tubal patency testing should be deferred.

Interpretation: Tubal spasm can cause false positive tubal block. The normal fallopian tube can be identified by the presence of longitudinal hypoechoeic lines along the tubal lumen which represent normal tubal plicae. Normal HSG does not exclude endometriosis or peritubal adhesions. Hydrosalpinx can be easily diagnosed. Peritubal adhesions cannot be diagnosed but could be suspected if the dye escaping through the fimbrial end is seen loculated near the fimbrial end. Salpingitis isthmica nodosa is diagnosed by the presence of nodularity of the proximal region of the tube. Even though PID is a contraindication for HSG, if done for a patient with tuberculosis, the tubes show a beaded appearance. When cornual block is seen (Fig. 8.3), it is important to make out whether the intramural portion of the tube is patent or not. If the intramural portion of the tube is seen and the block is ahead of it, a tubo-cornual anastamosis is feasible where as if the intramural portion is not visualized, the patient may need tubo-cornual implantation.

Falloposcopy and Salpingoscopy

These techniques are used for evaluating the endosalpinx. Salpingoscopy is visualization of the fallopian tube by introducing a rigid endoscope through the fimbrial end. This procedure can be performed at laparoscopy. The tubal lining up to the isthmio ampullary junction can be visualized. Falloposcopy is visualization of the proximal region of the fallopian tube by passing a fiber-optic device through the tubal ostia. This procedure thus needs a concurrent hysteroscopy.

With the advances in IVF procedures and its easy availability, the damaged tubes are being bypassed rather than being repaired.

Laparoscopy

In recent years laparoscopic equipment and surgical techniques have improved by leaps and bounds. It is usually the final investigation done in a woman complaining of infertility. If in the initial examination a pelvic pathology is suspected, laparoscopy should be considered early enough. Laparoscopy for purely diagnostic indications is rarely resorted to these days as most of the pathologies can be diagnosed by a transvaginal ultrasound. *If laparoscopy is decided upon for diagnosis, it should only be undertaken in a setup with full operational facilities.*

8.7 MANAGEMENT OF UNEXPLAINED INFERTILITY

When all the standard clinical investigations yield normal results in an infertile couple, the couple is thought to have unexplained infertility. The percentage of unexplained infertility in couples under investigation for infertility is reported as 10-15%. If laparoscopy too shows normal findings the prevalence falls to less than 10%. Spontaneous conception among these couples depends upon the duration of infertility. About 60% will conceive in another three years with expectant management if the duration of infertility is less than three years. In a young woman below 30 years it is reasonable to adopt this expectant line of management. However controlled ovarian hyperstimulation and IUI may be resorted to as monthly fecundity rates decrease with time, if the woman is more than 30 years because age of the female partner is the most important factor affecting success rate in infertility treatment.

Several drugs have been tried to treat unexplained infertility. A Cochrane review has revealed that the use of dopamine agonists in the absence of hyperprolactinemia and Danazol empirically, suspecting endometriosis has shown no increase in the fertility rates. On the contrary, treatment with clomiphene citrate[12] has been found to increase the odds of pregnancy compared to placebo. Oral ovulation inducers were found to be as effective as Gonadotropins in treating unexplained infertility.[11] However, certain studies have shown increased pregnancy rates per cycle with

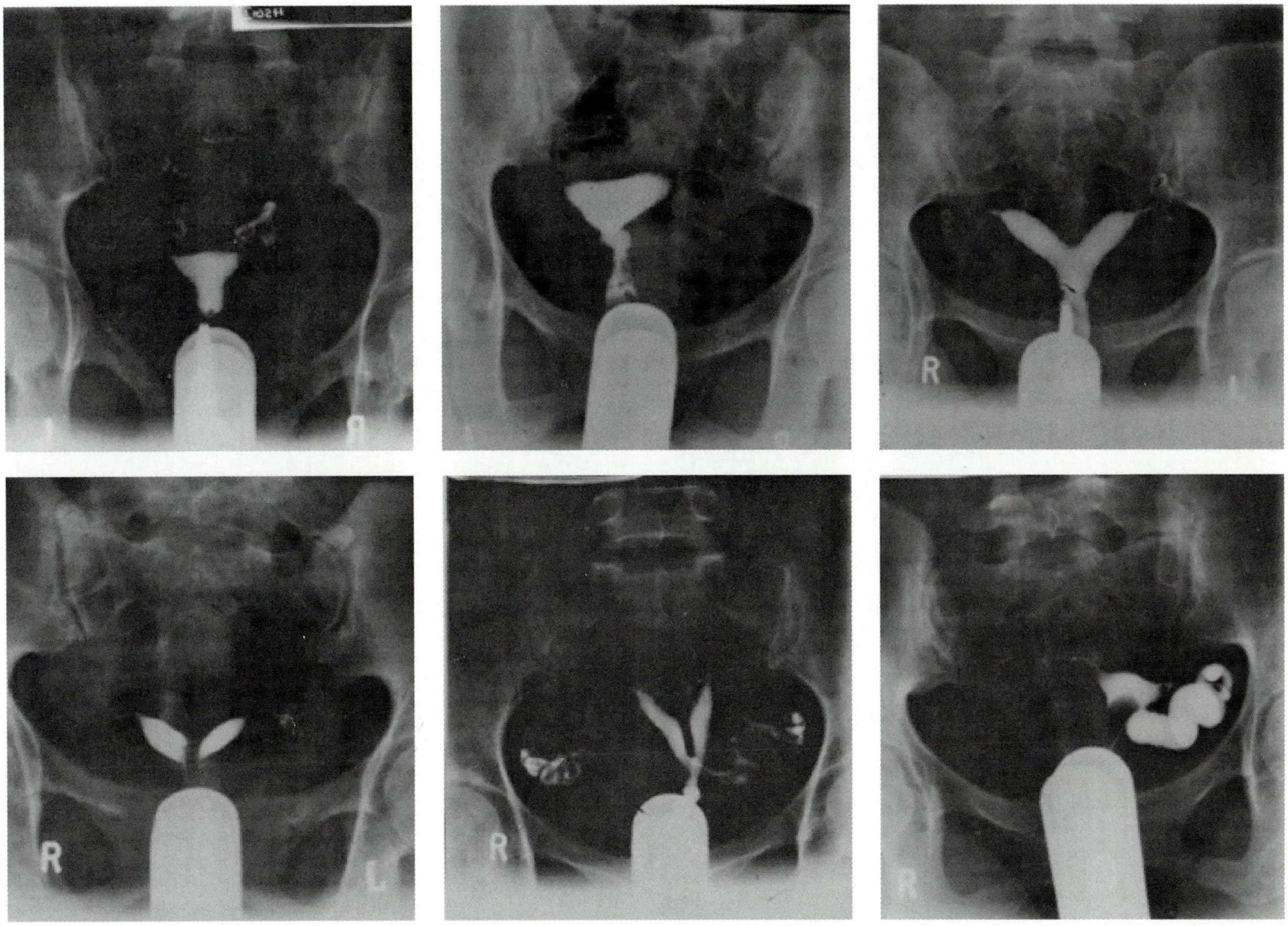

Fig. 8.3: Hysterosalpingogram: Normal HSG, bilateral cornual block, uterus bicornuate unicolis, uterus bicornuate bicolis, septate uterus and unilateral hydrosalpinx

gonadotropins and IUI compared to clomiphene citrate and IUI.[14] But there is concern about the increased risk of ovarian cancer with the use of ovulation inducing drugs in women with normal ovulation.

Super ovulation and IUI as well as other assisted reproductive technologies (ARTs) increase pregnancy rates in these women. The effect of ovarian stimulation alone is not as good as the two combined. The rationale of ovarian stimulation is to overcome the reduced ovarian reserve. Controlled ovarian hyperstimulation and IUI should be limited to three or four cycles following which the couple should be counselled for IVF.

Gonadotropin treatment without IUI should not be recommended. As already mentioned, all women undergoing ovulation induction should be monitored by ultrasound to ascertain the number of developing follicles and to avoid hyper stimulation and higher order multiple pregnancies.

8.7.1 Monitoring While on Super Ovulation

Monitoring should be done with TVS and serum estradiol levels. TVS should be done first in the post menstrual phase to evaluate the uterus, endometrium and the ovaries. If the endometrium is found to be thick in this phase of the cycle, it could be endometrial hyperplasia or polyp which has to be further evaluated and treated. Gonadotropins should be started at a lower dose of 75-100 IU/day if the woman is less than 30 years of age. For older women the starting dose can be 150-300 IU/day. This dose is maintained till day 7, when TVS is done and serum estradiol is measured. Depending upon the ovarian response, gonadotropin dose is increased by 50-100 IU/day. TVS and serum estradiol estimation are repeated daily. The follicle size increases by 1-2 mm/day. Maximal follicle diameter expected is 18-19 mm. At this size of the follicle the serum estradiol level expected is 150-250 pg/ml. PCOD patients are at higher risk of ovarian hyperstimulation syndrome (OHSS). When the estradiol level reaches 800-1000 pg/ml, the dose of gonadotropins should be reduced. If more than 4 follicles measuring 14 mm or more are seen in both ovaries, the gonadotropins should be stopped. An estradiol level of 1500-2000 pg/ml is also an indication to stop gonadotropins. When the follicle size reaches ≥18-19 mm, hCG 10,000 IU or recombinant GnRH 250 μg should be given subcutaneously or intramuscularly for follicular rupture. IUI should be timed 33-39 hours after hCG. Pregnancy test should be done at about 16 days after hCG injection. If appropriate estradiol levels and follicular size has reached, the same dose can be adopted in the next cycle also.

The response is unpredictable in PCOD patients. The multiple follicles could sometimes be resistant to treatment with gonadotropins. On the other side, some women are more prone for hyperstimulation syndrome as well. Pre-treatment with metformin and surgical ovarian diathermy has been found to decrease the incidence of hyperstimulation.

8.8 GONADOTROPIN THERAPY

Gonadotropin therapy carries remarkable success rate in patients with hypogonadotropic hypogonadism. Human menopausal gonadotropins (hMG) should be preferred to purified or recombinant FSH, since it contains both FSH and LH. Gonadotropins should be started at a low dose and increased according to the response.

8.8.1 Gonadotropin Preparations

There has been great improvement in the gonadotropin preparations over the years. The previously used gonadotropin preparations were from menopausal urine. They were a mixture of FSH and LH. Later purified and highly purified preparations were developed. They also contained a mixture of FSH and LH. The development of recombinant DNA technology led to the invention of recombinant FSH and LH preparations. The FSH produced by recombinant DNA technology has no LH or any other protein. This recombinant FSH is found to be superior because of a small increase in pregnancy rates compared to other preparations. The exogenously administered gonadotropins supplement the woman's endogenous gonadotropin in controlled ovarian hyperstimulation (COH). When given for pituitary failure it substitutes. FSH and LH act on the follicle, promoting follicular development. Hyperstimulation and life-threatening ovarian hyperstimulation syndrome (OHSS) are complications of such therapy.

8.8.2 Prevention of Premature LH Surge

In the present ART protocols, the endogenous gonadotropins are suppressed by giving either GnRH agonists or antagonists. The ovary is thus exclusively under the control of exogenous gonadotropins. GnRH analogue is administered in a non-pulsatile fashion to cause an initial flare up followed by downregulation of GnRH receptors, thus suppressing the pituitary. In ART, GnRH downregulation is done as a long or luteal downregulation protocol.

Long Downregulation Protocol

As follicular recruitment starts in the luteal phase of previous cycle, GnRH analogue is started on day 21 of the previous cycle. This long protocol significantly reduces premature leutinization and ovulation, thus lowering the rate of cycle cancellation. The incidence of OHSS is less, and more oocytes can be retrieved. Since the follicular maturation is exclusively on exogenous gonadotropins, the dose of gonadotropin required is more and so also is the cost. But this can be compensated by an improvement in the pregnancy rates and a decrease in the cycle cancellation rates.

Short Protocol

In the short protocol, GnRH is used at the commencement of the follicular phase so that the dose of gonadotropins and GnRH needed are less. The incidence of OHSS is more.

GnRH Antagonist Regimen

GnRH antagonists bind to receptors in pituitary and suppress the release of FSH and LH. Due to this antagonistic effect, they will not produce the flare up effect seen with agonists. Hence, they can be started concurrently with gonadotropins, so that additional time for downregulation is not needed. It suppresses more of LH than FSH. These GnRH antagonists are administered subcutaneously starting from day 7 and hence prevents premature LH surge. The incidence of OHSS is less when antagonists are used compared to long protocol.

8.9 TREATMENT OF HYPOTHALAMIC FAILURE

Hypothalamic failure is the reason for hypogonadism following cranial surgery, radiotherapy as well as in hypothalamic amenorrhea. Pulsatile GnRH administration using a mini-pump delivery system should be preferred over gonadotropin injections. GnRH at a dose of 75-100 ng/kg/pulse is given every 60-90 minutes. Since, the pituitary is under the GnRH control, OHSS is rare. Risk of multiple pregnancies is same as in CC induced cycle (8%). Cumulative pregnancy rate is 80% in 6 cycles. Ovulation can also be induced with gonadotropins which avoids the use of pump but with the disadvantage of increased risk of hyperstimulation syndrome.

8.10 ASSISTED REPRODUCTIVE TECHNOLOGIES (ARTs)

Assisted reproductive technologies include:

1. Oocyte retrieval
2. *In vitro* fertilization and embryo transfer (IVF-ET)
3. Gamete intrafallopian transfer (GIFT)
4. Zygote intrafallopian transfer (ZIFT)
6. Tubal embryo transfer (TET)
7. Intracytoplasmic sperm injection (ICSI)
8. Cryopreserved embryo transfer

GIFT, ZIFT and TET are not practiced at present because of the high success rates of IVF and ICSI.

8.10.1 Indications

1. Tubal factor infertility when surgical treatment fails or is not feasible
2. Anovulatory infertility not responding to ovulation induction
3. Unexplained infertility when COH and IUI is not successful
4. Immunological infertility when IUI fails
5. Male factor infertility when other treatment fails

8.10.2 IVF Procedure

Procedure for IVF is provided as a flow diagram in Figure 8.4.

Ovarian stimulation is different from that in COH and IUI in that more number of follicles are allowed to develop. Several oocytes are retrieved and fertilized in vitro. Healthy embryos are selected and transferred to the uterine cavity. The number of embryos developing depends on the number of embryos transferred. Excess embryos are cryopreserved for later use if required. Premature LH surge should be prevented which is achieved by administering GnRH agonists starting 7-8 days after ovulation in the previous cycle. GnRH agonists are given at a dose of 1 mg/day. Recently, GnRH antagonists are found to be more useful than GnRH agonists. Since folliculogenesis is under the control of exogenous gonadotropins, day of ovum retrieval can be chosen as desired.

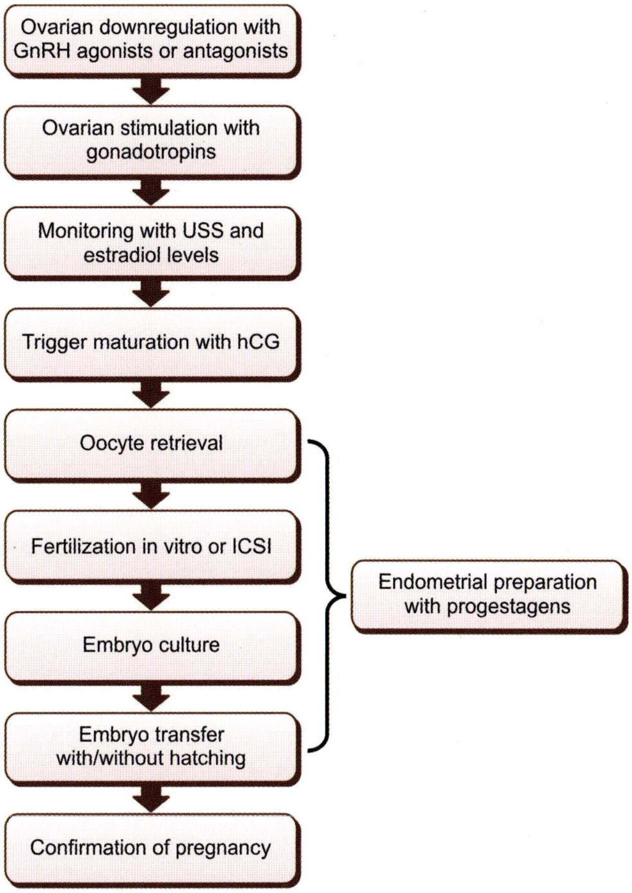

Fig. 8.4: Flow diagram of IVF

Oocyte retrieval: Oocyte retrieval is performed by transvaginal ultrasound guided approach under i.v. sedation. Prophylactic antibiotics should be given. The procedure should be done under sterile precautions to prevent contamination of the oocyte. The vagina should be cleaned by povidone iodine followed by sterile normal saline. Retrieval is done by a 16 gauge needle attached to the transvaginal probe. Follicular fluid is aspirated into a sterile pre-warmed culture tube. All the follicles are aspirated.

Even though transvaginal US guided aspiration of follicular fluid is a minimally invasive procedure, rarely complications can result. Needle injury can occur to bowel, bladder or major blood vessels like internal iliac or common iliac, which may require laparotomy and repair. Pelvic infection with tubo-ovarian abscess is also a rare complication.

Fertilization: The oocytes are fertilized in vitro or by ICSI.

Embryo culture: In natural conception, the fertilized ovum takes 2-3 days to reach the uterine cavity. By this time, the endometrium will be prepared by progesterone. 2-3 days after reaching the endometrial cavity, the embryo gets implanted. In ART protocol the embryo is allowed to grow in vitro and good quality embryos are selected. The embryos that have cleaved to 4-5 cells on day2 or 7-8 cells on day3 are assessed morphologically and good quality embryos are transferred.

The development of sequential culture media appropriate for embryo development at various stages has made extended culture of embryo until the blasotcyst stage feasible. In vitro culture to day-5 post retrieval allows them to be evaluated in their blastocyst stage at which the quality can be evaluated better. Symmetric blastomere sizes without multi-nucleation and less than 20% cytoplasmic fragmentations are considered good quality. By selecting the blastocysts for uterine transfer, the number of embryos transferred can be reduced (preferably one) without compromising the pregnancy rates. By reducing the number of embryos transferred, higher order multiple pregnancies can be minimized. The pregnancy rate for blastocyst[13] transfer is reported to be as high as 43.8%.

Embryo Transfer: The cultured embryo is transferred to the uterine cavity with the help of a catheter. Patients with tubal disease have high rates of ectopic pregnancy. Since multiple embryos are transferred, the rate of heterotopic pregnancies is also higher than in the general population. Patients having hydrosalpinx should have it removed before IVF, since embryotoxic substances can come from hydrosalpinx and reduce the success rate of conception.

Luteal Support

Luteal support is needed for ART cycles, because ovum retrieval can adversely affect granulosa function resulting in progesterone deficiency. Luteal support can be in the form of micronized progesterone vaginal suppository twice daily or progesterone vaginal gel.

8.10.3 Cryopreservation of Embryos

In ART cycles, excess embryos are produced than what is required for transfer. To avoid multiple-pregnancy, fewer embryos are transferred. The excess embryos can be cryopreserved and transferred in a natural unstimulated cycle. Since stimulation is not necessary, the cost of gonadotropins can be overcome in the cycle when cryopreserved embryos are transferred. The risk of OHSS can also be avoided. In one study, transferring frozen embryos at a later date increased the delivery rate from 26.8 to 50% with a twin pregnancy rate[14] of 7.6%.

In the future single embryo transfer and cryopreservation of the remaining embryos will be the standard of care.

8.11 CONCLUSION

It is important to understand that couples seeking medical help for infertility would be going through serious emotional trauma and hence a sympathetic and considerate attitude should be adopted while approaching them. The primary responsibility of the clinician is to alleviate anxiety and to put in a sincere effort to find out the root cause of infertility. Investigations should be prioritized in such a manner that the least expensive and most informative ones are done first. A definite, informed plan of management should be charted out for each couple. Investigations and management should be evidence based and should start with semen analysis. In the event of an abnormal report, it should be repeated after 70-75 days provided proper method of collection is ascertained. Abnormal semen parameters warrant clinical examination and further investigation before resorting to treatment. Routine imaging of the female partner should be done using TVS because a lot of abnormalities including small sub-mucus fibroids, polyps, intra-uterine adhesions, Mullerian anomalies, polycystic ovaries, endometriosis, PID, etc can be detected. Routine MRI should not be resorted to. Invasive investigations like D and C which carry the risk of PID should be avoided. An early decision for laparoscopy should be taken if a pelvic pathology is suspected at initial clinical evaluation. When laparoscopy is decided, it should be done only with operative facilities because if a pathology is identified it can be corrected simultaneously. Controlled ovarian hyperstimulation and IUI should be advised in unexplained infertility and after treatment of pelvic disease like endometriosis or PID before choosing IVF. In conditions like advanced endometriosis and PID, an early decision for IVF should be taken as age of the female partner is the most important factor determining success rate in ART cycles. Even though advances in the treatment modalities have improved success rates of infertility treatment, adoption should be advised whenever it is deemed appropriate.

REFERENCES

1. Hull, et al. Population study of causes treatment and outcome of infertility Br Med J 1985;291:1693-7.
2. Jayaprakashan K, Campbell D, Hopkisson K, Johnson I, Raine F. A prospective comparative analysis of anti Mullerian hormone, inhibin B and 3 dimensional ultrasound determinants of ovarian reserve in the prediction of poor response to controlled ovarian stimulation. Fertil Steril 2008 (ahead of print).

3. Clomiphene, Metformin or both for infertility in the polycystic ovary syndrome. Richard S, Leyro, MD, et al. New England J of Medicine 2007;356:551-6.
4. J Clin Endocrinol Metab 2007;92:3128-35.
5. Dunaif J. Nat Clin Pract Endocrinol Metab 2008;4(5): 272-83.
6. Rouzi AA, Ardaw MS. A randomized controlled trial of the efficacy of Rosiglitazone and Clomiphene citrate vs. Clomiphene citrate and Metformin in women with Clomiphene citrate resistant polycystic ovary syndrome. Fertil Steril 2006;85(2):428-35.
7. Ahmed Badawy, Abeer Mosbah, Magda Shady. Anastrozole or letrozole for ovulation induction in clomiphene-resistant women with polycystic ovarian syndrome: a prospective randomized trial. Fertil Steril 2008; 89(5):1209-12.
8. Felemban A, Tan SL, Tulandi T. Laparoscopic treatment of polycystic ovaries with insulated needle cautery; a reappraisal. Fertyl Steril 2000;73:266-9.
9. Naether OG, Fischer R. Adhesion formation after laparoscopic electrocoagulation of the ovarian surface in polycystic ovary patients. Fertil Steril 1993;60:95-8.
10. Ismajovich B, Lidor A, Confino E, et al. Treatment of minimal and moderate intrauterine adhesions (Asherman's syndrome). J Reprod Med 1985;30:769-72.
11. NP Johnson, et al. Gaps in the evidence for fertility treatment: An analysis of the Cochrane Menstrual disorders and sub-fertility group database; Human reproduction 2003;18 (5): 947-54.
12. Karlstrom PO, Bergh T, Lundkbist O. A prospective Randomized of artificial insemination versus intercourse in cycles stimulated with human menopausal Gonadotropins or Clomiphene citrate, Fertilsteril 1993;59:554.
13. Hackmon-Ram R, et al. Blastocyst-stage embryo transfer in patients who failed to conceive in three or more day 2-3 embryo transfer cycles: a prospective, randomized study. Fertil Steril 2004;81:567-71.
14. Tiitinen A, Halttunen M, Harkki P, Vuoristo P, Hyden-Granskog C. Elective single embryo transfer: the value of cryopreservation. Hum Reprod 2001;16:1140-4.

9 Polycystic Ovarian Syndrome

Sareena Gilvaz, B Presannakumari

9.1 INTRODUCTION

It was Stein and Leventhal who first described the association of anovulation, hirsutism and enlarged polycystic ovaries as a syndrome, which was later named after them. Over the years there have been many changes in the definition, pathophysiology as well as management of this syndrome. The possible long-term problems of this syndrome have also gained importance recently. PCOS is now recognized to be a very heterogenous condition, which is the single-most common endocrinological problem of women in the reproductive age group. The prevalence of the condition as defined by the 1990 National Institutes of Health (NIH) criteria, in unselected populations of women of reproductive age is between 6·5 and 8%.The importance of establishing a clear evidence-based diagnosis and management of PCOS appears to have clinical implications.

9.2 GENETICS

The finding of a familial clustering of the association of anovulation with polycystic ovaries has led researchers to look for a genetic basis for the disease. An X-linked dominant inheritance and an autosomal dominant inheritance pattern have been identified. The genetic expression is found to be modified by environmental factors. The present consensus is that PCOS is familial and the various aspects of the syndrome may be differentially inherited.

9.3 CLINICAL FEATURES

It is presently understood that the condition is one of chronic anovulation with a spectrum of manifestations. The presenting symptoms can be

1. Menstrual irregularities and infertility
2. Features of hyperandrogenism
3. Metabolic symptoms

9.3.1 Menstrual Irregularities and Infertility

Menstrual irregularities are seen to occur in 70% of women. The menstrual patterns associated with PCOS include:

a. **Oligomenorrhea:** Irregular infrequent periods is the common irregularity seen which may date from menarche or start later, in the third decade of life
b. **Secondary amenorrhea:** These women can also present with secondary amenorrhea which denotes a severe form of the disease.
c. **DUB:** Prolonged heavy menses can be seen in association with anovulation.
d. **Regular menstruation:** About 10-35% of patients present with regular menstrual cycles. This need not necessarily indicate ovulation, especially in the presence of other evidence of hyperandrogenism. There can be varying periods of regular ovulatory menses also

Due to the ovulatory disturbance, those who pursue conception can present with infertility. The high LH and androgen levels in PCOS women were thought to cause repeated miscarriage. However, recent evidence does not support the fact that the incidence of abortion in PCOS is high.[1]

9.3.2 Features of Hyperandrogenism

Androgens are produced in the females from the adrenals under the influence of ACTH and in the ovary under the influence of LH. The androgens produced are androstenedione, testosterone, DHEA and DHEAS. Approximately one half of testosterone in women is produced from the peripheral conversion of androstenedione and the other half is synthesized in the ovary and adrenals. About 66-78% of circulating testosterone is bound to sex hormone binding globulin (SHBG) and the unbound is mainly transported weakly associated with albumin. Only about 1% of total testosterone is entirely free. The fraction of testosterone that is unbound is inversely related to concentration of SHBG. The use of oral contraceptives containing estrogen increase SHBG and thus decrease free testosterone. SHBG is decreased in PCOS, thus increasing the level of free T (discussed below).

Hyperandrogenism will be seen in most women with PCOS. The raised LH level along with hyperinsulinemia cause increased production of androgens from the theca cells. Adrenal androgens will also be elevated in about 30% of these women. The clinical features of androgen excess are hirsutism, acne and alopecia. Hirsutism is the commonest presenting symptom of hyperandrogenism and will be seen in about 70% women with PCOS. These symptoms usually start a few years after menarche and progress later on. The most common method of evaluating the severity of hirsutism is by using the visual score based on the modified Ferriman and Gallwey scoring system. In this system, 9 body areas namely the upper lip, chin, chest, upper back, lower back, upper abdomen, lower abdomen, arms and legs are considered.[2]

Table 9.1: Modified Ferriman and Gallwey scoring of hirsutism

Score	*Hirsutism*
<8	No hirsutism
9-16	Mild hirsutism
17-25	Moderate hirsutism
> 25	Severe hirsutism

A score of 0-4 is given based on the density of terminal hair in these areas. A score of 0 represents absence of terminal hair whereas 4 denotes extensive terminal hair. A score greater than 8 is classified as having hirsutism. The grading is provided in Table 9.1. This rating scale has since been modified by some to include a total of 19 locations, with the 10 extra locations being: *sideburns, neck, buttocks, inguinal* area, *perianal* area, *forearm, leg, foot, toes* and *fingers*. Each area has its own specified definition of the 4 point scale.[3]

Hirsutism is noticed in over 65–75% of PCOS patients. The increase in facial hair in PCOS (Fig. 9.1) is seen around puberty and the rate of hair growth is gradual. The distribution is more over the side of the face, upper lip, chin and neck, and the abdominal hair is seen distributed between the mons and umbilicus. Hair growth over arms and legs are no longer considered androgen dependant. Hence the

Ferriman and Gallwey scoring system is modified excluding these areas.

For the biochemical evidence of hyper-androgenemia, free testosterone level (free 'T') is the best marker. Free 'T' is the testosterone which is not bound to the sex hormone binding globulin (SHBG). Free T is calculated by the formula- (T/SHBGx100). It is this free 'T' which acts on target tissues.

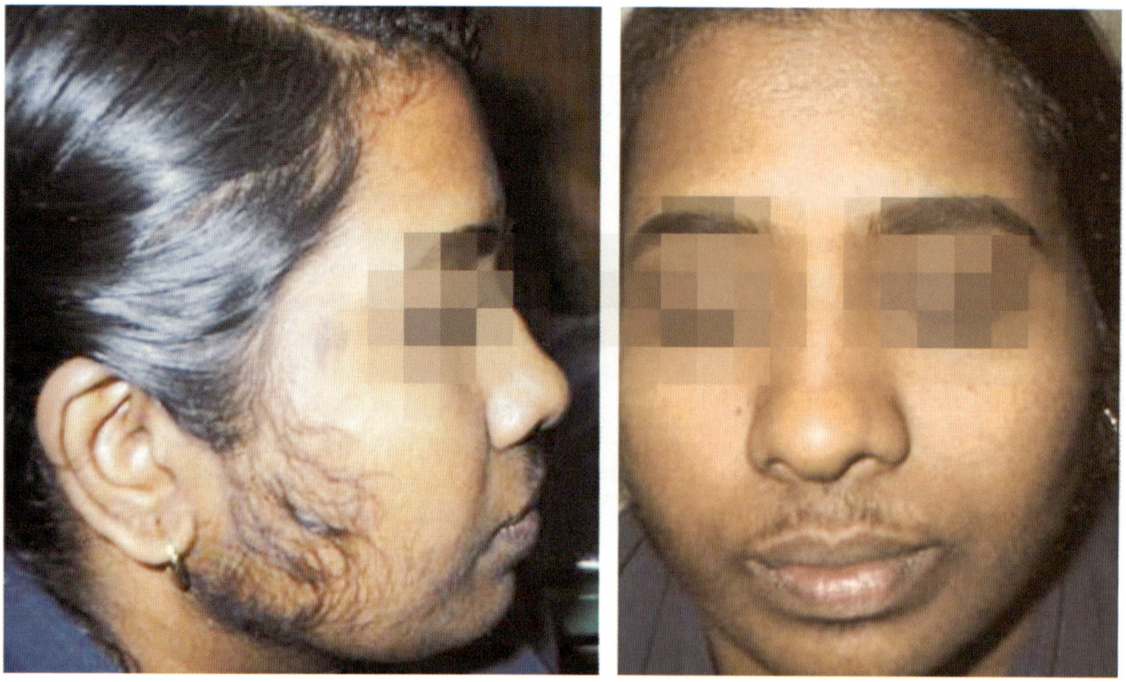

Fig. 9.1: Hirsutism in a patient with PCOS

In addition, androstenedione and dehydroepiandrosterone sulphate[4] (DHEAS) may also be elevated. Increased androgen level acts at the level of the hair follicle to result in acne which is seen in about 30%. Acne has been correlated with the increased levels of androgens. Acne is a more sensitive index of insulin resistance than hirsutism due to the longer period needed for expression of the latter. In spite of the presence of persistent hyperandrogenemia, other virilizing features are often not encountered. Features of virilization, like clitoromegaly and hoarseness of voice and alopecia are extremely rare in PCOS patients. Hence, women who have virilization should be investigated for other causes of androgen excess. It is also important to remember that measuring androgen level is particularly useful in women who do not show overt signs of hyperandrogenism.

9.3.3 Metabolic Symptoms

A group of abnormalities associated with insulin resistance was first described in 1988 by Dr Gerald Reaven who used the term syndrome X.[1] Since, then this syndrome has been addressed by several names and at present is called the metabolic syndrome.

Presence of 3 or more of the following metabolic abnormalities forms the criteria for diagnosing the metabolic syndrome.[5,6]

Obesity (BMI >25 kg/m^2) is seen in about 50% of women who have PCOS. Upper body obesity is characteristic of PCOS. The deposition of fat seen in normal women is more around the hips, buttocks and thighs giving a normal waist/hip ratio of < 0.85 (pear shaped). But in the obesity of PCOS, which is seen in over 30-60% of patients, the fat distribution is more central as evidenced by a high (> 0.85) waist/hip ratio (apple obesity). This fat is more sensitive to catecholamines and more metabolically active. This central obesity in patients with PCOS makes them more prone for the 'metabolic syndrome'. Peripheral aromatization of androgen to estrol is increased and is directly proportional to body weight.

Even in women who are not obese, the waist to hip ratio was found to be high. Insulin resistance and the resultant hyperinsulinemia are understood to be part of the disease and are thought to be contributing to hyperandrogenism. The most commonly used criteria in clinical practice and research is that described by the National Cholesterol Education Programme –Adult Treatment Panel III (NCEP-ATP III) [2] (Table 9.2). The fundamental components that define the metabolic syndrome include central obesity, hypertension, atherogenic dyslipidemia and impaired glucose tolerance or insulin resistance.

The data from the third National Health and Human Examination Survey III (NHANES III)[3] shows a high prevalence of the metabolic syndrome in the range of around

Table 9.2: Modified NCEP – ATP III, 2005 criteria for the diagnosis of metabolic syndrome

Risk factor	*Criteria*
Waist circumference	> 88 cm or 35 inches
Triglycerides	>150 mg/dL
High-density lipoprotein cholesterol	<50 mg/dL
Blood pressure	≥135/85
Fasting and 2-hour glucose utilizing an oral glucose tolerance test	>110–126 mg/dL and140–199 mg/dL

Sources: The Rotterdam ESHRE/ASRM-sponsored PCOS consensus workshop group2004; Apridonidze et al. 2005. Persons meeting three of the five criteria qualify for the diagnosis of the syndrome

50 % in these women between the ages 20 and 40. Hence the American Association of Clinical Endocrinology recommends routine screening for diabetes with GTT by the age of 30 for all women with PCOS [4] (Tables 9.3 and 9.4).

Table 9.3: The two hour glucose response to 75 gm oral glucose challenge test [5,6]

Normal	*Impaired glucose tolerance*	*Diabetes mellitus*
Fasting <100 mg/dL	100-125 mg/dL	≥ 126 mg/dL
2 hour <140 mg/dL	140-199 mg/dL	≥ 200 mg/dL

Table 9.4: Interpretation of the 2 hour insulin response

Peak insulin level
> 300 mIU/ml indicates severe hyperinsulinemia
150 - 300 mIU/ml—moderate hyperinsulinemia
100 - 150 mIU /ml—mild hyperinsulinemia

With the high prevalence of dyslipidemia in metabolic syndrome[7-9] most patients with PCOS would benefit from an evaluation of their lipid profile which is likely to show:

1. Reduced HDL cholesterol levels
2. Elevated triglyceride levels
3. Elevated LDL cholesterol levels
4. High LDL: HDL ratio[10]

This dyslipidemia is seen in both the lean and obese women with PCOS. Prolonged exposure to atherogenic dyslipidemia along with hypertension and hyperinsulinemia confers substantial risk of coronary artery disease.

Women with PCOS have substantially increased risk of developing impaired glucose tolerance and type II diabetes. About 40% of obese women with polycystic ovary syndrome have impaired glucose tolerance after a standard challenge with 75 g oral glucose. Excessive serine phosphorylation of the insulin receptor is thought to be the major reason for insulin resistance. *Acanthosis nigricans,* a cutaneous marker of insulin resistance characterized by patchy, velvety hyperpigmented skin changes in the neck, axilla or extensor aspect of joints is seen in some women with PCOS. It is reported that markers prothrombotic state and that of inflammation are high among these women. Endothelial dysfunction, probably caused by hyperinsulinemia occurs even in younger women with PCOS.

An association between epilepsy and PCOS has been recognized recently. This may be due to the effect of epilepsy or anti-epilepsy drugs on the endocrine centers in the brain.

9.3.4 Diagnostic Criteria

There was controversy prevailing regarding the diagnostic criteria of PCOS till recently. Originally the diagnostic criteria were based on clinical features only. With the evolution of biochemical methods, raised LH/FSH ratio was considered as one of the diagnostic criteria for PCOS. However, because of its inconsistency, this is no longer included as a criterion. Evaluation of ovarian morphology by ultrasound led to the ultrasound criteria for diagnosing the syndrome. However, it was understood that hyperandrogenism and chronic anovulation can be present without polycystic ovaries on ultrasound examination. For the sake of uniformity as well as to have an internationally agreed criterion for the diagnosis of PCOS, a joint consensus meeting of the American Society of Reproductive Medicine (ASRM) and the European Society of Human Reproduction and Embryology (ESHRE) was held in May 2003 at Rotterdam. A revised definition of PCOS (Table 9.5) was agreed upon at this meeting which is tabled below.

Table 9.5: Criteria for defining PCOS

ESHRE/ASRM (Rotterdam) 2003
To include 2 of the following after excluding other related disorders.
1. Clinical and/or biochemical signs of hyperandrogenism
2. Oligo-ovulation or anovulation
3. Polycystic ovaries
AES (Androgen Excess Society) 2006 criteria
To include all of the following
1. Hyperandrogenism
2. Ovarian dysfunction (Oligo/anovulation and/or polycystic ovaries)
3. Exclusion of related disorders

Source: The Rotterdam ESHRE/ASRM-sponsored PCOS consensus workshop group. Revised 2003 consensus on diagnostic criteria and long-term health risks related to polycystic ovary syndrome (PCOS). Hum Reprod 2004;19:41–7.

The recently held Thessaloniki ESHRE/ASRM meet at Greece (PCOS consensus workshop group 2007) has also endorsed this.

The principal features of PCOS include ovulatory dysfunction at the center with associated androgen excess and/or polycystic ovaries. Polycystic ovaries need not be present for the diagnosis of PCOS. Before confirming the diagnosis, exclusion of related disorders would mean ruling out other causes of androgen excess such as non-classical adrenal hyperplasia (NCAH) adrenal tumors, Cushing's syndrome, ovarian androgen secreting neoplasms, etc. Ovulatory dysfunction due to hypothyroidism, hyperprolactinemia as well as those due to intake of drugs should also be excluded.

9.3.5 Ovarian Morphology

Polycystic ovaries are commonly detected by ultrasound (Fig. 9.2), but this does not confirm the diagnosis of PCOS unless it is associated with the clinical and biochemical features which define the syndrome. Approximately 75% of anovulatory women will have polycystic ovaries. Polycystic ovaries are also observed in 8-25% of normally ovulating women as well as in 14% of women on oral contraceptives. The growth of the antral follicle gets arrested when they are less than 9 mm size, before the dominant follicle is recruited.

The presence of 12 or more follicles measuring 2-9 mm in diameter seen in at least one ovary, and/or an increased ovarian volume (> 10 cm^3) is considered to be the criteria of polycystic ovary. The follicles may be distributed at the periphery of the ovary in a 'pearl-necklace' pattern or scattered throughout the ovary. An ovary conforming to the normal volume may also be polycystic.

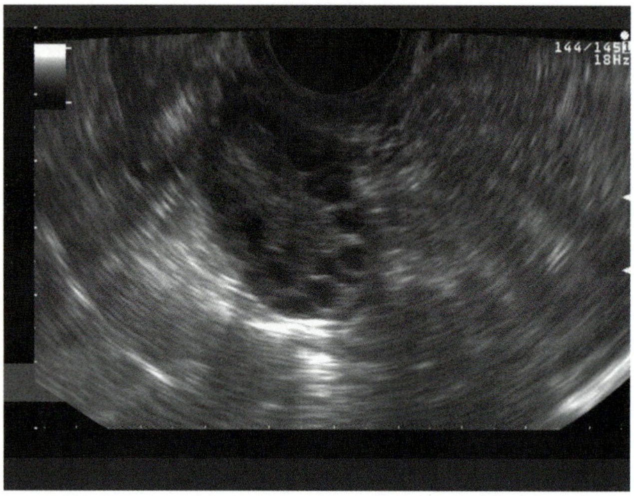

Fig. 9.2: Polycystic ovary on transvaginal ultrasound

9.4 DIFFERENTIAL DIAGNOSIS

PCOS has to be differentiated from other conditions which cause menstrual irregularities and hirsutism like non-classical adrenal hyperplasia, androgen secreting ovarian or adrenal tumors or Cushing's syndrome as well as other conditions which cause menstrual irregularity like hyperprolactinemia, hypothyroidism or premature ovarian failure. Typically women who have PCOS will have gradual onset of hirsutism which progresses slowly and features of virilization like clitoromegaly, or hoarseness of voice is very rare. Presence of features of virilization needs estimation of DHEA, DHEAS and testosterone as well as imaging studies of adrenal and ovary. Those who show features of Cushing's syndrome should have estimation of 24 hours cortisol level. 17 hydroxy progesterone will be significantly elevated in non-classical adrenal hyperplasia. Adrenal and ovarian tumors can be diagnosed by imaging. It should be kept in mind that functioning tumors of the ovary can be very small and hence can escape identification by ultrasound. History and clinical findings of hypothyroidism should be looked for in women who present with irregular menses and obesity. Estimation of TSH will clinch the diagnosis. Women who develop premature ovarian failure will have menopausal symptoms along with infrequent cycles followed by amenorrhea. They will have very high serum FSH level.

9.5 PATHOPHYSIOLOGY

PCOS is a spectrum of clinical disorders associated with insulin resistance, ovarian dysfunction, abnormal gonadotropin secretion and increased androgen production from the ovaries.

9.5.1 Altered LH/FSH Ratio and its Consequences

To begin with, there is an exaggerated pulsatile release of LH followed by ovarian steroidogenic enzyme dysregulation. The increased LH level stimulates the ovary to secrete increasing amounts of androgens namely testosterone and androstenedione from its stromal compartment.

In contrast to the high LH levels, the FSH levels would be low to normal which may be as a result of inhibitory feedback of estrogen on FSH,[11-13] supplemented with the effect of inhibin production from the polycystic ovaries. The increase in LH/ FSH ratio (≥ 2:1) is seen in 20-60% of women. It is also important to remember that this increase may not be seen in the other 40%.

Since the FSH level is not totally suppressed, new follicular growth will continue, but not to the point of full maturation and ovulation. As these follicles undergo atresia, they constantly add to the stromal compartment of the ovary.

The androgens elaborated from the stromal tissue namely testosterone suppresses the SHBG production by the liver, which in turn increase the circulating levels of free testosterone and estradiol.

In the ovary there is a relative aromatase defect secondary to FSH deficiency and the high intra-ovarian androgen rich environment impairs follicular maturation and cyclic production of estradiol and also induces follicular atresia.

Relation of LH to ovarian androgenic activity

- Increase in both free and total testosterone level as a direct effect of high LH.
- Androgen forming enzyme, CYP-17 dysregulation in the ovary making it more sensitive to LH.
- GnRH agonist treatment which suppresses the pituitary, effectively suppressing androgen production.

Though estradiol production from the ovary is not increased, free estradiol levels are raised because of the significant decrease in SHBG. Circulating estrone levels are also raised due to the peripheral conversion of androstenedione to estrone (Fig. 9.3). This persistent acyclic levels of estrogen, results in unopposed estrogenic stimulation of the endometrium placing these women at higher risk of developing endometrial hyperplasia and cancer in later life.

9.5.2 Insulin Resistance

50-70% of patients with PCOS have insulin resistance, and hyperinsulinemia appears to be the key to the pathogenesis of the syndrome. Due to insulin resistance there is a compensatory hypersecretion of insulin in response to glucose, and euglycemia is maintained at the expense of hyperinsulinemia. This insulin resistance is seen in both the lean and obese PCOS individuals.

Why insulin resistance?

Normally when insulin binds to its receptor, tyrosine residues on the receptor undergo phosphorylation to initiate insulin action. In PCOS, this process is altered in favor of serine phosphorylation which results in decreased insulin action within the cell. This accounts for the insulin resistance and the resultant hyperinsulinemia. The cause for the serine phosphorylation is uncertain but could presumably have a genetic basis.

Hyperinsulinemia and hyperandrogenemia (Fig. 9.4)

The association between hyperinsulinemia and hyperandrogenism dates back to the bearded diabetic woman reported by Archard and Thiers in 1921.

- Insulin and insulin like growth factor I (IGF-1) work with LH to directly stimulate the activity of the ovarian enzyme P450c 17 α which is pivotal in the production of androgens by the ovary.
- Insulin also inhibits hepatic synthesis of SHBG leading to increased free androgen.

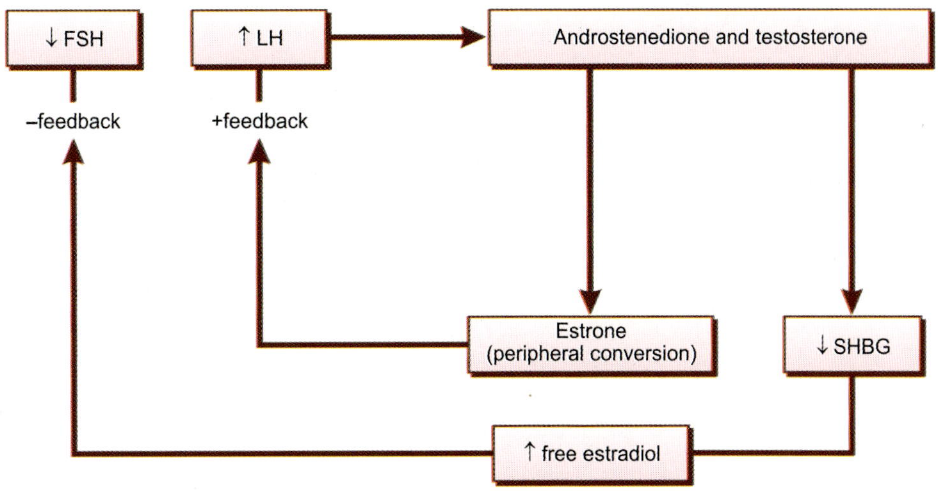

Fig. 9.3: Diagrammatic representation of pathophysiology of PCOS

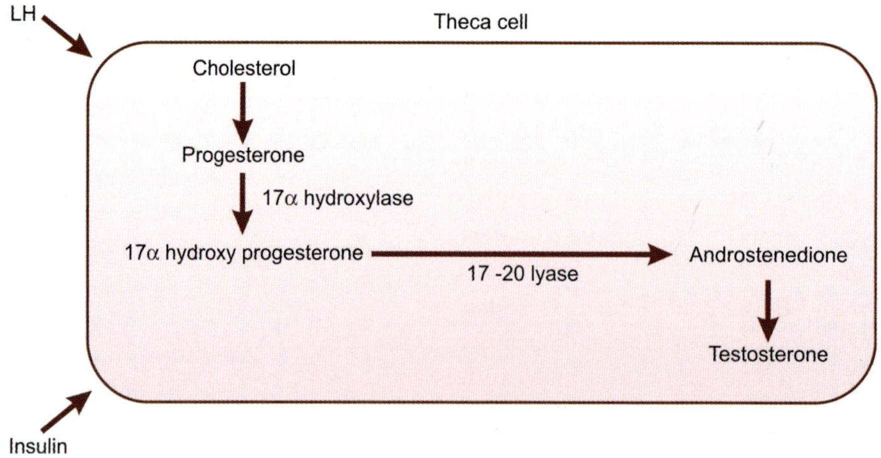

Fig. 9.4: Diagrammatic representation of the pathophysiology of hyperandrogenism in PCOS. Within the theca cells of the ovary, insulin and LH stimulates the cytochrome P450c 17 α activity resulting in increased 17 α hydroxylase and 17-20 lyase activity. It is these two enzymes which comprise the P450c 17 α complex

- The hyperandrogenism and insulin resistance are often associated with acanthosis nigricans which is clinically seen as a grey-brown velvety discoloration of the skin usually found at the nape of the neck, axilla, under the breasts and groin.
- The combination of hyperandrogenism (HA) insulin resistance (IR) and acanthosis nigricans (AN) has been termed the "HAIR- AN" syndrome.
- Hyperinsulinemia is associated with increased levels of Plasminogen Activator Inhibitor Type 1 (PAI-1). Raised PAI-1 levels increase the risk for coronary artery disease.
- Obesity is also another marker of insulin resistance. Insulin resistance combined with abdominal obesity is found to account for the higher prevalence of type II diabetes in later life.
- Therefore, administration of insulin-lowering drugs has been shown to improve insulin sensitivity, reduce androgen levels and restore ovulation.
- Evidence suggests that insulin resistance is the likely link between PCOS and the metabolic syndrome.

9.5.3 Endocrine Abnormalities

Instead of cyclic hormones in normal women, a steady state of gonadotropins and sex steroids will be seen in anovulatory PCOS women. The most commonly encountered marker is an increase in the serum testosterone[14] concentration. Androstenedione, dehydroepiandrosterone and 17- hydroxyprogesterone levels are also elevated in some women. DHEAS, which is exclusively secreted by the adrenal, is elevated in about 50% of anovulatory women with PCOS. Sex hormone binding globulin level will be less in these women due to the inhibitory effect of androgen on their production by the liver.

About 25% of these women will have mildly elevated prolactin levels also. This is explained to be due to the abnormal estrogen feedback to the pituitary.

9.5.4 Ovarian Defects

There is increasing evidence of ovarian abnormalities in the pathogenesis of PCOS. Folliculogenesis in polycystic ovaries is defective right from the gonadotropin-independent stages of development. Follicular recruitment, growth and selection of the dominant follicle are all deranged.

Studies have shown increased density of both resting and growing follicles in the ovary of PCOS women compared to normal women.[15,16] The early follicular development in the FSH independent stage is initiated by hyperandrogenemia.[17,18] Anti-mullerian hormone (AMH) synthesized by the granulosa cells of the growing follicle which inhibits growth of surrounding primordial follicles is found to be deficient in primordial and transitional follicles in PCOS.[19] This also enhances early follicular development.

Gonadotropin dependant follicular growth is prematurely arrested and selection of dominant follicles fails due to multiple factors in the intra ovarian environment such as:

- Elevated 5 alpha reductase activity in the small follicles.[20] This increases the active androgen levels in the follicle which inhibits the granulosa cell aromatase activity leading to reduced E_2 secretion.
- Low Activin A levels leads to low FSH secretion. This is augmented by high follistatin levels which binds activin and inhibits its action.[21]

- Defective inhibin biosynthesis[22]
- Premature responsiveness of the small follicles to high LH levels. This premature follicle luteinization promoted by hyperinsulinemia causes follicular arrest.[23]

Further, there is evidence that impaired oocyte signaling decreases granulosa cell proliferation and follicle growth, promoting accumulation of follicles with a PCO appearance. The oocyte secreted growth differentiation factor-9 (GDF-9) which promotes granulosa cell proliferation and preantral follicular growth[24] is found to be reduced in PCOS. Thus ovarian defects at various levels suggest a primary ovarian cause in the pathogenesis of PCOS.

9.5.5 Leptin and PCOS

Leptin is a 167 amino acid protein produced mainly in adipocytes. Insulin is a potent stimulator of leptin production. In PCOS this insulin stimulated leptin secretion is limited by the insulin resistance in the adipocytes. Furthermore the amount of visceral fat is more in PCOS and visceral fat has been shown to secrete less leptin[25] than subcutaneous fat (Vauhkonen *et al* 1998b, Van Harmelen *et al.* 1998). Leptin inhibits Neuropeptide Y, a hypothalamic neuropeptide which serves as an effector molecule in mediating the downstream effects of activation of central leptin receptors. Neuropeptide Y is a potent stimulator of food intake. The insulin resistance in PCOS which results in lower leptin levels inturn leads to higher Neuropeptide Y levels leading to decreased satiety signals in the hypothalamus, permitting further development of obesity (Jacobs & Conway 1999).

9.5.6 Long-term Consequences

Management of infertility was the main concern previously in women with PCOS. With the understanding of the fact that insulin resistance and the associated hyperinsulinemia is the key to the pathophysiology of the syndrome led to research about the long-term consequences of the syndrome. There is ample evidence that women with PCOS[26] are at a 7 time greater risk of developing type II diabetes in later life. The magnitude of the risk depends on prevalence of obesity and racial influences. This risk can be modified by altered lifestyle and diet. Even though the hyperandrogenic state and hyperinsulinemia predispose to adverse coronary artery events there is no evidence that mortality due to the same is more among these women on follow up studies. However in the Nurses' Health study cardiovascular mortality was higher in women who had irregular cycles compared to those with regular periods. This could probably have been a consequence of the associated polycystic ovaries.

The association of PCOS and endometrial, ovarian and breast carcinoma has also been the focus of interest. The endometrial hyperplasia associated with chronic anovulation in these women predisposes to the development of endometrial cancer. There is no evidence that women with PCOS are at increased risk of development of breast cancer.

Aim of treatment

- Reduce androgen level to correct hirsutism, improve lipid profile, etc.
- Improve insulin sensitivity so as to decrease insulin level and prevent development of diabetes
- Protect the endometrium from developing hyperplasia and malignancy
- Prevent the cardiovascular effects of altered lipid profile
- Ovulation induction if pregnancy is desired

9.6 MANAGEMENT

9.6.1 Investigation

Investigations are necessary for confirming the diagnosis of PCOS as well as for the further management of the problem. Laboratory testing should be individualized based on the patient's clinical manifestations. Estimation of serum LH and FSH which is widely practiced does not help in diagnosing PCOS. Since there is a wide range in the physiological levels of these hormones due to the pulsatile nature of their secretion, they can be in the normal range in women who have PCOS. Even if the ratio of these hormones is altered the management does not differ. Serum 17 hydroxyprogesterone level should be measured to exclude non-classical adrenal hyperplasia among adolescent girls presenting with irregular periods and hirsutism. For improving test sensitivity the sample should be drawn at 8 am. A value less than 2 ng/mL excludes congenital adrenal hyperplasia. If features of virilization are present, serum testosterone, DHEA and DHEAS should be estimated to exclude androgen secreting tumors. Testosterone level of > 60 ng/dL is considered abnormal. Levels > 200 ng/dl warrants evaluation for a possible ovarian or adrenal tumor. Elevated DHEAS in the presence of virilization needs evaluation of adrenal by CT scan. Serum cortisol level should be measured if there is clinical suspicion of Cushing's syndrome.

Ultrasound scan will reveal the nature of ovaries and help in diagnosing functioning tumors. If galactorrhea is present serum prolactin should be estimated to exclude hyperprolactinemia.

Since these women are at increased risk for developing type II diabetes and cardiovascular disease, screening for diabetes and estimation of lipid panel are indicated. A 2 hours GTT along with estimation of fasting and 2 hours insulin level should be done to assess hyperinsulinemia and insulin resistance.

The management of PCOS is based on the individual's concern, her marital status and fertility wishes. The woman may be concerned about a variety of problems like hirsutism, acne, menstrual problems, etc. Management should be aimed at the particular symptom. The clinician should aim at preventing the long-term consequences of PCOS like endometrial cancer, cardiovascular disease, diabetes mellitus etc, apart from managing the immediate concerns of the woman.

9.6.2 Weight Reduction

Obesity not only worsens the disordered ovarian function but also decreases the success of ovulation induction. Obesity increases insulin resistance. Weight loss also increases SHBG concentration, reduces testosterone concentration and androgenic stimulation of the skin, improves menstrual function and conception rates and reduces miscarriage rates. Weight reduction is more effective than Insulin sensitizers. Even after conception obesity adversely affects pregnancy by increasing the risk of pregnancy complications like pre-eclampsia, gestational diabetes and macrosomia. Weight reduction can overcome both short term as well as long-term consequences of PCOS. A modest weight reduction of 5-10% can lead to restoration of menstruation and ovulation. The Thessaloniki ESHRE/ASRM workshop has recommended weight loss as the first-line therapy in obese women with PCOS seeking pregnancy. There is no evidence that women who have normal body habitus will benefit from diet restriction and exercise. However, they should be advised to maintain body weight.

9.6.3 Lifestyle Changes

Promoting weight loss is difficult and requires effective counseling. Individual susceptibility to develop metabolic abnormalities among these women can be modified by environmental factors like change in dietary habits and increase in physical activity. Energy restriction is necessary for reducing weight but acute weight loss should not be encouraged for not only is it difficult to be sustained but also has adverse effects on reproduction.

Diet modifications

- Include more complex carbohydrate and fiber. Avoid simple sugars.
- Improve the quality of fat by avoiding saturated fat and increasing poly unsaturated oils
- Include ω3 oils
- Small more frequent meals
- Reduce alcohol intake

A low calorie diet along with an effective exercise regime should be incorporated into the lifestyle and should form the first line management in reducing weight. Regular exercise can maintain weight loss and improve mood.

9.6.4 Drug Treatment

Pharmacological agents which enhance satiety as well as those which inhibit the absorption of fat from the gastrointestinal tract can help in weight reduction. *Sibutramine* is a centrally acting drug which inhibits the reuptake of noradrenaline, serotonin and dopamine, enhancing satiety. However, caution should be exercised in prescribing the drug due to the possible side effects like dry mouth, paradoxical increase in appetite, etc. *Orlistat*, a pancreatic lipase inhibitor interferes with fat absorption from the intestine. Since its use can interfere with absorption of fat soluble vitamins also, multi-vitamin supplement which should include Vitamin A, D, E, K and beta-carotene should be co-prescribed.

9.6.5 Bariatric Surgery

For women with morbid obesity who do not respond to diet modification and medicines bariatric surgery should be considered. The weight loss achieved by surgery has been found to improve reproductive function.

9.6.6 Improving Insulin Sensitivity

Insulin resistance is seen in both lean and obese PCOS. The Glucose: Insulin ratio is an accurate index of insulin sensitivity in women with PCOS. A ratio of < 4.5 is found to be 95% sensitive and 85% specific in the diagnosis of insulin resistance.

Insulin sensitizers have been proved useful in the treatment of the metabolic aspects of PCOS. Women whose BMI is >35 and those who have insulin resistance would benefit from therapy with insulin sensitizers.

Metformin

Metformin, a biguanide derivative acts by:

1. Predominantly decreasing the hepatic glucose production
2. Improving the peripheral utilization of glucose

3. Decreasing intestinal glucose uptake
4. Decreasing lipolysis, thereby reducing the substrate for gluconeogenesis
5. Improving the lipid profile by decreasing the LDL and triglyceride and slightly increasing the HDL level[26]

It is advisable to start with a small dose (available strengths being 500 mg, 850 mg and 1000 mg) and then titrate up to the maximum dose of about 2000–2550 mg over several weeks depending on patient tolerance.

Side effects of metformin mainly include gastrointestinal symptoms such as anorexia, nausea, diarrhea, abdominal bloating and a peculiar metallic taste. The most serious side effect, though rare is lactic acidosis and it is best not to administer the drug to patients with renal or hepatic disease, cardiac failure or alcoholism as they are more prone to develop this problem. Hence, this drug should be started only after establishing normal renal and hepatic function and should be reviewed periodically while on treatment.

The greatest advantage of metformin is that when taken alone it does not cause hypoglycemia. Metformin is a *category B* drug in pregnancy.

Thiazolidinediones

The mechanism of action of these insulin sensitizers is by increasing the muscle insulin sensitivity and also by effecting the adipocyte gene expression through the peroxisome proliferator-activated receptors gamma (PPAR-γ). They decrease insulin resistance in the liver and cause decrease in free fatty acids, pre and postprandial glucose, insulin, triglycerides, LDL and increase HDL cholesterol. By decreasing insulin and androgen levels, and correcting anovulation, these drugs regularize menstrual cycle and decrease hirsutism. It seems that by modulation and attenuation of insulin resistance, thiazolidinediones can be used effectively to treat anovulation, infertility and hyperandrogenemia.

Rosiglitazone at a dose of 4 mg daily showed improved insulin sensitivity leading to menstrual regularity in most patients. But an increase in body weight has been noted[27] in the range of 0.5–4.5 kg.

Pioglitazone at a dose of 30 mg daily also improves insulin sensitivity with a decrease in triglyceride levels,[28] but with a disadvantage of weight gain.[29] Both these drugs have been placed as *category C* drug during pregnancy.

Troglitazone, another thiazolidinedione has been given up because of its hepatotoxicity.

Somatostatin, a hypothalamic peptide is being evaluated for its role in improving insulin sensitivity. The disadvantage is its short half life necessitating multiple daily injections. To overcome this disadvantage, a long acting analog of somatostatin, Octreotide-LAR has been developed, which need be given once in 28 days.

Insulin sensitizers (metformin and thiazolidinediones) aimed at lowering insulin levels have shown to improve menstrual irregularity and even induce ovulation. Long-term use of these drugs will prevent development of diabetes as well as coronary vascular diseases.

Treatment options to prevent metabolic syndrome

1. Lifestyle modification through increased physical activity and reduction in body weight especially a reduction in waist circumference represents the first line therapy.
2. A diet low in saturated fat, high in fiber, and low glycemic index carbohydrates is found suitable for women with PCOS.[12]
3. No single dietary composition has clearly proved ideal for women with PCOS.
4. The addition of insulin sensitizers like metformin and thiazolidinediones have greatly helped in reducing the morbidity associated with the metabolic syndrome and should be advised for women whose BMI is more than 35 and those with insulin resistance.

9.6.7 Reduction in Androgen Level

The androgen excess associated with PCOS has significant dermatologic, reproductive and metabolic consequences. Increased androgenic milieu is the cause for defective folliculogenesis. Androgen excess affects the lipid profile adversely resulting in increased LDL and decreased HDL levels. Dermatologic consequences of androgen excess are acne and hirsutism. Reducing androgen level is crucial for improving ovulation as well as lipid profile. There are several pharmacological options for achieving reduction in androgen levels.

Oral Contraceptives

The older generation COCs increase insulin resistance. However the low-dose COCs are found to have only a negligible effect on carbohydrate metabolism and long-term follow-up studies have shown no increase in the incidence of diabetes mellitus among low-dose pill users. Low-dose COCs containing ethinyl estradiol and anti-androgen cyproterone acetate may be preferred in PCOS patients to prevent the long-term adverse consequences of hyperandrogenism.

Mechanism of action of COC: COC pills suppress LH secretion and thereby reduce ovarian androgen production, increases SHBG levels thus reducing free testosterone and also inhibit 5 *α* reductase.

There are various combination pills with anti-androgenic effect available for the adolescent PCOS. These reduce the androgen related symptoms such as hirsutism and acne, in addition to the regulation of menstrual cycle. For this purpose the third generation COCs containing 30 μg ethinyl estradiol and 150 μg desogestrel (Novelon™, Intimacy plus 3™) which are androgen neutral should be prefered..

The antiandrogen, cyproterone acetate 2 mg with 35 μg ethinyl estradiol (Diane 35™, Krimson 35™) is another combination which can be preferred in PCOS patients with hirsutism and acne.

The latest in this category is a combination of estradiol 30 μg with 3 mg of drosperinone (Dronis 20™, Crisanta™, Yasmin™). Drosperinone is a spironolactone derivative with antiandrogenic and anti-mineralocorticoid effect.[27] The anti-mineralocorticoid effect reduces weight gain associated with COC use. Women should be counseled that the results of this treatment may not be appreciable until 6 months of initiating treatment. Therefore mechanical hair removal techniques with medication should be advised for best results.

Antiandrogens

When hirsutism and acne are the concern, antiandrogens are indicated. It should be emphasized that medical treatment cannot influence existing hair. They can only prevent further growth. Hence, existing hair should be treated with mechanical hair removing techniques like using depilatory creams like Eflornithine (inhibitor of ornithine decarboxylase enzyme) or by electrolysis.

Antiandrogens are frequently used in combination with oral contraceptives because their mechanism of action is different and hence the combined effect is additive. Flutamide, a non steroidal anti-androgen acts by inhibiting DHT binding to androgen receptor. Thus the drug suppresses androgen action and has been found to improve lipid profile. It is used at an initial dose of 250 mg/day and a maintenance dose of 125 mg/day. The addition of oral contraceptive has the added benefit of preventing pregnancy and unwanted teratogenicity due to the antiandrogens and it also reduces the irregular bleeding associated with anti-androgen use. Finasteride is another anti-androgenic drug which acts by inhibiting 5 α reductase, which is particularly potent in hair follicle.

Spironolactone is an aldosterone antagonist, competitively binds to aldosterone receptors in the kidney. Its effectiveness is due to the following mechanisms.

1. Competitive inhibition of DHT at the intracellular receptor level
2. Suppress testosterone biosynthesis
3. Improved peripheral conversion of testosterone to estrone
4. Inhibit 5 α reductase in the skin

The drug is used in a dose of 50-100 mg twice daily. Since this drug can increase serum K^+ level, this should not be administered to women with renal insufficiency.

Cyproterone acetate is a synthetic progestin with potent antiandrogenic properties. The mechanism of action is mainly by competitively inhibiting androgen action at the receptor level. The drug is administered in a reverse sequential regime—Cyproterone acetate 100 mg/day on days 5-15 and ethinyl estradiol 30-50 μg on day 5-26. The drug can also be used in small dose in combination with estrogen as COC (discussed above).

9.6.8 Endometrial Protection

The persistently high level of estrogen along with absence of progesterone in the anovulatory PCOS women can lead to endometrial hyperplasia and malignancy. Endometrial malignancy has been reported in very young women who have chronic anovulation. Whenever the endometrial thickness measures >15 mm, endometrial biopsy is mandatory to exclude hyperplasia and malignancy. The endometrial effects of unopposed estrogen can be prevented by administering progestagens in the second half of menstrual cycle.

Progestagen Therapy

All anovulatory women with oligomenorrhea or amenorrhea should be treated with progestagens for a minimum period of 10 days every month so as to induce regular withdrawal bleed. Even adolescent girls with PCOS and infrequent periods should be treated with progestagens. The preferred progestagen preparation is medroxy-progesterone acetate at a dosage of 5-10 mg/day for about 10 days every month. This helps in the shedding of an estrogen built-up endometrium thus preventing hyperplasia. For those with hirsutism and acne, combination OC pills containing antiandrogen should be preferred as mentioned earlier.

9.6.9 Management in Adolescent Girls

Irregular infrequent periods in the adolescent age group is widely regarded as due to the immaturity of the HPO axis. However, follow-up studies of adolescents who have oligomenorrhea revealed that a large proportion of these girls later on develop PCOS. The oligomenorrhea due to immature HPO axis will correct itself within 2 years of menarche. Otherwise these girls should be investigated and managed as PCOS. Counseling is very important and the girl as well as her parents need counseling. Obesity should be managed by lifestyle and dietary changes. If hirsutism and acne are the concern, it is better to manage these girls with COC containing cyproterone acetate and ethinyl estradiol, which will halt the progression of the disease and will reduce hirsutism. Minimum 6 months treatment is required for a clinically evident effect. It is better to advise mechanical hair removal as an initial procedure. Presence of severe hirsutism needs treatment with antiandrogens like finasteride or flutamide. Those who present with secondary amenorrhea or infrequent menses can be managed with medroxyprogesterone taken at least 10 days a month so that they will have regular endometrial shedding. Long-term use of insulin sensitizers like metformin is not recommended for use in adolescent girls for preventing the development of metabolic syndrome later in life, since there is no sufficient evidence to recommend metformin use in such a situation. However in adolescents with impaired glucose tolerance, other signs of insulin rsistance or a strong family history of type II diabetes, metformin use is warranted.

9.6.10 Management of Infertility

With the introduction of ovulation inducing agents, management of infertility in PCOS has shown great improvement in the past few decades. Weight loss is recommended as first line therapy in obese women with PCOS seeking pregnancy. Successful weight reduction has shown to regularize menstrual cycles, induce ovulation and achieve pregnancy.

Ovulation Induction with Clomiphene Citrate

Clomiphene citrate is an effective first line method of ovulation induction in both obese and lean PCOS individuals. It is used in the lowest dose required to bring about ovulation, followed by timed intercourse or IUI. If no ovulation is achieved even with doses up to 150 mg/day for 5 days, alternative strategies can be attempted by including metformin, dexamethasone, etc. Ideally up to 6 cycles can be tried (never more than 12 cycles). Women with elevated BMI, those with amenorrhea, marked hyperandrogenemia and insulin resistance are likely to be clomiphene-resistant.

Metformin

The use of insulin-sensitizing agents, such as metformin, in women with polycystic ovary syndrome has been widely studied. Suppression of insulin levels with metformin might reduce the hyperinsulinemia and hyperandrogenism. As a consequence, metformin was thought to improve both pregnancy and live birth rates. In the trials which compared Metformin with placebo and Metformin and CC with CC alone, there was an improved pregnancy rate in the group which took metformin.

A Cochrane review on metformin use before ART did not find evidence that metformin treatment before or during ART cycles improves live birth or pregnancy rates.

However recent adequately powered studies did not reveal significantly improved pregnancy rates[28] when Metformin – CC combination was compared with CC alone.

In another trial, when metformin was compared with CC it was found that metformin was not superior to CC as regards fertility rates. In the recently held Thessaloniki PCOS consensus workshop of ESHRE/ASRM 2007 with regard to the use of metformin for induction of ovulation, it was pointed out that metformin does not increase live birth rates above those observed with CC alone, in either obese or normal weight women with PCOS (Moll et al 2006;Legro et al 2007a) except perhaps in women with BMI >35 kg/m^2 and in those with CC resistance. Further, metformin treatment conferred no additional advantage when administrated to women with newly diagnosed PCOS and it does not appear to reduce the incidence of early pregnancy loss when continued in pregnancy. Hence the consensus regarding use of metformin in PCOS is to restrict its use to those patients with glucose intolerance.[29]

Glucocorticoids

Those women in whom the adrenal gland makes an important contribution to androgen excess as evidenced by elevated levels of DHEAS, dexamethasone 0.5 mg daily is added as an adjunct to CC from day 3 for 10 days. Since insulin resistance is usually associated, glucose level should be monitored while the women are on steroid therapy. Current evidence has questioned this therapy.

Aromatase Inhibitors

Aromatase inhibitors competitively inhibit aromatase enzyme which converts androgen to estrogen thereby reducing the circulating level of estrogens. Thus the negative feedback of estrogen on the hypothalamus is removed which results in increased secretion of FSH. Aromatase inhibitors usually cause monofollicular development and ovulation. Letrozole, the aromatase inhibitor in use at present, is given in doses of 2.5 mg from day 3 to day 7. This drug scores over CC in that there is a better endometrial receptivity and thickness (in the range of 6-9 mm [30,31]) compared to the thin endometrium of patients on CC.

GnRH Agonist

It has been found in randomized controlled trials, that the use of combination treatment with GnRH agonist and COC improves ovulation and pregnancy after discontinuation of treatment. The mechanism could be by decreasing LH level and thus the hyperandrogenism.

If ovulation induction is not successful with the above measures, there are two options.

1. To proceed with gonadotropin treatment with/without IVF
2. Laparoscopic Ovarian Drilling (LOD)

Gonadotropins

The major problem with induction of ovulation with FSH is the development of ovarian hyper-stimulation syndrome (OHSS),[32] which these patients are prone for. Hence, it is advisable either to resort to the low dose regimen which is the preferred protocol or start with high doses of FSH and rapidly reduce the dose once the dominant follicle appears.[33-35] Intense ovarian response monitoring is required and in the event of a hyper-response, cycle cancellation must be resorted to in order to avoid complications. If four or more follicles measuring more than 14 mm are seen it is advisable to stop administering gonadotropins. The recommendation of the 2007 Thessaloniki ESHRE/ASRM PCOS workshop is to withhold hCG administration in the presence of more than two follicles >16 mm, or more than one follicle >16 mm and two additional follicles >14 mm, to minimize the risk of multiple pregnancy and hyperstimulation syndrome.

An estradiol level more than 2500 pgm/ml is an indication of hyperstimulation. However, A Golan et al have shown that estimation of serum estradiol did not add to monitoring with ultrasound.

If pregnancy is still not achieved, the next step is IVF-ET. PCOS patients undergoing IVF is a major challenge due to the high risk of hyperstimulation syndrome. The use of GnRH agonists for desensitizing the pituitary before initiation of gonodotropin therapy is not recommended as it is associated with increased risk of OHSS and multiple pregnancy and is not seen to increase pregnancy rate.

In Vitro Maturation of Oocyte (IVM) and Intracytoplamic Sperm Injection (ICSI)

This concept of IVM helps avoid the use of gonodotropins with its associated side effects. Immature oocytes retrieved from the antral follicles are harvested in special culture media. After 24-48 hours, the cumulus is stripped and those oocytes that have progressed to metaphase II stage are fertilized using ICSI. Studies have reported an increased rate of miscarriage. Li et al revealed significant spindle and chromosomal abnormalities with IVM.[36] The safety of the method is to be established before its widespread use.

Laparoscopic Ovarian Surgery (Fig. 9.5)

For many years wedge resection of the ovary was the only treatment for PCOS. This was given up because of the extensive pelvic adhesions it produced and the increased incidence of premature ovarian failure. Today with laparoscopic access, we have a good alternative when medical treatment fails. Laparoscopic ovarian drilling (LOD) is free of the risks of multiple pregnancy and ovarian hyperstimulation with the added benefit of a fall in the serum concentrations of LH and testosterone.

The greater the damage to the surface of the ovary, the greater will be the risk of peri-ovarian adhesion formation. The more the number of punctures, the more will be the chance for premature ovarian failure. This has led Armar to develop a strategy of minimizing the number of diathermy points to four per ovary avoiding the hilum, for 4 seconds at 40 watts.[37] With this technique there was a low rate of adhesion formation, but the pregnancy rates were not satisfactory. Women with greatly enlarged ovaries need more ovarian reduction which can be achieved by increasing the number of punctures. LOD should not be offered for non-fertility indications. Even after LOD some women may need ovulation induction. Hence, if conception does not occur within 3 months clomiphene can be added and after 6 months gonadotropins may be tried.

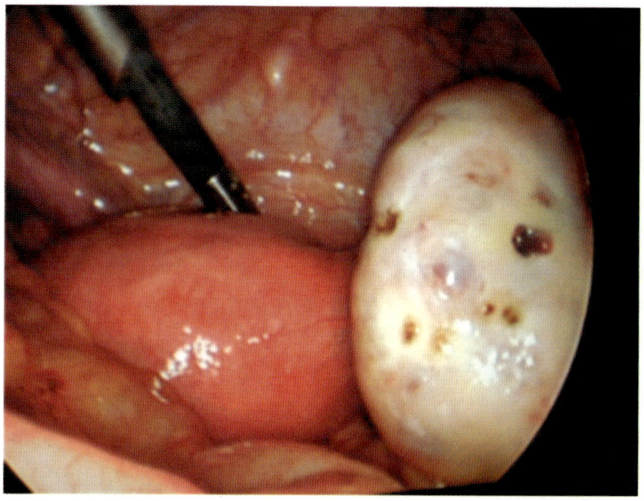

Fig. 9.5: Laparoscopic ovarian drilling

9.7 CONCLUSION

Polycystic ovarian syndrome refers to a spectrum of disorders which include chronic anovulation, hyperandrogenism, hyperinsulinemia and obesity. The prevalence of the disorder is on the increase, probably because of the increased identification or due to the altered lifestyle of the adolescent population. Previously, management of infertility was given priority. But the understanding that the condition is associated with or caused by insulin resistance has thrown light into the altered lipid profile and abnormal carbohydrate metabolism associated with the syndrome. The etiologic association of the unopposed estrogenic action and the development of endometrial hyperplasia and malignancy have also been understood. Hence, in the management of the condition, the priority is not only in treating the short-term problems like infertility, irregular menses or cutaneous manifestations of androgen excess, but also in preventing the long-term detrimental effects of the metabolic abnormalities and endometrial changes that stretch over the entire life span of the woman. A lot more has to be done in the preventive aspect of PCOS. Since the disease usually starts during adolescence, prevention of long-term problems should be addressed right from the beginning. For preventing endometrial hyperplasia, a progestagen should be administered to ensure regular withdrawal bleeding, especially for women who get very infrequent periods or have amenorrhea. For women with acne and hirsutism, long-term use of the newer low-dose oral contraceptives especially those containing drosperinone is promising. The abnormal lipid profile which is a consequence of hyperandrogenism should be prevented by improving insulin sensitivity. Weight reduction by lifestyle changes has an important role in achieving this. Insulin sensitizers like metformin should be preferred in PCOS women showing glucose intolerance or with BMI > 35 kg/m^2. The first line treatment of infertility is lifestyle changes to effect weight reduction. Ovulation induction should be initiated with clomiphene citrate. Aromatase inhibitors can be tried in women who fail to ovulate with CC. The management choices for those who do not conceive with oral ovulogens are induction with gonadotropins or LOD. ART should be resorted to as the final option. With advances in ovulogens and ART technologies, the problem of infertility among these women carry very good prognosis. Thus the overall health and long-term problems of women with polycystic ovarian disease should be the main concern.

REFERENCES

1. Reaven GM. Banting lecture 1988. Role of insulin resistance in human disease. Diabetes 1988;37:1595-607.
2. Expert Panel on Detection. Evaluation and Treatment of High Blood Cholesterol in Adults (Adult treatment Panel III).Executive Summary of The Third Report of the National Cholesterol Education Program (NCEP) JAMA. 2001; 285: 2486-97.
3. Ford ES, Giles WH, Dietz WH. Prevalence of the metabolic syndrome among US adults: findings from the third National Health and Nutrition Examination survey. JAMA 2002;287: 356-59.
4. American Association of clinical Endocrinologists. American Association of clinical Endocrinologists Position Statement on metabolic and Cardiovascular consequences of Polycystic Ovary Syndrome. Endocr Pract 2005;11:126-34.
5. Legro RS, Kunselman AR, Dodson WC, et al. Prevalence and predictors of risk for type 2 diabetes mellitus and impaired glucose tolerance in polycystic ovary syndrome: a prospective, controlled study in 254 affected women JC clin Endocrinol Metab. 1999;84:165-69.
6. World Health organization. Definition diagnosis and Classifications of Diabetes Mellitus and its complications. Report of a WHO consultation, Part 1: diagnosis and classification of diabetes mellitus Geneva: WHO; 1999.
7. Legro RS, Kunselman AR, Dunaif A. Prevalence and predictors of dyslipidemia in women with polycystic ovary syndrome Am J Med 2001; 111:607-13.
8. Dokras A, Bochner M, Hollinrake E, et al. Screening women with polycystic ovary syndrome for metabolic syndrome Obstet Gynecol 2005;106:131-37.
9. Apridonidze T, Essah PA, Iuorno MJ, et al. Prevalence and characteristics of the metabolic syndrome in women with polycystic ovary syndrome. J Clin Endocrinol Metab.2005: 90:1929-35.
10. Talbott E. Guzick D, Clerici A, et al. Coronary heart disease risk factors in women with polycystic ovary syndrome, Arterioscler Thromb VascBioll 1995;15:821-26.
11. Rexrode KM, Carey VJ, Hennekens CH, et al. Abdominal adiposity and coronary heart disease in women. JAMA 1998; 280:1843-48.
12. Marsh k, Brand – Miller J. The optimal diet for women with polycystic ovary syndrome? Br J Nutr 2005; 94:154-65.
13. Leblanc ES, Laws A. Benefits and risks of third generation oral contraceptives. J Gen Intern Med 1999;14:625-32.
14. Guido M, Romualdi D, Giuliani M, et al. Drospirenone for the treatment of hirsute women with polycystic ovary syndrome: a clinical endocrinological metabolic pilot study. J Clin Endocrinol Metab 2004;89:2817-23.
15. Webber LJ, Stubbs S, Stark J, Trew GH, Margara, R Hardy, K, Franks S. Formation and early development of follicles in the polycystic ovary. Lancet 2003; 362: 1017-21.

16. Maciel GA, Baracat EC, Benda JA, Markham SM, Hensinger K, Chang RJ, Erickson GF. Stockpiling of transitional and classic primary follicles in ovaries of women with polycystic ovary syndrome. J Clin Endocrinol Metab 2004;89:5321-27.
17. Vendola KA, Zhou J, Adesanya OO, Weil SJ, Bondy CA. Androgens stimulate early stages of follicle growth in the primate ovarian. J Clin Invest 1998;101:2622-29.
18. Gilling-Smith C, Willis DS, Beard RW, Franks S. Hypersecretion of androstenedione by isolated theca cells from polycystic ovaries. J Clin Endocrinol Metab 1994;79: 1158-65.
19. Stubbs SA, Hardy K, Da Silva-Buttkus P, Stark J, Webber LJ, Flanagan AM, Themmen AP, Visser JA, Groome NP, Franks S. Anti-mullerian hormone protein expression is reduced during the initial stages of follicle development in human polycystic ovaries. J Clin Endocrinol Metab 2005; 90: 5536-43.
20. Jakimiuk AJ, Weitsman SR, Magoffin DA. 5α-Reductase activity in women with polycystic ovary syndrome. J Clin Endocrinol Metab 1999;84:2414-18.
21. Norman RJ, Milner CR, Groome NP, Robertson DM. Circulating follistatin concentrations are higher and activin levels are lower in polycystic ovarian syndrome. Hum Reprod 2001;16:668-72.
22. Welt CK, Taylor AE, Martin KA, Hall JE. Serum inhibin B in polycystic ovary syndrome: regulation by insulin and luteinizing hormone. J Clin Endocrinol Metab 2002;87:5559-65.
23. Willis D, Watson H, Mason H, Galea R, Brincat M, Franks S. Premature response to LH of granulose cells from anovulatory women with polycystic ovaries: relevance to mechanism of anovulation. J Clin Endocrinol Metab 1998;83:3984-91.
24. Filho FLT, Baracat EC, Lee TH, Suh CS, Matsui M, Chang RJ, Shimasaki S, Erickson GF. Aberrant expression of growth differentiation factor-9 in oocytes of women with polycystic ovary syndrome J Clin Endocrinol Metab 2002;87:1337-44.
25. Morin-Papumen LC, Kovivumen RM, Ruokonen A, et al Metformin therapy improves the menstrual pattern with minimal endocrine and metabolic effects in women with polycystic ovary syndrome. Fertile Steril 1998; 69:691-96.
26. Bailey CJ, Turner RC. Metformin N Engl J Med 1996;334:574-79.
27. Belli SH, Graffigna MN, Oneto A, et al. Effect of rosiglitazone on insulin resistance, growth factors, and reproductive disturbances in women with polycystic ovary syndrome. Fertil Steril 2004;81:624-29.
28. Yki-Jarvinen H. Thiazolidinediones N Engl J Med 2004:351:1106-18.
29. DeLeo V, laMarca A, Petraglia F. Insulin – lowering agents in the management of polycystic ovary syndrome Endocr Rev 2003; 24:633-67.
30. Holzer H, Casper R, Tulandi T. A new era in ovulation induction. Fertil Steril 2006;85:277-84.
31. Mitwally MF, Casper RF. Aromatase inhibition: a novel method of ovulation induction in women with polycystic ovarian syndrome. Reprod Technol 2000;10:244-47.
32. Aboulghar MA, Mansour RT. Ovarian hyperstimulation syndrome: classifications and critical analysis of preventive measures. Hum Reprod Update 2003;9:275-89.
33. Hamilton-Fairely D, Kiddy D, Watson H, et al. Low dose gonadotropin therapy for induction of ovulation in 100 women with polycystic ovary syndrome. Hum Reprod 1991; 6:1095-99.
34. Meldrum DR Low dose follicle – stimulating hormone therapy for polycystic ovarian disease. Fertil Steril 1991;55: 1039-40.
35. Macklon NS, Fauser BCJM. Ovulation induction: step-up and step-down regimens. In: kempers RD, Cohen J, Haney AF, et al (Eds). Fertility and Reproductive Medicine: Proceedings of the XVI world Congress on Fertility and Sterility. San Francisco. New York Elsevier Science B.V; 1998:529-36.
36. Li Y, et al. Confocal microscopic analysis of the spindle and chromosome: Configurations of human oocytes matured in vitro. Fertil Steril. 2006;85:827-32.
37. Armar NA, Magarrigle HHG, HonourJW, Holownia P, et al. Laparoscopic ovarian diathermy in the management of anovulatory infertility in women with polycystic ovaries; Endocrine changes and clinical outcome. Fertil Steril 1990: 53:45-49.

10 Contraception

B Presannakumari

10.1 INTRODUCTION

The past two decades have seen significant advances in the field of contraceptive technologies. From 1960s, when the hormonal contraceptives were brought into the market, there has been a transition from high dose to low dose combined oral contraceptives, inert devices to the copper incorporated devices and hormone releasing intrauterine devices. Another breakthrough was the introduction of injectables and implants as contraceptives. Despite the widespread availability of a range of contraceptives, unintended pregnancies continue to be a major public health issue. Of the major lacunae one important aspect is lack of awareness among women as well as their misconceptions. The provider should be well versed with the efficacy of the various methods, possible health benefits, the side effects, as well as the health hazards resulting from pre-existing medical problems. The clinician should be able to match the user with the optimum contraceptive method. This chapter gives an account of hormonal contraceptives, intrauterine devices, barrier methods, fertility awareness based methods, emergency contraception as well as male and female sterilization.

10.2 EFFECTIVENESS OF METHODS

Choice of contraceptive mainly depends on the effectiveness in preventing unplanned pregnancy. Efficacy of a method is assessed by measuring the number of unplanned pregnancies that occur during a specified period of exposure when a contraceptive method is used. For most contraceptives, the effectiveness depends not only on the protection offered by the method itself, but also on how consistently and correctly the method is used. Consistent and correct or perfect use of the method gives the maximum effectiveness. There can be a wide range of effectiveness in the 'typical use' (usual experience) of the method. Efficacy can be expressed as:

1. ***Lowest expected (perfect use) failure rate*** is the failure rate which is determined by clinical trials among highly motivated subjects and hence will be comparatively less.
2. ***Typical failure rate*** is the failure rate in the usual experience, which will be higher. 'Typical use' applies when the contraceptive is not used correctly.

Contraceptive failure rates quoted in the text are derived from the National Survey of Family Growth (US), 1995. (Table 10.1)

Knowledge about the definitions used in assessing contraceptive efficacy is important in counseling couples. The two methods that are used to assess contraceptive efficacy are the pearl index and life table analysis. The *pearl index* is defined as the number of failures per 100 women years of exposure. One disadvantage of using the pearl index for assessing contraceptive effectiveness is that it is based on a specific exposure, usually one year and hence does not take into account the decline in the effectiveness over time. This is overcome by the use of life-table analysis. *Life-table analysis* calculates a failure rate for each month of use. A cumulative failure rate can then compare methods for any specific length of exposure.

10.3 WHO ELIGIBILITY CRITERIA

In order to make contraception safe for individuals with certain health conditions, WHO published recommendations about medical eligibility criteria on contraceptive use in the

Table 10.1: Percentage of women experiencing an unintended pregnancy during the first year of typical use and the first year of perfect use of contraception in the United States

Method	Percentage of women experiencing an unintended pregnancy within the first year of use	
	Typical use (%)	*Perfect use (%)*
No method	85	85
Sponge	-	-
Parous women	32	20
Nulliparous women	16	9
Diaphragm	16	6
Condom	-	-
Female (Reality)	21	5
Male	15	2
Combined pill/progestin-only pill	8	0.3
Evra Patch	8	0.3
NuvaRing	8	0.3
Depo-Provera	3	0.3
IUD	-	-
ParaGard (copper T)	0.8	0.6
Mirena (LNG-IUS)	0.2	0.2
Implanon	0.05	0.05
Female sterilization	0.5	0.5
Male sterilization	0.15	0.10

Source: Trussell J. Contraceptive efficacy. In Hatcher RA, Trussell J, Nelson AL, Cates W, Stewart FH, Kowal D. *Contraceptive Technology: Nineteenth Revised Edition.* New York NY: Ardent Media, 2007

year 1996, which was updated later in 2003, 2004 and 2008, based on the most up-to-date information available on the safety of different methods. Accordingly, there are four categories, i.e. 1 to 4 which are as follows:

1. A condition for which there is no restriction for the use of the contraceptive method.
2. A condition where the advantages of using the method generally outweigh the theoretical or proven risks.
3. A condition where the theoretical or proven risks usually outweigh the advantages of using the method.
4. A condition which represents an unacceptable health risk if the contraceptive method is used.

To cite an example, a woman who is known to have thrombophilia (e.g. Factor V Leiden; Prothrombin gene mutation; Protein S, Protein C and Antithrombin deficiencies) falls under Category 4 for prescribing combination oral contraceptive pill (the pill should not be used) whereas a woman who has BMI>30 kg/m^2 body falls under Category 2. For further details refer *Medical Eligibility Criteria for Contraceptive Use, WHO, 2004 and 2008 update.*

10.4 NATURAL METHODS OF CONTRACEPTION

Coitus interruptus is practiced by many couples. The method involves withdrawal of the penis before ejaculation. Even though not well studied, the method has a failure rate of 4 per 100 women in the first year. HIV transmission is also, to some extent, prevented by the method. Since deposition of semen in the external genitalia also can result in pregnancy, the penis should be withdrawn from the vagina and from the external genitalia.

Lactation Amenorrhea

Since prolactin inhibits gonadotropin secretion; ovulation is suppressed in women who completely breastfeed. This period can be variable among individuals. On an average ovulation suppression can be expected for 6 months in completely breastfeeding mothers and 3 months in partially breastfeeding mothers. Hence, contraceptive should be started appropriately.

Periodic abstinence is another widely practiced method of fertility control. Intercourse is avoided during the fertile period. Various methods are resorted to for calculating the fertile period. In a woman who has regular menstruation, the 9th to 19th day is considered to be the fertile period, during which coitus is avoided for preventing conception. 'Persona' is a battery operated monitor which is used to identify the fertile period based on urinary LH and estriol using disposable dipstick. This method can help reduce the number of days of abstinence. The annual pregnancy risk estimated is 6% with this method of determining safe period. Because sperm may survive for 5 to 7 days in the female genital tract there is a high failure rate for this method. The chance for pregnancies with aging gametes is high if failure occurs. But there is no evidence for increased incidence of congenital anomalies in the fetuses.

10.5 ORAL CONTRACEPTION

Understanding the physiology of ovulation led to the development of oral contraceptives (OC). It was Ludwig Haberlandt, Professor of Physiology (1920) who first demonstrated that ovarian extract could prevent pregnancy in mice. But the ovarian extract, *Infecundin* developed by him did not gain popularity because of the difficulty in obtaining the extract.

Russell E Marker, born in 1902 in Hagerstown, Maryland, a Chemist, dedicated several years of his career to isolate progesterone from plant source. Marker's search for a plant source took him to Texas where he found *Dioscoria mexicana*, from which he initially extracted *diosgenin* and later progesterone.

Carl Djerassi, a Belgian chemist who migrated to US in 1939 succeeded in synthesizing norethindrone from yam derived progesterone by removing the 19th carbon and made it orally active. A closely related compound norethinodrel was the first orally active progestational agent to receive a patent. This is developed by Frank Colton, a chemist working in GD Searle Company. Gregory Pincus, born in 1903 in New Jersey, was interested in developing an oral contraceptive. It was Pincus and Chang together who experimented with synthetic progestin and developed the contraceptive tablet which was later made available to women seeking contraception. The initial preparation was contaminated with 1% mestranol. The first oral contraceptive was marketed by Searle in the name *Enovid* in the year 1960, the components being 150 μg mestranol and 9.85 mg norethynodrel.

10.5.1 Pharmacology of Combined Oral Contraception (COC)

Estrogen or progesterone alone can be used as a contraceptive. Estrogen inhibits ovulation and progesterone induces changes in cervical mucus and endometrium. The side effects of both these hormones differ greatly but also overlap to some extent. As estrogen dose increases venous thromboembolism (VTE) risk also increases. Increase in progesterone dose alters lipid profile, increasing the atherosclerosis risk. Combining these two can reduce the risk by reducing the quantity of each of these hormones without compromising efficacy.

Estrogen Component

Estrogen secreted by the ovary is mainly estradiol. It is the most potent estrogen but is not orally active. A major breakthrough in the discovery of COC was the introduction of ethinyl estradiol (EE) in 1938. Addition of an ethinyl group to estradiol made it orally active. Ethinyl estradiol is a very potent oral estrogen and is more common of the two forms of the estrogen used in COC. The other estrogen used is 3-methyl ether of ethinyl estradiol-mestranol. The most serious side effect of estrogen is VTE which is dose related. The initial pill used contained high doses of estrogen, as high as 150 μg. There was a very high incidence of VTE at this dose. The estrogen dose was gradually decreased in the later pills from 50 to 30 μg and the latest pills have only 15 μg. *The critical dose above which there is a significantly increased risk of VTE is 50 μg.*

Progesterone Component

Ethinyl substitution of testosterone resulted in the discovery of ethisterone, an orally active derivative having progestational effect. The removal of 19th carbon from ethisterone changed the major hormonal effect from that of an androgen to that of a progestational agent, at the same time not destroying the oral activity. This resulted in the discovery of 19-nortestosterone derivatives. These derivatives have mainly progestational effects but minimal androgenic as well as anabolic effects as well. Norethindrone was the initially discovered 19-nortestosterone derivative. The various 19-nortestosterone derivatives are:

- Norethindrone
- Norethynodrel
- Norethindrone acetate
- Ethynodioldiacetate

- Lynestranol
- Norgestrel and Levonorgestrel, the active isomer of norgestrel

The newer progestins

The unfavorable effects of the older progestagens on the lipid profile as well as the decrease in carbohydrate tolerance led to the search for better progestational compounds with favorable metabolic effects. The newer progestins, Desogestrel, Gestodene and Norgestimate are less androgenic. They increase the level of sex hormone binding globulins and thus reduce free testosterone concentrations to a greater extent than the older progestagens. This difference is of clinical value in the treatment of hirsutism and acne. Because of their decreased androgenicity, they are predicted to have favorable effects on the cholesterol lipoprotein profile.

Drosperinone is a spironolactone analogue with progestational acivity. When used in a dose of 3 mg along with ethinyl estradiol the contraceptive efficacy is similar to other formulations. It has antiandrogenic activity which is useful in treating women with hirsutism and acne, especially those associated with PCOS. Because of its anti-mineralocorticoid activity, drosperinone will not cause weight gain, but necessitates monitoring serum potassium level. Women who have abnormal liver, renal or adrenal function should avoid using this combination.

The common definitions used in epidemiologic studies to refer to the different formulations are listed below.

Low dose COC: products containing <50 μg EE

First generation oral contraceptive: COCs containing > 50 μg EE.

Second generation oral contraceptive: COCs containing levonorgestrel, norgestimate and other members of the norethindrone family and 20, 30 or 35 μg EE.

Third generation oral contraceptive: COCs containing desogestrel or gestodene with 20 or 30 μg EE.

Sequential pill: In the sequential pill, to mimic the natural cycle, the initial pills of the cycle were estrogen alone and the rest were estrogen and progesterone combinations. Use of estrogen alone carries the risk of endometrial hyperplasia and hence the sequential pills are no longer used.

Triphasic pill: In the triphasic pill, both hormones are used but the dose is altered to mimic the natural cycle without compromising efficacy. Thus, the total dose of hormone can be reduced thereby reducing side effects.

Newer formulations

1. Cyproterone acetate and EE
2. Combination of drosperinone and EE
3. Pills containing 15 μg of EE available in the USA by the name Minesse.

10.5.2 Mechanism of Action

Combination pill is given daily for 21 days starting from the first day of the cycle. After a withdrawal bleed, in the subsequent cycle it can be started within the fifth day of withdrawal bleed. The estrogen component of the pill inhibits FSH release and follicular development. This contributes significantly to the contraceptive effect. Estrogen gives stability to endometrium and prevents break through bleeding. It potentiates the action of progesterone by increasing the intracellular progesterone receptors. Progestagen suppress LH surge and prevents ovulation even if follicular growth has occurred. Since the progestagen dose is more than estrogen, the effect on the cervical mucus and endometrium will be dominated by progestagen making it hostile for implantation.

10.5.3 Efficacy

The clinician should be knowledgeable about the failure rate of the different formulations. When counseling couples, the clinician's anecdotal experience is insufficient. The most commonly referred publication is that of Trussel J et al.[1] (Table 10.1) The annual perfect failure rate (lowest expected) of combined pills is quoted as 0.3%.

Typical usage (usual experience) is associated with a failure rate of 8% during the first year.

Metabolic effects of COC (Table 10.2)

Even with a lowest expected failure rate of 0.1%, combination oral contraceptive pills are not widely used by women. Hormonal contraceptives are used only by 25% of women in the developed countries. In India, it is used by only 8% of women. This is mainly attributed to the fear of cardiovascular diseases and cancer. Careful screening based on family history, past medical history and investigations wherever necessary, will help prevent cardiovascular disease to a great extent.

Cardiovascular Risk

Venous thromboembolism

Estrogen in the COC causes an increase in the production of clotting factors such as factor V, VIII, X and fibrinogen, resulting in hypercoagulability of blood and an increased

Table 10.2: Metabolic effects of hormonal contraceptives

Estrogen component	*Progestagen component*
• Risk of venous thrombosis is adversely affected in a dose related manner. Risk is more in women who have inherited abnormalities of coagulation. It is more in current users and decline with increase in duration of use. OCs with 20 μg estrogen has lower risk compared to 30-40 μg. Critical dose above which VTE significantly increases is 50 μg. • Acting on the renin-angiotensin system, it can increase blood pressure. • Minimal effect on carbohydrate metabolism. The low dose pill has no clinically significant effect on insulin sensitivity. • High dose OCs can cause cholestasis.	• Risk of venous thrombosis was reported to be higher among women who use 3rd generation progestin products. However, studies have shown that this increase reported is not clinically significant and may be a reflection of biases and confounders. • Adverse effect on lipid profile is in a dose dependent manner. The risk is more among smokers and hypertensives. Products containing desogestrel or gestodene have less adverse effect. • Insulin sensitivity is significantly affected. With low-dose formulations the effect is minimal.

risk of venous thrombosis. Estrogen induced thrombosis is dose related. The original preparations which contained 80-100 μg EE were associated with a six-fold increased risk of venous thrombosis. However, the use of 20 and 30 μg EE pills have only mild pro-coagulant activity. The risk is increased only in current users of COC. Past usage of COC is not associated with an increased risk.[2] It has been clearly documented that the risk decreases with increased duration of use. *With the introduction of low-dose formulations and avoidance of COC use in high risk patients, a marked reduction in venous thrombosis was documented.*

Use of COC markedly increases the risk of thrombosis in women with inherited abnormalities of coagulation. The risk factors mainly include:

1. Factor V Leiden mutation
2. Other inherited thrombophilias
   a. Protein C deficiency
   b. Protein S deficiency
   c. Anti-thrombin III deficiency
   d. Prothrombin gene mutation
   e. Anti-phospholipid antibody syndrome
3. Smoking more than 10 cigarettes a day increase the risk of thrombosis among COC users
4. Hypertension
5. Age >35 and
6. Overweight

Thrombophilia screening should be done before prescribing hormonal contraceptives, for women who have a past history of venous thromboembolism and for those who give history of venous thrombosis in a close family member. The impact of smoking on the risk of venous thrombosis is less than that of arterial thrombosis.

The risk of venous thrombosis can be significantly reduced by:

1. Avoiding COC in high risk groups
2. By using a low dose formulation (<50 μg EE)

It was noted in the WHO Collaborative study of Cardiovascular Disease and Steroid Hormone Contraception that the use of desogestrel or gestodene increases venous thrombosis risk by 2.6 times compared to levonogestrel. However, this inference is controversial because pills containing desogestrel or gestodene were less androgenic and hence thought to be better, so that clinicians preferentially prescribed these to older and high risk women while the second generation pills were prescribed to younger healthier women. The Transnational Case Control Study did not find a difference in the incidence of venous thrombosis[3] between second and third generation pills. Hence, *it was concluded that the difference in the incidence of VTE reported between the second and third generation pills could be small or not clinically meaningful or was a reflection of biases and confounders.*

Progestagen only OCs does not increase venous thrombosis.

Arterial thrombosis can cause myocardial infarction and stroke. The risk of arterial thrombosis mainly depends on abnormal lipid profile, hypertension and smoking. The lipid profile is adversely affected by the progesterone component. Theoretically, the type of progesterone influences the risk of myocardial infarction and stroke. Studies have noted a statistically significant reduction in the risk of myocardial infarction and stroke in women who used the third generation oral contraceptives (containing desogestrel). A WHO study concluded that the risk of myocardial infarction and stroke are increased only among women who smoke or are hypertensive. *The risk is extremely low with the use of low dose formulations among healthy nonsmoking women.*

Carbohydrate metabolism

Insulin sensitivity is affected mainly by the progestagen component. The effect of estrogen on lipid metabolism, hepatic enzymes and the level of unbound cortisol can also cause derangement of carbohydrate metabolism. The effect of low dose pills on carbohydrate metabolism is so minimal that it has no clinical significance. Hyperglycemia associated with COC is completely reversible. Low dose pills can be used in women who had gestational diabetes. There is no effect even on overt diabetics with the use of low dose pill. Hence *low dose pills can be thought to have no significant adverse effect on carbohydrate metabolism.*

Liver

High dose estrogen containing COCs precipitate cholestasis and pruritus. Hence, they are contraindicated in patients with acute or chronic cholestatic liver disease. However, previous hepatic disease is not a contraindication for use, provided the woman has recovered from the acute phase. Hepatocellular adenomas can be caused by the use of COCs. The risk is related to the duration of use and the dose of estrogen. However, the low dose preparations have not been found to increase the incidence of hepatic adenomas.

Other metabolic effects

Fear of weight gain is a major problem affecting compliance to COC. The present day low dose preparations have not been shown to increase weight significantly. Studies have shown that weight gain is identical in the placebo group[4] as well. Women should be given assurance in this regard. Advice about diet and exercise also should form a part of counseling.

Recently introduced COCs containing drosperinone as the progestagen does not increase weight as it is an aldosterone analogue and hence does not cause sodium and water retention.

Nausea and breast discomfort may be disturbing in some women, but gradually disappear over a few months of use. These are also much less among the low-dose pill users.

Chloasma (facial pigmentation) is a side effect of COC but it is rare among low dose pill users.

Mental depression is very rarely encountered in women using COCs. This may be due to estrogen interfering with the synthesis of tryptophan and can be reversed with pyridoxine treatment. However, it is better to stop treatment if depression is diagnosed.

Estrogen component of COC increase the level of SHBG (sex hormone binding globulin) levels. The increased SHBG level increases binding of testosterone and consequently decreases free testosterone level.This causes an improvement in acne and hirsutism. COCs containing cyproterone acetate markedly improve hirsutism due to peripheral anti androgenic effect. Drosperinone also has anti-androgen effect but to a lesser degree than cyproterone acetate.

High dose COC suppresses functional ovarian cyst but low dose preparation has no such effect. Hence, functional cyst is encountered in women using low dose pill.

Oral contraceptives and its effect on pituitary

Even though estrogen stimulates prolactin secretion and hypertrophy of pituitary lactotrophs, prolactin secreting pituitary adenomas are not affected by OC use. Oral contraceptives were thought to cause secondary amenorrhea but studies have shown that incidence of amenorrhea on discontinuing the pill is 0.7-0.8%, which is equal to the incidence of spontaneous amenorrhea. Since there is no relation between COC use and amenorrhea, women who have not menstruated for 12 months following stoppage of the drug should be evaluated for secondary amenorrhea.

10.5.4 Oral Contraceptives and the Risk of Cancer

The risk of breast cancer in oral contraceptive users is an important concern for women and is an essential reason for the reduced popularity of COC as a contraceptive.

Breast Cancer

There had been extensive studies over the past few decades to determine the association of oral contraceptive use and the risk of breast cancer.[5] The study result of the National Institute of Child Health and Human Development is reassuring. The relative risk estimated was 1 and 0.9 for current and past users compared to non-users respectively. COC use will not increase the risk of breast cancer in patients with a positive family history.[6] In a meta-analysis of 54 studies, it was concluded that the relative risk of breast cancer in the current COC users is 1.07. The incidence of benign breast diseases like fibrocystic disease of the breast is reduced by COC use. This reduction is noted among women using low dose pills also.

Endometrial Cancer

Oral contraceptive use gives protection against endometrial cancer. Use for at least 10 months decreases risk of endometrial cancer by 50%. The protection lasts several years after discontinuation of use.

Ovarian Cancer

COC use protects against ovarian cancer also. The risk of developing epithelial ovarian cancer is reduced by 40% compared to non-users. The protection increases with duration of use and lasts 20 or more years after stopping medication. Use of COC even for 3-6 months causes this reduction in incidence. But with 10 years of use the reduction in risk reaches 80%. This protection is observed among high-risk women (positive family history) also. Hence, it can be used for reducing the risk among women who are carriers or suspected carriers of familial ovarian cancer genes.

Oral contraceptives and the risk of cancer

- Relative risk of breast cancer in COC users is only 1.07. However, OC pill users should undergo regular breast examination.
- There is a 50% reduction in risk of endometrial cancer among women who use COC for at least 10 months
- There is an 80% reduction in risk of ovarian cancer among women who use COC for 10 years. The risk is reduced even among women who have a positive family history
- There is a significant increase in the risk of adenocarcinoma of cervix in COC users. Hence, it is mandatory that COC users should undergo yearly Pap test

Cervical Cancer

In contrast to ovarian cancer and endometrial cancer it has been found that invasive cervical cancer is increased in women who use COC. This could be due to the lack of protection from human papilloma virus by not resorting to barrier methods rather than the direct effect of COC on cervical epithelium. It has also been argued that invasive cervical cancer[7] is identified more among COC users due to the more frequent pap smears taken from them. The incidence of adenocarcinoma of cervix has been found to be increased among young women over the past few decades. Hence, it was concluded that COC use increases the risk of adenocarcinoma cervix. Therefore, it is mandatory that COC users should undergo yearly Pap test.

10.5.5 Contraindications for Use

History of thromboembolism, thrombophilias, active liver disease, cardiovascular disease and migraine with aura are absolute contraindications for COC use.

Migraine: Migraine headache with aura is a risk factor for stroke. COC should not be prescribed for such women. Migraine headache without aura is not a contraindication if the woman has no other risk factors for stroke.

Absolute contraindications

- Arterial or venous thrombosis
- Ischemic heart disease
- Valvular heart disease
- Active liver disease
- Polycythemia
- Porphyria
- Migraine with aura
- Sickle cell anemia
- Collagen vascular disease

Hypertension: Estrogen in COC can cause a worsening of hypertension by interfering with renin angiotensin mechanism. But low dose COC can be used in women with hypertension who are not smokers and without target organ damage. Previous history of pregnancy induced hypertension is not a contraindication for COC, provided the BP is normal after delivery.

Diabetes: Oral contraceptives can be used in women with well controlled diabetes and younger than 35 years without end organ damage.

Low-dose COCs are not contraindicated in women who had gestational diabetes as there is no evidence that low dose COC increase the incidence of diabetes.[8]

Uterine fibroids: Fibroids are not a contraindication for low dose COC use. Although most of the studies do not show increase or decrease in the size of leiomyomata, the Nurses' Health Study reported a slightly increased risk myoma growth when COCs were used in early teenagers.[9] It has been reported that there is a reduction in menstrual bleeding with low dose pills.

Elective surgery: High dose COC pills should be stopped 4 weeks before elective surgery due to the risk of VTE. At present there is no data whether the continuation of low

Relative contraindications

- Obesity
- Smoking
- Hypertension
- Breast cancer
- Diabetes mellitus
- Elective surgery
- Seizure disorder
- Gallbladder disease
- Hypercholesterolemia
- Uterine leiomyoma
- Cholestasis of pregnancy

dose COC right up to the date of major surgery increases the risk of thrombosis. However, it is prudent to stop even the low dose COC before major elective surgery which necessitates immobilization. However, it need not be discontinued before short surgical procedures which do not necessitate much immobilization.

Seizure disorder: Several anti-epileptic drugs are enzyme inducers and hence may interfere with drug metabolism. This can decrease the contraceptive efficacy. Even though higher dose estrogen products may overcome this effect, there is no evidence for this. It is better to advise other methods of contraception to these women. Injectable progesterone only contraceptives and intrauterine devices are better options for them.

Cholestasis of pregnancy: Cholestasis of pregnancy is considered a contraindication for COC use. The low dose formulation seems to be safer for women with history of cholestasis of pregnancy.

Sickle cell disease: COCs are contraindicated in sickle cell disease as they may promote sickling crisis. Depot medroxy progesterone acetate is found to have an inhibitory effect on sickling and hence should be preferred in patients with sickle cell disease. Low dose OC pills have not been reported to cause adverse effect in patients with sickle cell diseases.

Gallbladder disease: COCs are contraindicated in patients with gallbladder disease as it can precipitate symptoms.

Heart disease: COC should not be used in patients with cardiac failure, atrial fibrillation or clotting factor abnormality. Progestagen only pill can be used in patients with clotting factor abnormality.

Collagen vascular disease: SLE is a contraindication for COC use as estrogen can exacerbate vascular disease of SLE. Progestagen only pill is preferred. Patients in remission and without renal involvement may however be given COCs.

Hyperlipidemia: Is not an absolute contraindication for low dose COC. However, women with triglyceride level more than 250 mg/100 ml should not be given low dose COC. Women, who are smokers or have vascular disease and dyslipidemia, also should not be given hormonal contraception.

Smokers: Women over 35 years who smoke should not be given COCs.

Hepatic disease: Active liver disease is a contraindication for COC. If the liver function is normal, prior hepatic disease in not a contraindication.

Hemorrhagic disorders: Hemorrhagic disorders and anti-coagulant therapy are not contraindications for COC.

Obesity: Healthy obese women may use low dose OC. Women who are overweight have an increased failure rate with the low dose pill. Increasing the estrogen dose to 50 μg will lower the failure rate but will increase the risk of VTE. However, the failure rate is much less compared to other contraceptive methods and hence may be used.

Prolactin secreting adenomas: Microadenomas are not a contraindication for COC.

Ulcerative colitis: Women with ulcerative colitis can have COC as the drug is absorbed in the small intestine and will not interfere with the severity of ulcerative colitis.

10.5.6 Inadvertent Use of Oral Contraceptive during Conceptive Cycle

There is no reliable evidence implicating COC and cardiac anomalies, NTD, limb reduction anomaly or even virilization. The risks of these anomalies were not greater than the general population risk of 2-3%.

10.5.7 Fertility after withdrawing COC

Studies have suggested a slight delay in fertility after stopping COC. This may be due to the continuing suppressive effect on the pituitary. The interval between stopping COC and conception was 13 months or greater in 24.8% of prior COC users whereas after removal of IUD it is 12.4%. There is no increase in spontaneous miscarriage after stopping COC. Also there is no increased incidence of congenital anomalies in pregnancies following discontinuation of COCs.

10.5.8 Breastfeeding

There is a decrease in quantity and quality of milk production in COC users. The progestational component can reach the baby in significant amounts but an 8 year follow-up study did not show any decreased intelligence or abnormal psychological behavior in children who were breastfed by mothers who were on COC.[10]

10.5.9 Timing of Initiation

Initiation of ovulation after delivery is not predictable. The resumption of ovulation among non breastfeeding women has been documented as early as 7 weeks. A significant number of non breastfeeding women ovulated even before 7 weeks postpartum. Hence, it is advisable to start contraception as *early as third postpartum week in women who are not breastfeeding*. Women who fully breast feed will not ovulate until at least 10 weeks postpartum but most fully breastfeeding women do not ovulate till almost 6 months. Hence, in such women, it is advisable to delay contraception till 6 months postpartum. However, women who breastfeed partially might ovulate earlier. Hence, it is advisable to initiate contraception 6 weeks postpartum. After abortion contraception can be started immediately which will also take care of the abnormal bleeding following abortion. Ovulation can resume 2-3 weeks after abortion and the first period can be ovulatory.

Considering the adverse effect of COC on lactation, the progestagen only mini pill should be preferred in breastfeeding women. Due to the adverse effect of estrogen on the coagulation profile, initiation of COCs should be delayed even if the woman is not lactating. However, the mini pill can be started 4 weeks after delivery as it has only positive effect on lactation. Women who had gestational diabetes are at increased risk of developing diabetes if they are on progesterone only pill. Hence, these women should be advised other methods of contraception.

10.5.10 Use of OC in PCOD

Women with PCOD, oligo-ovulation and hyper androgenic features like hirsutism and acne should be treated with low dose estrogen COC. Adolescent girls with PCOD and hirsutism should be advised COC. Preparations which contain antiandrogens like cyproterone acetate or drosperinone should be preferred for these girls due to their beneficial effect on hirsutism and acne. Drosperinone has the advantage of anti-mineralocorticoid activity, so that weight gain is less. Fear of impairment of growth of such girls on COC is not supported by evidence.

10.5.11 Choice of Pill

Current evidence indicates that the low dose preparation containing 30 μg or 20 μg of ethinyl estradiol is as efficacious as high dose preparation. Risk of VTE and stroke are much less with the low dose preparation. Hence low dose preparations should be preferred. Triphasic pills were designed to reduce the total dose of hormones. The present low dose monophasic pill contain almost same amount of hormones as triphasic pill and hence low dose monophasic pill is the preferred one.

Women with hirsutism and acne will benefit from COCs containing cyproterone acetate or drosperinone as the progestagenic component. The antiandrogenic effect of cyproterone is more than that of drosperinone. Women with hypertension without target organ damage can be given COC containing drosperinone, since it has antimineralocorticoid activity.

Women who are not hypertensive, diabetic or smokers can use low dose pills till menopause. Women with breakthrough bleeding while on low dose pills, can be reassured that the bleeding will subside within 3-4 months. If she continues to have breakthrough bleeding she can be changed to a pill with slightly higher dose of estrogen. This can also be tackled by conjugated equine estrogen along with OC. Taking the pill on the same time everyday can also reduce the incidence of break through bleeding. There is no evidence that break through bleeding is associated with decreased efficacy. Breakthrough bleeding can also occur after many months of OC use due to progesterone induced decidualization.

10.5.12 Method of Pill Taking

It is better to start the pill on the first day of menses to ensure immediate protection in the first cycle of pill use. If the pills are taken on the same time every day, the incidence of breakthrough bleeding is less. Taking the pill at a fixed time can make it a habit so that compliance can be improved.

Missing pills can interfere with contraceptive efficacy. However, missing one or two pills in a cycle have not been proven to decrease efficacy. Even if ovulation occurs, the effect of progesterone on cervical mucus and endometrium prevents conception. Nevertheless it is safer to be more conservative in advising patients, as there can be individual variations in the pill free interval that can result in ovulation. If the woman misses one pill she should take the pill as soon as she remembers and then take the rest as usual. Back-up contraception is not needed in this situation. If she misses 2 pills in the first week, she should take two pills each in the next 2 days but needs back-up contraception for the next 7 days, as ovulation can occur. Whereas if she misses 2 pills in the third week, she can start a new package without resorting to back-up contraception since she is anovulatory in that particular cycle by using pills in the previous 2 weeks. During an episode of gastroenteritis absorption can be erratic and it is advisable to use backup contraception for at least 7 days even if no pill is missed.

10.5.13 Amenorrhea while on OC Use (Absence of withdrawal Bleed)

This is due to the atrophic endometrium as a result of the predominant progesterone effect. Low dose estrogen pills are commonly associated with amenorrhea. For women who are concerned about the absence of withdrawal bleeding, the addition of extra estrogen in the form of conjugated estrogen at a dose of 1.25 mg/day for 21 days along with OC can bring forth withdrawal bleeding.

Table 10.3: Drugs increasing COC failure

• Carbamazepine
• Felbamate
• Nevirapine
• Phenobarbitol
• Rifabutine
• Rifampicin
• Vigabatrine
• Ethosuximide
• Griseofulvin
• Troglitazone

10.5.14 Drug Interaction

It is believed that the effectiveness of COC is reduced by ampicillin, metronidazole, quinolones and tetracycline. However studies have shown that even though antibiotics can alter excretion of COC, plasma levels of COC are unchanged and there is no evidence that antibiotics interfere with contraceptive effectiveness. Drugs that stimulate liver metabolism can increase COC failure. A list of such drugs is given in Table 10.3.

It is better to choose alternative contraception for women taking these medications. Progesterone only contraceptives can be preferred in such women.

As OC is thought to potentiate the action of diazepam, chlordiazepoxide, tricyclic anti depressants and theophylline, lower doses of these agents may be sufficient for COC users. On the contrary, because of increased clearance, larger dose of acetaminophen and aspirin are needed for COC users (Table 10.4).

10.5.15 Alternative Routes of Administration

Oral contraceptives can be used vaginally in women who have nausea and vomiting due to other causes. It has been found to be as effective as oral use.

10.5.16 Non-contraceptive Benefits of COC

Apart from the protection from ovarian cancer and endometrial cancer, COC use has several non contraceptive benefits.

Table 10.4: Drug interactions of COC

Drugs potentiated by COC	*Drugs rapidly cleared*
Diazepam, chlordiazepoxide	Acetaminophen
Tricyclic antidepressants	Aspirin
Theophylline	

Oral contraceptives protect against ascending infection of pelvic organs by organisms in the lower genital tract. Probable reasons could be thickening of cervical mucus and decreased menstrual bleeding which reduces movement of pathogens up to the tubes and reduction in quantity of menstrual effluent which is a culture medium for these pathogens. Lower genital tract infections are not prevented. Oral contraceptive use causes extension of columnar epithelium from endocervix to ectocervix. This is the mechanism for the association of chlamydial cervicitis with OC use. Even though chlamydial infections are reported to be more with COC use, tubal infertility is not reported to be higher. There is no relation between HIV seropositivity and COC use. Contraceptive efficacy may be decreased by anti-retroviral drugs through its effect on drug metabolism and by causing diarrhea and vomiting. For polygamous women, barrier contraception should be advised along with OC.

COCs are beneficial in athletes. Eating disorders are common among athletes which can cause decrease in bone mineral density (BMD). COC user can improve BMD. The progestagen component increases ventilation as in pregnancy which might improve exercise tolerance. COC use can be tailored to the exercise schedule, by changing the periodicity of withdrawal bleed. Women can decrease the frequency of periods and at the same time have withdrawal bleeding at their choice. The pill marketed as 'Seasonale' is an extended cycle regimen which is used continuously for 4 months.

Ectopic pregnancies are also prevented, unlike IUD. The incidence of benign breast disease is less among COC users. Even though the incidence of functional ovarian cyst is reduced with high dose pills, the low dose pills do not have this benefit. Endometriosis, dysmenorrhea and menorrhagia are less in COC users. COC use has been found to improve BMD. Incidence of fractures in postmenopausal women is less in prior COC users than among non users. OCs can also be used for treating conditions like:

1. Dysfunctional uterine bleeding
2. Dysmenorrhea not responding to analgesic and anti prostaglandins
3. Endometriosis for preventing progression as well as recurrence after surgery when fertility is not desired
4. Mittelschmerz
5. Premenstrual syndrome
6. Acne and hirsutism: Preparations containing cyproterone acetate are preferred
7. Amenorrhea (HRT)
8. Functional ovarian cyst
9. BRCA carriers

10.5.17 Factors Affecting Compliance

Side effects are an important factor affecting compliance with COC. The usual side effects are nausea, vomiting, breakthrough bleeding, and absence of withdrawal bleeding, weight gain and breast tenderness. Non-compliance can be overcome by counseling or by changing over to a different product.

Fear about breast cancer is one of the important reasons for non compliance. The patient should be given the realistic figure of breast cancer risk. Inadequate instruction leads to improper pill use and failure. Failure adversely affects pill use. Hence patient counseling is an important factor before prescribing COC. Counseling often has 6 elements, or steps enlisted by the 'GATHER' approach. Each letter in the word GATHER stands for one of these elements - Greet, Ask, Tell, Help, Explain and Return. (Family Planning and Population Unit, Department of Reproductive Health and Research, World Health Organization). Women should be given advice regarding how to take the pill, what to do if pills are missed, how it works, about failure rate, return of fertility after stopping and how events like vomiting and diarrhea episodes can affect efficacy. The warning signs of serious problems should be clearly explained.

With the introduction of low dose COC, hormonal contraception carries less risk with many non contraceptive benefits as well. Starting of hormonal contraception after taking a proper history, clinical examination and performing relevant investigations, can render COC risk negligible. From an individual point of view, COC use improves overall health. The clinician's responsibility is to provide the necessary information to couples and help them make their choice.

10.6 OTHER METHODS OF HORMONAL CONTRACEPTION

10.6.1 Progestagen only Contraceptives

Progestagen alone can be used as contraceptive in various forms:

1. Mini pills
2. Progestagen incorporated IUD
3. Implants
4. Newer delivery methods like vaginal rings, patches and gel preparations

Dose of progestagen varies in the different methods. The mechanism of contraceptive action of progestagen only contraception depends upon the dosage of steroid administered. High doses like depot injections inhibit ovulation. Low doses also might inhibit ovulation, which may not always be consistent. Whatever be the route administered, progestagen thickens the cervical mucus making it impermeable to sperms. The effect of progestagen on the endometrium makes it hostile for implantation.

10.6.2 Minipills

The minipill is a progestagen only pill containing lesser amount of progestagen than in the COC. Minipills are recommended for women who have contraindications for estrogen use like diabetes with vascular complications, severe SLE and cardiovascular disease. Currently it is recommended for lactating women since it will not affect the quantity and quality of milk secretion. They are also preferable for those above 40 years of age. It can also be recommended for women who cannot tolerate estrogen because of its side effects.

Mechanism of action: The main mechanism of action is thickening of cervical mucus making it impermeable and changes in the endometrium which prevents implantation. Gonadotropins are not consistently suppressed. Hence ovulation might occur. Contraceptive efficacy is less than COC. Failure rates 1.1– 9.6/100 women year in first year of use.

Pill use: Presently, 0.075 mg desogestrel (Cerazette) is available as minipill. This is more effective than levonorgestrel. Other preparations available include:

- Norethindrone 350 μg
- LNG 30 μg

Changes in cervical mucus start 2-4 hours after taking the pill and diminishes within 22 hours. Hence after 24 hours the effect on cervical mucus nearly vanishes. Hence, it is imperative that the pill be taken the same time everyday.

Ovulation occurs in 40% of cases. Pill should be taken continuously and a back up method should be used for the first two days. If there is an incidence of GI upset or if the pills are forgotten back up method should also be used for two days after the pills have been restarted. If the pill taking is delayed for 3 hours or more, then also a back up method should be used.

Advantage: Because of the smaller dose of progesterone, the metabolic effects are not significant. Lipid levels are not significantly affected. Return to fertility is immediate after stopping the drug. As ovulation is not suppressed in most women, they can expect to have regular periods.

The WHO case control study and Transnational Case Control Study did not find increased risk of stroke, venous thromboembolism or myocardial infarction in minipill users.

Minipill can be used in women with previous history of thrombosis.

Disadvantage: In 10% of women short irregular periods and even amenorrhea can occur. Because of the unpredictable bleeding, compliance to pill taking is a problem. Another major side effect is development of follicular cysts. The androgenic activity of levonorgestrel can cause acne. The incidence of ectopic pregnancy is higher in minipill users than COC users. It has been noted that there is a 3-fold increase in diabetes mellitus when minipill is used by lactating women with a history of gestational diabetes.

Drug interaction: Patients on chronic medications which cause increased liver metabolism like carbamazepine, phenobarbitone, rifampicin, etc. should avoid minipill.

Non-contraceptive benefits: Even though all the non contraceptive benefits of COC do not apply to minipill, the risk of PID is less due to the effect on cervical mucus. The protection against endometrial cancer is greater than that of COC.

10.6.3 Vaginal and Transdermal Estrogen and Progesterone Contraception

Vaginal Methods

Hormonal contraception through vaginal route has several advantages. By avoiding the first pass through the liver, there is less impact of estrogen on blood clotting. Another advantage is improved compliance achieved by avoiding the need for daily drug intake. The vaginal route avoids the interference with absorption due to vomiting. Contraceptive efficacy of 'typical use' is superior to oral contraceptive.

Vaginal contraceptive rings are available for short term (1 week) as well as for long term use (1 year). The *Nuva ring* is a combined estrogen-progestagen contraceptive ring for use vaginally. It is a flexible soft transparent ring made of ethylene-vinyl acetate co-polymer in which 3-ketodesogestrel (etonogestrel) and ethinyl estradiol are impregnated. The device is 4 mm thick and 54 mm in diameter. It releases 15 μg ethinyl estradiol and 120 μg of 3-ketodesogestrel. The ring can be inserted by the woman herself and removed after 3 weeks. The subsequent ring should be inserted 1 week later after the withdrawal bleed. Ovulation is effectively suppressed and the failure rate is <1%. Vaginal method ensures more circulating level of hormones and hence they have less episodes of irregular bleeding compared to COC. If the ring is removed for 3 hours, back up method should be resorted to for 7 days. The ring can be kept in the vagina in any position. Vaginal infection should be treated before insertion.

The contraceptive vaginal ring

- Easy to insert
- Contraceptive efficacy is same as COC
- Contraindicated in situations where COC is contraindicated
- Cycle control is better than COC
- Efficacy is not affected by gastrointestinal upset
- Easy to use by the woman herself

Transdermal Contraception

Combination hormonal contraceptives are available as transdermal patches marketed as Ortho-evra. It is a 4.5 cm^2 patch with three layers. The outer polyester layer provides support, the middle layer contains hormones and the inner layer is a polyester liner which has to be removed before application. The patch contains 750 μg ethinyl estradiol and 6 mg of norelgestromine. It delivers 20 μg EE and and 150 μg of norelgestromine. The patch can be applied to upper outer arm, buttock or back but not over the breast. Norelgestromine is metabolized to levonorgestrel in the body.

The patch should be applied every 3 weeks with a one week patch free interval. Each new patch is to be applied on clean dry skin without applying lotion or cream and each time the site should be changed.

Clinical trials have shown that the failure rate is common among overweight women. Common adverse effects are breast tenderness, nausea, and headache and skin irritation. Incidence of breakthrough bleeding is reported to be more among patch users compared to COC users. The patient can have her routine physical activities including water related activities.

Contraceptive efficacy is better than COC. The contraceptive patch and vaginal ring are contraindicated in situations where COCs are contraindicated.

10.6.4 Contraceptive Implants

Contraceptive efficacy of COC, patches and vaginal rings are affected by inconsistent use or interference with absorption. This is overcome by injectables and implants. Implants are sustained release systems made of silastic tubing permeable to steroid molecules inside which progestagen source is kept.

Implant contraception is preferred in:

1. Women with estrogen related side effects
2. Women who are non compliant with OC pill taking

Table 10.5: Contraindications of contraceptive implants

Absolute contraindication	*Relative contraindication*
• Acute liver disease	• Heavy cigarette smoking women >35 years of age
• Active thrombosis	• Previous ectopic pregnancy
• Breast cancer	• Diabetes mellitus
• Benign and malignant liver disease	• Hypercholestrolemia • Gallbladder disease • Patient taking enzyme inducers

3. Those who prefer coitus unrelated method of contraception
4. Those with contraindication for IUD and who cannot tolerate IUD
5. Those who have medical disorders like sickle cell anemia.

Contraindications (Table 10.5)

Mechanism of action: The mechanism of action is mainly by inhibition of ovulation. Cervical mucus changes and endometrial changes also contribute to contraceptive effect. Since etonogestrel concentrations are not affected by body weight the failure rate is not high in obese women.

Advantages: Efficacy of implant is not affected by compliance as only a one-time motivation is required. Aborption is not affected by factors like vomiting. The efficacy is very high and is comparable to sterilization, with a pearl index of 0.01. A three year follow-up of women who had Implanon[11] did not report any failure. Unlike contraceptive injection, fertility is rapidly reversible after removal and pregnancy outcomes are within normal limits. Probably risk of endometrial and ovarian cancers are less in implant users.

Disadvantages: Reports about change in weight in Norplant users are variable. In a five year follow-up of Norplant users, no increase in BMI was reported.

Irregular menstruation is one of the common side effects seen in implant users. Depression, mood changes, anxiety, etc. are also rarely encountered.

Mastalgia can occur due to fluid retention but it wears off in a few months. Symptomatic treatment with evening prim rose oil is very effective. Galactorrhea also has been reported in some implant users. Severe galactorrhea warrants prolactin estimation.

Acne is a common complaint due to the androgenic activity of levonorgestrel. Acne in Implanon users are less than in Norplant users because etonogestrel is less androgenic than levonorgestrel. Local treatment with clindamycin gel and avoiding fatty food and chocolates are effective in reducing acne.

Unlike COC, progesterone only contraceptive can cause formation of follicular cysts. These cysts regress spontaneously. However if they enlarge and produce symptoms, a neoplastic cyst should be suspected and managed accordingly.

Types of Implants

Norplant

Norplant consists of 6 rods, each one measuring 34 mm in length and 2.5 mm in outer diameter. Each rod has 36mg of levonorgestrel.

Jadelle: The six rod system is replaced by the two rod system known as jadelle or Norplant II.

Implanon (Fig. 10.1)

Implanon is a single flexible rod 4cm long and 2 mm in diameter containing 68 mg of 3 ketodesogestrel or etonogestrel, releasing 67μg of hormone/day which is under trial. Serum concentration of the drug which inhibits ovulation will be achieved within 8 hours. Contraceptive efficacy is found to be excellent in the trials.

Factors that contraindicate hormonal contraception should be excluded by careful history and physical examination. Patient should be informed about the possible side effects, method of insertion and removal. An informed consent should be taken. The device should be inserted on the first day of the period. Back-up contraception is advised for insertions after fifth day of menses. Implants can be inserted in the immediate postpartum period. In non breastfeeding women insertion should be within third postpartum week and in breastfeeding women within the third postpartum month. The non dominant upper inner arm

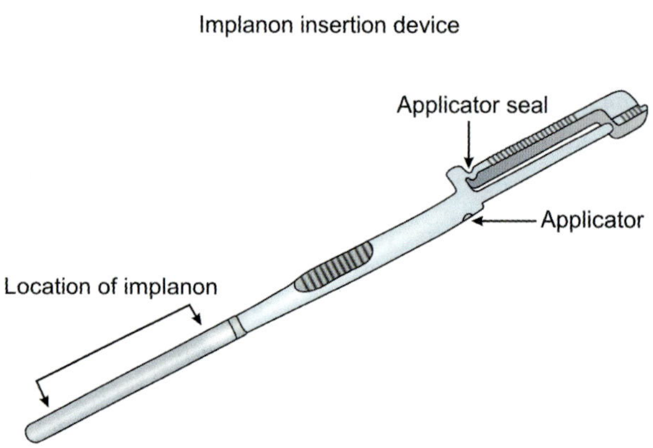

Fig. 10.1: Implanon in the insertion device

is the ideal site as it is easily accessible with minimum exposure.

Technique of Implanon Insertion and Removal

Implanon is a single rod available in a pre-loaded applicator. The arm is positioned by rotating 90° laterally. A point 6-8 cm superior and lateral to the medial epicondyle of the humerus, which lies between the triceps and biceps muscle, is identified. After giving local anesthesia the insertion needle and obturator cannula is pushed directly under the skin. By lifting the skin with the obturator the applicator is turned 90° in either direction. The needle is slowly pulled out of the skin keeping the implant under the skin. After the procedure the implant can be verified by palpating the skin. The patient should be taught to palpate the implant and she should be given a user card.

Removal can be done as an office procedure under local anesthesia.

10.7 INJECTABLE CONTRACEPTIVES

Injectable contraceptives include:

- Depot progestagen only
- Depot progestagen and estrogen combination

Depot progestagen only contraception: Depot medroxy progesterone acetate (DMPA) is the widely used progestagen only contraceptive. It is being extensively used in countries like Indonesia, Thailand, Sri Lanka and Mexico since 1960. The preparation contains micro crystals of MPA suspended in aqueous solution. It is available as injection of 150 mg, which is to be given intramuscularly every three months. The intramuscular injection should be deep using the Z track technique and the injection site should not be massaged. DMPA is one of the most effective methods of contraception available. As with implant contraception it is not user-dependant. The depot produces a higher peak of progesterone so that the suppression of ovulation is more than that in implant users.

Mechanism of Action

Apart from the effect on cervical mucus and endometrium, DMPA maintains high level of progesterone so that ovulation is suppressed. Since FSH suppression is not as effective as that with COC, some amount of follicular growth and estrogen production occurs. This estrogen production is sufficient enough to prevent vaginal and breast atrophy. The first injection should be given within the first 5 days of menstruation, to ensure effective contraception. There is a significant chance of failure if the injection is given after the fifth day of menstrual cycle. If pregnancy occurs after having had injection, there is a significant risk of intrauterine growth restriction. Back up method should be given for 2 weeks if the injection is delayed more than 5 days of menstruation. Contraceptive efficacy is better than any other temporary method of contraception or even sterilization, with a pearl index of 0.3. (Even though the lowest expected failure rate of COC is 0.3, on typical use it reaches 7.6 due to factors like lack of compliance, interference with absorption, interaction with other drugs, etc.).

Advantages

It is advantageous in women who are epileptic, as high progesterone level raises the seizure threshold. It can be used in women with sickle cell disease as it can reduce the episodes of sickling crisis. Due to the absence of estrogen it can be given to women with congenital heart disease and those with previous history of VTE. It is not contraindicated in women with hypertension and diabetes mellitus. Because of the positive impact on lactation it can be given to lactating women. It has also been found that there is no adverse effect on infant growth and development. As in COC users, women on DMPA also have decreased endometrial cancer risk. Regarding ovarian cancer risk data are controversial. However, WHO collaborative study did not find any difference in the risk of ovarian cancer among DMPA users.[12] DMPA use has no relation to the incidence of breast cancer or cervical cancer. Incidence of PID is less due to the effect on cervical mucus.

Disadvantages

Irregular vaginal bleeding is the most common problem. Bleeding, even though not heavy, will be irregular and unpredictable. The bleeding episodes will gradually subside and become very less within 1 year. At the initial period if the woman finds the bleeding unpleasant and does not respond to anti-prostaglandins, a short course of estrogen in the form of 1.25 mg of conjugated estrogens for 7 days will be effective. If still severe a three months course of COC can be given. An alternative treatment is with 50 mg mifepristone every 2 weeks which will increase the endometrial estrogen receptors and hence reduce breakthrough bleeding. Amenorrhea develops in 50% of women, by one year and 80% of women by 3 years. Depression, fatigue and decreased libido is also reported but not confirmed with placebo controlled trial. Studies addressing the effect on weight gain have given contradictory results with some reporting a marginal increase of 4 kg. Anaphylactic reaction has very rarely been reported but this may be due to the inert substances present in the injection. A large case control study showed a marginal increase in breast cancer in the first 4 years of use. Carcinoma cervix has not been found to be increased in DMPA users.

Metabolic effects

A slight decrease in HDL cholesterol, increase in total cholesterol and an elevation in glucose tolerance has been reported. There is a definite decrease in bone mineral density, which will be reversed after discontinuation.

Reversal of fertility after discontinuation[13]

Reversal of fertility is not as prompt as seen after removal of implants. The delay in conception can be as late as 9 months after the last injection. But after 18 months, the pregnancy rates are same as that with COC use.

Depo-SubQ Provera

A new low dose DMPA preparation in the name Depo-SubQ Provera 104 is approved for subcutaneous use. The total dose is (104 mg) 30% less than that of DMPA intramuscular preparations. Its contraceptive efficacy is reported to be excellent with no pregnancy reported in phase 3 trials. The advantage is earlier return to fertility (mean-30 weeks) compared to DMPA.[14] Other progestagen only injectable contraceptive available is

1. NET–EN: Norethindrone enanthate 200 mg IM every 2 months

Short term injectable combination hormonal contraceptives available are:

1. Lunelle: Cyclofem: 25 mg MPA and 5 mg estradiol cypionate monthly.
2. Mesigyna: 50 mg NET-EN and estradiol valerate monthly

10.8 NONHORMONAL ORAL CONTRACEPTIVE PILL

Centchroman is a non steroidal, nonhormonal birth control pill developed by the **Central Drug Research Institute** of **India (CDRI).** The drug is marketed as **Saheli**. The failure rate is only 1.63% which is not much higher than oral contraceptive pills. This drug has undergone extensive clinical trials and is presently used for the management of DUB also.

10.8.1 Method of Action

The drug is a selective estrogen receptor modulator (SERM). Centchroman suppresses the estrogen receptors in ovaries, uterus and breasts but it stimulates the estrogen receptors in bones. Hence, while acting as a contraceptive, it prevents cancer of breast and uterus and improves bone density. The contraceptive action is by increasing the movement of the fertilized ovum through the tube so that it reaches the uterus too early for implantation.

10.8.2 Dose

It is available as 30 mg tablets and should be taken twice a week in the first 3 months and weekly thereafter. The first pill should be taken on the 1st day of periods. An additional contraceptive should be used for the first month as there is delay in the achievement of the effect of contraception.

Advantages

- No adverse effects unlike hormones on blood coagulation, lipid profile and liver functions.
- Less expensive compared to COC
- Rapid return of fertility on stoppage
- Highly effective

10.9 INTRAUTERINE CONTRACEPTIVE DEVICE (IUD)

Intrauterine contraceptives are in use for about 100 years. The first IUD was a pessary developed by Hollweg in Germany. It used to be self introduced, needless to say with very high infection rates. Later on different substances in different shapes were used to make IUD. Two such devices were the Graffenberg ring and the Ota ring. Both had very high expulsion rates and hence did not gain popularity. In the 1970s Dalcon shield was introduced, which was a device with multifilament tail. This tail provided a pathway for bacteria which led to a high incidence of PID and the device went into disrepute.

10.9.1 The Modern IUD

It was Jaime Zipper of Chile, who found out that copper acted locally on the endometrium. Howard Tatum developed the T shaped IUD and incorporated copper as suggested by Zipper. Since, then several types of copper incorporated IUDs were used and the latest of this is Cu T 380A containing 380 mm^2 of exposed surface area of copper. The letter A stands for arm. Copper wire is wound around the arms and the stem. The lifespan of 380A is 10 years.

10.9.2 Types of IUD

Unmedicated IUD: The Lippy's loop which was in use in the 1970s was a polyethylene device impregnated with barium. The severe menorrhagia, pelvic pain and high expulsion rate associated with Lippy's loop led to the search for a better device.

Copper IUD: The copper IUD frame is made up of polyethylene impregnated with barium sulphate which makes it radiopaque. The copper IUD enhances prostaglandin production and various enzymes in the endometrium. Copper is spermicidal and decreases sperm motility. It also prevents implantation by producing inflammation in the endometrial cavity. Symptoms of pain and bleeding were much less and the effectiveness was far more due to the added effect of copper. Due to the T shape, expulsion rate was also less.

Cu 7: This device is shaped like the number 7 and containing copper wound round the stem was in vogue during the 1970's and 80's but was later withdrawn from the market due to the high expulsion rates.

Cu T 200: The first generation copper T had 200 mm^2 area of copper wound around the vertical limb of the device.

Multi-load 375: To increase the life span, more copper was added. Multi-load 375 has 375 mm^2 of copper wire wound around the vertical stem. The device is serrated so that expulsion is less. The method of application is easier than the other devices. The limbs need not be loaded in the applicator so that it can be inserted by a no touch technique.

Cu T 380 A (Fig. 10.2): It has 380 mm^2 of exposed surface area of copper. 176 mg of copper is wound around the vertical stem and the copper sleeves in the horizontal arm have 66.5 mg of copper. The stem has a 3 mm ball at the end, which prevents the perforation of the cervix. A polypropylene monofilament is tied through the ball in the stem which helps in detection and removal. The IUD frame is made of polyethylene impregnated with barium sulphate.

Cu T 380 Ag: This device is identical to copper T 380 A. The copper wire in the stem has a silver core which prevents fragmentation. The life span of copper is also increased by silver. The performance is similar to Cu T 380 A.

Cu T 380 slim line: This device is also like 380 A, but the copper sleeve is placed at the end of the horizontal limb. This helps in easy loading of the device in the applicator.

Hormone releasing IUD: Levonorgestrel-Intra Uterine System (LNG-IUS) and progestasert are the two hormone releasing IUDs. LNG-IUS (Mirena; Fig. 10.3) is a T-shaped device which contains 52 mg levonorgestrel dispersed in poly-dimethyl-siloxane. The mechanism of contraceptive action is by inhibiting implantation, sperm capacitation, penetration and survival. LNG-IUS produces an increase in the serum concentration of progestin but only about half of that achieved with Norplant. Hence ovulation is partially inhibited. As other progesterone contraceptives, cervical mucus is thickened creating a barrier to sperm penetration. The device releases 20 µg/day of levonorgestrel initially, but progressively declines to reach half of the initial rate after 5 years. Hence, it is approved for 5 years of use. The effect may probably last for 10 years. The device effectively reduces menstrual loss and is a treatment modality for menorrhagia. Hence it can be preferred as a contraceptive for women with menorrhagia. Pelvic infection rate is less among LNG-IUS users.

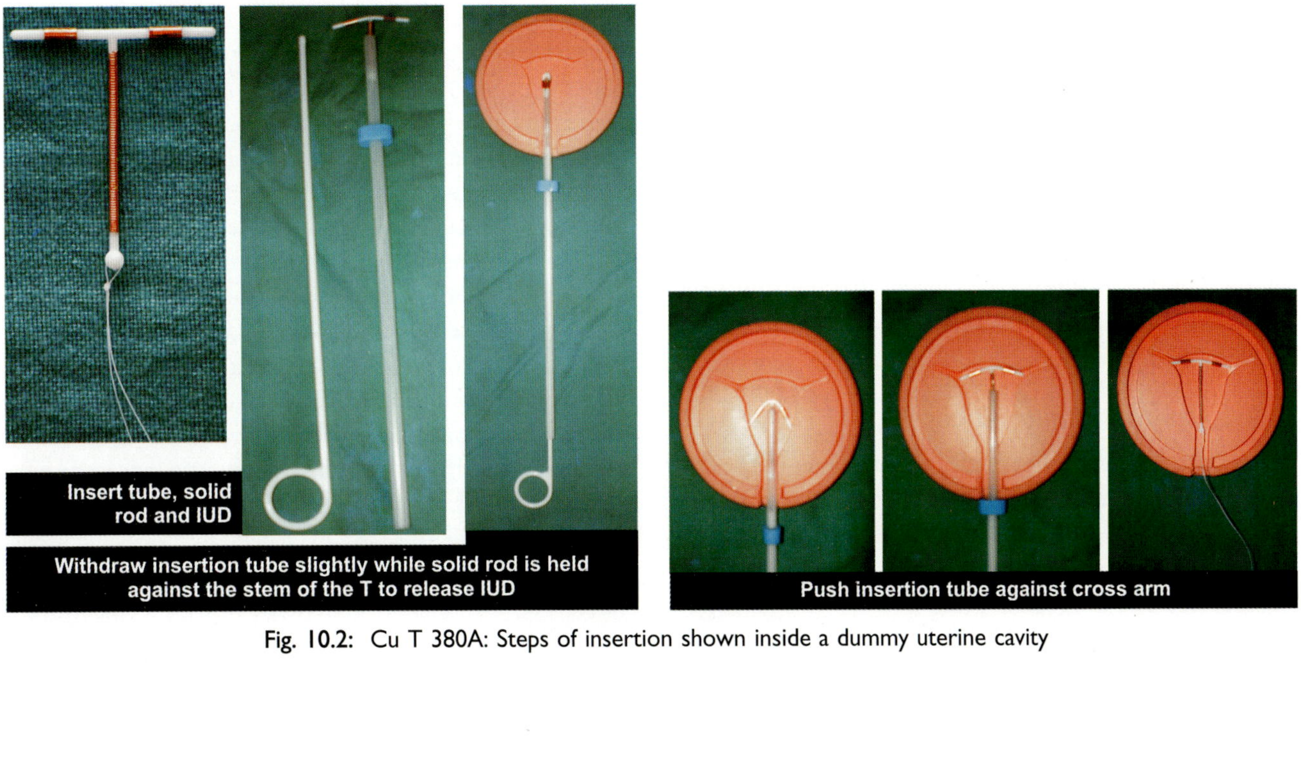

Fig. 10.2: Cu T 380A: Steps of insertion shown inside a dummy uterine cavity

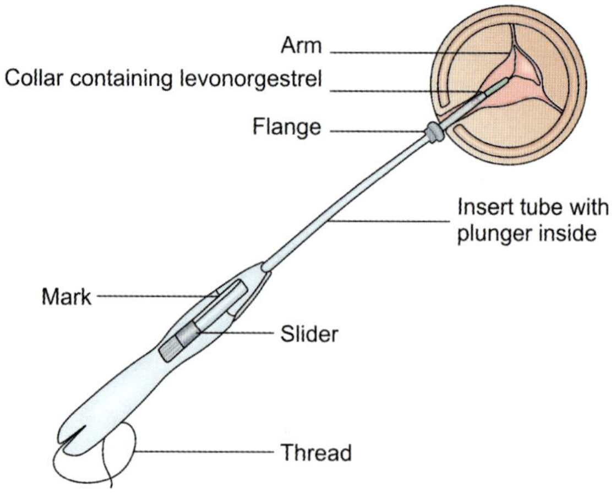

Fig. 10.3: Mirena intrauterine device shown inside a dummy uterine cavity with the slider pulled completely back. The device is T shaped. The IUD is placed high in the fundus

10.9.3 Reversal of Fertility After Use

Following removal, fertility is rapidly restored. Even though IUD has been blamed to cause increased incidence of PID, studies have not shown much increase in infection rates. Following removal fertility has not been found to be decreased.

10.9.4 Expulsion

Expulsion rate was higher for Lippy's loop and Cu7. Cu T 200 also had high expulsion rate. Cu T 380 Ag and Cu T 380 slimline has much less expulsion rate. Cu T 380 A has been found to be superior to all other IUDs considering failure rate, expulsion rate and efficacy. This is the most widely used intrauterine device at present.

10.9.5 Frameless IUDs

Frameless IUDs are presently marketed as Flexyguad, Cu Fix and Gyne Fix. It consists of 6 copper sleeves containing 330 mm^2 of copper strung on a nylon thread (prolypropelene) which is knotted at the end. The knot is pushed in to the myometrium with the help of a notched needle thus fixing the needle in the myometrium. The insertion needs experienced hands, but the expulsion rates are very low.

10.9.6 Contraceptive Efficacy

Failure rate and expulsion rate of the previous IUDs were higher. Failure rate of the modern device i.e Cu T 380A is reported as 0.8 (typical use) and 0.6 (perfect use).

A Cochrane review has shown that progestagen incorporated IUDs have the same effectiveness as copper IUDs containing >250 mm^2 Cu, but more effective than copper IUDs containing $\leq$ 250 mm^2 Cu. Since the presently used device which is Cu T 380A contains 380 mm^2 of Cu whose contraceptive efficiency is same as LNG-20 IUS and discontinuation rate for the later is more due to amenorrhea, the former should be preferred as contraceptive and the latter reserved as a treatment modality for menorrhagia.[14] The Cu T 380A IUD is a good reversible contraceptive choice for parous as well as nulliparous women. It has excellent contraceptive efficacy similar to LNG-20 IUS. Ectopic pregnancies are not *significantly* higher among IUD users contrary to the widespread belief. Proper history taking and examination before insertion should be given importance. Conforming to proper technique of insertion is important in reducing perforation and preventing pelvic infection. Incidence of pelvic inflammatory disease is related to pre-existing PID as well as introduction of infection while insertion.

Contraindications for IUD use
- Uterine anomalies
- Presence of PID
- Sexually transmitted diseases
- Myomas distorting uterine cavity
- Undiagnosed genital bleeding
- Women on anticoagulants and inherited abnormalities of coagulation (progestagen incorporated IUDs are not contraindicated)
- Immunocompromised women

10.9.7 IUD Insertion

Patient Selection

Proper patient selection is important in the success of IUD use. IUDs are not the contraceptive of choice for women who are prone for pelvic inflammatory disease. These women can have barrier method of contraception along with IUD. Age and parity are not important for selecting patients for IUD. Nulliparous women with monogamous relation can resort to IUD contraception. Patients with menorrhagia should be counseled that there can be an increase in menstrual bleeding after IUD insertion. Women on anticoagulant and those with bleeding disorders should not be chosen for copper IUD, but progestagen incorporated IUD may be resorted to. IUD is not a good choice for women who have uterine anomalies like bicornuate or septate uterus, myomas which distort the uterine cavity and those who have allergy to copper, immunologically suppressed patients and those with Wilson's disease. Even heart disease patients who are at risk for endocarditis can have IUD, but insertion should be under prophylactic antibiotic coverage. IUD is not contraindicated in women with diabetes.

Patient Counseling

Prospective IUD users should be counseled about the following factors:

1. Contraceptive effectiveness begins immediately after insertion.
2. The first few periods after insertion can be longer and heavier but can be reduced with the use of drugs like anti-fibrinolytic agents and anti-prostaglandins.
3. If the woman has menorrhagia, she would benefit from hormone releasing IUD.
4. Following insertion, there is a slightly increased risk of pelvic infection in the first few months.
5. Additional use of condom can prevent sexually transmitted infections.
6. Ectopic pregnancies are more common when pregnancy results from failure of IUD. Hence she should report early if the period is missed or has irregular bleeding/ pain abdomen.
7. The IUD can get spontaneously expelled or can escape into the abdomen: the woman should be taught to palpate the string of the IUD and advised to report if it is not felt.

Timing

IUDs can be inserted after delivery, spontaneous miscarriage or induced abortion or after menstrual period. Expulsion rates are high if inserted immediately after vaginal delivery. Hence, after delivery, insertion can be advised between 4 and 8 weeks (WHO). An IUD can be inserted during Cesarean. It is safer to fix the IUD with an absorbable suture material to the fundus of the uterus. IUD insertion in lactating women[15] is not reported to carry increased risk of perforation. Insertion immediately after menstrual period ensures that it is not inserted into a pregnant uterus. Since copper IUD is an interceptive (preventing implantation) it can be inserted even in the mid-menstrual phase or as a post-coital contraceptive. Since routinely ovulation is not monitored, it is better to advise insertion soon after periods.

Pre-insertion Examination

A speculum examination and bimanual examination is mandatory to exclude infection and associated conditions like myomas, adnexal masses, etc. The size and position of the uterus should be carefully ascertained. Vaginitis and bacterial vaginosis should be treated before insertion.

Technique of IUD Insertion

Insertion of an IUD is a minor procedure which takes only a few minutes and does not require anesthesia as it causes only minimal discomfort. Very rarely, the uterine manipulation can cause parasympathetic stimulation resulting in bradycardia and cardiac arrest. Hence it is prudent to keep atropine ready and to monitor the patient's pulse during the procedure. After inserting a speculum, the anterior lip of the cervix should be caught with a Volsellum forceps. If the uterine length is more than 9 cm it is not advisable to insert IUD.

Pain and discomfort can be reduced by the injection of local anesthetic on either side of the cervix below the 3'o clock and 9'o clock positions. After giving local anesthetic, 2-3 minutes should be given for the anesthetic to take its action. The uterine cavity is sounded and the length should be measured. If the uterus is acutely retroflexed or ante flexed, care should be taken to prevent perforation during insertion.

The IUD is taken out from the sterile wrapper. The horizontal limbs are folded and tucked into the applicator just enough to hold the device during insertion. The horizontal limbs can even be tucked into the applicator without removing it from the sterile wrapper before starting the procedure, but this requires training. The movable flange on the applicator should be twisted and kept in the same plane as the horizontal arm. The portion of the applicator ahead of the movable flange should conform to the length of the uterine cavity sounded earlier. The device with the applicator and the solid rod inside is introduced into the upper part of the uterine cavity till it touches the fundus. Keeping the solid rod in place, the applicator is withdrawn so that the 'T' will unwind and occupy the upper portion of the uterine cavity. The device is gently pushed upwards so that the horizontal limbs occupy the fundal region of the uterus. The solid rod, followed by the applicator is removed. The string is trimmed leaving 2-3 cm length from the external os.

After insertion, it is usual to experience mild abdominal cramps, but if distressing cramps occur, it can be alleviated by oral mefenamic acid. The patient should be cautioned about having heavier periods in the first few months and advised to take anti-fibrinolytic agent if necessary. She should have her first check-up preferably after the next periods, to confirm the device is in place.

10.9.8 Method of Insertion of LNG IUS

The device is available in pre-sterilized package with the IUD inside the applicator. The packet is opened under sterile precautions. Keeping the arms of the devise horizontal, the slider is pushed as far forwards as possible. Holding the slider steady, the strings are pulled down so that the horizontal arms are drawn in to the applicator. The strings are pulled and fixed in to the notch at the bottom of the inserter. The flange is moved in such a way that the portion ahead will conform to the length of the uterine cavity. The applicator with the device in situ is inserted in to the uterine cavity till the flange is about 2-3 cm from the cervix. The slider is pulled back till it reaches the mark. The arms will unwind and occupy the uterine cavity. After waiting for a few seconds for the arms to completely open, the device is further advanced till the flange touches the cervix. Thus the horizontal arms are made to occupy the fundal region and then the applicator is removed. The thread is trimmed leaving about 4 cm from the external os.

10.9.9 Side Effects

Ectopic pregnancy: A WHO multicentric study showed that IUD users are 50% less likely to have ectopic pregnancy compared to those not using contraception. Pregnancies in IUD users are more likely to be ectopic. This has to be kept in mind when women present with irregular periods or missed periods while on IUD use. Levonorgestrel IUD can be preferred for women with previous history of ectopic pregnancy.

Irregular bleeding, menorrhagia and cramps: Irregular bleeding, menorrhagia and abdominal pain are complained of by women following IUD insertion. These complaints abate by 2-3 months. Pain as well as bleeding can be relieved by anti-prostaglandins like mefenamic acid and anti-fibrinolytic agent like tranexamic acid.

Pelvic infection: IUD related bacterial infection is understood to be due to contamination of the uterine cavity during insertion. Hence it is important to observe aseptic precautions during insertion. The insertion related infections are due to polymicrobial flora from the vagina. Infections which occur later on are not related to IUD. Like hormonal contraceptives, IUD will not prevent infection. However, progestagen incorporated IUD does not increase the pelvic infection rate. Valvular heart disease is not an absolute contraindication for IUD. It can be inserted under antibiotic prophylaxis. Amoxicillin 2 gm, 1 hour before insertion and removal can be used as a prophylactic antibiotic. However, the American Heart Association[16] does not recommend antibiotic prophylaxis for IUD insertion or removal. If there is an evident pelvic infection in an IUD user, the device should be removed under broad spectrum antibiotic cover. Certain studies have reported high incidence of HIV among copper T users. HIV positive couple should be advised additional barrier contraception also. A good option for them is to have dual contraception with LNG IUS and one of the barrier methods. Unilateral pelvic abscess with gram positive Actinomycetes is rarely reported. Actionomycetes are part of normal vaginal and gastrointestinal flora. If there are signs of infection like a pelvic mass or uterine tenderness, IUD is to be removed after starting penicillin group of antibiotics which should be continued for one month.

Perforation of Uterus

Perforation of uterus usually occurs at the time of insertion. Acutely ante-flexed and retroflexed uteri are more prone for perforation. Puerperal uterus is also more prone for perforation due to the small size. Adhering to correct method of insertion will minimize perforation.

10.9.10 Contraindications

1. Uterine anomaly like bicornuate uterus is a contraindication because of high failure rate.
2. Active PID. IUD should not be inserted in the presence of active PID.
3. Women having menorrhagia and/or dysmenorrhea
4. Women on anticoagulant therapy
5. Pregnancy
6. Immunocompromised women
7. Fibroid uterus with distortion of the uterine cavity.

10.9.11 Pregnancy with IUD in situ

With IUD *in situ*, ectopic pregnancy has to be ruled out with transvaginal ultrasound. Presence of intrauterine pregnancy and the location of IUD should be ascertained. In the presence of intrauterine pregnancy if the woman wishes to continue the same, IUD should be removed and the pregnancy may be permitted to continue as there is no reported increase in the risk of septic abortion or congenital anomalies of the fetus, though there is a fourfold increase in the incidence of preterm labor.[17,18] In the case of infection in pregnant uterus with IUD, the device should be removed under broad spectrum antibiotic cover and the pregnancy has to be terminated.

10.9.12 Missed IUD

If the IUD thread is missing the possibilities could be:

1. The thread might have coiled into the cervical canal
2. The thread might have broken and fallen off
3. The device with the thread would have escaped into the peritoneal cavity
4. The device and the thread would have been expelled

The presence of the thread in the cervical canal can be made out and recovered by inserting and hooking out using a small mosquito forceps. If the thread can be recovered, the IUD need not be removed. If the thread cannot be located in the cervical canal the IUD can be searched for in the uterine cavity by transvaginal ultrasound scan. The presence of IUD in the uterine cavity or myometrium can be made out clearly with TVS.

If the device is not seen in the uterus its presence in the peritoneal cavity cannot be made out by ultrasound. Hence an X-ray abdomen should be taken to confirm or exclude the presence of the device. Copper IUDs which have escaped into the peritoneal cavity should be removed as it can cause adhesions and even perforations into the bowel lumen. This can be accomplished laparoscopically. Through the laparoscope, the device can be located by searching the region where there is omental adhesion.

10.10 BARRIER METHODS OF CONTRACEPTION

Even though barrier method of contraception is one of the oldest methods with high contraceptive failure rate, presently there is a renewal of its importance in view of its effectiveness in preventing transmission of STDs. Barrier methods like condom and diaphragm prevent STDs and pelvic inflammatory disease (PID). The role of condom in prevention of HIV transmission is being given great epidemiological importance. Prevention of PID has the important beneficial effect of reducing tubal infertility and ectopic pregnancies. Studies have shown that women who have never used barrier contraceptives are twice as likely to develop cancer of the cervix, implying that HPV infection also can be prevented using this method.

10.10.1 Diaphragm

The diaphragm was a popular method before COCs and IUDs came into the market. It has a 'typical use' failure rate of 12%. Consistent use of diaphragm is associated with a reduced incidence of PID but HIV transmission cannot be prevented completely.

Diaphragm is available in 3 sizes ranging from 65 to 105 cm. It is used in such a way as to cover the cervix and the upper anterior vaginal wall. It has to be inserted about 6 hours before intercourse and should be removed 6 hours later. The disadvantage is that it is coitus dependent and has high failure rate.

10.10.2 Cervical Cap

Cervical cap is as effective as the diaphragm but more difficult to use. The efficacy can be improved by using spermicides. The device should be introduced into the vagina and applied to the cervix in such a way as to cover it. As the diaphragm, it should be used before each act of intercourse and should be left in place for a minimum 8 hours. The method is not popular because of the high failure rate.

10.10.3 Contraceptive Sponge

This is a device which releases spermicide in a sustained release manner. It is available as *Today,* which is a polyurethane disc impregnated with 1g of non-oxynol-9. The sponge should be kept in the vagina for 24 hours. The failure rate is higher than diaphragm or condom.

10.10.4 Male Condom

Recently, the condoms have gained popularity due to its efficacy in preventing STDs especially HIV transmission. Nevertheless HPV transmission is not believed to be prevented, because it is spread through skin contact. Condoms made of latex, polyurethane and silicon rubber are available. Condoms should be advised if one of the partners is HIV positive. For effective contraception in HIV couple, condom should be used along with another contraceptive which has very low failure rate *(Belt and brace method).*

The failure rate quoted for typical use is 15%, which decreases to a much lower value with perfect use.

10.10.5 Female Condom

Female condoms are made of polyurethane. It is also an effective barrier for STIs. The device is a pouch which lies in the vagina. It has an inner ring at the closed end which overlies the cervix and an external ring which extends outside the vagina. The device should be used about 8 hours before intercourse and should be in place for about 6 hours after intercourse. With proper use the efficacy is similar to diaphragm and cervical cap.

10.10.6 Spermicidal Agents

Jellies, creams, foams, foaming tablets are used as vehicles for chemical agents which inactivate sperm. These have very high failure rate of approximately 20-25%. Excepting rare incidents of allergic reactions, there are no serious side effects.

10.10.7 Contraceptive Vaccines

Evolution of contraceptive vaccine sounds attractive as an alternative to the presently available methods of contraception. A wide variety of molecules are being studied. These include the following:

- Vaccines targeted at gamete production—GnRH and FSH.
- Vaccines targeted at gamete function—sperm antigens and zona pellucida.
- Vaccines targeted at gamete outcome-hCG.

The vaccines that target gamete production, even though effective has the disadvantage of causing sex steroid production and impotency. Vaccines targeted at sperm function like sperm antigens and zona pellucida proteins are exciting choices. Two sperm antigens SP-10 and PH-20 are being experimented in laboratory animals. Zona pellucida antigen can inhibit fertility, but there is no convincing evidence that it will not cause harmful effects in the ovary. The hCG vaccine under trial by the WHO task force on vaccines for fertility regulation is based on a portion of the β subunit of hCG-the carboxyterminal peptide. This vaccine had undergone phase II clinical trials in humans.

10.11 CONTRACEPTIVE OPTIONS AMONG WOMEN WITH MEDICAL DISORDERS (TABLE 10.6)

When selecting contraceptive method for women with chronic medical disorders, the contraceptive risk should be weighed against the risk of pregnancy complicating the underlying medical disorder. The contraceptive prescribed should be the one having the least risk relating to her specific disease process, at the same time having the greatest efficacy. The decision should be taken in consultation with the physician managing the woman. Hence by a team approach, the contraceptive protection can be optimized, minimizing her risk along with planning for future pregnancies.

10.12 EMERGENCY CONTRACEPTION

Emergency contraceptives, otherwise called morning-after pills are drugs taken after coitus for prevention of pregnancy. The exact mechanism of post-coital contraception is not fully known. These drugs act either by preventing ovulation or implantation. It is a method to prevent pregnancy in women who have unprotected sexual intercourse and can be used in situations like rape, unplanned intercourse or when a birth control method fails. Since these act to prevent ovulation or implantation they are medically and legally considered as forms of contraception. It can also be considered as abortifacients as these act after fertilization.

10.12.1 Types of Emergency Contraception

Several types of emergency contraceptive regimes are available which include:

1. **The Yuzpe regime** was the originally discovered emergency contraceptive regime. In this regimen, a combination of estrogen and progestagen (0.2 mg EE and 2 mg levonorgestrel), usually 2 doses of 2 Ovral pills each at 12 hour interval should be taken within 72 hours of coitus. The method was poorly tolerated due to nausea and vomiting as a result of the high dose of hormones. Failure rate was very high with this regimen.
2. **Levonorgestrel:** In the year 1999, FDA approved levonorgestrel emergency contraceptive pill (Plan B). The dose comprises two tablets of 750μg of levonorgestrel to be taken 12 hours apart. In 2006, the FDA approved non-prescription license for the drug to be used for women 18 years or older. A WHO randomized trial found it to be very effective with a failure rate of 1.1%. Nausea and vomiting occur much less frequently compared to the Yuzpe regime. A single dose of 1.5 mg is as effective as 2 doses of 0.75mg. It has been found to be effective even up to 5 days after intercourse but with a slightly higher failure rate.
3. **IUD:** An intrauterine device inserted into the uterine cavity within 7 days after an unprotected intercourse prevents pregnancy by interfering with implantation. It is more effective than hormonal methods of post-coital contraception. If the patient wants long-term contraception, the device can be left in place.
4. **Mifepristone** used in a dose of 200 mg prevents implantation and hence can be used as an emergency contraceptive.[19] It has been proved recently that even 10 mg dose inhibits ovulation.

10.12.2 Mechanism of Action

The Yuzpe regime and the levonorgestrel pill works by delaying ovulation and affecting sperm or egg transport through fallopian tube. IUDs and mifepristone interfere with implantation.

10.12.3 Effectiveness

The levonorgestrel regime is reported by the FDA to have 89% effectiveness. Various reports state that Yuzpe regimen has an effectiveness[20] ranging between 47% and 74%. A

Table 10.6: Considerations for contraceptive choice in women with medical conditions

Medical condition		*COC*	*Progestin only*	*Injectable or implant progestin contraception*
Cardiac lesions	Complicated congenital and acquired valvular lesions	Contraindicated – increased risk of thrombosis	Not contraindicated	Not contraindicated
	Uncomplicated valvular disease	Acceptable with risk. Low dose estrogen formulations preferred	Not contraindicated	Not contraindicated
	Hypercoagulable state associated with cardiac valvular disease	Contraindicated	Not contraindicated	Not contraindicated
Current or previous venous or arterial thrombosis		Contraindicated	Acceptable with risk, but should be avoided if current DVT	Acceptable with risk, but should be avoided if current DVT
Known thrombophilia		Contraindicated	Acceptable with risk	Acceptable with risk
Coronary artery disease		Contraindicated	Acceptable with risk	Acceptable with risk
Hypertension		Contraindicated	Acceptable with risk	Acceptable with risk
Diabetes mellitus	Type I or II without vascular disease	Acceptable with risk, choose the lowest dose of progestin	Acceptable with risk	Acceptable with risk
	Type I or II with vascular sequelae	Contraindicated	Acceptable with risk	Acceptable with risk
	Prior gestational diabetes	Lowest dose estrogen progestin combination to be preferred	Contraindicated if breastfeeding	No contraindication
Hyperlipidemia		Contraindicated	Acceptable with risk	Acceptable with risk
Sickle cell disease		Contraindicated	Not contraindicated	Not contraindicated
Seizure disorders		Not contraindicated, but may require higher dose formulations	Not contraindicated, but will have high failure rate	Preferred due to decrease in seizure frequency; but higher failure rate to be anticipated
Migraine with aura		Contraindicated	Acceptable with risk	Acceptable with risk
Active liver disease		Contraindicated	Contraindicated	Contraindicated
CIN		Acceptable; higher risk for progression to cancer; hence yearly Pap test	Not contraindicated	Acceptable with risk
Prolactinoma		Not contraindicated	Not contraindicated	Not contraindicated

combined estimate from three trials reported an effectiveness of 83% for 10 mg of mifepristone[19] taken up to 120 hours after intercourse.

Counseling

Patient should be counseled about the effectiveness of the various methods, the common side effects and the fact that her period may get delayed even if pregnancy has not occurred. In the event of failure, if pregnancy continues no particular adverse effect has been reported following the use of Yuzpe regime or levonorgestrel.

10.12.4 Adverse Effects

Common adverse effects are nausea, vomiting and abdominal pain. Delayed period and irregular bleeding are other side effects.

10.13 FEMALE STERILIZATION

Female sterilization is intended to be a permanent method of contraception. Due to its permanent nature it is important to obtain an informed consent from the couple. The couple, especially young and those with no or 1-2 children should be provided with information about alternative highly effective long term temporary methods of contraception. Laws relating to norms for sterilization procedure are different in different nations and should be followed. For making sterilization procedures safe, WHO has made recommendations depending upon the medical fitness of women. On the basis of medical eligibility four categories have been defined by WHO which are:

Accept (A): There is no medical reason to deny sterilization to a person with this condition.

Caution (C): The procedure is normally conducted in a routine setting, but with extra preparation and precautions.

Delay (D): The procedure is delayed until the condition is evaluated and/or corrected. Alternative temporary methods of contraception should be provided.

Special (S): The procedure should be undertaken in a setting with an experienced surgeon and staff, equipment needed to provide general anesthesia, and other back-up medical support. For these conditions, the capacity to decide on the most appropriate procedure and anesthesia regimen is also needed. Alternative temporary methods of contraception should be provided, if referral is required or if there is any delay otherwise.

For example, a woman who had severe pre-eclampsia, eclampsia, severe ante partum or postpartum hemorrhage, puerperal sepsis or prolonged rupture of membranes falls under Category D. For further details refer: *Medical Eligibility Criteria for Contraceptive Use, 2004 And 2008 Update, WHO.*

10.13.1 History

It was James Blundell in 1823 who proposed tubectomy as a method of sterilization. It is not known whether he actually performed the procedure. The first report of tubal ligation was published by Samuel Lungren of Toledo in the year 1881. The procedure was ligating the tube at the time of cesarean section. Madlener (1910) described the Madlener technique which had very high failure rates. The method which is popularly adopted at present is the Pomeroy's method which was described by Ralph Pomeroy, a physician in New York (1929). This method became popular in the 1960s. The vaginal method of sterilization was discovered later but was given up due to the high infection rate. With the advent of laparoscopic procedures in 1970, laparoscopic sterilization greatly replaced mini-laparotomies and thus sterilization became a day-care procedure.

10.13.1 Efficacy of Sterilization

The failure rate of sterilization greatly varies depending upon the method used and the skill of the surgeon. Up to 50% of the failures are due to technical errors. Technical errors are more frequent following use of silastic rings and clips. Ectopic pregnancies occur more frequently following tubal occlusion. Bipolar tubal coagulation is more likely to result in ectopic pregnancy than mechanical occlusion with silastic ring or clips. Approximately 1/3rd of pregnancies that occur among women after tubal sterilization are ectopic. But overall, the risk of ectopic pregnancy in sterilized women is lower than in women who have not undergone sterilization. Sterilization failures are more among women younger than 35 years and among women who breastfed after sterilization. The reason may be the influence of low fecundity among these women.

One of the benefits of sterilization is the decreased incidence of ovarian malignancy. The Nurses' Health Study indicated that there is 67% reduction in the risk of ovarian cancer among women who had tubal sterilization.

10.13.2 Counseling for Sterilization

Before deciding on sterilization women should be made aware of the nature of the surgery, it's possible consequences as well as the alternatives like temporary methods of contraception. Patient should also be informed about the chance of failure of the particular method adopted and the possibility of recanalization. It should be emphasized that even though sterilization is intended to be permanent, it cannot be guaranteed to prevent intrauterine or ectopic pregnancy and that failure can occur even several years after the procedure.

Common procedures include:

- Tubal sterilization at the time of cesarean
- Postpartum minilaparotomy within 7 days of vaginal delivery
- Interval minilaparotomy
- Laparoscopy
- Hysteroscopy

Tubal sterilization at the time of cesarean has no added risk except a slight increase in the duration of surgery. In developing countries where there is a high rate of neonatal mortality, it is better to postpone sterilization to a later date as an interval procedure. Minilaparotomy after vaginal delivery is a comparatively easier procedure because the uterus is an abdominal organ and the tubes can be easily reached through an incision in the abdomen placed 2 finger-breadths below the fundus. During interval sterilization, the uterus will be a pelvic organ hence the tubes can be approached by short suprapubic transverse incision placed 2 finger-breadths above the pubic symphysis. Mini-laparotomy can be performed as an outpatient procedure under local anesthesia and sedation.

10.13.3 Pomeroy's Method

In the classical Pomeroy's method (Fig. 10.4) a loop of the tube, preferably the isthmial region is ligated with a single absorbable suture and excised. About 1-2 cm of the isthmial region of the tube is caught with Babcock's forceps and ligated with plain catgut and the loop is cut at about 5 mm from the ligature so that a small portion, about 0.5-1 cm of the tube is removed. As sequelae, the ends will retract causing discontinuity. The failure rate reported is 0.5. There are several modifications for the method, like repeat ligation of the cut ends or coagulation of the cut ends. When the procedure is performed during puerperium, it is preferable to double ligate the tube, as there is an increased risk of hemorrhage from the cut end due to the enlargement and increase in the vascularity during pregnancy. In modified Pomeroy's method, after excision of the loop of the tube, the cut ends are ligated separately. Care should be taken during the procedure to avoid mesosalpingeal injury which can cause hemorrhage. This method is otherwise called *Parkland hospital technique*. Failure rate following this method is less than the classical Pomeroy's method.

The isthmial region is preferred for the following reasons:

1. Failure rate is less as the chance of neo-fimbria formation is low in the isthmial region
2. Success of recanalization is more as the isthmial region can be anastomosed without much luminal disparity
3. The interference with the ovarian blood supply is less compared to partial salpingectomy.

10.13.4 Irwing's Method

The isthmial portion is dissected from the mesosalpinx and is cut and both ends ligated separately. The medial end is then buried in the posterior wall of the uterus. No failure rate is reported with this method. Since the procedure requires a larger incision and longer time, this is not usually followed.

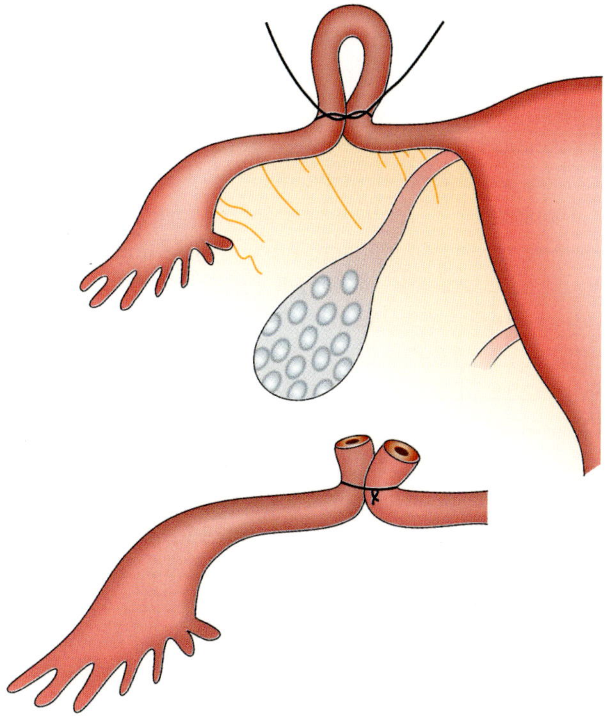

Fig. 10.4: Pomeroy's method of sterilization. A loop of the isthmial region of the fallopian tube is ligated with absorbable suture and excised

10.13.5 Uchida Technique

In this method, a portion of the isthmial region of the tube is separated from the mesosalpinx and is cut and buried in the broad ligament. No failure rate is reported with this method also.

10.13.6 Laparoscopic Sterilization

The advantage of laparoscopic sterilization is that hospital admission is not required and, the patient can be discharged a few hours after the procedure. The woman can return to normal activities within 24 hours.

The incision is very small and the discomfort is slight. Laparoscopy gives the opportunity to visualize the pelvic organs as well as the abdomen for abnormalities. The disadvantage of the procedure includes:

- Need for expensive equipment
- Special training required for performing the procedure
- Risk of injury to bowel or great vessel which could be fatal
- Laparotomy may rarely be necessary to tackle complications.

Any of the following methods could be resorted to for performing laparoscopic sterilization:

1. Occlusion by mechanical means using either silastic rings or clips

2. Occlusion by bipolar electrocoagulation
3. Occlusion and transection by unipolar electrocautery
4. Occlusion or partial resection using electrocautery

The procedure is preferably done under general anesthesia. In situations where general anesthesia is not feasible, it can be done under local infiltration anesthesia.

Laparoscopic sterilization can be done by either single-puncture or double-puncture method. The umbilical trocar should be inserted with the patient in the dorsal position, after creating pneumoperitoneum. In the single-puncture method, the telescope and the instrument are inserted through the same cannula through different channels. In the double-puncture method, the telescope is inserted through an umbilical port and the applicator is inserted through a second trocar site, usually a few centimeters above the pubic symphysis. The fallopian tube should be identified by tracing the fimbrial end so that inadvertent application on the round ligament can be avoided. The ring is applied to a loop of the isthmial region of the tube with the help of an applicator. The applicator is designed to grasp a loop of the tube and release the silastic band on to the loop. Mesosalpingeal bleeding is one of the common complications which can occur during the procedure. This can be prevented by catching hold of the tube alone avoiding the mesosalpinx. If the bleeding occurs after the application of the band, placement of an additional band will be necessary. If bleeding still continues, it should be controlled by electrocoagulation. Abdominal cramps may be experienced by the woman post-operatively. Application of local anesthetic on to the tube through the cannula before applying the falope ring (Fig. 10.5) or clip prevents the pain. Falope ring application destroys a greater portion of the tube compared to the application of the clip. The Hulka-Clemens spring clip consists of two plastic jaws made of lexan hinged by a metal pin. The jaws have teeth on the opposing surfaces. After application, a stainless-steel spring is pushed over the jaws to hold them closed over the tube. The spring destroys only 3 mm of the tube. In the event of accidental dislodgement of the clip into the peritoneal cavity, it should be retrieved. The Filshie clip is made of titanium lined by silicon rubber. Incomplete or incorrect application results in failure. Since, it destroys only a very small portion of the tube, recanalization can be achieved with very high success rates.

Gas embolism is a rare complication which can occur as with any other laparoscopic surgery. The chance of embolization is high if air is used for distending the abdomen. Carbon dioxide should be preferred, as even if it gets into the circulation, carbon dioxide is immediately converted to bicarbonate and hydrogen ions and will not exist in the gaseous state.

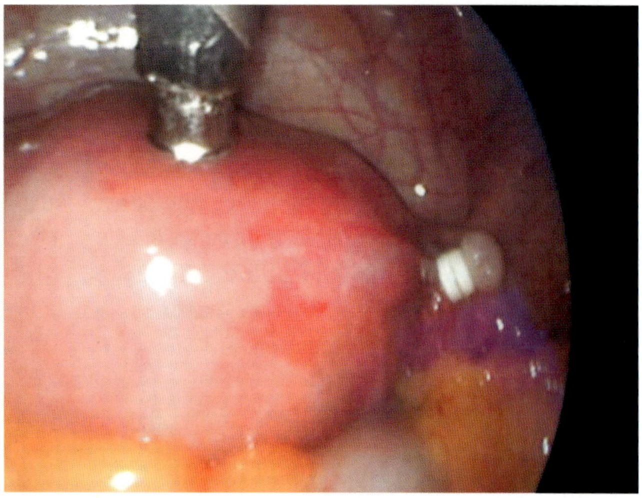

Fig. 10.5: Falope ring in the isthmial region of the tube

Long-term Complications

Post ligation syndrome: Symptoms like abdominal pain, dyspareunia, dysmenorrhea, exacerbation of premenstrual symptoms, etc. have been attributed to the procedure. However, available literature does not support this contention. These symptoms may be a manifestation of regret about having undergone the procedure.[21,22]

Ectopic pregnancy is recognized to be higher among sterilization failures.

10.13.7 Changes in Menstrual Function after Sterilization

Studies have reported conflicting findings about alteration in menstrual function following tubal ligation. When some studies reported increase in the incidence of dysmenorrhea and increased frequency of menstruation following tubal ligation, others have reported no change in menstrual function.

10.13.8 Reversibility

The need for reversal of sterilization arises usually following demise of children or after remarriage. The success rate of reversibility depends upon the method of sterilization. Tubal occlusion with Filsche clip and Hulka clip which damages minimal length of the tube carries the best success after reversal. Pomeroy's method and bipolar coagulation destroys a greater length of the tube and hence the success rate is less than following Filsche or Hulka clip. Partial salpingectomy as a method of sterilization should not be practiced as it has high failure rate as well as almost nil success rates after reversal. The fimbrial end and the ampullary region of the tube are essential for successful pregnancy following recanalization.

Using microsurgical techniques the success rate in expert hands for reversal can be 70-80% if the sterilization method adopted was clips or rings. The pregnancy rate following recanalization depends upon the length of the tube which should be 4 cm or more for optimal results.

10.13.9 Hysteroscopic Sterilization

Sterilization can be achieved hysteroscopically by inserting a micro-insert consisting of stainless steel inner coil and Nickel-Titanium alloy outer coil (ESSURE) into the fallopian tube. The device is introduced through the operating channel of a hysteroscope and guided to the fallopian tube through the tubal ostia. Tubal occlusion can be documented by hysterosalpingography 3 months after the procedure. The patient should be advised contraception till tubal occlusion is documented. The efficacy of the device is 85-90%. However since it causes a fibrotic reaction in the tube including its intramural portion, reversibility is a matter of concern.

10.14 MALE STERILIZATION

Vasectomy is a safer and easier method compared to female sterilization because the vas can be approached without opening the abdomen. After vasectomy the absence of sperm should be documented 3 months following the procedure.

10.14.1 Method

The widely accepted method is the no-scalpel technique perfected by Li Shunqiang (China). The procedure requires few instruments and is less invasive.

Failure rate following vasectomy[23] is less than female sterilization. It is reported to be 9 per 1000.

Complications and sequelae

Hematomas and infection can occur rarely as a complication of vasectomy. Most men develop sperm antibodies following vasectomy. There are no adverse effects on sexual function even though adverse psychological sequelae have been reported. Though animal studies have reported accelerated atherosclerosis after vasectomy, no such risk is reported among men. Vasectomy will not change the risk of HIV transmission.

10.14.2 Reversibility

Eventhough vasectomy reversal is easier than tubal recanalization, pregnancy rates are lesser than successful tubal recanalisation. Pregnancy rate reported is 50%. This could be due to sperm antibody formation.

10.15 CONCLUSION

Family planning could bring more benefits to more people at less cost than any other single technology now available to the human race (UNICEF). The search is still on for an ideal contraceptive. Combination estrogen-progestagen contraception is highly effective with added non-contraceptive benefits like reduction in the incidence of endometrial, colorectal as well as ovarian cancer. The combination oral contraceptive pill, patch as well as vaginal ring offer excellent contraceptive efficacy although all of them increase the risk of venous thrombosis and thrombo-embolism. The reported increased incidence of breast cancer associated with COC is actually an exaggerated figure. Proper history taking and adequate counseling should be given importance before prescribing COC so that the gap between 'typical use' and 'perfect use' failure rates is minimized. Investigations should be resorted to whenever necessary. The low dose COCs are comparatively safe and can even be prescribed to women with uncomplicated diabetes and hypertension. COC containing drosperinone, which does not cause water and salt retention, has the added advantage of not causing weight gain. The clinician's mind set should be changed to promote a positive attitude among women for adopting COC as an effective contraceptive which in turn can contribute to overall health of women. Implanon, which will be launched shortly, might prove to be an effective contraceptive, as it is less user dependent. 1.5 mg levonorgestrel is the most effective hormonal emergency contraception. The present day intrauterine devices containing more than 250 mm^2 of copper have much less failure rate as well as side effects compared to the older generation devices. Cu T 380 A as well as LNG-IUS provide effective contraception. LNG-IUS has the added advantage of reducing menstrual blood loss. The greatest advantage of barrier methods of contraception is the prevention of transmission of STIs including HIV. Contraceptive efficacy of barrier methods, when used consistently, can be improved with the concurrent use of spermicides. Male and female sterilization provide permanent contraception. Vasectomy, (especially no-scalpel) causes less morbidity compared to female sterilization. Considering hospital stay as well as reversibility, laparoscopic sterilization using clips is superior to using Falope ring, coagulation with bipolar cautery or Pomeroy's method. Widespread use of contraceptives has greatly reduced the morbidity associated with termination of pregnancies. Research is continuing towards the development of contraceptive vaccines, vaginal rings and non-toxic spermicidal agents which will prevent HIV transmission.

REFERENCES

1. Trussell J. Contraceptive efficacy. In Hatcher RA, Trussell J, Nelson AL, Cates W, Stewart FH, Kowal D. Contraceptive Technology: Nineteenth Revised Edition. New York NY: Ardent Media, 2007.
2. Vessey MP, Mcpherson K, Johnson B. Oxford Family Planning Association Study. Lancet, 1977;2(8041):731-3.
3. Suissa S, Spitzer WO, Rainville B, Cusson J, Lewis M, Heinemann L. Recurrent use of newer oral contraceptives and risk of venous thromboembolism. Hum Reprod 2000;15:817.
4. Coney P, Washenik K, Langley RGB, DiGiovanna JJ, Harrison DD. Weight change and adverse event incidence with low dose oral contraceptive: two randomized placebo-controlled trials. Contraception 2001;63:297.
5. Marchbanks PA,McDonald JA.Wilson HGoral contraceptives and the risk of breast cancer N Engl J Med 2002; 342:2025-32.
6. Kahlenborn C, Modungo F, Potter DM, et al. Oral contraceptive use as a risk factor for premenopausal breast cancer: a meta-analysis Mayo clin Proc 2006;81:1290-302.
7. Brinton LA, Reeves WC, Brenes MM, Herrero R. Oral contraceptive use and risk of invasive cervical cancer. Int J Epidemo 1990;19:4.
8. Kjos SL, Peters RK, Xiang A, Thomas D. Contraception and the risk of type 2 diabetes in Latino women with prior gestational diabetes. JAMA 1998;280:533.
9. Chiaffarino F, Parazzini F, La Vecchia C, et al. Use of oral contraceptives and uterine fibroids; results froma case-control study. Br J Obstet gynaecol 1999;106:857.
10. WHO, special programme of Research Development and research training in human reproduction, Task Force on Oral contraceptives, Effects of hormonal contraceptives on milk volume and infant growth, Contraception 1984;30:505.
11. Croxatto HB et al, a multicentre efficacy and safety study of the single contraceptive implant implanon. Implanon study group, Hum Reprod 1999;14:976.
12. Weiderspass E,Adami HO, Beren JA, et al. Use of oral contraceptives and endometrial cancer. WHO Collaborative study of neoplasia and steroid contraception. Int J Cancer. 1991;49.
13. Lee P. Shulman, Carolyn L. Westhoff Return to Fertility After Use of Reversible Contraception. Contraception 2006; 70:3-10.
14. French R, Van Vliet HHAAM, Cowan F, Mansour DD, Hughes DD, Robinson AA, Proctor TT, Summerbell CC, Logan S, Helmerhorst FM, Guillebaud J. Hormonally impregnated intrauterine systems (IUSs) versus other forms of reversible contraceptives as effective methods of preventing pregnancy. Cochrane Database of Systematic Reviews 2004, Issue 3. Art. No.: CD001776. DOI: 10.1002/14651858.CD001776.pub2.
15. Chi J, Potts M, et al. Performance of the T Cu -380A device in breastfeeding and non breastfeeding women. Contraception 1989;39:603.
16. Dajani AS, et al. Prevention of bacterial endocarditis: Recommendations of American Heart Association. JAMA 1997;277:1794-801.
17. Atrash HK, Frye A, et al. Incidence of morbidity and mortality with IUD in situ in the 1980s and 1990s. Proceedings from the 4th International Conference on IUDs. Butterworth-Heinmann, Boston, 1994. p76.
18. Layde PM, Goldberg MF et al. Failed intrauterine device contraception and limb reduction deformities: a case control study. Fertil Steril. 1979;31:18.
19. Piaggio G, Heng Z, von Hertzen H, Bilian X, Linan C. Combined estimates of effectiveness of mifepristone 10 mg in emergency contraception. Contraception 2003;68(6): 439-46.
20. Trussell J, Ellertson C, von Hertzen H, Bigrigg A, Webb A, Evans M, Ferden S, Leadbetter C. Estimating the effectiveness of emergency contraceptive pills. Contraception 2003; 67 (4): 259-65.
21. Wilcox LS Martinez-Schnell B, Peterson HB, Ware JH, Hughes JM, Menstrual function after tubal sterilization, Am J Epidemiol 1992;135:1368.
22. Peterson HB, Jeng G, Folger SG, Hillis SA, Marchbanks PA, Wilcox LS, for the U.S. collaborative Review of sterilization Working Group, The risk of menstrual abnormalities after tubal sterilization. U.S. Collaborative Review of Sterilization Working Group, New Engl J Med 2000;343:1724.
23. Jamieson DJ, The US Collaborative Review Of Sterilization Working Group. The risk of pregnancy after vasectomy. Obstett Gynaecol. 2004; 103:848.

11 Menopause

B Presannakumari

11.1 INTRODUCTION

Menopause is the permanent cessation of menstruation which occurs as a result of loss of ovarian activity. It is a retrospective diagnosis made when 12 months have elapsed after the final menstrual period. The word menopause is derived from the Greek words 'menos' meaning month and 'pausis' meaning cessation. Menopause is possibly an evolutionary adaptation to prevent child bearing in the older age group. Life expectancy continues to increase and has reached 82 years for women in developed countries. Most women thus live more than one third of their lifetime after menopause. The age at menopause is predominantly genetically determined and over the years has seen only a minimal increase. Mothers and daughters experience menopause almost at the same age. Natural menopause usually occurs between the ages 45 and 55. Average age is estimated to be 50.7. Menopause occurs early in undernourished women, those on vegetarian diets and also among smokers. It seems to be affected by chemotherapy, radiation, surgery on the ovary, hysterectomy etc whereas race, socioeconomic status, age of menarche etc have no role in determining the age at menopause.

Premature menopause is defined as menopause occurring at an age less than two standard deviations below the mean estimate for the reference population. In developing countries, due to the absence of reliable data, menstruation ceasing before the arbitrary cut-off value of 40 years is considered premature menopause. The marked decrease in hormone production after menopause affects several systems in the body.

11.2 HORMONAL EVENTS AT MENOPAUSE

Menopause is primarily ovarian failure. The female child is born with 1-2 million follicles and at menarche owing to apoptosis, the number decreases to 400,000. The transition from normal ovulatory cycles to complete cessation of menses is gradual. The hormonal changes start about 2-8 years prior to menopause, referred to as menopausal transition. As the number of follicles reaches 25000, FSH and LH levels start increasing due to the decreased inhibin production from the ovary. Thus, inhibin is a marker of ovarian follicular competence. There is no failure of hypothalamopituitary ovarian axis during this period. The pituitary continues to secrete FSH and LH in increased quantities due to the absence of negative feedback from the ovary. At menopause, all the follicles will be depleted due to apoptosis resulting in failure of estrogen, progesterone and inhibin from the ovary. Since the ovarian stroma continues to function, androgen production is not affected. After menopause there is a 10-20 fold increase in FSH and 3–fold increase in LH. The maximal level of FSH and LH is reached 1-3 years after the last period. This is followed by a gradual decline. Since the half-life of LH is short and the negative feedback by inhibin on LH is negligible, the LH level is not as high as that of FSH. Peripheral conversion of androgen from ovary and adrenals results in increased levels of estrone which in turn is partly converted to estradiol. Postmenopausal level of estradiol is 10-20 pg/ml and the circulating level of estrone is higher than in premenopausal women. Androstenedione to estrone ratio will increase which causes mild hirsutism and central obesity. Gradually, the ovarian stroma and adrenal undergo exhaustion resulting in decreased production of androgen and consequently estrogen. The different phases of transition from normal ovulatory period to menopause and postmenopausal years are defined as follows by WHO (1994):

Menopausal transition is the period before the final menstrual period when variability occurs in the menstrual cycle. This variability can be in the form of skipped periods followed by bleeding which may be above normal or frequent periods occurring once in every 15-20 days.

Perimenopause includes the period beginning with the first clinical and endocrinological features of the approaching menopause (e.g. vasomotor symptoms, menstrual irregularity) and ending 12 months after the last menstrual period.

Climacteric is the phase in the aging of women marking the transition from the reproductive to the non reproductive phase. This phase incorporates perimenopause as well as a longer variable period before and after perimenopause.

Climacteric syndrome refers to the symptoms which occur during the climacteric period. All women need not experience these symptoms.

Premenopause refers to 1-2 years immediately before menopause or the whole of the reproductive period prior to menopause.

Postmenopause is the period after 12 months of spontaneous amenorrhea irrespective of whether the menopause is induced or spontaneous. However, if a woman presents with bleeding after 6 months of amenorrhea it should be considered worthy of investigation for postmenopausal bleeding.

Induced menopause is defined as cessation of menstruation which follows surgical removal of both ovaries or iatrogenic ablation of ovarian function, e.g. chemotherapy or radiotherapy.

A functional staging system of reproductive aging was developed by the Reproductive Aging Workshop (STRAW) held in 2001 (Fig. 11.1). Reproductive aging is divided into 7 stages according to STRAW (–5 to +2). –5 begin with menarche and +2 is late menopause. The menopausal transition is divided into 2 stages: early –2, and late –1. These stages are characterized by elevated FSH level. The duration of these stages have individual variation. In –2 stage, the menstrual cycles remain regular but the length changes with a decrease in the interval between periods. In stage-1 (late menopausal transition) there can be skipped periods. Menopausal symptoms like hot flashes, sleep disturbances etc can be experienced in this stage. The +1 stage corresponds to early postmenopausal period and includes the first 5 years following the final menstrual

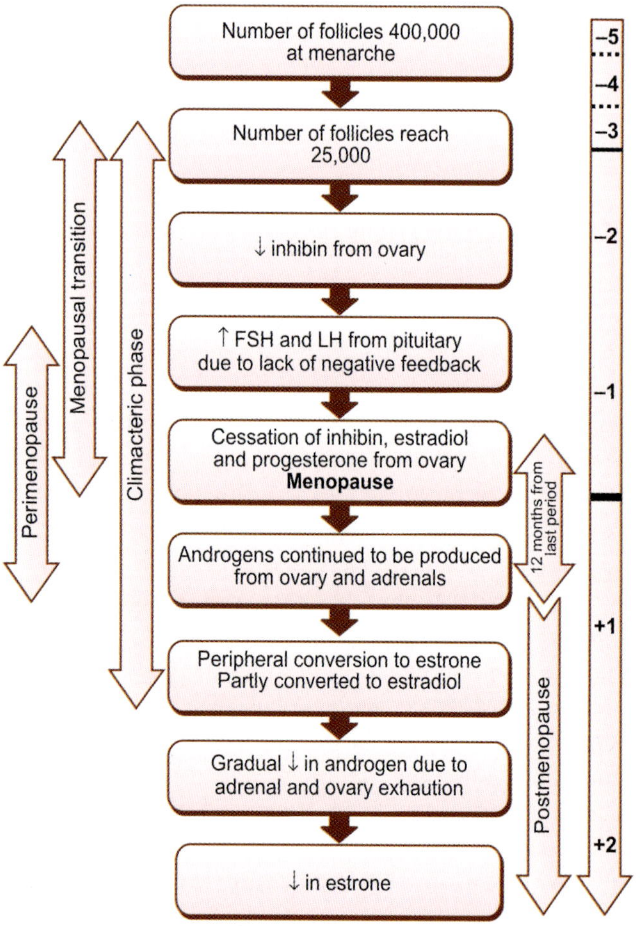

Fig. 11.1: Hormonal events of menopause. Stages of reproductive aging (STRAW) are schematically represented on the right side

period. The +2 stage is late postmenopause, which begins 5 years after the final menstrual period and continues until death.

11.3 SYMPTOMS OF PERIMENOPAUSE

Estrogen withdrawal at menopause has short-term and long-term consequences. In surgical menopause, all these events are more dramatic contributing to exaggerated effects of hormone withdrawal. The common symptoms of perimenopause are:

- Irregular, infrequent or scanty periods
- Vasomotor symptoms- night sweats, hot flashes
- Insomnia, mood swings, fatigue, depression, irritability, headache, poor concentration, mental confusion, disorientation, memory lapse
- Vaginal dryness
- Changes in libido
- Urinary symptoms—urgency, burning micturition, incontinence and frequent urinary tract infections
- Skin itching, skin eruptions, hair loss and hair thinning
- Weight gain

It is estimated that about 85% of women experience more than one symptom including hot flashes and night sweats. The vasomotor symptoms which are due to withdrawal of estrogen last for usually 1 year and rarely for above 5 years. The combination of symptoms and their severity differ between individuals.

Hot flashes are the commonest symptom of menopause. The classic symptom is periodic attacks of body heat which typically starts in the face and spreads all over the body. This is followed by an episode of sweating. The exact mechanism of hot flashes is not well understood. Nor-adrenergic, serotoninergic or dopaminergic activation may be the triggering factor. Since these symptoms are known to occur in women who had their pituitary glands removed, LH and FSH cannot be thought of as the causative factor. Estrogen withdrawal may be the triggering factor. This is implicated due to the fact that women having Turners syndrome will not experience hot flashes in spite of very low levels of estrogen, whereas it seems to occur when they are treated with estrogen and withdrawn.

11.4 LONG-TERM HEALTH PROBLEMS OF MENOPAUSE

Cessation of progesterone production has no significant clinical effects, but it can cause lack of protection from endometrial proliferation, hyperplasia and cancer. However, estrogen withdrawal is attributed to the occurrence of long term health problems. Since menopause and aging occur simultaneously, it is difficult to distinguish the effect of aging from that of menopause.

Long-term health problems attributed to menopause are listed below:

- Osteoporosis
- Cardiovascular diseases
- Poor muscle power and tone
- Skin wrinkling
- Urogenital symptoms

11.5 MANAGEMENT OF MENOPAUSE

11.5.1 Management of Perimenopausal Symptoms

Menopause can be very challenging for many women, more so when they have surgical menopause. Women reach menopause without having had adequate knowledge about it. There is a need for educating them about how to adjust with this changing phase of life. Cessation of ovulation and menstruation is actually a physiological adaptation preventing pregnancy and child birth at an age when a woman is not physically fit for it. Understanding this truth will help women to adopt a positive attitude towards menopause. Menopause should not be considered as a disease and unnecessary medication should be avoided.

Management of Vasomotor Symptoms

Lifestyle modification

Lifestyle changes like drinking cold liquids, avoiding triggers like hot drinks and spicy foods, staying in cold rooms, etc. may partially obviate the need for medications. Relaxation and paced respiration are techniques which have been found to have beneficial effects in reducing the severity and frequency of vasomotor symptoms. Regular exercise, cessation of smoking and maintaining body weight helps to reduce vasomotor symptoms. Regular exercise has a key role in the maintenance of health of postmenopausal women. Exercise has the following several advantages even though it may not alleviate the vasomotor symptoms significantly.

- Prevents osteoporosis
- Decreases the risk of heart disease
- Increases vital capacity
- Keep muscles strong and joints moving, preventing arthritis and maintaining balance
- Helps maintain weight and indirectly decreases the risk of diabetes and hypertension
- Increases endorphin and hence creates a better feeling of well-being

Walking is a good exercise. Low impact aerobics can also be undertaken.

Hormone therapy (HT)

Estrogen therapy is the most effective treatment for vasomotor symptoms. Presently, the most important indication for systemic estrogen therapy is the occurrence of unpleasant hot flashes which are distressing and causing sleep disturbance. The lowest effective dose should be used for the shortest duration to control the symptoms in order to avoid the adverse effects of hormone therapy. For many women, a low dose of conjugated estrogen 0.3 mg daily or transdermal estradiol 0.025 mg weekly is effective. Women who have not had hysterectomy should be given progestin (2.5 mg) also. For most women, a few months to one year of treatment may be enough to control the symptoms. Those who continue to have symptoms after this period can be offered hormones for a maximum period of 4-5 years. Bone mineral density will also be taken care of. Treatment up to 4-5 years is not seen to increase the risk of breast cancer. Estrogen dose should be reduced gradually before stopping as sudden withdrawal can precipitate vasomotor symptoms.

When a woman has contraindications for estrogen use, a higher dose of progesterone (Medroxyprogesterone acetate, MPA 20 mg/day or megesterol acetate 20 mg twice daily) alone can be advised.

Tibolone

This is a synthetic progestagen with estrogenic, androgenic and progestagenic properties. An international multi disciplinary panel of experts – The International Tibolone Consensus Group, formed the opinion that tibolone is effective in relieving vasomotor symptoms, mood disorders, vaginal atrophy and urogenital symptoms and improves sexual well-being. Tibolone is as effective as estrogen in preventing bone loss and does not increase mammographic density. Since it does not induce endometrial proliferation it can be used alone as a period-free HT.[1]

Other Medications

Antihypertensives

The antihypertensive drug clonidine has also been found to be effective in relieving hot flashes due to its effect on neurotransmitter pathways. Clonidine can be used in a dose of 0.1-0.2 mg or as weekly transdermal patch which delivers 0.10 mg/day.

Antidepressants

Since serotonin and nor epinephrine are involved in hypothalamic thermoregulation, drugs which inhibit their uptake have been tried for the alleviation of vasomotor symptoms. Even though their role is not established by large randomized studies, smaller studies have shown beneficial effects. Selective Serotonin Reuptake Inhibitors (SSRI) have been studied in randomized placebo controlled trials and found to be effective. They have the added advantage of relieving anxiety and improving mood. A selective nor-epinephrine reuptake inhibitor, venlafexine has been extensively studied for the treatment of vasomotor symptoms. Extended release venlafexine has been found to decrease vasomotor symptoms by 61%, in one study. These drugs can be preferred for patients who have contra-indications for hormone therapy.

Anticonvulsants

Gabapentin, an anticonvulsant has been found to reduce frequency and severity of hot flashes in a placebo controlled study.

Nutritional and vitamin supplementation

Phytoestrogens are plant products with a phenolic structure similar to estrogens. They act as estrogen receptor modulators. Among phytoestrogens, Isoflavones contained in soy and red clover has been extensively studied for the relief of vasomotor symptoms. Studies have shown only a small effect in reducing vasomotor symptoms with their use. Vitamin E and black cohosh have also been found to minimally reduce hot flashes. Indian menopause Society recommends that a diet rich in phytoestrogens should be started in all families for women of all ages. There are no randomized controlled trials on the use of extracts or capsules of phytoestrogens for relief of menopausal symptoms or prevention of osteoporosis.

Management of vaginal atrophy and urogenital symptoms

Estrogen receptors are abundant in the urethra, bladder and vagina. Estrogen withdrawal causes changes in the urethra and vagina. The reduction in collagen and decrease in muscle fibers in the pelvic floor make them more prone for urinary tract infections, urinary incontinence as well as burning, itching and discomfort in the vulvovaginal area. Lack of estrogen can lead to alteration of vaginal flora, predisposing to colonization with pathogenic bacteria, which also can cause urinary tract infection.

Vaginal atrophy and urogenital symptoms respond to local estrogens. Vaginal administration of low dose of 17β estradiol is effective in relieving urogenital symptoms. It can be used daily in the first 2 weeks, followed by twice a week for 12 months.

The preparations used for urogenital symptoms and vaginal atrophy are:

- Conjugated equine estrogen cream
- Estradiol vaginal tablet
- Estradiol vaginal ring which releases 7.5 μg of estradiol daily

If the woman has vasomotor symptoms also, systemic estrogens may be preferred.

Management of psychological symptoms

Even though depression, cognitive impairment and memory loss have been associated with menopausal age, menopause cannot be solely attributed as its causative factor.[1] A longitudinal study of postmenopausal women, Massachusetts Women's Health study could not associate menopause with depression.[2] Hormone replacement therapy (HRT) was previously believed to improve memory and prevent onset of Alzheimer's disease. A few studies reported improvement of verbal memory after estrogen use. The WHIMS study [women's health imitative memory study] which is a supplementary study to the WHI study examined the relationship between HRT and dementia in women older than 65 years. It was observed that there is a higher incidence of Alzheimer's disease in women taking CEE/MPA, the reason for which could not be explained. Before arriving at a conclusion, HRT use during the menopausal transition period for the improvement of psychological symptoms need to be studied further. However, in the presence of classical menopausal symptoms, depression will improve with hormone therapy.

11.5.2 Osteoporosis and Management

Osteoporosis is a skeletal disorder characterized by compromised bone strength predisposing to an increased risk of fracture (NIH, Consensus statement 2000).

Osteoporosis is an important health hazard of the post-menopausal women due not only to the symptoms but also to the risk of fractures. Estrogen withdrawal causes increase in osteoclast activity which result in bone resorption, decrease in bone mass and change in micro architecture of skeleton which predisposes the postmenopausal women to an increased risk of fracture, but at variable rates. Of the 50% of trabecular bone loss and 30% of cortical bone loss occurring during the lifetime of a woman, about half is lost during the first 10 years after menopause. This loss is affected by several factors. There are modifiable and non-modifiable risk factors as listed in Table 11.1.

Measurement of Bone Density

Bone mineral density testing (BMD) can be used to diagnose osteoporosis and sort out women who are at risk for fractures so that they can be treated. BMD strongly correlates with bone strength. Dual energy X-ray Absorptiometry (DXA) is the preferred method of testing of BMD. DXA uses ionizing radiation to measure BMD in grams per square centimeter. Using DXA, BMD is usually measured in the lumbar spine (Fig. 11.3): hip (Fig. 11.2): or in the non-dominant forearm in case of severe obesity or hyperparathyroidism. BMD is expressed as Z-score or T-score. Z-score represents the difference in standard deviation between the patient's BMD and the mean BMD of a healthy young adult. T-score represents the difference in standard deviation between the patient's BMD and the mean BMD of age matched reference population. Based on WHO criteria (Table 11.2) patients are classified into normal when T-score ≥ -1, osteopenia if the T-score is between –1.1 and –2.4, osteoporosis if the T-score is ≤ -2.5 and severe osteoporosis if the T-score is ≤ -2.5 with history of fragility fracture.

Quantitative ultrasound (QUS) of peripheral skeletal sites e.g. heel, can be used as a potential screening method for selecting patients for DXA as the device used is portable and small as well as free of ionizing radiation. Quantitative

Table 11.1: Risk factors for development of osteoporosis

Modifiable	*Non-modifiable*
• Decreased calcium and vitamin D intake • Smoking • Sedentary lifestyle • Medical disorders like hypothalamic amenorrhea, hyperthyroidism, hyperparathyroidism, chronic renal disease • Medical disorders needing corticosteroid therapy	• Age • Race • Small body frame • History of fracture • Early menopause • Oophorectomy before menopause

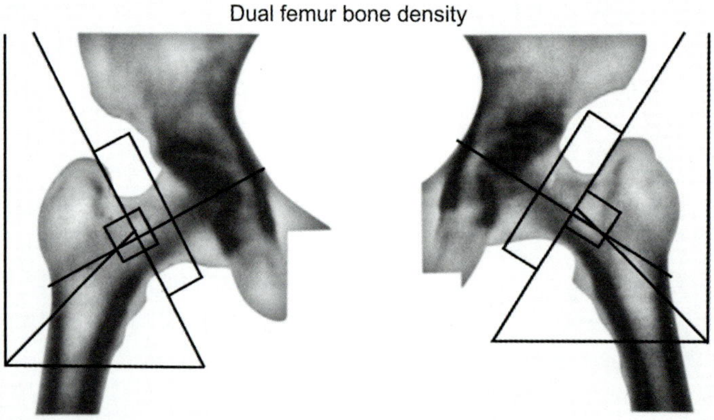

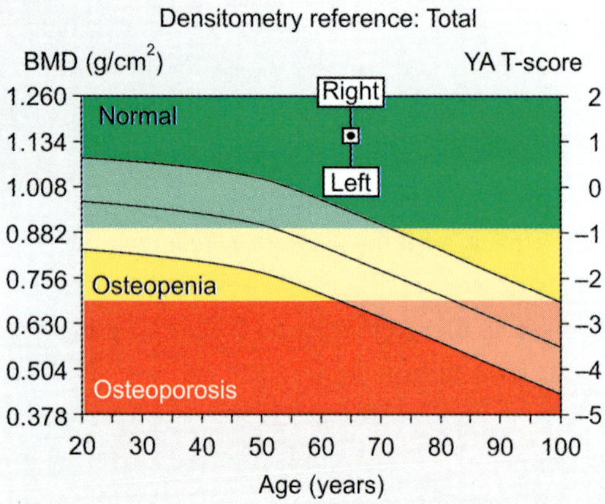

Image not for diagnosis

Region	BMD[1] (g/cm²)	Young-adult[2,7] T-score	Age-matched[3] Z-score
Neck			
Left	1.035	0.0	1.9
Right	1.053	0.1	2.0
Mean	1.044	0.0	1.9
Difference	1.018	0.1	0.1
Total			
Left	1.140	1.1	2.7
Right	1.142	1.1	2.7
Mean	1.141	1.1	2.7
Difference	0.002	0.0	0.0

Fig. 11.2: DXA report (femur neck) of a 69-year-old lady. T-score is 0.0. This patient is considered normal according to WHO criteria

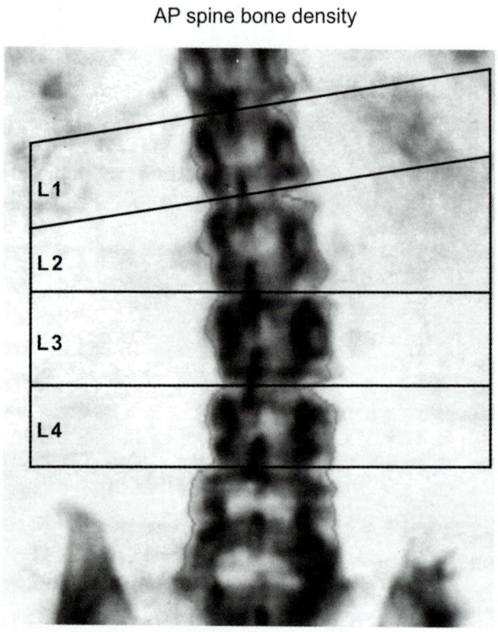

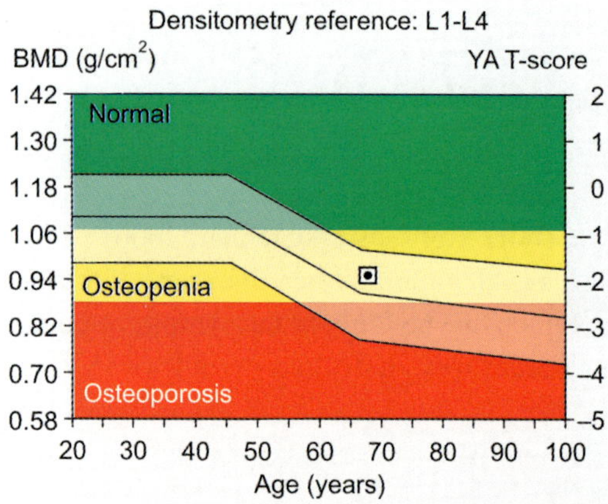

Region	BMD[1] (g/cm²)	Young-adult[2,7] T-score	Age-matched[3] Z-score
L1	0.854	−2.3	0.0
L2	0.854	−2.9	−0.6
L3	1.080	−1.0	1.3
L4	1.065	−1.1	1.1
L1-L4	0.968	−1.8	0.5

Fig. 11.3: DXA report (spine) of a 65-year-old lady. T-score is −1.8. She is considered osteopenic according to WHO criteria

Table 11.2: WHO assessment of fracture risk and its application for screening for postmenopausal osteoporosis (Geneva, WHO 1994)

Classification	*T-score*
Normal	≥-1
Osteopenia	between -1.1 and -2.4
Osteoporosis	≤-2.5
Severe osteoporosis	≤-2.5 with history of fragility fracture

computed tomography can also be used to asses BMD, but uses more radiation and is more expensive than DXA.

Indications for BMD Testing

BMD testing should be considered in any woman who is at risk of fracture. It is ideal to do BMD testing for all women aged 65 and older regardless of the risk. Even if she is younger than 65, if there is at least one risk factor for osteoporosis, BMD should be done. The guideline given by the International Society for Clinical Densitometry (ISCD) is given below:

1. Women aged 65 years and older
2. Postmenopausal women younger than 65 years with risk factors for osteoporosis
3. Women during the menopausal transition with clinical risk factors for fracture, such as low body weight, prior fracture, or high risk medication use
4. Adults who have fragility fracture
5. Adults who have a disease or condition associated with low bone mass or bone loss
6. Adults taking medication associated with low bone mass or bone loss
7. Anyone being considered for pharmacologic osteoporosis therapy
8. Anyone being treated for low bone mass to monitor treatment effect
9. Anyone not undergoing therapy in whom evidence of bone loss would lead to treatment

Prevention of Osteoporosis

According to Prof Charles E Dent 'senile osteoporosis is a pediatric disease'. Peak bone mass (PBM), achieved at around the age of 25 (Fig. 11.4) depends upon healthy lifestyle during the bone forming years through good nutrition, adequate calcium and vitamin D intake and physical activity. But according to recently acquired evidence, factors during fetal life can also affect peak bone

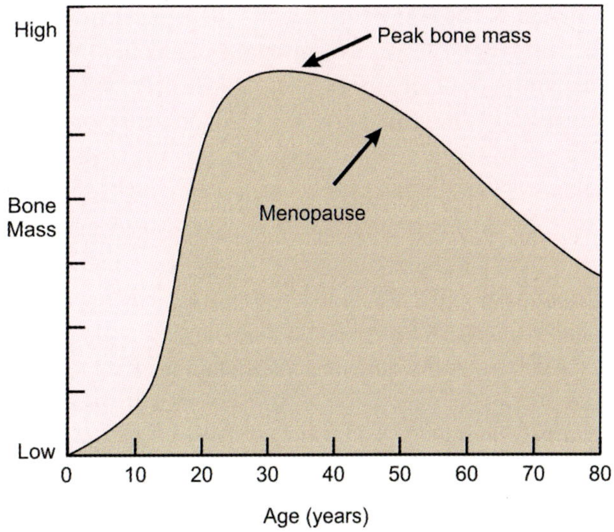

Fig. 11.4: Trend in normal BMD over years

mass. Low parental birth weight, cigarette smoking, suboptimal vitamin D during pregnancy, thin maternal skin-fold etc. adversely affect fetal bone mineral content. Bone loss starts soon after attaining PBM. Maximizing PBM and reducing rate of bone loss are important aspects of osteoporosis prevention. After menopause there is accelerated bone loss. Maintaining good nutrition and adequate physical activity throughout life goes a long way in preventing osteoporosis in later life.

Role of Diet and Exercise

Modification of risk factors is an important aspect of prevention and treatment of osteoporosis. Understanding of bone metabolism and turnover is important for clinicians in planning treatment and educating patients. Bone is a metabolically active organ which undergoes constant remodeling. Osteoclasts resorb bone and form small pits where osteoblasts deposit bone. When these two processes are balanced, there is no net loss of bone mass. After menopause withdrawal of estrogen causes increased osteoclastic activity and bone resorption. The higher the peak bone mass achieved, the lesser will be the probability to develop osteopenia or osteoporosis later in life. There are several factors which affect peak bone density. Calcium and vitamin D intake and exercise during childhood are important factors. Calcium intake in pregnancy also has an important role in the prevention of osteoporosis of the mother as well as the fetus later in life. Excessive alcohol intake, cigarette smoking, sedentary lifestyle, and lack of estrogen can adversely affect bone density. Hence clinicians should give importance in educating women about the role of diet, exercise and cessation of smoking.

Calcium is necessary for several biochemical processes in the body. Bone serves as a reservoir of calcium. Whenever calcium is deficient in the diet, it will be mobilized from the bone. Parathyroid hormone maintains this homeostasis. It is an important factor necessary for the absorption of calcium from the intestine as well as it's deposition in the bone. Even though vitamin D is synthesized in the body from precursors by sunlight, it should be supplied in the diet to fully meet the demand since most women are not exposed to sufficient sunlight everyday.

There is sufficient data confirming the effect of calcium in reducing the rate of bone loss in postmenopausal women. Women should receive 1000-1500 mg of Calcium and 400-800 IU of vitamin D daily. Vitamin D is a key regulator of calcium absorption and bone mineralization. If this cannot be met by diet, it should be supplemented.

Weight bearing exercises significantly improve BMD of postmenopausal women, who have osteopenia or osteoporosis. Minimum of 30 minutes of physical activity such as brisk walking on almost all days of the week will be enough. Swimming is inferior to brisk walking in improving BMD. An exercise program must be incorporated into the lifestyle and should be continued lifelong due to the chronic nature of bone loss in older women.[3]

Pharmacotherapy

When to Advise Pharmacotherapy?

Treatment should be decided after assessment of fracture risk using T-score and clinical risk factors. The guideline which is widely followed is that of the US National Osteoporosis Foundation. The recommendation is to treat postmenopausal women when the T-score is less than –2, in the absence of risk factors and in the presence of risk factors even if the T-score is less than – 1.5.

Role of Hormone Therapy (HT)

It has been clearly shown that hormone therapy protects bone mass by decreasing osteoclastic activity. The protection lasts as long as hormone therapy is continued and stops on discontinuation of therapy. The standard bone protective dose was estimated as estradiol 2 mg, conjugated equine estrogen 0.625 mg and transdermal patch of 50 µg. Low dose CEE/MPA (0.3/1.5 mg) was later found to be sufficient in increasing bone density (Women's HOPE Study). Over the past thirty years, HRT used to be prescribed as a panacea for all the menopausal problems even at the risk of an increase in the incidence of breast cancer. Lifelong hormone replacement was advised to prevent osteoporosis.

The increase in breast cancer risk associated with HRT became an important concern. In order to study the effect of hormone replacement on breast cancer risk, the million women study was undertaken. The study enrolled more than a million women from 1996 to 2001. When the study results were published in 2003 in the Lancet, clinicians as well as women were surprised to know that long-term use of HRT significantly increases the risk of breast cancer—18-20/1000 women after 10 years of use. The relative risk of breast cancer was significantly raised for current users of estrogen-only preparations, estrogen-progestogen combinations and tibolone. However, the magnitude of the relative risk of breast cancer varied significantly between these three HRT types ($p < 0{\cdot}0001$) and was substantially greater in users of estrogen-progestagen[4,5] combinations than other preparations; the relative risk being 2.0 in the case of estrogen-progestagen combination users and 1.3 among estrogen alone users and 1.45 among tibolone users.

The effect of HRT on osteoporosis, menopausal symptoms and heart disease[6] were studied in another large randomized controlled trial—The WHI study (Women's Health Initiative study). The WHI study was a randomized controlled trial which addressed health issues consequent to hormone replacement. The study enrolled 16000 women aged between 50 and 79 years. The major measures analyzed in the study were prevention of heart disease, prevention of fractures and the risks associated with estrogen-progestin treatment. The study made out that there is a significant increase in BMD and reduction in hip fractures in women who received HRT compared to placebo. But contrary to what was thought earlier, after 5 years of follow-up it was noted that there was a 29% increase in the incidence of heart disease and 41% increase in the incidence of stroke among hormone users. (See Table 11.3) Thus, HRT became unpopular as a drug for the prevention of osteoporosis. This led to a drastic decrease in prescribing HRT for the prevention and treatment of osteoporosis. The American Heart Association does not recommend HRT for the same. Whether the findings of

Table 11.3: Observations of WHI study

- 41% increase in stroke
- 29% increase in heart attacks
- Doubling of venous thromboembolism
- 26% increase in breast cancer
- 37% reduction in colorectal cancer
- 1/3rd reduction in hip fracture
- 24% reduction in total fracture
- No difference in total mortality

the WHI study holds good to the younger postmenopausal women or for other formulations or modes of estrogen is unknown. A later report of the WHI study found out that the excess of cardiovascular events occurred only in women starting estrogen and progesterone about 20 years after menopause. For those who started within 10 years of menopause such events were seen to be less. *Hence, for healthy women in the early menopausal years with vasomotor symptoms as well, HRT should be preferred.*

Alternative Therapies (Table 11.4)

1. **Bisphosphonates:** Bisphosphonates have evolved as the best anti-osteoporotic agents available. They specifically inhibit bone resorption by incorporating in osteoclasts which are then induced to undergo apoptosis. This reduced osteoclastic activity consequently improves bone strength and reduces fracture risk. They are very effective in prevention as well as treatment of osteoporosis. The preparations used are listed in Table 11.4. Oral bisphosphonates are relatively poorly absorbed, and hence should be taken in an empty stomach, with no food or drink to follow for the next 30 minutes. The commonest side effect is esophagitis which is responsible for the poor tolerance. Hence, the patient should be advised to remain upright for about 30 minutes after taking the drug. Alendronate and Risidronate need to be taken weekly. Ibandronate is a monthly preparation and Zolendronate is administered annually as an intravenous drip. Intravenous formulations though available are not prescribed due to the unpleasant side effect of osteonecrosis of the jaw.
2. **Teriparatide:** Recently, teriparatide, a recombinant parathyroid hormone analogue has been shown to be effective in osteoporosis. It is paradoxically a bone building agent, which acts by stimulating osteoblasts, thus increasing their activity. Thus, teriparatide increases BMD, improves bone strength and reduce fracture risk. Headache is a common side effect of the drug. Animal studies have documented increased incidence of osteosarcoma in mice. The preparation available is synthetic human 1-34 parathormone produced by mRNA genetica. It is used mostly as treatment in patients with established osteoporosis, those with particularly low BMD or several risk factors for fracture or cannot tolerate the oral bisphosphonates. It is given as 20 μgm injection as a daily dose using a pen-type injection device. After completing a course of therapy (18-24 months), treatment may be continued using an anti-resorptive agent like one of the bisphosphonates.
3. **Calcitonin:** Calcitonin can be used as a nasal spray for the treatment of established osteoporosis. It is reported to be useful in reducing vertebral fractures rather than non vertebral fractures. It has an added analgesic effect also.
4. **Selective estrogen receptor modulators (SERM):** SERMs are a group of compounds having both estrogen agonistic and antagonistic action depending upon the tissues. Raloxifene is a SERM which is approved for use for the prevention and treatment of osteoporosis. It has estrogenic action on bone and lipids, but anti-estrogenic action[7,8] on breast and endometrium.

   One disadvantage of raloxifene is the aggravation of hot flashes in some women. Raloxifene use is also associated with a three fold increase in the risk of venous thromboembolism. Hence, it should not be prescribed for women with past history of venous thromboembolism or for women at risk for stroke. The long-term safety of this drug has not yet been proven. Before prescribing, the risk-benefit balance should be considered.

Table 11.4: Drug treatment of osteoporosis

1. **Bisphosphonates**
   a. Alendronate: 35-70 mg weekly
   b. Risidronate: 35 mg weekly
   c. Ibandronate: 150 mg monthly
   d. Zolendronate: 5 mg IV infusion yearly
2. **Parathyroid analog**
   Teriparatide: 20 μg/day SC
3. Calcitonin: 200 IU/day intranasally, 100IU/day SC
4. **SERM**
   Raloxifene: 60 mg/day

Choice of Therapy

a. **Women in the immediate postmenopausal period:** This group of women may otherwise need estrogen for treatment of vasomotor symptoms. Since the lowest dose of estrogen is enough for skeletal protection, the treatment of vasomotor symptoms with estrogens will take care of bone density also. The protective effect of estrogen on bone lasts only as long as treatment is continued and dissipates quickly over a period of one year of discontinuation of therapy. Androgenic progestagens augment the effect of estrogen.

b. **Women between menopause and 65 years:** If the woman has identifiable risk factors, BMD should be tested and management should be planned based on

BMD. If there are no risk factors prevention of osteoporosis by diet and lifestyle changes only need be considered. However, most women will have their BMD tested. Management then will depend on the BMD.

c. **Women aged 65 or older:** As mentioned earlier, women older than 65 years should have their BMD tested. If the T-score is ≤ -2.4, therapy is indicated. Even though estrogen offers excellent bone protection in these women, it cannot be advised, in the background of the adverse effects brought out by the WHI study. Bis-phosphonates should be the first choice for these women. Alendronate 10 mg daily/70 mg weekly or risidronate 5 mg daily/35 mg weekly is preferred. If the patient, even though above 65, has no identifiable risk factors, markers of bone turnover (serum alkaline phosphatase, urinary excretion of hydroxyproline and calcium) should be measured. If the markers are well below the reference level, recommending calcium, vitamin D and exercise is enough. BMD should be tested every 2 years and pharmacotherapy recommended accordingly.

d. **Women who have sustained an osteoporotic fracture:** Treatment is indicated if a fracture had already occurred, irrespective of BMD. A baseline BMD should be taken to monitor therapy. If BMD is above –3, bis-phosphonates are still the choice of treatment. If the T-score is –3 or lower, therapy with teriparatide is advised.

Monitoring Therapy

Response to therapy should be ascertained by repeating DXA, once every 2 years. If the BMD remains stable or improves, it is an acceptable response. A worsening of BMD should prompt investigations for contributing factors. Bisphosphonates should be continued until there is no further increase in BMD. Afterwards the drug may be discontinued, but the patient should be monitored with markers of bone resorption at 3 month interval and therapy should be restarted if there is an increase in any of the markers.

11.5.3 Cardiovascular Diseases and Management

A woman's risk of dying due to heart disease is estimated to be more than 10 times that of breast cancer or genital tract cancer. Women are more prone to develop cardiovascular disease after menopause. The incidence of cardiovascular disease depends upon several modifiable and non-modifiable risk factors.

Familial tendency for cardiovascular disease is a non-modifiable risk factor. Modifiable risk factors include obesity, smoking and sedentary lifestyle. Medical conditions like diabetes, hypertension and hypercholesterolemia increase the risk for heart disease. Women are somewhat protected from developing cardiovascular disease till menopause by endogenous estrogen. Hence, it was assumed that replacing estrogen by hormone therapy after menopause can prevent or decrease the risk of cardiovascular events. The older observational studies reported a beneficial effect of HRT on cardiovascular diseases. The Postmenopausal Estrogen Progesterone Interventional (PEPI) trial (1987-90) was a 3 year trial to study the effect of estrogen therapy on factors that affect a woman's risk of heart disease. The factors studied were HDL, systolic blood pressure, fibrinogen and insulin level.[9] 875 postmenopausal women aged 45-64 years were given CEE + MPA.

The study result showed significantly greater increase in HDL, no increase in blood pressure and no weight gain. Hence, it was assumed that HRT protects women from cardiovascular disease. The Nurses' Health Study was another observational study among 122,000 women using either estrogen or progesterone alone or both. This study also concluded that, there is a decrease in the risk of coronary artery disease in women using HRT (CEE/MPA).

The PEPI trial was a short duration trial which could not prove whether these changes can reduce the incidence of heart attacks and strokes. To address these issues, the WHI trial was started. Contrary to the results of the above observational studies the WHI study observed an increase in heart attack during the early stages of HRT. Hence, the study concluded that older women with cardiovascular disease who are not on HRT should not be given hormone therapy.

The publication of the Heart and Estrogen Replacement Study (HERS), a prospective randomized placebo-controlled clinical trial, found that the use of estrogen plus progestin in women with existing heart disease did not show any improvement in outcome. The overall outcome of HERS, both at 5 and 7 years, did not show difference in the incidence of myocardial events in women with preexisting coronary artery disease, between HRT users and placebo group. Moreover there was an increase in cardiovascular events in the first year and a decrease overtime. This may be due to an adverse effect of HRT in women who are already at risk. Estrogen therapy was also associated with venous thromboembolism and gallbladder disease. *Hence, it was proved that there is no role for hormone therapy in the secondary prevention of coronary artery disease.*

Even though the WHI and HERS study gave the aforementioned facts, it was criticized as well. The estrogen used in the study was CEE and the progesterone was MPA. The effects of transdermal estradiol and other estrogen preparations may be different. Moreover, the average age of women who participated in this trial was 63. A later report of the WHI showed that the excess of cardiovascular events occurred in women who started hormones 20 years after the menopause. The incidence of adverse cardiovascular events in women who started estrogen within 10 years of menopause was less. Older women might have already developed atherosclerotic plaques which promote platelet aggregation and clot formation. It was found later that women who had started hormones early but discontinued due to the adverse events reported, actually had a 42% decrease in adverse coronary events, 28% decrease in breast cancer, 41% decrease in colorectal cancer, 27% decrease in deaths and 20% decrease in global index pathology. *If women started using HRT during perimenopausal period, it can be assumed that there may be beneficial effects as a consequence of the effect of estrogen on lipid profile and endothelium.*[7]

WISDOM (Women's International Study of Long Duration of Estrogen use after Menopause) study was another study started in 1989 as a 10 year long trial to study the effect of long-term HRT use. However, it was stopped just one year after starting, due to the 'scaring results' of WHI. According to this study, there was a notable reduction in the incidence of osteoporotic fractures[8] while there was no significant difference in cardiovascular events, stroke or cancer.

Dramatic changes happened with the acquisition and publication of these two studies. Presently HRT is not recommended for the purpose of preventing cardiovascular events. American Heart Association (AHA) guidelines clearly state that HRT or SERMs should not be used to prevent heart disease not only because it fails to give protection from heart disease but also due to the fact that it potentially increases its incidence. Instead, AHA recommends lifestyle changes to control weight, increased physical activity, moderate alcohol intake, refrain from smoking and reduce sodium intake. Diet should include adequate vegetables and fruits, but less of fat.

Physical activity recommended by AHA for women is minimum 60-90 minutes of brisk walking preferably on all days of the week. Diet should contain adequate quantities of ω3 fatty acids which can be met with by taking oily fish twice a week. Women who have coronary vascular disease should take 850-1000 mg of EPA (eicosapentaenoic acid) acid or DHA. Those who have high triglyceride levels should take 2-3 gm of the same. Low dose aspirin therapy is recommended for all women above 65 years and high risk women should take a higher dose of 325 mg/day. LDL level should be maintained at <70 mg%. If cholesterol lowering drugs are needed, these should also be given.

11.5.4 Breast Cancer and Management

Breast cancer is the leading cause of death in women and is one of the most common cancers in women. Early menarche, late menopause and family history are identified as its risk factors. Oophorectomy and term pregnancy before the age of 30 reduce the risk. Prolonged estrogen exposure increases the risk of breast cancer. As mentioned previously, the WHI study and Million Woman's study observed significant increase in the risk of breast cancer among HRT users. The WHI study results showed a 25% increase in breast cancer risk. Use of tamoxifen or raloxifene reduces the risk by 50%. However, tamoxifen and raloxifene increases the venous thromboembolism risk. Raloxifene has the disadvantage of precipitating hot flashes, while tamoxifen stimulates endometrium resulting in hyperplasia.

Early detection of breast cancer should be emphasized. Routine mammography screening is advised for women older than 50 years. Women should be taught monthly breast self examination. HRT should not be prescribed for women who are at high risk for breast cancer. Prophylactic tamoxifen therapy can be thought of in women who are at high risk for breast cancer. However, they should be on regular follow-up for endometrial pathology.

11.6 HORMONE THERAPY (TABLES 11.5 AND 11.6)

With the understanding of the fact that replacing estrogen after menopause is not natural and brings about dangerous side effects, 'hormone replacement therapy' has become simply 'hormone therapy'. Menopause should be considered as a natural transition and not a disease. Unnecessary and dangerous medications should be avoided.

Women should be counseled to have a positive attitude towards menopause as mentioned earlier. Osteoporosis, heart disease and other chronic health problems develop as a result of not just menopause, but also due to the aging process. Proper diet and regular exercise should be given preference.

Hormone therapy is presently indicated in the following instances.

1. For the treatment of vasomotor symptoms
2. For the treatment of genitourinary symptoms.
3. For women who had their ovaries removed at a very young age.

Table 11.5: HT has not been shown to

• Cure urinary incontinence • Help moodiness or depression • Improve sexual desire or responsiveness • Prevent heart disease • Improve memory • Prevent Alzheimer's disease

Table 11.6: Hormone therapy regimes

1. Full replacement
   Estrogen
   - Conjugated Equine Estrogen: 0.625 mg
   - Micronised estradiol: 1 mg
   - Estradiol valerate: 2 mg
   - Ethinyl estradiol: 0.05 mg
   - Estradiol patch: 0.05 mg

   Progesterone
   - Medroxy progesterone 2.5 mg or 5 mg daily
   - Micronised progesterone 100 mg daily
2. Half replacement
   Estrogen
   - CEE: 0.3 mg
   - Micronised estrogen: 0.5 mg
   - Estradiol patch: 0.025 mg

   Progesterone
   Medroxyprogesterone:1.5 mg
3. Estrogen-progesterone combination
   Cyclic (along with estrogen)
   - Medroxyprogesterone: 5 to 10 mg from d1 to 14 of each month
   - Norethindrone
   - Micronised progesterone 100 mg morning and 200 mg in the evening

   Continuous combined
   - 0.625 mg CEE + 2.5 mg MPA
   - 0.05 mg EE + 1 mg norethindrone acetate
   - Micronised estradiol (0.5 mg) + norethindrone acetate (2.75 mg) transdermal patch, twice weekly

4. Can be used for the prevention and treatment of osteoporosis if started in the early postmenopausal years among healthy women.

When to start treatment?

Treatment should be started soon after menopause. If symptoms develop prior to menopause hormone therapy can be started before menstruation ceases. Those who develop premature menopause should be started on hormones without delay.

How long to be given?

The *lowest possible dose* should be advised for the *shortest period* needed to achieve the desired effect. A Cochrane review has found that low dose estrogen along with 1 mg norethisterone or 1.5 mg medroxyprogesterone is enough if given as treatment for hot flashes.[9]

For the treatment of menopausal symptoms, maximum 5 years treatment is usually recommended. However, for those who continue to have symptoms and have no contraindication for hormone use, treatment may be continued for longer periods. Women who have premature menopause need a larger dose for a longer period, till the average age of menopause and even a few years ahead if there are no contraindications for hormone use. Women who are on hormone treatment should have breast examination every 6 months and mammogram every year.

The preparations available are listed in Table 11.7.

11.6.1 Patient Counseling

Proper counseling before initiating HT is necessary for optimal outcome as well as to avoid litigation issues. Potential risks should be weighed against benefits. Medical jargons should be avoided and explanations given should be comprehendible. All types and routes of hormone administration and the advantages as well as disadvantages of each should be explained. The patient should be provided information regarding the risk of breast cancer, stroke, VTE, CHD etc and advantages of reduction in menopausal symptoms, colorectal cancer and bone fracture. All available treatment options should be explained.

Information given should include:

1. Route of administration
2. Types of HT available

Table 11.7: HT and related preparations

Oestrogens	Conjugated equine estrogens (CEE) 17β estradiol Estradiol valerate Estrone
Progestogens	Progesterone Progesterone analogues a. Didrogesterone b. Medroxyprogesterone c. 19 nortestosterone derivatives-norethisterone, norethisterone acetate, levonorgestrel
Gonadomimetics	Tibolone (progestagenic, estrogenic and androgenic components)
SERMs	Raloxifene, tamoxifen
Phytoestrogens	Natural estrogens obtained from plant food

Table 11.8: Benefits and risks of HT

Benefits	Risks
• Relief of menopausal symptoms • Protection against osteoporosis and fracture-lost bone may be regained	• Increased incidence of breast cancer Background risk increase by 2/1000 if used for 5 years 6/1000 if used for 10 years
• Reduction of adverse cardiovascular events if started in the early menopausal women who are healthy (controversial) • Takes care of urogenital atrophy • Decreased colon cancer incidence	• Increased incidence of thromboembolism • Increased incidence of endometrial carcinoma (if progesterone is not added) • Coronary artery risk if started several years after menopause (controversial)
• Limits age related thinning and shrinkage of skin • Decreased weight gain	• Stroke • Bleeding (HOPS trial) • Cholelithiasis

3. Duration of therapy planned
4. Potential benefits and risks (Table 11.8)
5. Pattern of vaginal bleeding depending upon the type of HT

11.6.2 Pretreatment Assessment

Before starting on hormones, women should be evaluated to exclude contraindications for hormone use listed in Table 11.9. In the presence of contraindications, alternate therapy should be considered. If uterus is present progesterone should be added. In hysterectomised women estrogen alone need be given.

Half dose replacement is preferred in patients with high triglyceride levels. In the presence of mood changes and bloating progestogen dose can be reduced to half.

Table 11.9: Contraindications of HT

Absolute contraindications	Relative contraindications
• Active hepatic disease	• Chronic liver disease
• History of thrombosis	• Severe hypertriglyceridemia
• History of breast cancer	• Endometriosis
• Undiagnosed vaginal bleeding	• Proven coronary heart disease or a recent event
• Previous myocardial infarction	
• Previous stroke	
• History of pulmonary embolism	

11.7 CONCLUSION

Quality of life and health issues of postmenopausal women are important, because most women live one third of their life after menopause. Estrogen deprivation and aging causes important short-term problems like vasomotor symptoms and long-term ones like osteoporosis and cardiovascular disease. A smooth transition through menopause needs counseling which should include advice about the need for regular exercise, proper diet and medications whenever necessary. Vitamin D and calcium may need to be supplemented. Peak bone density which is an important factor determining bone density after menopause is achieved in the mid 20's. The two important factors which influence the peak bone density are exercise and nutrition. Adequate intake of calcium and vitamin D should start in the early life itself. In this respect, diet and exercise during childhood and adolescence should be given proper emphasis. For the treatment of established osteoporosis, bisphosphonate is the drug of choice. Menopausal symptoms, especially hot flashes are better treated by estrogen implants/oral estrogen in hysterectomised women and estrogen and progesterone in non hysterectomised women. Problems related to urogenital atrophy can be treated by local estrogens. However, those who continue to have recurrent cystitis should be treated with oral hormones. Women who undergo premature menopause need a larger dose of estrogen which should be continued till the age of natural menopause and even beyond if needed for 5 to 10 years. Results from the WHI study should not be a deterrent for advising hormones in the treatment of menopausal symptoms in women who do not have contraindications for hormone use. Treatment should be started early, before the age of 60, preferably around the time of menopause. Hormone treatment started early has been found to reduce the incidence of cardiovascular events. Estrogens should not be prescribed for the secondary prevention of cardiovascular disease. The dose, route and preparation used should be individualized. The lowest dose should be prescribed for the shortest period needed. Women who are on hormones should have periodic breast examination and yearly mammogram to detect breast cancer which is higher in hormone users compared to non-users. Lifestyle modification, proper diet and medications whenever necessary can add life to the postmenopausal years of a woman rather than years to her life.

REFERENCES

1. Kenemansa P, Speroff BL,Tibolone. Clinical recommendations and practical guidelines. Report of the International Tibolone Consensus Group, Journal of the European menopause and andropause society 2004;51:21-8.
2. Avis NE, Brambilla D, McKinlay SM, Vass K. A longitudinal analysis of the association between menopause and depression. Results from the Massachusetts Women's Health study. An Epidemiology 1994;4:214.
3. Zehnacker CH, Bemis-Dougherty A. Effect of weighted exercises on bone mineral density in post-menopausal women. A systematic review. J Geriatr Phys Ther 2007;30(2):79-88.
4. Valerie Beral, Emily Banks, Gillian Reeves, Diana Bull and on behalf of the Million Women Study Collaborators. Breast cancer and hormone replacement therapy: the Million Women Study. The Lancet 2003;362(9392):1330-1.
5. Toine Lagro-Janssen, Walter W Rosser, Chris van Weel. Breast cancer and hormone replacement therapy: up to general practice to pick up the pieces. The Lancet 2003; 362(9382):414-5.
6. Writing group of the Women's Health Initiative investigators. Risks and benefits of estrogen plus progesterone benefits in healthy postmenopausal women. Principle results from the women's health initiative randomized control trial. JAMA 2002;288:321-33.
7. Taranta A, Brama M, Teti A, et al. The selective estrogen receptor modulator raloxifene regulates osteoclast and osteoblast activity *in vitro*. Bone 2002;30(2):368-76.
8. Meunier PJ, Vignot E, Garnero P, et al. Treatment of post-menopausal women with osteoporosis or low bone density, with raloxifene. Raloxifene study group. Osteoporos Int 1999;10(4):330-6.
9. Effects of estrogen or estrogen/progestin regimens on heart disease risk factors in postmenopausal women. The Postmenopausal Estrogen/Progestin Interventions (PEPI) Trial. The Writing Group for the PEPI Trial. JAMA. 1995 6;274(21):1675-6.

12 Endometriosis

B Presannakumari

Endometriosis is a chronic benign disease which can cause severe pain and infertility, resulting in significant reduction in quality of life.

12.1 DEFINITION

Endometriosis is defined as the presence of endometrial glands and stroma outside the lining of the uterine cavity. This disease is commonly found in women of child bearing age group.

12.2 PREVALENCE

The prevalence of endometriosis is on the increase than it was 100 years back. This is attributed to several factors.

- The number of pregnancies the present day woman undergoes is less compared to that of previous decades.
- Women defer child bearing to later years than previously.
- The introduction of laparoscopy has made possible detection of even the milder forms of endometriosis.

The current prevalence of endometriosis is estimated to be 10%.[1]

12.3 EPIDEMIOLOGY

Several large epidemiological studies were done to get an insight into the disease. Endometriosis is found in women of all ethnic groups, but is reported to be less prevalent among African and more among East Asians compared to Caucasians. Among women presenting with infertility[2, 3] it is reported to be present in 20-30%.

Prevalence of endometriosis among women presenting with pelvic pain is as high as 40-50%. Early menarche, long duration of menstrual flow, low parity, presence of mullerian anomalies etc are all risk factors for endometriosis.

12.4 ETIOLOGY

The exact etiology of endometriosis is not yet known. More than one mechanism is at work in most patients (Table 12.1). Many theories have been put forward ever since the disease was discovered by Rokintansky in 1860. No single theory explains the occurrence of endometriosis in all the sites.

12.4.1 Coelomic Metaplasia Theory

Meyer (1909) postulated that the coelomic epithelium has the potential to undergo metaplasia to endometrial tissue in later life. This explains the occurrence of endometriosis in the pelvic peritoneum. Till recently there was no data to support this theory. A recent study in mice showed that endometriosis of the ovarian surface can occur as a result of metaplastic differentiation induced by activation of an oncogenic K-ras gene.

12.4.2 Induction Theory

This theory supplements the coelomic metaplasia theory. The theory proposes that endogenous, biochemical or immunologic factors can induce undifferentiated cells to transform to differentiated endometrial tissue. The evidence for this theory was originally derived from experiments in rabbits. Later, it was demonstrated that endometriotic tissue can be induced on ovarian surface epithelium in *in vitro* culture of ovarian tissue.

12.4.3 Transplantation Theory

Sampson (1920s) postulated that endometriosis is caused by growth of transplanted endometrial cells from the uterine cavity through the fallopian tube. There is no doubt about the occurrence of retrograde menstruation. Menstrual blood is seen in the peritoneal cavity of 80-90% of women. In women who had tubal sterilization peritoneal fluid contains menstrual effluents in only 15%. The fact that endometriotic lesions are commonly seen in the dependent areas of the pelvis, the anterior and posterior peritoneal pouch, the uterosacral ligaments, the lower part of the posterior surface of uterus and the posterior aspect of the broad ligaments goes in favor[4,5] of the spill theory.

The points against this theory are that the cells found in endometriosis are not the same as that found in the endometrium, and that it does not explain the occurrence of endometriosis in premenarchal girls and postmenopausal women.

12.4.4 Lymphatic and Vascular Embolization

Lymphatic and vascular embolization explains the presence of endometriosis in distant sites like lung, pleura, brain, umbilicus, retroperitoneal space, vulva, vagina, cervix, lower extremity etc to which lymphatic and vascular communications are present.

12.4.5 Immunological Theory

It was Bleicher (1987) who postulated that altered immune function may be the reason for the discrepancy between the frequency of retrograde menstruation and the frequency of endometriosis. The understanding that the peritoneal fluid of women with endometriosis has increased levels of macrophages, lymphocytes, cytokines and growth factors points towards an intricate link between endometriosis and the immune system.

Immune system alteration results in a failure to remove ectopic endometrial cells from the body. This can cause

Table 12.1: Etiology of endometriosis

1.	Coelomic metaplasia theory
2.	Transplantation theory
3.	Lymphatic and vascular embolization
4.	Immunological theory
5.	Genetic basis
6.	Progesterone resistance
7.	Environmental factors

infiltration and growth of endometrial cells. A subclinical inflammation is identified in the peritoneal cavity in pelvic endometriosis, as evidenced by the increased secretion of Tumor Necrosis Factor-α (TNF-α), which might probably facilitate pelvic implantation of ectopic endometrium. Growth factors and angiogenic factors secreted by macrophages and adhesion molecules such as integrins favor adhesion and growth of endometrial cells. Subsequent invasion may be modulated by matrix-metalloproteinases. Whether these immune reactions have a real causative role or they merely reflect a passive reaction to the presence of endometrial implants is not known.

12.4.6 Genetic Basis

The recognition that clustering of endometriosis is seen in families, concordance is seen among monozygotic twins, a similar age at onset of symptoms is seen among sisters and increased prevalence of endometriosis is seen in first degree relatives has led us to think that endometriosis might have a genetic basis. It was Simpson et al who proposed a genetic basis for the occurrence of endometriosis (1980). Genetic studies have identified a susceptibility locus on chromosome 10q26, but the inheritance could be polygenic in nature.

12.4.7 Progesterone Resistance

The most recent theory is that endometriosis could be due to progesterone resistance. Impaired regulation of matrix metalloproteinase due to decreased responsiveness to progesterone may be the implicating factor. This forms the basis of treatment of endometriosis with the anti-progesterone, mifepristone.

12.4.8 Environmental Factors

Reproductive health and infertility may have links with environmental factors. Environmental factors including nutrition, exposure to video display terminals and environmental toxins like dioxins are being studied as the etiological factors for endometriosis. Recent research has shown a genetic mechanism to explain the link between dioxin and endometriosis. Transcripts of a dioxin induced gene (CYPIA1) is reported to be significantly higher in endometriotic tissue.[6] The data on this is insufficient at present.

12.5 SITES OF ENDOMETRIOSIS

The most commonly affected sites (Table 12.2) of endometriosis are the pelvic peritoneum and the pelvic organs like the ovary, fallopian tube, pouch of Douglas (POD), uterosacral ligament, ureter, urinary bladder and rectovaginal septum. There is a wide variation in the severity and progression of the disease among individuals. The lesions can be present in a variety of types. There can be multiple petechial or reddish lesions, dark powder burn or gunshot lesions, dark brown or bluish puckered lesions, nodular lesions or small cystic lesions containing jelly like material. The ovarian lesions can be surface lesions or cyst formations. The cystic lesions are commonly known as endometriomas or chocolate cysts. Endometriomas usually contain thick chocolate like fluid. Rarely may it be thin dark brown fluid or straw colored fluid. These lesions are usually unilocular but can also be multilocular. As the disease progresses, adhesion formation and scarring occur. The ovaries will adhere together and to the surface of the uterus and pouch of Douglas. The tubes also will be involved in the adhesions. Later the POD would be obliterated by these adhesions as well as by adhesion with the rectosigmoid. In the most severe situation, the uterus and the adnexa will be completely buried in the adhesions.

Table 12.2: Sites of endometriosis

Pelvic sites	*Extra pelvic sites*
Ovary	Lung
Fallopian tube	Pleura
Pelvic peritoneum	Umbilicus
Surface of uterus	Vulva
Uterosacral ligaments	Lower extremities
Urinary bladder	Episiotomy scar
Rectovaginal septum	Abdominal scar
Rectum	Brain

Infiltrating endometriotic lesions can extend more than 5 mm below the peritoneum. These deeply infiltrating lesions can involve the uterosacral ligaments, rectovaginal septum, the vaginal walls, rectosigmoid and the ureters. Ureteric obstruction occurs usually due to kinking as a result of scarring but rarely could it be due to endometriotic infiltration. Ureteric obstruction resulting in hydroureter and hydronephrosis is very rare.

Rare Sites of Endometriosis

Occasionally endometriosis can occur in areas like lung, pleural cavity, brain, umbilicus (Figs 12.1A and B), vulva, vagina, appendix, small intestine, etc. Lymphatic and vascular embolization explains the presence of endometriosis in these sites. Rarely endometriosis is seen in episiotomy and laparotomy (hysterotomy or cesarean) scars. Implantation of endometrial tissue explains such occurrence.

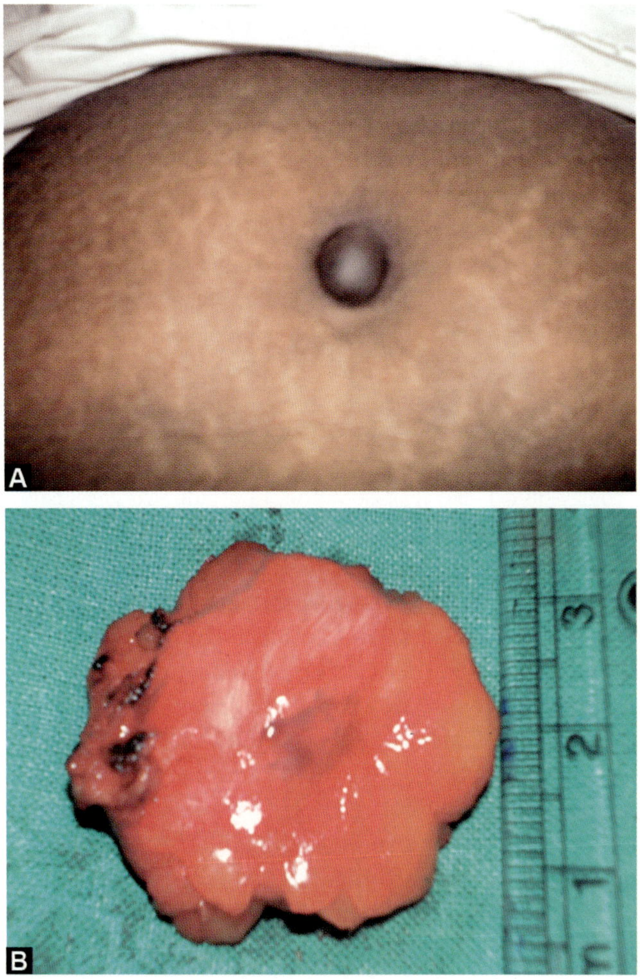

Figs 12.1A and B: Endometriosis of the umbilicus (A). 28-year-old lady, para I presented with pain around the umbilicus during periods since 2 years. Amenorrhea was induced for 3 months with danazole, during which period there was no pain. Excision of the lesion with reformation of the umbilicus was done. Excised specimen of scar endometriosis at cesarean section scar (B) of a 26-year-old lady who presented with pain at the site of cesarean scar in relation to menstruation. CT scan showed the lesion to be in the outer aspect of rectus sheath in close relation to it. The lesion was excised along with the attached part of the rectus sheath

12.6 STAGING OF ENDOMETRIOSIS

Classification of endometriosis dates back to as early as 1921. Several classifications existed ever since endometriosis was discovered. None received wide spread acceptance. All classification systems are based on the pelvic inspection findings. Pain, which is the predominant symptom, has poor correlation with the stage of the disease. Samson classified endometriosis into three grades. Acousta et al proposed a classification for endometriosis, under which endometriosis was classified into mild, moderate and severe. This classification was based on the site of lesion, size of endometrioma, presence of adhesions and presence of scarring.

Acousta's Classification of Pelvic Endometriosis

I. Mild
   a. Fresh lesions in the anterior and posterior cul-de-sac and pelvic peritoneum
   b. Surface implant on ovary with mild endometrioma or small endometrioma
   c. No peritubal adhesions

II. Moderate
   a. Endometriosis involving one or both ovaries with several surface lesions with scarring, retraction and small endometrioma.
   b. Minimal periovarian adhesions associated with ovarian lesions.
   c. Minimal peritubal adhesions associated with ovarian lesions.
   d. Superficial implants in the anterior or posterior cul-de-sac with scarring and retraction. No sigmoid invasion.

III. Severe
   a. Endometriosis in one or more ovary with endometrioma of size > 2 cm.
   b. Endometriosis in one or more ovaries bound down by adhesions.
   c. One or both tubes bound down by adhesions or obstructed by endometriosis
   d. Obliteration of cul-de-sac by adhesions of endometriosis
   e. Thickening of uterosacral ligaments by cul-de-sac lesions from invasive endometriosis
   f. Significant bowel or urinary tract involvement

AFS classification: Since then several modifications came. The American Fertility Society[7] designed a classification for endometriosis which was published in 1979 in the journal of fertility sterility.

The classification is based on a presumed natural history of disease progression. The flexibility in point allowed in this classification system permits any case to be categorized including situations where the normal chronology of disease progression varies. The classification includes anatomic diagnosis which helps to document the surgical exploration findings.

According to AFS, endometriosis is classified into mild, moderate, severe and extensive disease considering the following factors.

a. Presence, extent and type of lesion (red/white/black)
b. Presence of adhesions involving peritoneum, ovary and tubes
c. Presence of unilateral or bilateral disease
d. Size of endometriomas

An anatomic drawing for documentation was included along with the cumulative score.

However, it was later understood that the arbitrary point scores were not accurately reflecting the actual likelihood of fertility. Hence it was revised.

Revised AFS classification: AFS classification was revised in 1985 and later in 1996 to overcome the shortcomings in the original classification. In this revised classification, the extensive disease category was eliminated. Three dimensional assessments which differentiated superficial from deep lesions were included. A distinction was also made of dense adhesions.

Patients with complete obliteration of cul-de-sac were included in the severe disease category. Because of the varied appearance of endometriosis, there can be differences in interpretation which can affect staging.

Biochemical activity of the lesion can be predicted from its appearance. Reddish petechial implants are biochemically more active than dark brown implants. Black powder burn implants are older lesions and biochemically least active.

Revised ASRM Classification of Endometriosis (Table 12.3)

Table 12.3: American Society for Reproductive Medicine revised classification of endometriosis (reproduced with permission from ASRM)

Endometriosis	*<1cm*	*1-3 cm*	*>3 cm*
Peritoneum			
Superficial	1	2	4
Deep	2	4	6
Ovary			
R superficial	1	2	4
Deep	4	16	20
L superficial	1	2	4
Deep	4	16	20
Posterior cul-de-sac	**Partial**	**Complete**	
Obliteration	4	40	
Adhesions	*<1/3 enclosure*	*1/3- 2/3 enclosure*	*>2/3 enclosure*
Ovary			
R filmy	1	2	4
Dense	4	8	16
L filmy	1	2	4
Dense	4	8	16
Tube			
R filmy	1	2	4
Dense	4*	8*	16
L filmy	1	2	4
Dense	4*	8*	16

*If the fimbriated end of the fallopian tube is completely enclosed, change the point assignment to 16. Stage I (Minimal) – 1-5 Stage II (Mild) –6-15 Stage III (Moderate) 16-40 Stage IV (Severe) > 40 Denote appearance of superficial implant types as red [(R) red, red-pink, flame like, vesicular blobs, clear vesicles], white [(W), opacifications, peritoneal defects, yellow-brown], or black [(B) black, hemosiderin deposits, blue]. Denote percent of total described as R_%.W_% and B_%. Total should equal 100%. (Figs 12.2 to 12.5)

Reference: Revised American Society for Reproductive Medicine Classification of Endometriosis: 1996 Fertility and Sterility May 1997;67:5817-821.

Additional Endometriosis.......
To be used with normal tubes and ovaries

Associated Pathology.......
To be used with abnormal tubes and/or ovaries

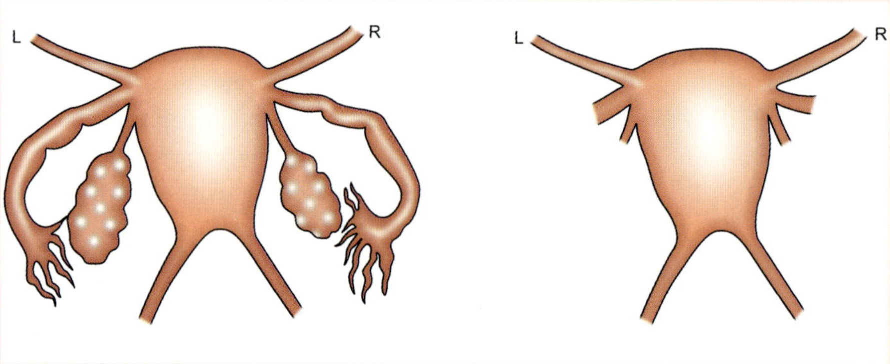

Examples and Guidelines

Stage I (Minimal)

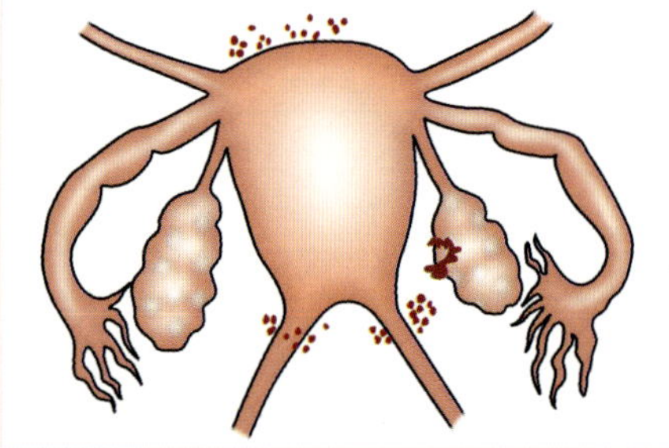

PERITONEUM		
Superficial Endo	1-3 cm	2
R OVARY		
Superficial Endo	<1 cm	1
Filmy Adhesions	<1/3	1
TOTAL POINTS		4

Stage II (Mild)

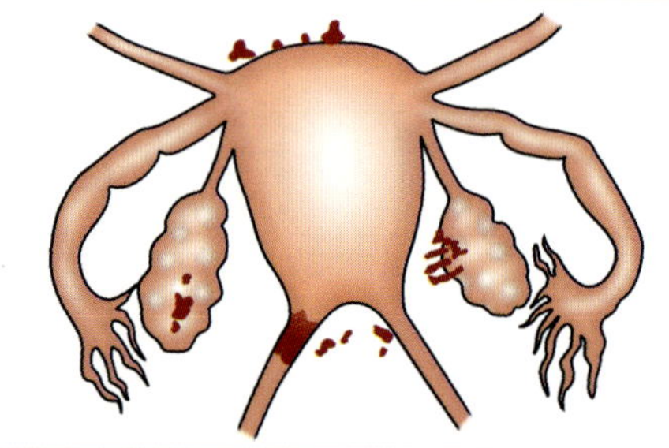

PERITONEUM		
Deep Endo	>3cm	6
R OVARY		
Superficial Endo	<1cm	1
Filmy Adhesions	<1/3	1
L OVARY		
Superficial Endo	<1cm	1
TOTAL POINTS		9

Stage III (Moderate)

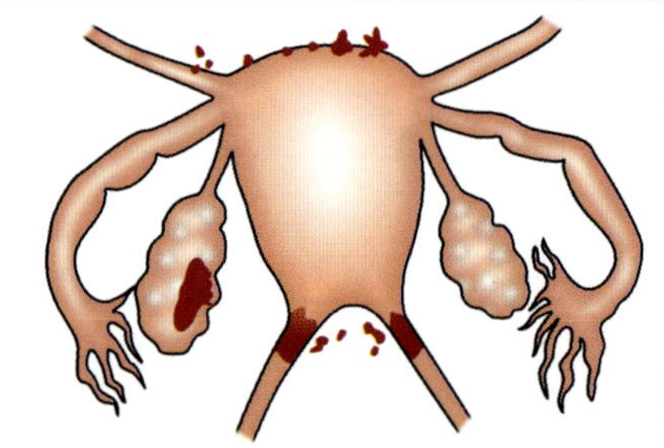

PERITONEUM		
Deep Endo	>3cm	6
CUL-DE-SAC		
Partial Obliteration		4
L OVARY		
Deep Endo		
TOTAL	1-3cm	16
		26

Stage III (Moderate)

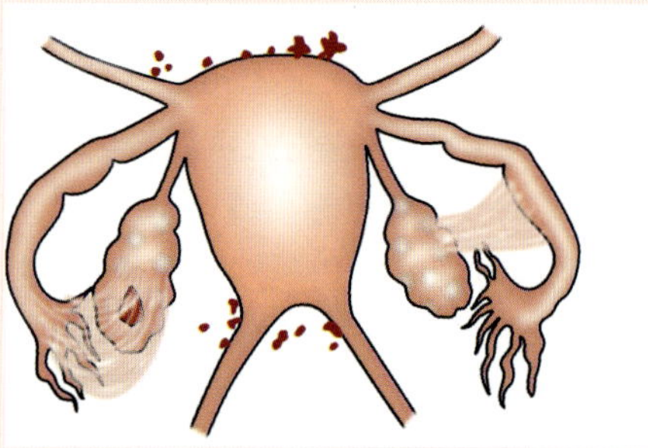

Stage IV (Severe)

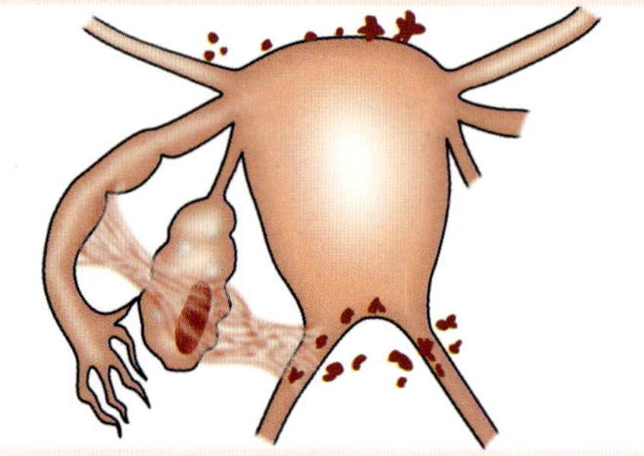

Stage IV (Severe)

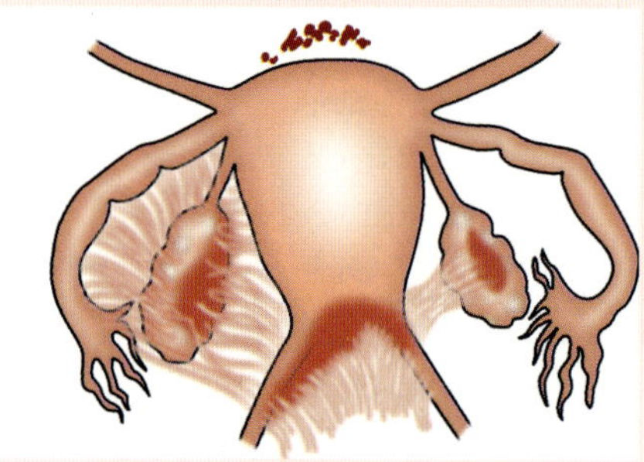

Contd...

Contd...

PERITONEUM			PERITONEUM			PERITONEUM		
Superficial Endo	> 3cm	4	Superficial Endo	>3cm	4	Deep Endo	>3cm	6
R TUBE			L OVARY			CUL-DE-SAC		
Filmy adhesions	< 1/3	1	Deep Endo	1-3cm	32	Compl obliteration		40
R OVARY			Deep Adhesions	<1/3	8	R OVARY		
Filmy adhesions	< 1/3	1	L TUBE			Deep Endo	1-3 cm	16
L TUBE			Dense Adhesions	<1/3	8	Dense adhesions	< 1/3	4
Dense adhesions	< 1/3	16	TOTAL POINTS		52	L TUBE		
L OVARY						Dense adhesions	> 2/3	16
Dense Endo	< 1cm	4				L OVARY		
Dense adhesions	< 1/3	4				Deep Endo	1-3 cm	16
TOTAL POINTS		30				Dense adhesions	>2/3	16
						TOTAL POINTS		114

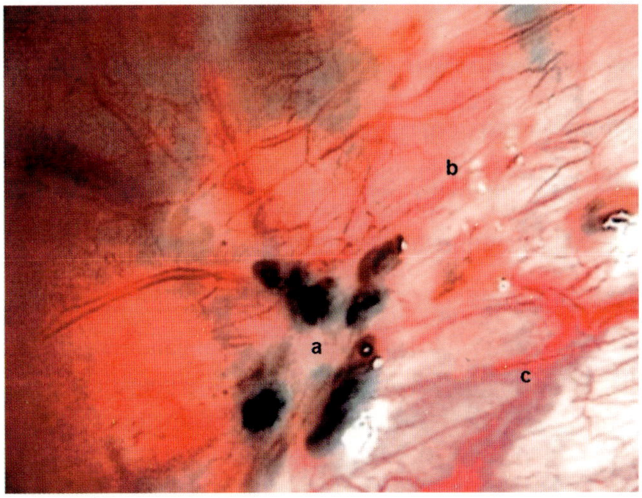

Fig. 12.2: Laparoscopic picture showing black lesions. *Courtesy: KJK Hospital, Trivandrum*

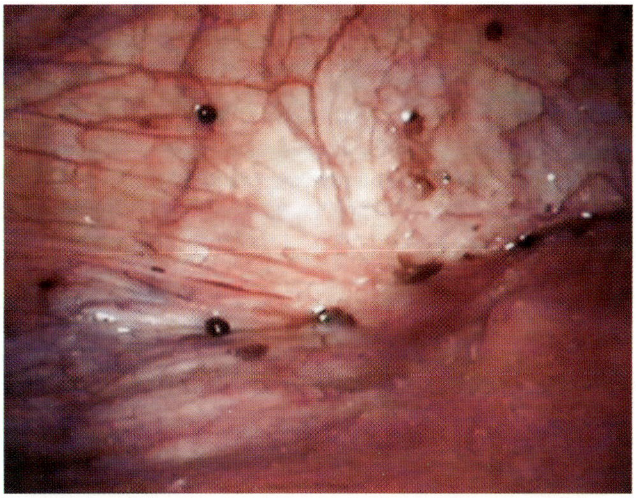

Fig. 12.3: Laparoscopic picture showing powder burn appearance. *Courtesy: KJK Hospital, Trivandrum*

A new classification system based on the AFS classification and the historical aspects is being developed, called Endometriosis Fertility Index (EFI). Based on the scores ranging from 0-10, fertility[8] can be predicted.

12.7 CLINICAL FEATURES

12.7.1 Symptoms

Pelvic endometriosis causes severe symptoms like

a. Dysmenorrhea
b. Infertility
c. Pelvic pain
d. Deep dyspareunia
e. Cyclical dyschezia
f. Dysuria
g. Cyclical hematuria
h. Ovulation failure
i. Mass abdomen

Factors causing infertility in endometriosis

- Anatomic distortion caused by adhesions
- Activation of inflammatory and immunologic responses-increased monocyte and natural killer activity causing sperm/egg/embryo destruction
- Leuteinized unruptured follicle syndrome
- Altered endometrial receptivity
- Impaired sperm function
- Poor oocytes quality

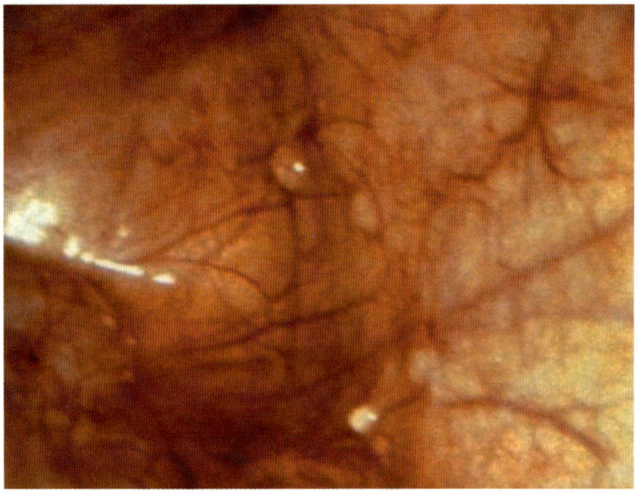

Fig. 12.4: Laparoscopic picture showing jelly like lesions
Courtesy: KJK Hospital, Trivandrum

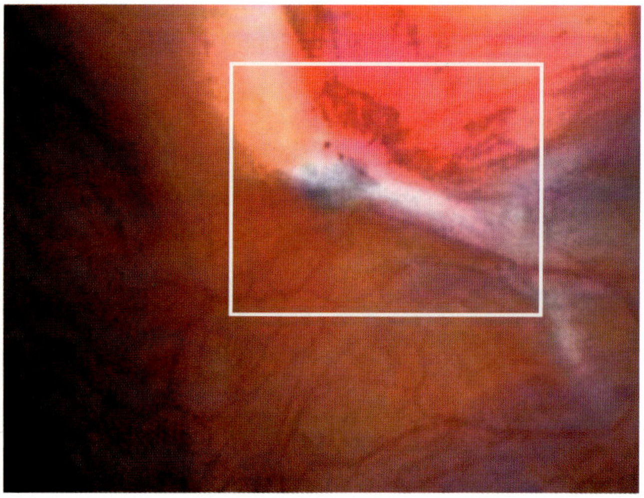

Fig. 12.5: Laparoscopic picture showing white lesions due to scarring

The symptoms depend on the location and the depth of the lesion. The commonest symptom of endometriosis is severe dysmenorrhea, which is commonly seen in women with lesions in the uterosacral ligament and obliteration of the pouch of Douglas. Pain typically starts just before menses and continues throughout the duration of menstrual flow and even after menses (triple dysmenorrhea). The woman can have continuous pelvic pain.

There can be associated ovulation pain, deep dyspareunia, dysuria or dyschezia. Referred pain to the flanks, low back or the thighs can also be present. However, there can also be endometriosis without much pain.

Another common complaint is infertility, which is associated with AFS stages III and IV. When the disease is AFS stage I or II, it is doubtful whether it can be attributed solely to endometriosis or is a coincidence in the presence of other causes of infertility. There are several factors contributing to infertility in endometriosis. Most important factor is anatomic distortion caused by adhesions which results in mechanical blockage of sperm-egg union. This is the cause in moderate and severe disease. Women with mild disease also are reported to have reduced fertility compared to those who do not have the disease. Activation of immunologic and inflammatory responses by the endometriotic deposits has been pointed out as the cause in such patients. Increased monocyte and natural killer cell activity can cause sperm or egg destruction. Luteinized unruptured follicle syndrome (LUF) has been reported as another etiological factor. Altered endometrial receptivity, impaired sperm function, embryotoxicity, oocyte toxicity and poor oocyte quality are all blamed to be contributing to infertility, but data are insufficient.

The symptoms of extrapelvic endometriosis depend on the site of lesion. It could be cyclical pain at episiotomy site, abdominal wound or umbilicus during periods. Endometriosis of pleura can cause pleuritic pain. Lung involvement can present as hemoptysis.

12.7.2 Signs

General examination and abdominal examination are usually unremarkable. Endometriomas are usually not palpable per abdomen. But rarely there can be large endometriomas which can reach up to the level of the umbilicus.

Speculum examination: Pelvic endometriosis causes nodularity of the uterosacral ligaments and POD, but these are usually not seen on speculum examination. Rarely, they may be seen as bluish nodules in the region of the uterosacral ligaments and the POD. Endometriotic infiltration may appear as a reddish irregular area in the upper vagina which can mimic vaginal neoplasm.

Bimanual examination: Tenderness on bimanual examination is a characteristic feature of endometriosis. The findings on bimanual examination depend upon the presence of lesions in the pelvis. The mild and moderate disease may not produce any signs on bimanual examination. A careful and systematic rectovaginal examination can make out indurations in the POD, uterosacral ligament or rectovaginal septum. Tender nodules can be palpated in the uterosacral ligaments and POD, which can be better appreciated if the examination is done during or immediately after periods.

12.8 DIAGNOSTIC MODALITIES (TABLE 12.4)

Ultrasound: Ultrasound can diagnose endometriomas. Endometriomas typically have ground glass appearance with thick walls. Restricted mobility of the uterus and adhesion of the ovary to the uterus can be made out at TVS.

CT/MRI: MRI is the best imaging modality for identifying endometriomas. It can detect small implants (as small as 3 mms) which are not detected by ultrasound. MRI can distinguish benign from malignant lesions when there is an adnexal mass,[9] with excellent sensitivity and specificity.

IVP or Barium enema may be needed in selected cases to map the extent of the disease.

Biochemical markers of endometriosis: CA-125 has been used as a biochemical marker of endometriosis. CA-125 level in the peripheral blood is elevated in moderate and severe disease. However, this marker is non specific as it is found to be increased in other conditions like ovarian and colon cancer, liver disease, pelvic inflammatory disease and even during menstruation in the absence of endometriosis. Hence, its diagnostic utility is limited.

Several other serum protein markers are being investigated for the diagnosis of endometriosis. Tissue inhibitor of metalloproteinase 1 is found to be decreased in peritoneal fluid and serum of women with endometriosis. Other markers which are being investigated include intercellular adhesion molecule 1, tumor associated trypsin inhibitor, soluble human leukocyte antigen 1 and C-reactive protein.

Laparoscopy: Laparoscopic visualization is the gold standard in the diagnosis of endometriosis. It should be done in suspected cases by an experienced laparoscopic surgeon, in centers with operative laparoscopic facilities. Laparoscopy gives magnified view of the entire abdomen and pelvis, so that even subtle lesions can be diagnosed. When gross disease is not seen at laparoscopy, subtle lesions should be looked for in the POD, inferior surface of ovary, peritoneum of the ovarian fossa, posteroinferior surface of the uterus etc. Pelvic organs should be mobilized with an instrument like grasper, so that lesions in the posterior wall of a retroverted uterus and the posterior wall of ovary and ovarian fossa can be visualized. Early lesions can be seen as papillary excrescences or vesicles and the color can be bright red or lighter shades of red. Long standing dormant and healed lesions can be seen as fibrosis which appears whitish. Advanced active lesions can appear in a variety of colors like black, brown, red or green caused by degradation of heme. Visualization of endometriosis by an experienced laparoscopic surgeon is sufficient for diagnosis. Treatment can be instituted immediately.

Table 12.4: Diagnostic modalities

• Laparoscopy	Definitive diagnosis
• Ultrasound	Diagnose endometrioma
• CT/MRI	Diagnose deep infiltrating endometriosis
• CA-125	Only prognostic significance

One specific manifestation of endometriosis is ovarian endometrioma or chocolate cyst. The name is due to the chocolate like material inside the cyst. They are formed by invagination of ectopic endometrium from the surface of the ovary into the cortex.

Histological confirmation: It is ideal to obtain histological confirmation at the time of laparoscopy/laparotomy. If there is peritoneal disease alone, visual inspection is enough for diagnosis. But endometriomas, especially when they are >3-4 cm in size, should have biopsy confirmation to exclude the rare occurrence of malignancy.

Speculum examination
- Bluish nodules in the vagina over uterosacral ligament
- Infiltrative lesion in upper vagina

Bimanual examination
- Retroverted fixed uterus
- Nodular uterosacral ligament
- POD nodularity
- Cystic adnexal mass
- Thickened rectovaginal septum

12.9 MANAGEMENT (FIG. 12.6)

12.9.1 Prevention

So far no strategy to prevent endometriosis has evolved. The only thing which can be done is to treat the disease once it is diagnosed. If diagnosed in adolescents, long-term hormonal treatment should be advised to prevent the progression of the disease. Since a familial tendency has been identified, the younger sister of a woman diagnosed with endometriosis can be advised to complete family early, so that her fertility may not be affected by endometriosis developing later.

12.9.2 Patient Counseling

Endometriosis is a chronic benign condition which has a high recurrence rate after medical or conservative surgical

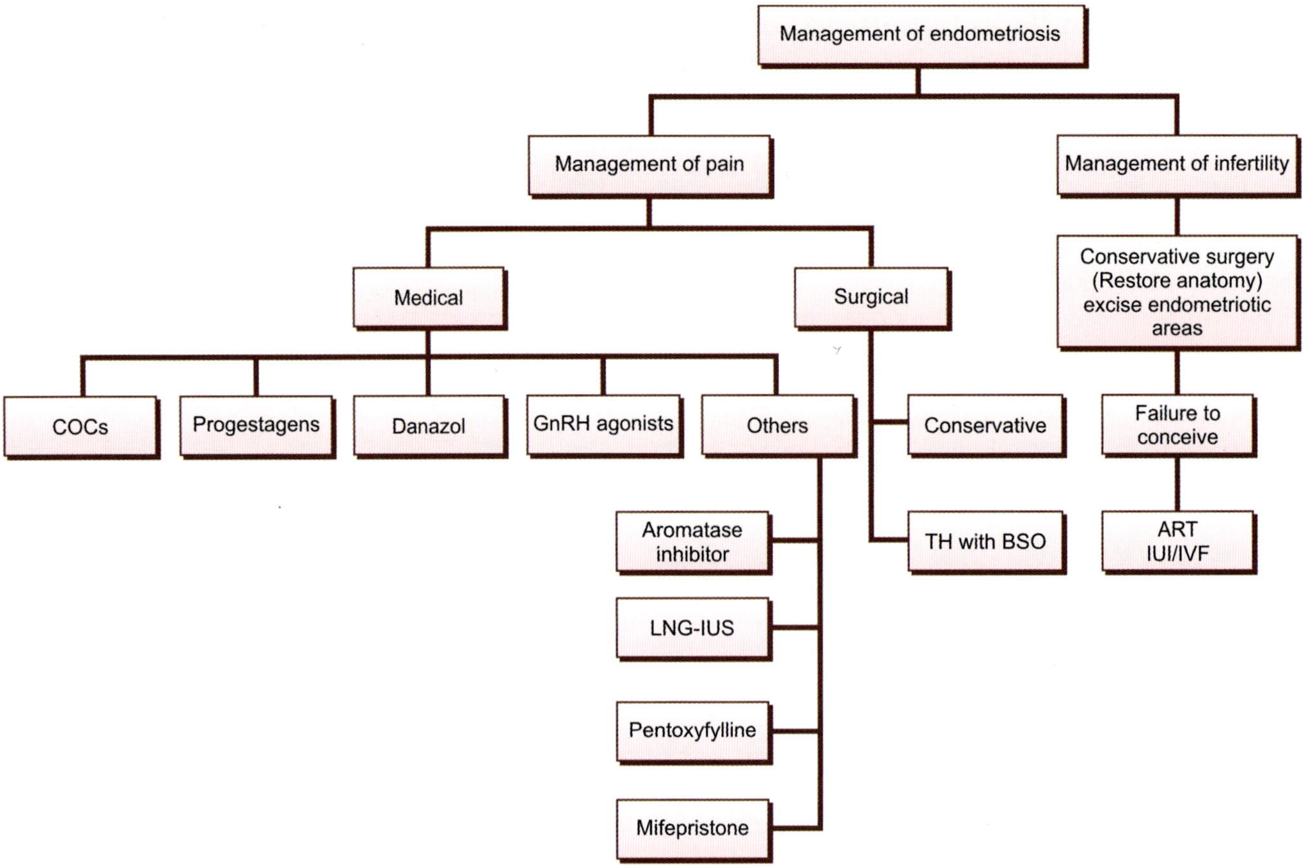

Fig. 12.6: Management algorithm of endometriosis

treatment. Hence women should be properly counseled at the time of diagnosis about the expected outcome with regard to pain relief and restoration of fertility. The chances of recurrence should always be emphasized. Women should be involved in decision making as to the choice of treatment and its duration.

The aim of management is to

i. alleviate symptoms, the most important ones being pelvic pain and dysmenorrhea
ii. restore fertility

12.9.3 Medical Management

NSAIDs are widely used for pain relief in endometriosis, but its usefulness in relieving pain is not satisfactory. The disadvantage is the antiovulatory effect when used mid-cycle and gastric ulceration due to repeated use.

Hormonal treatment: Medical management of endometriosis is principally by temporarily causing atrophy of endometriotic areas with hormones (pseudopregnancy state) or by causing extreme hypoestrogenism through pituitary suppression (pseudo menopause).

Hormones employed are:

1. Combined oral contraceptive pills (COCs)
2. Progestagens—Medroxy progesterone acetate, Dydrogesterone
3. Gestrinone
4. Danazol } Causes pituitary suppression
5. GnRH agonists } Causes pituitary suppression

COCs: The treatment of endometriosis with combination of estrogen and progesterone was introduced by Kistner in 1959. The combination pill causes decidualization of endometrial tissues. Currently low dose preparations are available.[10]

A pill containing 30 µg ethinyl estradiol and 150 µg of levonorgestrel can be given continuously to achieve amenorrhea. Relief of pelvic pain and dysmenorrhea is reported to occur in 60-95% of the patients. Compared to other methods of medical management COCs are less costly and can be used for longer periods. Even if given cyclically, COCs prevent recurrence of endometriosis.

Progestagens: Progestagens cause initial decidualization followed by atrophy of endometrium. They can be used for long-term treatment to alleviate pain because of their low cost and lesser side effect profile compared to Danazole or GnRH. Medroxy progesterone acetate is the most commonly used progestagen. It can be started at a dose of 30 mg/day and increased based on clinical response. The dose is adjusted to cause amenorrhea. Women whose fertility has to be preserved, can be administered dydrogesterone during the luteal phase only. Newer progestagens like desogestrel are now being studied.

The main side effects are weight gain, bloating sensation due to fluid retention and breakthrough bleeding due to hypoestrogenism. A short course of estrogen (7 days) can take care of breakthrough bleeding. Rarely, mood changes and depression are reported.

Levonorgestrel intrauterine system (LNG-IUS): In studies involving small number of women, LNG-IUS[11] was found to reduce dysmenorrhea, pelvic pain and dyspareunia significantly. Symptom control is found to be maintained for about 3 years.

Gestrinone: Gestrinone, a 19 nortestosterone derivative has androgenic, anti progestagenic, antiestrogenic and antigonadotrophic properties. Hence, it can be used for the treatment of endometriosis as it causes cellular inactivation and degeneration of implants. It is used at a dose of 2.5 mg twice a week. Amenorrhea occurs in most of the patients. The side effects are mainly due to its androgenic action, which includes muscle cramps, weight gain, acne, seborrhea and irreversible voice change. It is found to be as effective as GnRH in relieving pelvic pain.

Danazol: Danazol has action on the hypothalamus, ovary and endometrium, the main action being suppression of GnRH from the hypothalamus. Because of the high androgenic and very low estrogenic environment produced, danazol causes atrophy of the ectopic endometrium. The dose is 600-800 mg/day. But this high dose may not always be required to cause amenorrhea. Hence, a logical strategy is to start with 400 mg/day and increase the dose by 200 mg to achieve amenorrhea.

The adverse effects of danazol are due to the androgenic and hypoestrogenic state. The reported side effects are weight gain, fluid retention, acne, oily skin, hirsutism, voice change, hot flushes, atrophic vaginitis, reduced libido, muscle cramps and emotional instability. However, danazol has the advantage of causing gain in bone mineral density.

Since danazol is metabolized in the liver, it should not be given to patients with altered liver function. As danazol causes fluid retention, it is contraindicated in women with congestive cardiac failure and impaired renal function. Liver function and renal function should be tested before prescribing danazol. The effectiveness of low dose danazol[12] administered vaginally is being evaluated because of its reduced side effect.

Gonadotropin releasing hormone (GnRH) agonists: Administration of GnRH analog cause an initial flare up of gonadotropin production from the pituitary followed by pituitary suppression. Pituitary suppression produced causes suppression of ovarian function and extreme hypoestrogenic state which leads to atrophy of endometriotic lesions.

GnRH agonists available are leuprorelin, buserelin, nafarelin, histerelin, goserelin, triptorelin etc. Being peptide hormones, these cannot be administered orally and should be given intramuscularly, intranasally or subcutaneously. The hypoestrogenic state produced causes side effects due to estrogen deficiency which include hot flushes, vaginal dryness, reduced libido and reduction in bone mineral density. The reduction in bone mineral density is an important concern. If used for under 6 months, the lost bone will be regained in the next 12 months. More than 6 months of usage can cause irreversible bone loss.

Add-back Therapy

The use of COC along with GnRH analog prevents bone loss associated with GnRH treatment alone, without compromising pain relief. Moreover, the addition of COC takes care of other hypoestrogenic side effects of GnRH.[13] If add-back therapy is given, GnRH can be continued for about 2 years.

Drawback Therapy

In drawback therapy, GnRH is started at a high dose, which is given for 1 month, followed by a lower dose for the next 5 months. This regime causes less loss in bone mineral density.

A Cochrane review has reported that both pseudo-pregnancy state induced by COC and pseudo menopause induced by danazol and GnRH[14] are equally beneficial in relieving pain. The choice should be made by considering the side effect profile and the patient's choice. The duration of treatment depends upon the drug used, response to treatment and side effects. COC and medroxy progesterone acetate can be used for a long time. Danazol and GnRH cannot be used for more than 6 months. Along with add-back therapy GnRH treatment can be continued for 2 years or more.

Aromatase inhibitors: The latest addition to the drugs used for suppression of ovarian function is letrozole. Letrozole being an aromatase inhibitor inhibits production of estrogen causing extreme hypoestrogenic state and consequent atrophy of the endometriotic areas. The major disadvantage is significant loss of bone mineral density. Combination of letrozole and norethisterone or desogestrel has been shown to be effective, but the disadvantage is symptom recurrence after cessation of therapy.[15] *Hormonal treatment causes temporary atrophy of the ectopic endometrium, but the primary pathology is not treated by these drugs. The altered anatomical relations of the ovary, fallopian tube and uterus also are not corrected by hormones.* But for temporary pain relief, hormonal treatment can be resorted to.

Emerging Medical Therapies

Emerging medical therapies include GnRH antagonists, anti-progestagen-mifepristone, TNFα inhibitors, angiogenesis inhibitors and matrix metalloproteinase inhibitors. No clinical trials have been performed yet for angiogenesis inhibitors, matrix metalloproteinase inhibitors and antivascular endothelial growth factor. Limited data are available about mifepristone as a potential treatment option.

Pentoxyfylline, a phosphodiesterase inhibitor has anti-inflammatory properties. It has been found to be effective in improving pregnancy rates when given to patients with endometriosis in small scale randomized trials.

Conservative surgery

- Release of adhesions
- Excision of endometriotic nodules
- Coagulation and vaporization of peritoneal implants
- Excision of chocolate cysts >3 cm in diameter
- Drainage and coagulation of chocolate cysts < 3 cm in diameter

Empirical Treatment of Pain

There are clinicians who think that laparoscopy is a hazardous procedure. GnRH, progestagens or danazol can be used in clinically diagnosed endometriosis without laparoscopic confirmation. The recommendation is to give the above second line drugs for 6 months followed by NSAIDs or COCs. If symptoms recur, the above second line drugs can be restarted. However, there are no randomized controlled trials to compare this with laparoscopic surgery.

12.9.4 Surgical Management

Endometriosis diagnosed at laparoscopy should be surgically treated at the same time. In all clinically suspected cases, consent should be obtained preoperatively.

Surgical management involves excision/coagulation of endometriotic areas, surgical management of chocolate cysts, release of adhesions and restoration of anatomy. Severe disease in women who have completed family can be treated by bilateral ovariotomy.

Preoperative Treatment

It was previously thought that a 3 month course of medical treatment before surgery reduces vascularity and increases ease of surgery. But evidence does not support this contention.

Conservative management: Laparoscopic surgery is the preferred conservative surgical management. The aim is to destroy the endometriotic tissue, either by excising or by coagulating. Superficial coagulation will destroy the active lesion, but leaves the treated tissue and the underlying fibrosis. Hence, endometriotic areas should be excised. Different energy sources can be used laparoscopically.

Electrical energy: The commonly used is monopolar electrical energy, for excising endometriotic areas.

Ultrasound energy is used in harmonic scalpel to achieve precise cutting and excision under lower temperature. Thus, heat damage to the adjacent tissue can be reduced. Harmonic scalpel is free from the risk of insulation failure.

CO_2 and KTP laser creates highly focused visible light, which can be used for precise cutting.

Surgical Management of Ovarian Endometriosis

Superficial lesions can be coagulated. Endometriomas measuring < 3 cm can be aspirated, irrigated and coagulated. Larger endometriomas measuring > 3 cm should be completely removed. This can be achieved in a single sitting or in two sittings, especially when the endometriomas are very large. In the single sitting, the wall of the endometriomas should be completely excised after draining the contents. In the double sitting, initially the endometriomas can be drained and the patient treated with GnRH agonist. In the second sitting, the wall of the endometriomas should be excised (Fig. 12.7). Cystectomy has the disadvantage of removing ovarian follicles along with the cyst wall. Based on current evidence, pain and subfertility were improved more by cystectomy than by fenestration and coagulation.[16]

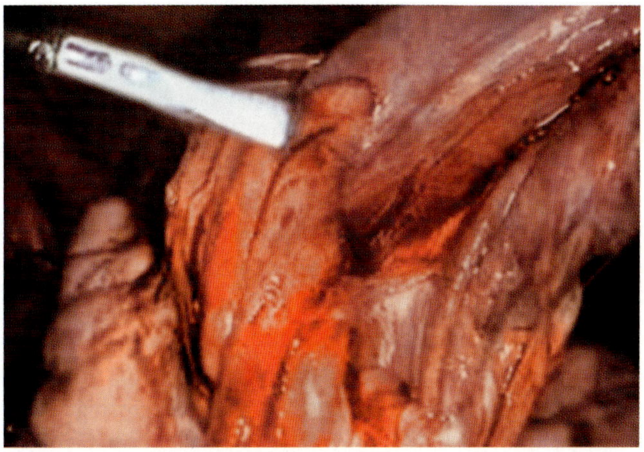

Fig. 12.7: Laparoscopic picture of excision of endometriotic cysts

Adhesiolysis

Endometriosis related adhesions should be released carefully. Release of adhesions will restore the anatomy, which is important for conception. Pharmacological agents routinely used for preventing adhesions have not been proved to be effective in endometriosis.

Postoperative Hormonal Treatment

GnRH analogs given for 6 months postoperatively after conservative surgical treatment can delay recurrence of pain for more than 12 months. In a small randomized control trial it was found that LNG-IUS inserted after laparoscopic surgery for endometriosis[17]associated pain, significantly reduced the risk of recurrent dysmenorrhea.

12.9.5 Recurrence

Medical, surgical (conservative) or combination treatment will not cure the disease. Hence, recurrence is common unless both ovaries are removed. Recurrence is seen two months to several years after initial surgery. In most situations, it will be difficult to differentiate between recurrent and persistent disease as microscopic implants may be missed at surgery. *The most important factor deciding recurrence is completeness of initial surgery.* There is no convincing evidence that treatment with GnRH or ovarian hormones before or after conservative surgery has significant effect in decreasing recurrence. The number and size of cysts also has no effect on recurrence rate. Deep infiltrating endometriosis, especially of the rectovaginal septum is the one which is usually missed at laparoscopy, thereby resulting in incomplete treatment. A careful rectovaginal examination can diagnose the disease.

12.9.6 Nonconservative Management

For patients who had several recurrences or treatment failures, nonconservative surgical treatment is the only option to relieve symptoms. Removal of both the ovaries is the definitive treatment as exposure to ovarian hormones is the implicating factor in the causation of the disease. Since both ovaries need to be removed, hysterectomy also is usually done. With the wide spread availability of ART procedures, the option of retaining the uterus for surrogacy is an option. Surgery in these women with severe endometriosis is fraught with the risk of injury to ureter, urinary bladder and rectosigmoid, especially if they had previous conservative surgical attempts. Ureteric injury can be minimized by ureteric stenting. In some situations when there are severe adhesions, the ureter may have to be skeletonized which can lead to avascular necrosis of ureter and urinary fistula. Even after hysterectomy and bilateral salpingo-oopherectomy, completeness of the removal of ovary may not be absolute. Rarely endometriomas have been reported to occur after presumed definitive surgery.

12.9.7 Management of Rectovaginal Endometriosis

Rectovaginal endometriosis is a deep infiltrating disease which causes severe symptoms. Excising rectovaginal endometriotic nodules is a challenge for laparoscopic surgeons. The risk involved is a possible injury to rectosigmoid and ureter which can cause fistulas. Dissection of the rectosigmoid from the vagina and cervix can injure the bowel which may require a temporary colostomy. Women presenting with rectovaginal nodule should be counseled appropriately prior to surgery. The possibility of bowel injury should be discussed with the patient preoperatively. When there are severe adhesions, ureteric catheterization may be required before surgery as there will be distortion of anatomy so that identification of ureter would be difficult.

Rectosigmoid is separated from the posterior vaginal wall and the cervix. If the upper part of the posterior vaginal wall is infiltrated, the vaginal wall should also be removed. The endometriotic nodules are shaved off from the bowel, avoiding injury to the bowel. If part of the bowel wall is also involved and need to be removed, a disc resection of the bowel can be done and the bowel closed with sutures. In case a large area of the bowel is involved, a segmental resection of the bowel may need to be done. A multidisciplinary approach may be needed. Urologist and colorectal surgeon may have to be involved in such situations.

12.9.8 Laparoscopic Uterine Nerve Ablation (LUNA)

LUNA involves cutting or coagulating about 1.5 cm of uterosacral ligament which contains the nerve supply to the uterus. It is done for pain relief as an additional procedure along with excision of endometriotic areas. The effect of LUNA on alleviating dysmenorrhea associated with endometriosis is questionable.

12.9.9 Presacral Neurectomy

Presacral neurectomy, which interrupts the nerves supplying the uterus in the presacral region, has been found to effect pain relief in women who have central pelvic pain. It can be done through the laparoscope also. The peritoneum over the sacral promontory is incised, taking care not to injure the presacral artery and vein. The nerve tissue in front of the sacral promontory is removed. 90% relief of pain has been reported after the procedure. Rarely, urinary retention and constipation can follow the procedure, but usually these will resolve over about 2 months. It can be resorted to as a last option when other treatment modalities fail.

12.9.10 Treatment of Endometriosis Associated with Infertility

Clearly there is no role for medical management of the endometriotic nodules, if the woman presents with infertility. While on medical management, due to the hormonal suppression, conception is prevented. Moreover, medical management cannot reverse the adhesions caused by the disease. *Since infertility in endometriosis is mainly due to the anatomical distortion caused by adhesions, surgical management is preferred.* Surgical management entails release of adhesions, restoring anatomy and excising endometriotic lesions (laparoscopic picture of excision of endometriotic cysts). There is evidence that surgical treatment of even minimal or mild endometriosis improves fertility.[18] Pregnancy rate in the treated group was 48% against 35% in the expectantly managed group in one randomized controlled trial.

Pregnancy rate after the surgical treatment of endometriosis depends upon the stage of the disease to which it is inversely related. The reported pregnancy rate after treatment of moderate and severe disease is 50%. If at laparoscopy, extensive disease is encountered, it is better to advise IVF without wasting time since conception is expected to be very remote.

Postoperative hormonal treatment has no effect on pregnancy rate. It will only delay the time to conception. After conservative surgery, controlled ovarian hyperstimulation and IUI should be advised. When this fails to achieve pregnancy, IVF should be preferred to repeat surgery. Whether endometriosis affects pregnancy rate adversely in IVF cycles is a controversial issue, with some studies reporting that there is no effect, whereas others report that it is less in women with endometriosis.[19]

A Cochrane review states that treatment with GnRH agonists for 3-6 months before IVF increases the pregnancy rates. If large endometriomas are present, it should be excised before IVF to improve access to ovum, to reduce infection and to exclude malignancy. Use of sclerosing agents instilled into the endometriomas after ultrasound guided aspiration is an alternative treatment. IVF pregnancy rate reported after such treatment is 57%.

12.10 ADENOMYOSIS

Adenomyosis is defined as the presence of endometrial glands and stroma deep in the myometrium associated with myometrial hyperplasia and hypertrophy. It is a common gynecological disorder, the data on the prevalence of which is not clearly known due to the lack of criteria for diagnosing the condition.

12.10.1 Pathology

The normal boundary between the endometrial basal layer and myometrium will be disrupted. The endometrial glands invade the myometrium resulting in myometrial hyperplasia and hypertrophy (Fig. 12.9). The disease is usually diffuse involving the entire myometrium or rarely localized to an

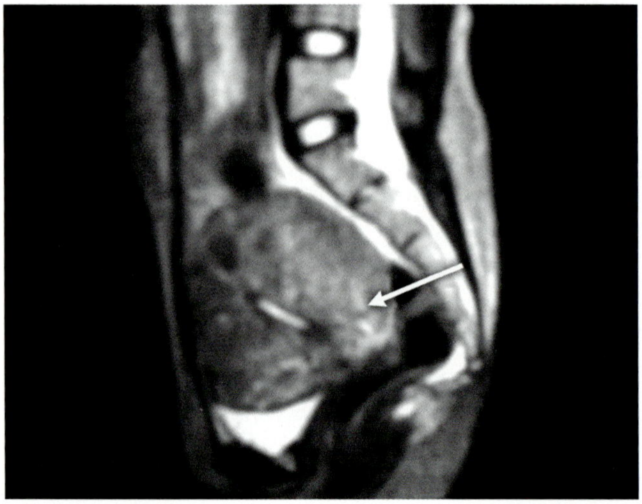

Fig. 12.8: MRI picture showing adenomyosis. Note the uniformly enlarged uterus (arrow). The uterus measured 22 cm, which is rare in adenomyosis

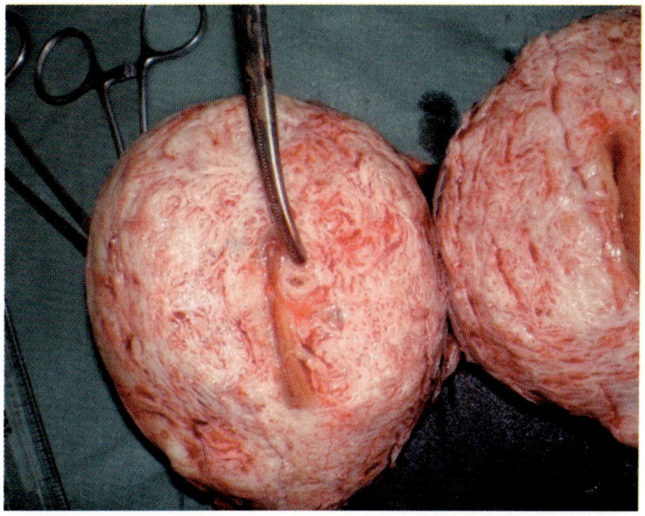

Fig. 12.9: Cut open specimen of uterus showing diffuse adenomyosis involving the whole of the myometrium. The artery forceps points towards a small cystic space in the myometrium which is characteristic of adenomyosis. The patient was a 45-year-old parous lady who presented with severe menorrhagia and anemia

area when it is called an adenomyoma. The symptoms of adenomyosis and the response to treatment depend on the depth of myometrial invasion. Siegler and Canilien divided endometriosis into 3 grades: 1, 2 and 3 depending on whether the involvement is in the inner 1/3rd, middle 1/3rd or the entire myometrium. Adenomyosis is also classified into mild, moderate and severe depending on the number of endometrial islands noted on histologic examination.

12.10.2 Prevalence

The exact prevalence is difficult to estimate as there are no strict criteria for its diagnosis by ultrasound. An analysis of 1334 hysterectomy specimens revealed that adenomyosis was present in 25%. The prevalence in hysterectomy specimens was reported to range from 10 to 25%.

12.10.3 Risk Factors

Repeat sharp curettage after abortion was found to increase the risk of adenomyosis, whereas endometrial curettage in the non pregnant stage has not been found to increase the risk. Adenomyosis has been shown to be significantly associated with pelvic endometriosis and infertility. In multiparous women, adenomyosis is found to be more which could be due to viable endometrium getting displaced into the myometrium. Endometrial hyperplasia has been found to be associated with adenomyosis.

12.10.4 Symptoms

Adenomyosis is thought to be associated with menorrhagia, dysmenorrhea, dyspareunia, chronic pelvic pain etc. However, Berghat et al did not observe any significant association between adenomyosis and these symptoms.

12.10.5 Diagnosis

Adenomyosis is characterized by uniform enlargement of the uterus. However, it can be mistaken for myomas. Imaging by ultrasound is the widely used diagnostic tool (Detailed discussion in Chapter 25: Ultrasound in Gynecology). The uterus would appear to have a heterogenous echo texture which differentiates it from the focal masses of myoma. On Doppler examination, adenomyosis will show diffuse vascularity whereas the vascularity of the myoma will be more at the periphery. Usually, enlargement of the uterus with adenomyosis involves one wall of the uterus (mostly the posterior), but it could be localized as well. It is difficult to distinguish localized adenomyosis from a myoma. In such situations, MRI is the imaging technique of choice since it provides better diagnostic capability due to the increased spatial and contrast resolution (Fig. 12.8).

12.10.6 Management

As adenomyosis is usually seen to involve the uterine wall diffusely, surgical treatment options are limited. Localized adenomyosis can be excised if symptomatic. Fertility might improve after local excision of adenomyosis. GnRH treatment might relieve symptoms temporarily. However, GnRH cannot be given long-term due to its adverse effect of causing extreme hypoestrogenic state. The disease will recur after stopping treatment. In patients with only moderately enlarged uterus, levonorgestrel intrauterine system can be tried. Uterine artery embolization is an option if menorrhagia is the concern for women who have completed their family. For those who are concerned with infertility, *in vitro* fertilization and embryo transfer to a gestational carrier is an option.

12.11 CONCLUSION

Endometriosis is an enigmatic disease, the exact etiology of which is not yet established. Pain and infertility are the major symptoms. Since affected women are usually in the younger age group and are often infertile, conservative treatment is the option. Laparoscopy is the preferred technique for diagnosis and treatment. Excision of all endometriotic areas, including endometriotic cysts and release of adhesions is the basis of conservative treatment. When infertility is not an issue, pain can be managed by treatment with COCs, progestogens, danazol or GnRH agonists. All these modalities relieve pain almost to the same extent. Recurrence rate is high after medical, surgical or combination treatment. If the disease recurs and infertility is the issue, IVF should be preferred to repeat conservative surgery. When there are multiple treatment failures, the final definitive treatment is bilateral oophorectomy with/without hysterectomy. Deep infiltrating endometriosis, especially of the rectovaginal septum is a challenge to the surgeon. Multidisciplinary input from colorectal surgeon and urologist may be needed in such situations. In the coming years, with better understanding of the etiology of endometriosis, supported by well designed randomized controlled trials on treatment modalities, clinicians will have a clearer view of effective treatment regimes.

REFERENCES

1. MP Vessey, L Billard-Mackintosh and R Painter. Epidemiology of endometriosis in women attending family planning clinic BMJ 1993;306:182-4.
2. TA Mahmood and A Templeton. Prevalence and genesis of endometriosis. Hum Reprod 1991;6(4):544-9.
3. B Eskenazi, ML Warner. Epidemiology of endometriosis. Obstet Gynaecol Clin North Am 1997;24(2):235-58.
4. MJ Blumenkrantz, N Gallagher, RA Bashore, H Tunckhoff. Retrograde menstruation in women undergoing peritoneal dialysis. Obstet Gynaecol 1981;57(5):667-70.
5. J Halme, MG Hammond, JF Hulka, SG Raj, LM Talbert. Retrograde menstruation in healthy women and in patients with endometriosis. Obstet Gynaecol 1984;64(2):151-4.
6. Heimler I, Rawlins RG, Owen H, Hutz RJ. Dioxin perturbs, in a dose and time-dependent fashion, steroid secretion, and induces apoptosis of human luteinized granulosa cells. Endocrinology 1998;139:4373.
7. Classification of endometriosis. Fertil Steril 1979;32:633-4.
8. Adamson GD, Pasta DJ. Pregnancy rates can be predicted by validated endometriosis fertility index. Fertil Steril 2002; 77(Suppl):S48.
9. Mawhinney RR, Powell MC, Worthington BS, Symonds EM. Magnetic Resonance Imaging of benign ovarian masses. Br J Radio 1988;61:179-86.
10. Harada T et al. Low dose oral contraceptive pill for dysmenorrhoea associated with endometriosis: A placebo-controlled, double-blind, randomized trial. Fertil Steril 2007.
11. Gomes MK, et al. The levonorgestrel-releasing intrauterine system and endometriosis staging. Fertil Steril 2007; 87(5):1231-4.
12. Razzi S et al. Efficacy of vaginal danazol treatment in women with recurrent deeply infiltrating endometriosis. Fertil Steril 2007;88(4):789-94.
13. Sagsveen M, Farmer JE, Prentice A, Breeze A. Gonadotrophin-releasing hormone analogues for endometriosis: bone mineral density. Cochrane Database Syst Rev 2003;(4):CD001297.
14. Prentice A, Deary AJ, Bland E. Progestagens and anti-progestagens for pain associated with endometriosis. Cochrane Database of Systematic Reviews 2000, Issue 2. Art No: CD002122. DOI: 10.1002/14651858.CD002122.
15. Remorgida V, et al. Letrozole and norethisterone acetate in rectovaginal endometriosis. Fertil Steril 2007;88(3)724-26.
16. Prentice A, Deary AJ, Bland E. Progestagens and anti-progestagens for pain associated with endometriosis. Cochrane Database of Systematic Reviews 2000, Issue 2. Art No: CD002122. DOI:10.1002/14651858.CD002122.
17. Yap C, Furness S, Farquhar C. Pre and postoperative medical therapy for endometriosis surgery. Cochrane Database Syst Rev 2004;(3):CD003678.
18. Marcoux S, Maheux R, Berube S and the Canadian Collaborative Group on Endometriosis. Laparoscopic surgery in infertile women with minimal or mild endometriosis. N Engl J Med 1997;337:217-22.
19. Sallam HN, Garcia-Velasco JA, Dias S, Arici A. Long-term pituitary down regulation before in vitro fertilization for women with endometriosis. Cochrane Database Sys Rev 2006;(1):CD004635.

13 Leiomyomata of the Uterus

B Presannakumari

13.1 INTRODUCTION

Leiomyomas (myomas) are benign estrogen dependent tumors which arise from the myometrium. They are the most common benign uterine tumors among women of reproductive age group. Even though only 50% of women with myomas are symptomatic, they are one of the most common causes of morbidity among women due to the variety of symptoms which they can cause and they form the most common reason for surgical intervention in women. Severity of symptoms depends upon the site, size and number of myomas as well as the presence of degenerative changes.

13.2 EPIDEMIOLOGY

Myomas occur mainly in the reproductive age group. They are rare in the adolescent age group, the incidence peaking in the pre-menopausal years, and declining after menopause. Clinically apparent myomas are seen in 25% of all women. Among women aged over 40 years, the prevalence is 30-40%. There is racial difference in the incidence with an increased incidence observed among Africans and other dark skinned races. It is lesser among Caucasians. A random sample review of medical records of women screened by sonography, reported that the prevalence of myoma among

African women is 60% by 35 years and 80% by 50 years of age. Among Caucasian women the prevalence is 40% by 35 years and almost 70% by 50 years.

13.3 ETIOLOGY

There is clear evidence that these tumors are estrogen dependent. This is supported by the fact that GnRH agonist treatment causes significant reduction in the size of myomas. The action of hormones on myoma is mediated by local growth factors such as epithelial growth factor, vascular endothelial growth factor, transforming growth factor and interleukin B. On hormone signals, these factors act on the myoma to increase its size. Each myoma develops from a single cell. The factor determining the transformation of a single cell into a myoma is not yet clear. Familial clustering of myomas have been reported. Myomas are 4-5 times more common in first degree relatives of women with myoma. These myomas with familial prevalence behave differently. However no particular gene involved in the causation has been clearly identified. Myomas were observed to occur more among atomic bomb survivors. Chromosomal changes like duplications, deletions and translocations are common in myoma cells. The most commonly observed cytogenetic abnormality is deletion of chromosome 7.

Leiomyoma cells have been found to have elevated transcriptional response to estrogen.[1] The increased responsiveness is thought to have a genetic basis. Polymorphism of gene CYP17 located on chromosome 7 which codes for P450 C17 α enzyme is thought to be responsible for the difference in the incidence seen among different races.[2] Another gene polymorphism involved is Catechol o-methyl transferase which converts a metabolite of estrogen (2 hydroxy estradiol) to a more mitotic estradiol (2 methoxy estradiol) creating a high estrogenic milieu.

Reides' syndrome is a rare syndrome characterized by multiple myomas in the skin and the uterus. Parity, cigarette smoking and oral contraceptive use protects against development of myomas.

13.4 SYMPTOMS

About 50% of myomas are asymptomatic. The exact reason why a myoma becomes symptomatic has not been clearly delineated. It could be dependent upon the site and size of myomas. Some women remain asymptomatic in spite of having very large myomas. Myomas can present with a variety of symptoms which include

1. Menstrual symptoms
2. Pelvic pain
3. Pressure symptoms like urinary frequency and bowel disturbance
4. Intervention with reproductive function. Myomas can interfere with reproductive function contributing to subfertility, abortions, pre-term labor, malpresentations, increased need for cesarean section, postpartum hemorrhage, etc.

13.4.1 Menstrual Abnormalities

The usual menstrual abnormality encountered is menorrhagia. About 30% of women with myomas have abnormal bleeding. Submucous and intramural myomas are the usual types associated with menorrhagia. The bleeding can sometimes be severe enough to produce anemia. The following factors are supposed to be causes for menorrhagia:

1. Increased endometrial surface area
2. Increased vascularity of uterus
3. Intervention with uterine contractility
4. Endometrial ulceration over submucosal myoma
5. Compression of venous plexus and congestion of endometrium and myometrium

Submucous myomas and polyps can cause inter menstrual bleeding. Myomatous polyps protruding out through the external os can cause continuous and profuse bleeding.

Dysregulation of growth factors which have direct effect on vascular function and angiogenesis can also result in these abnormalities.

13.4.2 Pelvic Pain and Pressure Symptoms

Pelvic pain and discomfort are the common symptoms of leiomyoma. However, the same symptoms can be complained of by women without myoma.

Myoma impacted in the pouch of Douglas can cause tenesmus and constipation. Those located in the anterior wall of the uterus can irritate the bladder and cause urinary frequency. Cervical myoma can cause retention of urine. To start with, the retention will be premenstrual due to the enlargement of the uterus in the premenstrual phase. As the myoma enlarges, the symptom will become persistent. Presence of myoma can cause distortion of urethrovesical junction causing difficulty in initiating micturition and incomplete bladder emptying. Large myomas that fill the pelvis can cause difficulty in urination, defecation as well as dyspareunia.

Complications occurring in myoma can result in acute pain. Pedunculated subserous myoma can undergo torsion resulting in severe pain. Very rarely, a fundal subserous pedunculated myoma can cause torsion of the uterus as well. Red degeneration which usually occurs during pregnancy can also cause pain. Broad ligament myomas might press on the sciatic nerve to cause radiating pain to the leg.

Submucous myomas produce severe dysmenorrhea.

13.4.3 Mass Abdomen

Sometimes myomas may attain very large size and the patient might present with the symptom of mass abdomen.

13.5 IMPACT OF MYOMA ON REPRODUCTIVE FUNCTION

Most myomas will not interfere with fertility or affect pregnancy outcome. According to the American Society of Reproductive Medicine, myomas[3] are associated with infertility in 5-10% of women. However, presence of myoma may not be the sole cause for infertility. When other causes are excluded, myomas may be responsible for infertility in only 2-3% of women. There were no studies which estimated the proportion of normal fertile women who have myoma. Unless there is a prospective study of women who are diagnosed to have myoma to assess their rate of conception, risk of abortion and pregnancy outcome, we cannot establish the role of myoma in causing subfertility and influence on pregnancy outcome.[4,5] Submucous and intramural myomas might interfere with implantation

Intramural myomas might interfere with endometrial blood supply and have a negative effect on nidation.[6,7]

Myomectomy, either by conventional abdominal route or laparoscopically is reported to be associated with improved pregnancy rates.[8,9]

It is reported that pregnancy rate in patients who underwent hysteroscopic myomectomy were comparable to control groups without myomas.[10]

There is evidence of improved outcome when submucous myoma and intramural myoma were removed in women undergoing ART.

Miscarriage

Myomas have been thought to cause first and second trimester miscarriage and recurrent pregnancy loss. The pre and post myomectomy abortion[11,12] rates were reported as 41% and 19% respectively in one study on 1941 women who underwent myomectomy. However no prospective studies are available. It is logical to advise myomectomy for patients who have submucous as well as intramural myomas that distort the uterine cavity. There is no sufficient evidence that purely intramural or subserous myomas are associated with miscarriage.

Late Pregnancy Complications

Red degeneration is the commonest complication of myoma in pregnancy. The incidence is reported as 5%. The effect of pregnancy on myoma growth is unpredictable. Some myomas increase in size while others will decrease or remain the same. Most myomas will not increase in size, but will get flattened out leaving an impression that it has reduced in size.

The presence of myomas usually will not cause unfavorable pregnancy outcome. While certain studies reported no difference in the incidence of preterm labor, PROM, IUGR, antepartum hemorrhage, postpartum hemorrhage, retained placenta, etc, certain other studies showed increased incidence of preterm delivery (19.2% vs. 12.7%), placenta praevia (3.5% vs. 1.8%) and postpartum hemorrhage[13-15] (8.3% vs. 2.9%). Cesarean section incidence was found to be higher in women with myoma, particularly large ones compared to those without (26% vs. 12%).

Several studies have reported increased incidence of preterm delivery among women with myomas. There is no evidence that myomas cause intrauterine growth restriction.

Postpartum Complications

Postpartum hemorrhage is reported to be higher among women who have very large myomas. However, certain studies reported no increase in the incidence of postpartum hemorrhage. Decreased uterine contractility is the likely cause for postpartum hemorrhage. Emergency obstetric hysterectomy is also higher among women who have very large myomas located near the placenta. Retained placenta does not appear to be related to myoma status. During the puerperium the blood supply to uterus is greatly reduced from that during pregnancy, resulting in ischemic degeneration of uterine myomas. The ischemic changes provide the favorable environment for the growth of anaerobic organisms leading to puerperal endometritis. Submucous myomas, even if large might become polypoidal and present as a mass in the vagina. Occasionally these may get expelled per vagina, sometimes needing surgical intervention.

13.5.1 Malignant Transformation

Leiomyomata are not considered precursor lesions of leiomyosarcoma. Leiomyosarcoma is thought to arise de novo.With widespread use of ultrasound, myomas are usually diagnosed in asymptomatic women. Women will be anxious to know whether these tumors can become cancers. There is no evidence that leiomyomas can undergo malignant change. In a retrospective analysis of hysterectomy done for myomas, it was found that one leiomyosarcoma was diagnosed in one million hysterectomies for leiomyoma. It was also made out that the mean age of presentation of leiomyosarcoma is 55 years and most of the patients presented with postmenopausal bleeding. Curettage was positive for malignant cells in almost all these patients. Hence removing every asymptomatic myoma for fear of sarcomatous change is unjustified. However, when a diagnosis of myoma is made in a particular lady by imaging, one cannot be sure whether a myoma is leiomyosarcoma or not. Hence when adopting a conservative management, follow-up is essential. Women with myomas which are seen to have rapid growth and increased vascularity should be advised surgery.

13.6 RARE COMPLICATIONS OF MYOMA

13.6.1 Polycythemia

Myomas rarely elaborate erythropoietin and cause polycythemia which resolves following hysterectomy.

13.6.2 Benign Metastasizing Myoma

Myoma like lesions can be seen in the lungs in women with uterine myoma.

13.6.3 Intravenous Leiomyomatosis

Intravenous leiomyomatosis is a rare smooth muscle proliferation that arises from the uterus and extends into the inferior vena cava and ultimately into the right heart. The histology of the lesion resembles that of leiomyoma of the uterus. Even though the tumor is benign, the hemodynamic effects due to its presence in the IVC necessitate its removal.

13.6.4 Peritoneal Leiomyomatosis

Peritoneal leiomyomatosis (Fig. 13.1) is a rare condition in which multiple benign smooth muscle tumors are seen diffusely over the peritoneal and omental surfaces of women in the reproductive age. It has a benign course. They occur as a result of metaplasia of sub-peritoneal mesenchymal stem cells to smooth muscle, fibroblast or myofibroblast under the influence of estrogen and progesterone. The cases reported in the literature occurred in the child bearing age group. Even though they appear as grossly malignant, the histology is benign and patients will have a favorable clinical outcome. Since the source of estrogen has to be removed, management is total abdominal hysterectomy, bilateral salpingo-oophorectomy and removal of all gross disease. Removal of the source of estrogen will cause regression of unresected tumor masses.

13.7 DIAGNOSIS OF MYOMA

Myoma is usually diagnosed from the symptoms and clinical signs. Clinical examination reveals a firm enlarged uterus. Single myoma causes uniform enlargement and multiple myomas cause irregular enlargement. Small submucous myomas even though symptomatic may escape diagnosis by bimanual examination. Pedunculated subserous myomas may be mistaken for adnexal masses.

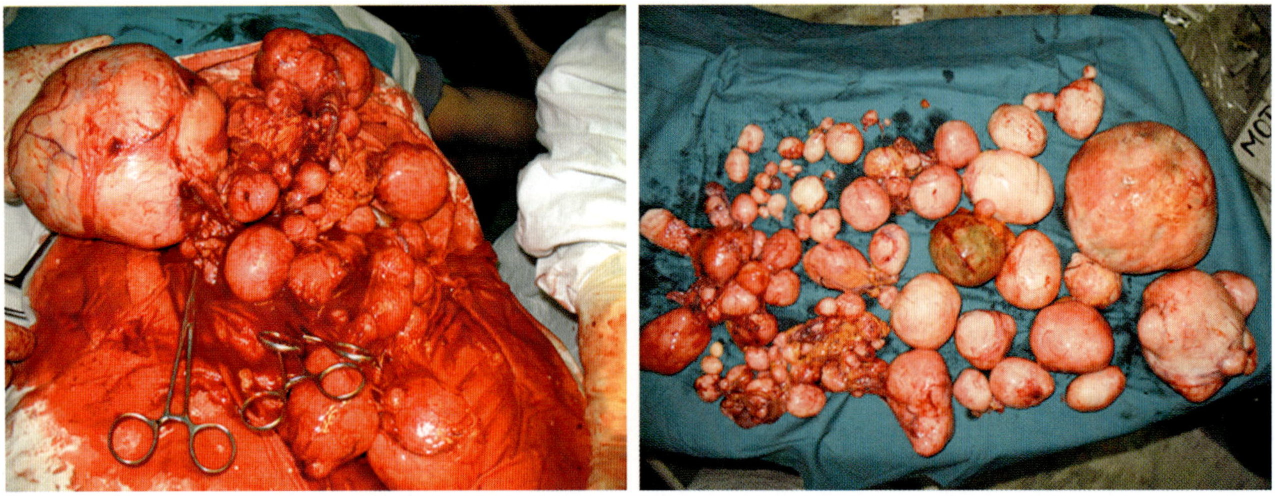

Fig. 13.1: Laparotomy picture showing multiple myomas studded over the peritoneal surface of omentum and bowel-peritoneal leiomyomatosis. The removed myomas are shown on the right side

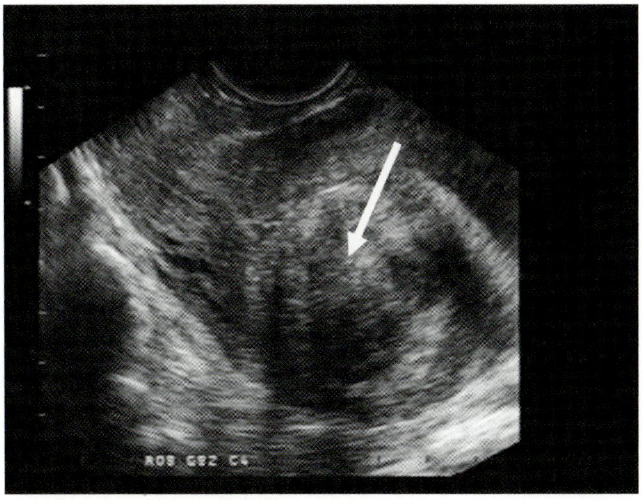

Fig. 13.2: TVS showing type II submucous myoma

13.7.1 Ultrasound

Ultrasound is a simple, rapid and relatively less expensive, side-effect free imaging modality to visualize myoma. Both TVS and TAS may have to be resorted to. Very large myoma extending to the abdomen should be evaluated by TAS. Myomas are usually hypoechoeic compared to the myometrium. TVS helps to evaluate myomas confined to the pelvis (Fig. 13.2). TVS is useful in diagnosing submucous myomas as small as 4-5 mm in size. Both TVS and TAS are used to identify position, size and number of myomas which are important before proceeding to myomectomy.

13.7.2 Sonohysterography

Submucous myomas can be clearly delineated by sonohysterography which will also help in making out the size and width of attachment of myoma. This information is important in planning hysteroscopic removal of myoma. Bleeding, discomfort and infection are the common complications of this procedure.

13.7.3 Doppler

Doppler examination might show different types of blood flow in myoma—high resistance as well as low resistance. Hence it will not help to differentiate between leiomyoma and leiomyosarcoma. However, in myoma the pattern of distribution of vessels will be different. Vessels in a myoma can be imaged around the periphery and the central area will be less vascular. In adenomyosis, vessels could be seen distributed equally throughout the lesion. This can be used to select patients for MR imaging which is the confirmatory imaging modality for adenomyosis.

13.7.4 MRI

MRI is more precise than ultrasound in the identification, mapping and counting of myomas and distinguishing myoma from adenomyosis.

13.7.5 CT

CT is less accurate than MRI, however CT angiography is useful in the evaluation of patients before uterine artery embolization.

13.7.6 Hysteroscopy

Hysteroscopy is resorted to in diagnosing very small myomas and distinguishing it from other lesions like intrauterine adhesions.

13.7.7 Hysterosalpingography

Hysterosalpingography used to be done for the diagnosis of submucous myomas. With the evolution of hysteroscopy and ultrasound, hysterosalpingography has no significant role in diagnosing leiomyomas.

13.8 CLASSIFICATION OF MYOMA

Myomata are classified according to the relation of myoma to the myometrium, endometrium and serosa.

1. *Intramural myoma (Fig. 13.3):* These are situated in the myometrium, but as they grow these can become partly subserous or submucous. The compressed myometrium around the myoma will form a pseudocapsule.
2. *Submucous myoma:* Myomas situated in close proximity to the endometrium are submucous. These are the most

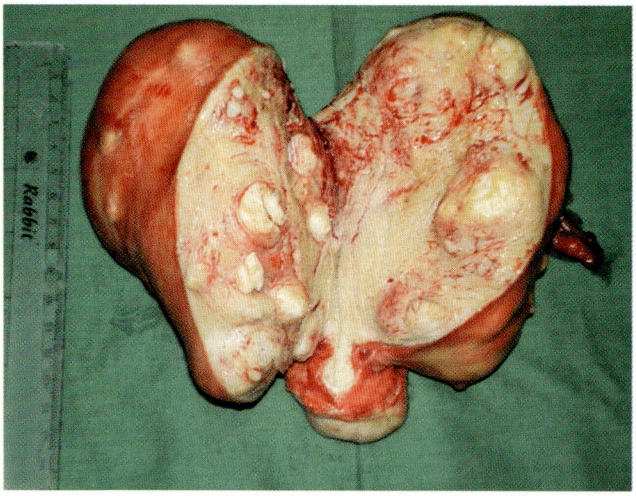

Fig. 13.3: Cut open specimen of uterus showing multiple intramural myomas. The patient was a 38-year-old multiparous lady who presented with dysmenorrhea and backache

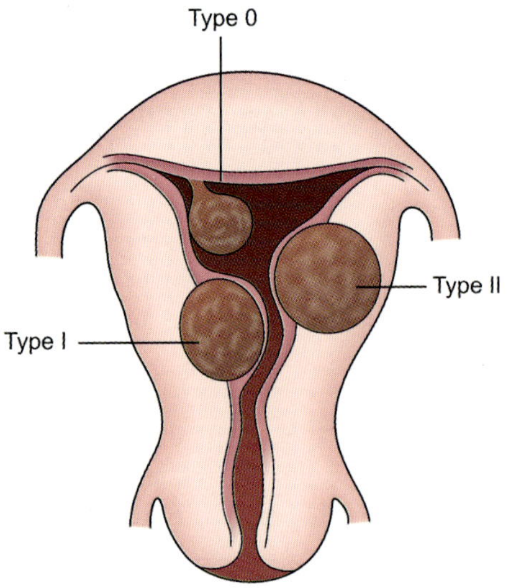

Fig. 13.4: Types of submucous fibroids (European Society of Hysteroscopy)

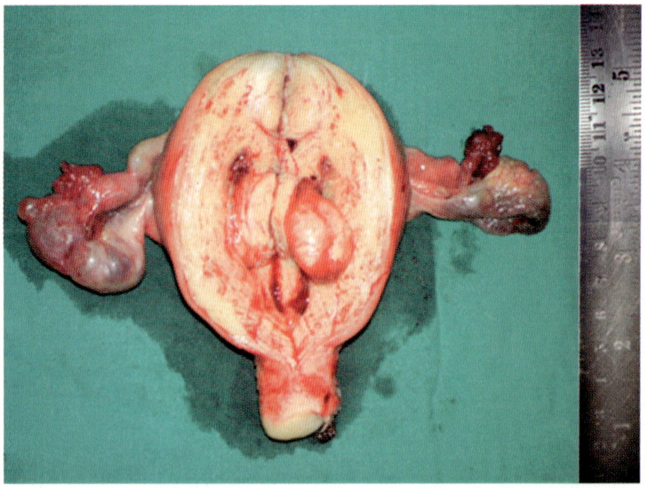

Fig. 13.5: Pan hysterectomy specimen with the uterus bisected to show type I submucous myoma in a 46-year-old lady who presented with severe menorrhagia and dysmenorrhea

symptomatic myomas. They can cause menorrhagia, dysmenorrhea, infertility and miscarriage. Extension of myoma into the uterine cavity can be of varying degrees. The portion protruding into the cavity is important in deciding the type of surgical treatment. Submucous myomas are classified by the European Society of Hysteroscopy into the following types (Fig. 13.4).

Type 0: These are pedunculated submucosal myomas located entirely in the uterine cavity

Type I: >50% of the myoma will be in the uterine cavity and <50% in the myometrium (Fig. 13.5).

Type II: >50% in the myometrium

In the classification described by Donnez et al an additional Type III is described where there are more than 2 submucosal and intramural myomas.

3. *Subserous myoma:* These are located beneath the covering peritoneum. They can grow into the peritoneal cavity and get pedunculated (Fig. 13.6). Sometime they may get attached to other intra-abdominal structures and attain blood supply from these structures. Gradually they become detached from the uterus and become wandering myomas or parasitic myomas. Myomas originating from the lateral wall can grow in between the leaves of the broad ligament to become a pseudo-broad ligament myoma. A true broad ligament myoma is one which arises in the broad ligament and is not continuous with the body of the uterus. Broad ligament myomas can also grow retroperitoneally. Myomas arising from the posterior aspect of cervix can grow between the rectum and vagina to reach the level of the perineal body. Anterior cervical myomas can grow anteriorly pushing the bladder upwards and anteriorly.

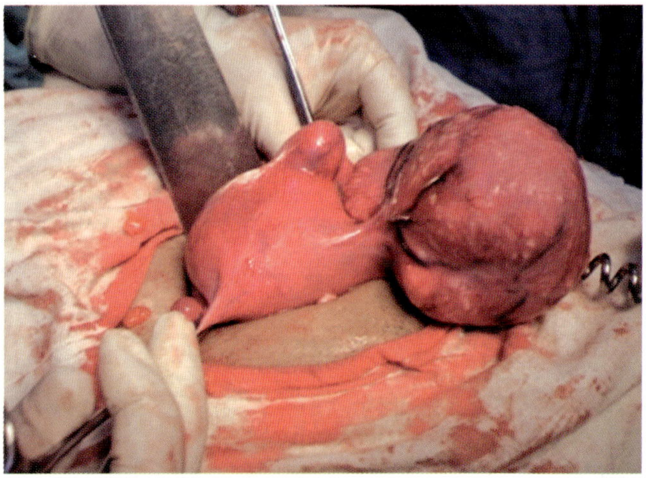

Fig. 13.6: Subserous pedunculated myoma arising from the anterior and lower aspect of uterine body. Patient presented with frequency of micturition

4. *Polypoidal:* Myomatous polyps can arise from the cervix and project into the vagina or even outside as a polyp (Fig. 13.7). Polyp arising from the fundus also can extrude out through the cervical canal and present as mass in the vagina which can be mistaken for chronic inversion of the uterus. The identification of cervical ring around the pedicle differentiates fibroid polyp from chronic inversion of the uterus. A uterine sound can be passed between the mass and the cervical rim if the mass is a polyp, whereas the sound cannot be passed in chronic inversion. Ultrasound examination also will help in differentiating between the two.

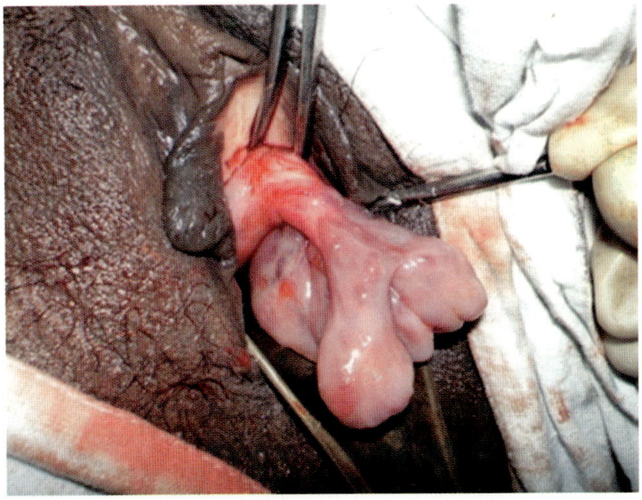

Fig. 13.7: Pedunculated polypoidal myoma arising from the anterior lip of cervix which presented as a mass extruding through vagina in a 42-year-old lady

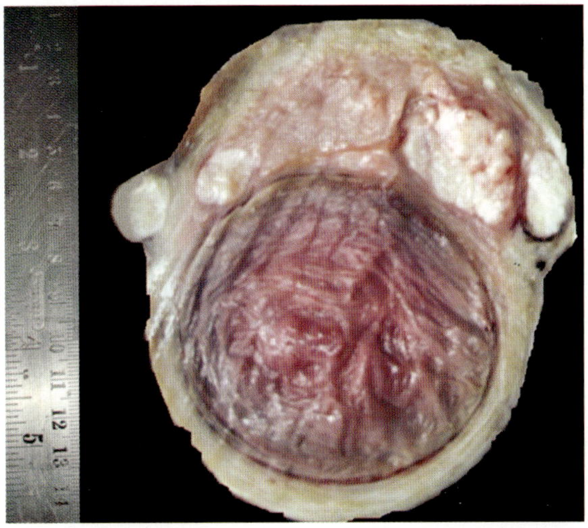

Fig. 13.8: Cut section of myoma showing red degeneration

13.9 DEGENERATIONS

Myomas can undergo various types of degenerations mainly due to lack of blood supply.

1. *Hyaline degeneration:* It is the commonest degeneration found in myoma. Smooth muscle of myoma is replaced by hyaline material.
2. *Cystic degeneration:* Cystic degeneration usually follows hyaline degeneration.
3. *Red degeneration:* It is common during pregnancy. It is a hemorrhagic infarction which involves the entire lesion (Fig. 13.8).
4. Calcification.

13.10 MANAGEMENT OF MYOMA

With widespread use of ultrasound, even a small myoma which is totally asymptomatic can be diagnosed. However, only symptomatic myomas and those which are bigger than 12 week size need to be removed. ACOG recommends removal of only symptomatic myomas.

13.10.1 Medical Treatment

GnRH Analog

GnRH induced artificial menopause causes inhibition of gonadal steroid secretion. Consequently, the vascularity and size of myoma will be reduced. The efficacy of GnRH treatment was evaluated in a systematic review of all the randomized controlled trials. The advantages as well as disadvantages of GnRH treatment were studied. It was found that as a result of GnRH pre-treatment more myomas could be dealt with laparoscopically. If a midline incision is planned due to the large size of a myoma, it can be avoided by preoperative GnRH treatment. Likewise, for women who needed hysterectomy, the vaginal route could be made feasible by achieving reduction in the size of myoma. GnRH treatment for a short period of 4 weeks prior to hysteroscopic myomectomy reduces the size and vascularity so that there will be reduction in bleeding as well as operating time. In the case of a severely anemic patient, the amenorrhea produced by GnRH will give sufficient time for building up the hemoglobin level.

However, GnRH treatment has disadvantages also. It is contented that prior GnRH treatment will make enucleation of myoma difficult. As myoma size is decreased smaller ones will go unnoticed so that it will escape removal, resulting in re-growth after surgery.

It is advisable to treat patients with GnRH prior to hysterectomy for large myomas, so that more hysterectomies can be done laparoscopically, vaginally or through a low transverse incision. It cannot be advised as a definitive treatment for symptomatic myomas in young patients, as long-term treatment causes side effects of hypoestrogenism like osteoporosis and hot flushes which can be minimised by estrogen-progestin add-back treatment. Another disadvantage is that when treatment is stopped, myoma will grow and attain the original size with the reappearance of symptoms.

Antiprogesterone: Mifepristone

Mifepristone (RU 486) given continuously at a dose of 25-50 mg daily is reported to cause shrinkage of uterine myomas, the effect being similar to GnRH therapy. Even though amenorrhea will be produced estrogen suppression will be less profound than that with GnRH therapy. Efficacy of low dose (5-10 mg) mifepristone,[16] for long-term is being evaluated for the treatment of myoma.

13.10.2 Expectant Management

Asymptomatic myomas do not need surgical intervention provided they are not very big. However, the diagnosis should be certain and the patient should be periodically reviewed. Rapid growth of leiomyoma should arouse suspicion of the possibility of leiomyosarcoma and should be intervened.

13.10.3 Myomectomy

Enucleation and removal of myoma, leaving the uterus for child bearing function was pioneered by Victor Boney in the 19th century. Myomectomy carries greater risk of primary and reactionary hemorrhage as well as post-operative adhesion formation compared to hysterectomy. Hence, it is usually preferred for women who wish to conserve their childbearing function. However, with the evolution of methods to reduce hemorrhage and post-operative adhesion formation, it can be preferred over hysterectomy even for women who have completed family depending on patient's choice. When myomas are diagnosed in infertile women, other causes of infertility should be evaluated before deciding on myomectomy. Most patients with myomas might conceive spontaneously. There is evidence that submucous myomas and myomatous polyps adversely affect fertility. Intramural myomas which distort the uterine cavity may be thought to interfere with fertility. Evidence on this is conflicting. Subserous myomas appear to have no effect on fertility.

Even though there are several treatment options for myomas, they have their limitations. Laparoscopic myomectomy is limited by the size and number of myomas and needs great surgical expertise. Only small submucous myomas can be removed by hysteroscopic surgery. Uterine artery embolization also is not recommended for very large myomas. It has the disadvantage of chronic vaginal discharge, premature ovarian failure as well as adverse influence on fertility.

While proceeding with myomectomy, due to uncontrollable hemorrhage, very rarely hysterectomy may have to be resorted to. Hence routinely, the patient's informed consent for hysterectomy should be obtained. However with proper planning and adequate precautions to reduce intraoperative hemorrhage, hysterectomy is seldom necessary.

For optimal outcome the following factors are important:

1. Careful preoperative mapping of myomas
2. Measures to reduce hemorrhage
3. Minimize adhesion formation

Preoperative Mapping of Myoma

Preoperative mapping of myoma with ultrasound or preferably with MRI will help in planning the incision on the uterus as well as removing all the myomas, which will reduce recurrence.

Measures to Reduce Hemorrhage

Myomas cause compression of surrounding myometrium to form a pseudo-capsule. Even though the myoma is not vascular, the surrounding myometrium will be more vascular due to the compression of venous plexus by the myoma. Enucleation of the myoma by cutting the pseudocapsule can lead to profuse hemorrhage. This can be reduced in several ways.

GnRH depot administered 3 months before surgery causes shrinkage of the myoma as well as vascularity. However, several disadvantages of such therapy have been put forward by researchers. Enucleation of myoma is reported to be difficult following GnRH therapy. Another disadvantage attributed is that myomas made smaller by GnRH therapy are likely to be missed during myomectomy. Still GnRH[17] pre-treatment can be resorted to achieve reduction in the size of myoma in situations where the myomas are very large so that it can be removed either vaginally or laparoscopically or through a low transverse incision if laparotomy is deemed necessary. Preoperative uterine artery embolization can be done in the presence of large myoma, when heavy bleeding which is likely to risk conversion to hysterectomy is anticipated.

Injection of vasopressin into the myometrium significantly reduces intraoperative hemorrhage. 20 U of the drug diluted in 20 ml normal saline can be injected into the surface of the myoma before incising the capsule.

Antifibrinolytic agent like Tranexamic acid has also been tried in an effort to reduce intraoperative hemorrhage. Even though it was found to be effective in reducing postoperative blood loss, there was no significant reduction in intra-operative blood loss.

Other agents tried are oxytocin, MESNA and vaginal mesoprostol. However, a Cochrane review has not found significant evidence.

Use of electrocautery for cutting the capsule and enucleation of the myoma causes less blood loss than the use of scalpel. There is limited evidence from a few RCTs that misoprostol, vasopressin, bupivacaine plus epinephrine, tourniquet and MESNA may reduce bleeding during myomectomy. However, there is no evidence that oxytocin and morcellation have an effect in intraoperative blood loss. There is need for adequately powered RCTs to shed more light on the effectiveness of different interventions in reducing blood loss during myomectomy.[18]

Minimize Adhesion Formation

Use of synthetic suture material rather than catgut for suturing the myoma bed can minimize adhesion formation. Suturing the serosal layer with base-ball sutures may reduce adhesion formation as it buries all raw surfaces. During surgery, drying of tissue should be avoided by irrigation. Bowel surfaces should be covered with moist mops.

Surgical Technique

Prophylactic antibiotics as well as thromboprophylaxis should be considered as in any other surgery. A No. 8 Foley catheter should be inserted in to the uterine cavity before the procedure and methylene blue injected so that inadvertent entry into the cavity can be clearly detected.

Conventional myomectomy demands great surgical skill so as to reduce hemorrhage, accurate reconstruction of the uterus to regain anatomic normalcy, as well as to reduce adhesion formation and recurrence. The abdomen can be opened through Pfannenstiel or Maylard incision. Large myomas which extend above the umbilical region need vertical incision. It is advisable to resort to a vertical incision for repeat myomectomy also due to the possible presence of bowel adhesions. After opening the abdomen, the pelvic organs should be carefully inspected and the anatomic distortion should be assessed. The uterus with the myoma should be exteriorized. The bowel should be packed with a moist mop. A myoma screw may be used to deliver the uterus. It is preferable to remove the myomas through anterior and midline incisions. Posterior incisions were traditionally avoided for fear of adhesion formation. A posterior myoma may be reached through an anterior hood incision, avoiding entry into the uterine cavity. However, with the advent of synthetic suture materials and improved surgical techniques as mentioned earlier, adhesions are much less. Hence, a posterior myoma need not be approached through an anterior incision transecting the uterine cavity. It can very well be removed through an incision on the posterior wall of the uterus and the uterine incision meticulously closed using polyglactin 910 sutures.

The capsule of the myoma is incised with cautery and the blood vessels should be caught with artery forceps and coagulated to reduce hemorrhage. The plain of cleavage can be reached by pulling on the myoma. Further enucleation can be done with fingers. All bleeding points are coagulated and the myoma bed closed in multiple layers without leaving dead space. In case the cavity is entered, it should be repaired. As mentioned earlier it is preferable to insert base-ball sutures for the outermost layer which includes the myometrium and serosa. While incising the capsule and suturing, care should be taken not to occlude the intramural portion of the fallopian tube.

Laparoscopic Myomectomy

Laparoscopic myomectomy has the advantage of short hospital stay, fast recovery, less postoperative pain and less adhesion formation. The number and size of myomas which can be removed laparoscopically depends upon the expertise of the surgeon. The surgeon needs expertise in endoscopic suturing. Subserous, large submucous and intramural myomas can be removed laparoscopically. It is doubtful whether removal of subserous and intramural myoma will improve fertility. However, their removal will prevent later enlargement of myoma and distortion of the uterine cavity. Large myomas can be removed by using a morcellator.

Rupture uterus in pregnancy and labor following laparoscopic myomectomy is reported to be more, when compared to open myomectomy (>1%). This is attributed to inadequate repair of uterine incision endoscopically. With multi-layer suturing of the uterine incision, scar rupture following laparoscopic myomectomy also is much less.

A Cochrane review has found no difference in fertility outcome between women who had laparoscopic myomectomy compared to those who had myomectomy[19] by laparotomy.

Hysteroscopic Myomectomy

Hysteroscopic myomectomy is the treatment of choice for women who have submucous myomas or myomas causing menstrual complaints, infertility or recurrent pregnancy loss. Myomas with <50% intramural component can be considered for hysteroscopic removal. Type 0 myomas and Type I myomas <3 cm diameter are the ideal ones for hysteroscopic removal. Larger myomas, more than 4 cm in size can be made smaller by preoperative treatment with GnRH. Routine preoperative administration of GnRH analog for 4 weeks prior to the procedure decreases vascularity and improves visualization thereby reducing operating time.

Monopolar current is usually used for the procedure. Hence, the distention medium should be a non-electrolyte solution like 1.5% glycine, sorbitol or mannitol. Absorption of large quantities of glycine can lead to pulmonary edema especially in elderly patients. Bipolar instruments are presently available which helps to perform surgery in saline medium.

Recurrence of Myoma

The reported recurrence rate of myoma is as high as 50% in 5 years. Whether this represents re-growth of existing tumor or growth of small tumors missed at initial surgery or new myomas has not been established. Large myoma at initial surgery, presence of multiple myomas, increased penetration into the myometrium and residual tissue after initial removal are factors associated with increased recurrence[20] rate.

13.10.4 Uterine Artery Embolization (UAE)

Embolization of the uterine artery used to be practiced as a treatment for postpartum hemorrhage as well as post-surgical bleeding. Inspired by the relief of myoma related symptoms in women who underwent uterine artery embolization for postpartum hemorrhage Ravina et al first introduced the procedure for treating women with symptomatic myomas[21] as an alternative to hysterectomy in the year 1995. Myomectomy is the standard of care for treating symptomatic myomas in women who wish to preserve childbearing function.

Diagnosis of myoma should be confirmed before embolization. Since infection is a complication of the procedure, pelvic infection is a contraindication. Allergy to contrast media and impaired renal function are also contraindications.

Procedure

Under radiologic guidance, a catheter is passed through the femoral artery and the uterine arteries are reached. The uterine arteries are catheterized selectively and embolized with non-spherical polyvinyl alcohol particles. Since this has the disadvantage of aggregation and subsequent recanalization of the embolized uterine artery, gelatin coated trisacryl microspheres were developed which has the advantage of more uniform embolization of perimyoma plexus.

Analgesia

Pain, during and after the procedure is side effect, but is reported to have individual variations. Pain control can be achieved by epidural analgesia or by opiates along with non-steroidal anti-inflammatory drugs.

Side Effects and Complications

Postembolization syndrome: This is a recognized complication of the procedure. It is characterized by low grade fever, malaise and discomfort which are usually observed from 3 to 7 days after embolization. Usually it will subside by itself. At times it can be severe.

Infection: Serious infection necessitating intervention is seen to occur in 1-2% of patients after the procedure.

Myoma extrusion: Submucous myomas will get extruded out through the cervix spontaneously. Rarely minor surgical assistance may be needed for removal.

Amenorrhea: Amenorrhea following embolization occurs in about 1% of the patients. The incidence is more among women nearing menopause. The reason may be premature menopause due to the effect on the ovary.

Efficiency

Improvement of menorrhagia is reported to range from 83-92%. Mean myoma volume reduction reported is 42-64%.

Two recent trials compared the usefulness of UAE with hysterectomy. One is the REST trial (Randomized controlled trial of Embolization vs. Surgical Treatment for myomas). Quality of life after one year follow-up was the same for both UAE as well as hysterectomy. There was a highly significant reduction in the duration of hospital stay as well as pain in the group who had UAE.[21] The other is the EMMY trial (EMbolization vs hysterectoMY for symptomatic uterine myoma disease). This was a prospective randomized multicentric trial which compared UAE with hysterectomy. There were no significant differences with regard to symptom control or incidence of major or minor complications. Re-interventions in the form of hysterectomy or hysteroscopic removal of necrotic myoma[22] were needed following UAE in a few patients. One death occurred due to sepsis.

Fertility after Uterine Artery Embolization

According to present guideline UAE should not be advised for women who have not completed family. However pregnancy has been reported following UAE. Rupture uterus in pregnancy following UAE is also a concern.

13.10.5 Laparoscopic Myolysis

Laparoscopic myolysis using Nd:YAG laser evolved as a method of treating symptomatic myomas in the 1980s. Later bipolar coagulation was developed as an alternative to the use of laser. Myolysis[25] is found to be effective in causing shrinkage and reduction of vascularity of myoma with subsequent alleviation of symptoms. The method can be resorted to in treating women with symptomatic myomas. However the evidence on the effectiveness of myolysis is limited.

13.10.6. MR Guided Focused Ultrasound (MRgFUS)

High intensity focussed ultrasound is directed under MR guidance to achieve ablation of myoma without producing harm to overlying organs or skin. Even though it has the advantage of non-invasiveness, the high cost of MRI is a disadvantage. Preliminary data are encouraging. Successful reduction[23] in fibroid related symptoms was reported in 79.3% of treated women. MRI guided laser ablations as well as radiofrequency ablation are also under trial.

13.10.7 Hysterectomy for Myoma

For symptomatic women who have completed childbearing, hysterectomy may be considered as definitive treatment. Before deciding on an alternative treatment modality like uterine artery embolization, this option should be discussed with the patient. The route of hysterectomy, vaginal, abdominal or laparoscopic depends upon the size, site and number of myomas. The size can be reduced by pre-operative treatment with GnRH as discussed earlier. The type of surgery also depends upon the skill of the surgeon.

Hysterectomy should be anticipated to be difficult in the following situations:

1. Large cervical myoma
2. Broad ligament myoma
3. Large myoma which grows retroperitoneally or into the rectovaginal septum
4. Associated endometriotic adhesions and pelvic inflammatory disease
5. Prior myomectomy because of adhesions with bowel, bladder, etc.

After entry into the abdomen, anatomy should be delineated. The uterus along with the myoma should be delivered out of the incision. If it is difficult to deliver the uterus out, cutting and clamping the round ligaments will make the uterus more mobile. All adhesions should be released. Enucleation of large myomas will make hysterectomy easier. In the case of broad ligament myoma and cervical myoma injury to the ureter should be avoided by enucleation of the myoma (Figs 13.9A and B) preferably after ligating the uterine vessels. In the presence of posterior cervical myoma, there is risk of injury to rectosigmoid. This can be avoided by incising the recto-uterine peritoneum as high as possible and pushing the rectosigmoid with the attached peritoneum downwards. Cervical myoma should be enucleated after bisecting the uterus. Anterior cervical myomas will push the bladder upwards. Bladder injury can be avoided by identifying the uterovesical peritoneum and pushing the bladder down.

13.11 SMOOTH MUSCLE TUMOR OF UNCERTAIN MALIGNANT POTENTIAL (STUMP)

The majority of uterine smooth muscle tumors can be classified into clearly benign tumors or obviously malignant with atypical nuclear features and a high mitotic index. However, there remains a group of tumors with intermediate degree of mitotic activity and nuclear atypia. These are termed smooth muscle tumor of uncertain malignant potential which is a variant of leiomyoma and cannot be grouped

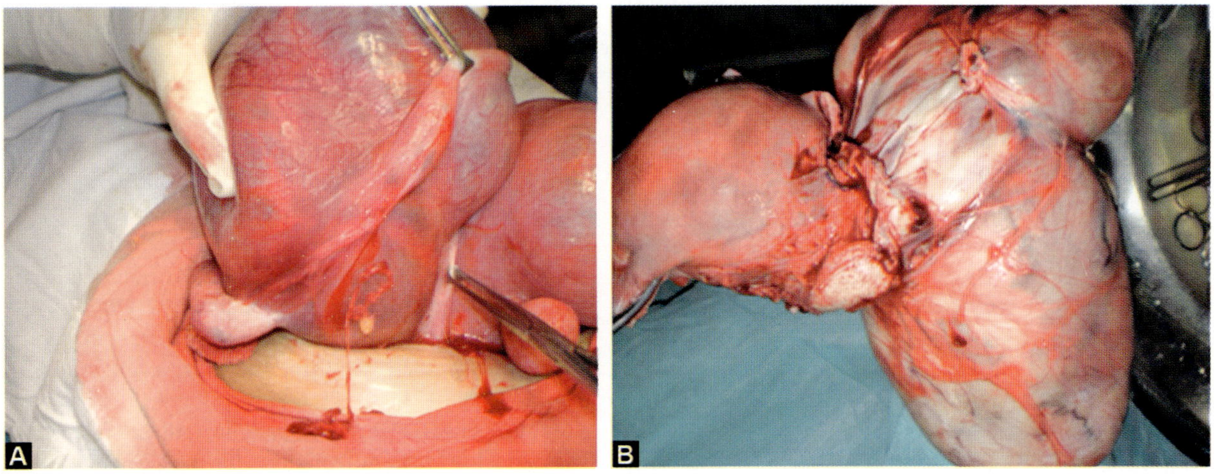

Figs 13.9A and B: Opening the peritoneum after cutting the round ligament to remove a broad ligament myoma in order to avoid injury to the ureter (A). Hysterectomy specimen with the broad ligament fibroid is seen (B)

either under leiomyoma or leiomyosarcoma. Tumors with 5-10 mitoses/10 high-power fields and with mild or moderate cellular atypia as well as those with 2-4 mitoses/10 high-power fields and severe cellular atypia are classified as tumors of uncertain malignant potential. The histology is usually characterized by coagulative tumor necrosis. It can be considered as a low-grade malignant neoplasm. Only a few cases are reported in the literature. The clinical course is unpredictable. After surgery, it might metastasize to distant sites several years later. Hence, long-term follow-up is advised. No consensus on mode of the treatment and adjuvant therapy has yet been reached.

13.12 CONCLUSION

Myomas are the commonest benign tumors of the uterus occurring in the childbearing age group. 30% of the women within the age group of 35 years will have myomas. 50% of women with myoma would be asymptomatic. The commonest symptoms are abnormal bleeding and pressure symptoms. Abnormal bleeding due to small myomas(<12 weeks size) can be treated by medications or by LNG IUS insertion. Those who do not respond can be treated by surgery. Submucosal and intramural myomas which distort the uterine cavity can compromise fertility. Hence, surgical intervention is indicated in women who have infertility or repeated abortions. Most myomas will not cause problems during pregnancy. Only symptomatic myomas need surgical intervention. Leiomyosarcoma is thought to occur *de novo* and is not due to malignant transformation of leiomyoma. Women who have leiomyosarcoma usually presents as post menopausal bleeding. However, it can occur in the child bearing age group as well. Since they cannot be conclusively diagnosed by imaging modalities, rapid increase in the size of a myoma should arouse a suspicion of leiomyosarcoma and should be taken for surgical intervention. Fearing sarcomatous change, small asymptomatic myomas need not be treated. Other than myomectomy and hysterectomy, there are several treatment options available for symptomatic myomas. Medical treatment with GnRH is not advised as a definitive treatment for young women. Its use is in reducing the size of myoma so as to alter the route and type of surgery. UAE has evolved as an alternative to surgical treatment. Other non-invasive treatment options like MRgFUS need sophisticated equipment. Treatment of myomas should be based on the patient's choice, her symptoms, need for childbearing as well as equipment and expertise available.

REFERENCES

1. Andersen J, DyReyes VM, Barbieri RL, et al. Leiomyoma primary cultures have elevated transcriptional response to estrogen compared with autologous myometrial cultures. J Soc Gynecol Investig 1995;2:542-51.
2. Al-Hendy A, Salama SA. Ethnic differences of estrogen receptor-a polymorphism is associated withhigher prevalence of uterine leiomyomas in black Americans. Fertil Steril 2006;86:686-93.
3. Practice Committee of the American Society for Reproductive Medicine. Myomas and reproductive function. Fertil Steril 2004; 82(Suppl. 1).
4. Casini ML, Rossi F, Agostini R, et al. Effects of the position of myomas on fertility. Gynecol Endocrinol 2006;22:106-09.
5. Richards PA, Richards PD, Tiltman AJ. The ultrastructure of fibromyomatous myometrium and itsrelationship to infertility. Hum Reprod Update 1998;4:520-5.
6. Check JH, Choe JK, Lee G, et al. The effect on IVF outcome of small intramural myomas not compressing the uterine cavity as determined by a prospective matched control study. Hum Reprod 2002;17:1244-8.
7. Hart R, Khalaf Y, Yeong CT, et al. A prospective controlled study of the effect of intramural uterine myomas on the outcome of assisted conception. Hum Reprod 2001;16: 2411-7.
8. Bulletti C, Ziegler D, Levi Setti P, et al. Myomas, pregnancy outcome, and in vitro fertilization. Ann NY Acad Sci 2004;1034:84-92.
9. Fernandez H, Sefrioui O, Virelizier C, et al. Hysteroscopic resection of submucosal myomas in patients with infertility. Hum Reprod 2001; 16:1489-92.
10. Shokeir TA. Hysteroscopic management in submucous myomas to improve fertility. Arch Gynnecol Obstet 2005;273:504.
11. Buttram Jr. VC, Reiter RC. Uterine leiomyomata: etiology, symptomatology, and management. Another retrospective study reported a reduction in abortion rate following myomectomy. Fertil Steril 1981;36:433-5.
12. Li TC, Mortimer R, Cook ID. Myomectomy: A retrospective study to examine reproductive performance before after Human Reprod 1999;14:1735-40.
13. Coronado GD, Marshall LM, Schwartz SM. Complications in pregnancy, labor, and delivery with uterine leiomyomas: a population-based study. Obstet Gynecol 2000;95:764-9.
14. Qidwai GI, Caughey AB, Jacoby AF. Obstetric outcomes in women with sonographically identified uterine leiomyomata. Obstet Gynecol 2006;107:376-82.
15. Davis JL, Ray-Mazumder S, Hobel CJ, et al. Uterine leiomyomas in pregnancy: a prospective study. Obstet Gynecol 1990;75:41-4.
16. Eisinger SH, Fiscella J, Bonfiglio, et al. Open label study of ultra low-dose mifepristone for the treatment of uterine leiomyomata. Eur J Obstet Gynecol Reprod Biol 2009;142(2): 215-8.

17. Lethaby A, Vollenhoven B, Sowter M. Pre-operative GnRH analogue therapy before hysterectomy or myomectomy for uterine myomas. Cochrane Database of Systematic Reviews 2001;Issue 2. Art. No.: CD000547. DOI:
18. Ongnyuy EJ, Wiysonge CS. Interventions to reduce haemorrhage during myomectomy for myomas. Cochrane Database of Systematic Reviews 2007, Issue 1. Art. No.: CD005355. DOI: 10.1002/14651858.CD005355.pub2.
19. Grifiths A, D'Angelo A, Amso N. Surgical treatment of myomas for subfertility. Cochrane Database of Systematic Reviews 2006, Issue 3. Art. No.: CD003857. DOI: 10.1002/14651858.CD003857.pub2.
20. Hanafi M. Predictors of leiomyoma recurrence after myomectomy. Obstet gynaecol 2005;105:877-81.
21. Uterine-Artery Embolization versus Surgery for Symptomatic Uterine Myomas. The New England Journal of Medicine 2007;356:360-70.
22. P. Burn. J McCall, R Chinn, J Healy. Embolization of uterine myomas. British Journal of Radiology 1999;72:159-61.
23. Volkers NA, Hehenkamp WJ, Birnie E, et al. Uterine artery embolization versus hysterectomy in the treatment of symptomatic uterine myomas: 2 years' outcome from the randomized EMMY trial. Am J Obstet Gynecol 2007;196(6):519. e1-e11.
24. Hindley J, Gedroyc, WM, Regan L, et al. MRI guidance of focused ultrasound therapy of uterine fibroids: early results. Am J Roentgenol 2004;183:1713-9.
25. Donnez, et al. Laparoscopic myolysis. Human Reproduction Update 2000;6(6):609-13.

14 Benign Vulvar Conditions

B Presannakumari

14.1 INTRODUCTION

Most vulvar lesions occur commonly in postmenopausal women with itching and soreness being the major symptoms. Depending upon gross changes occurring in the vulva, several conditions had been described previously. These are leukoplakia, lichen sclerosus et atrophicus, atrophic and hyperplastic vulvitis and kraurosis vulvae. Later it was noticed that malignancies rarely occur in these conditions. Malignant changes can be predicted by the presence of cellular atypia at biopsy of the lesion. However, if there is associated lichen sclerosus, risk of malignancy is more (5%).[1] In 1966, Jeffcoat coined the term chronic vulvar dystrophy to include all these conditions, as the epithelial changes in these conditions are variable and interchangeable. To make management simple, the International Society for the Study of Vulvar Diseases (ISSVD) recommended a new system to study such vulvar lesions. The ISSVD[2] recommended that the term dystrophy be replaced by 'non-neoplastic epithelial disorders of the skin and mucosa (Table 14.1).'

14.2 NON-NEOPLASTIC EPITHELIAL DISORDERS OF THE SKIN AND MUCOSA

Non-neoplastic epithelial disorders of the skin and mucosa include:

1. Lichen sclerosus
2. Lichen planus
3. Squamous hyperplasia
4. Other vulvar dermatoses

14.2.1 Lichen Sclerosus

Lichen sclerosus usually occur in postmenopausal women and prepubertal girls but can occur at any age. The

Table 14.1: Classification of preinvasive vulvar disease

Squamous VIN	
• VIN 1	Mild dyskaryosis
• VIN 2	Moderate dyskaryosis
• VIN 3	Severe dysplasia, undifferentiated type (warty/bowenoid)
	Severe dysplasia, differentiated
• VIN 3	Type (basaloid)
Non-squamous VIN	
Paget's disease	
In situ melanoma	
Other conditions that may be premalignant	
Lichen sclerosus	
Lichen planus	
Squamous hyperplasia	

Source: JM Kirwan, JJO Herod Premalignant vulvar lesions. Current Obstetrics and Gynecol. 2002:12:90-96

symptoms are pruritus, dyspareunia and burning sensation. Decrease in subcutaneous fat is characteristic, leading to small labia minora and labia majora. The clitoris shrinks with loss of clitoral hood and the vulval outlet will become constricted. The affected area will be thick parchment like and whitish, often with cracks. The lesion is usually symmetrical often extending to the perianal area. Biopsy confirms the diagnosis. Since invasive lesion is seen associated in about 5% of these women, all suspicious areas should be biopsied. The condition is not usually associated with HPV infection. The etiology is unknown. An autoimmune etiology due to antibodies against a component of skin has been suggested. Antibodies to extracellular matrix protein-1 have been detected in women who have lichen sclerosus.[3]

Treatment is with administration of topical steroids. Initially a potent steroid like 0.05% Clobetasol can be used.[4,5] A less potent topical steroid can be continued long-term as maintenance therapy. Vulvectomy is advised only if associated VIN or invasive lesion is present. Follow-up is essential due to its association with malignancy.

14.2.2 Lichen Planus

Lichen planus is an inflammatory condition of the vulva. It can also be part of a widespread disease. Symptoms are pruritus, burning sensation, ulceration and dyspareunia. Signs include violaceous papules on the labia majora and genitocrural folds. Malignancy is usually not an association. Application of topical steroids is the treatment of choice. If no relief occurs, oral steroids can be advised.[6]

14.2.3 Squamous Hyperplasia

Squamous hyperplasia is a thickened hyperkeratotic lesion occurring usually as discrete lesions. It commonly presents as pruritus vulva. The condition arises due to constant scratching in response to irritants like vaginal discharge. Biopsy of the lesion helps to exclude malignancy. Management should comprise alleviation of aggravating factors. Local corticosteroid ointments will suffice as treatment.

14.2.4 Other Vulvar Dermatoses

Seborrheic dermatoses, cherry hemangiomas and allergic conditions also can occur in the vulval skin.

14.3 VULVAR INTRAEPITHELIAL NEOPLASIA

As in the case of cancer of the cervix, recognition of the premalignant lesions offer an opportunity for prevention of vulval carcinoma.

Four major premalignant conditions were described previously.

1. Erythroplasia of Queyrat
2. Bowen's disease
3. Carcinoma *in situ* simplex
4. Paget's disease

In the year 1986, the International Society for the Study of Vulvar Disease (ISSVD) coined the term vulvar intraepithelial neoplasia (VIN) to include all these conditions, as they are gross variants of the same disease process. The Society's 8th World Congress in the year 2006 revised this classification.[6] Based on cellular differentiation, nuclear abnormalities, maturation disturbances and mitotic activity, VIN is graded as VIN I, VIN II, and VIN III. In VIN I, the changes are seen in the lower third of the epithelium. In VIN III, these changes are seen all through the epithelium while VIN II lies in between these two. In the presence of HPV infection, perinuclear halo and other changes of viral infection like displacement of the nuclei by viral protein, thickened cell borders, binucleation and multinucleation are common. HPV 6 and 11 are seen in association with vulvar condyloma whereas HPV 16 is detected in > 80% of VIN. Other types of HPV infection associated with VIN are 18, 33 and 39.

There are two types of invasive cancers of the vulva (Table 14.2). The one which occurs in younger women is recognized to occur from the precursor lesion VIN and is associated with HPV infection. These tumors are multifocal and carry better prognosis. In 40% of these women,

Table 14.2: Preinvasive vulval cancer–characteristics based on age

Younger age	*Older age*
HPV 16 association	No association with HPV infection
CIN association	Lichen sclerosus association
Multifocal disease	Unifocal disease
Keratinizing (well-differentiated VIN III)	Higher risk for squamous carcinoma
Smoking history strong association	
Warty or bowenoid	

premalignant conditions of the cervix are seen associated. The other type occurring in older women is usually unifocal, carries a poor prognosis and is usually seen in association with lichen sclerosus. Hence, lichen sclerosus also may possibly be regarded as a premalignant condition. Paget's disease is a non-squamous intraepithelial lesion of the vulva which can at times be invasive as well.

14.3.1 Incidence

Over the past few decades, there has been an increase in the incidence of VIN. Epidemiological studies have revealed that this cannot be attributed to increased detection rates by clinicians, but is due to an actual increase secondary to the higher incidence of HPV infection. The mean age of VIN has also decreased from 60 to 35. The incidence is very high among women who are immunocompromised either due to an HIV infection or due to the use of immuno-suppressant drugs as in renal transplant recipients.

14.3.2 Natural History of VIN

VIN carries about 10-15% risk of progression to invasive cancer.

14.3.3 Prevention

As HPV is associated with a very high proportion of VIN, vaccination against HPV goes a long way in preventing VIN and invasive cancer of the vulva as in the case of cancer of the cervix. Currently, a vaccine targeted at HPV 6, 11, 16 and 18 is available in the market (Gardasil™).

14.3.4 Clinical Features

The most common symptom is burning sensation in the vulvar region. Itching and dyspareunia may also be complained of. Sometimes the woman might notice the abnormal area on self-examination. VIN can be asymptomatic in some women so that the diagnosis might be incidental.

14.3.5 Diagnosis

The vulva should be carefully examined when women present with symptoms like itching, soreness or dyspareunia. It is ideal that a dermatologist also be present for the examination. On gross appearance the pattern can be of different types. Usually the lesions appear as raised hyperkeratotic areas. The disease can affect any region of the vulva. In about 81%, the labia are affected; the perineum is involved in 41% and the clitoris in 5%. The perineal lesions are most likely to progress to invasive disease.

Careful colposcopic examination of the vulva is advised to locate the abnormal area so that a biopsy can be targeted. Locating the abnormal area by painting with toluidine blue has currently been replaced by colposcopic examination.[7] The abnormal area can be located by the presence of abnormal vascular pattern. Identification of abnormal vascular pattern is the criterion for identifying invasive disease as in the case of cancer of the cervix. High grade lesions can appear as white, red or gray papillomatous areas. Biopsy and histological examination is the only method of distinguishing between invasive disease and VIN. Hence biopsies should be taken from all the abnormal areas. Large lesions can be managed by excision biopsy and primary closure of the wound.

14.3.6 Management

Proper management of VIN is important in preventing invasive cancer of the vulva. It should be kept in mind that a certain proportion of women who have VIN will progress to invasive lesion. Also, an occult invasive lesion can co-exist with VIN. Since, VIN associated with HPV infection occurs in younger women, psychosexual aspects should be considered before deciding on the type of surgery.

Surgical Management

The two modes of surgical management usually adopted are:

1. Excisional treatment
2. Ablative treatment

Excisional treatment

The type of excisional treatment depends on the size, site as well as the age of the patient. Excision of the abnormal area gives the opportunity to have histopathological examination. Underlying invasive disease is reported in about 10-20% at histopathological examination. Wide local excision should be preferred for younger women. Since VIN lesions usually extend to a depth of about 2 mm, a 3 mm deep excised tissue should be ensured. It is also important to remove 5 mm of grossly disease free margin.[8] After excision, recurrence is common (up to 35%). Hence, long-term follow- up is required. Extensive disease can be managed by skinning or superficial vulvectomy. For recurrent VIN III lesions too, superficial vulvectomy is the treatment of choice. In the case of Paget's disease, the histological abnormality extends beyond the margin of the gross lesion so that surgical excision is likely to leave positive margins causing recurrence. Hence wide excision is advised. Since recurrent Paget's disease too remain *in situ*, they can also be treated by a repeat wide excision.

Ablative treatment

VIN can be treated by laser vaporization. It has the advantage of treating large areas of the vulva without resorting to skin grafting.[9] However, ablative treatment gives lesser cure rates than excisional treatment. The failure of laser ablation is due to the inadequate destruction of deeper areas like the skin appendages. Laser ablation should be preferred in younger women as mutilation is minimal. Lesions involving the periclitoral and periurethral regions can be treated by ablation. Laser excision, a more difficult procedure gives the opportunity for histopathological examination.

Photodynamic Therapy

Photodynamic therapy is a new treatment modality which uses light of an appropriate wavelength along with a photosensitizer 5-aminolevulinic acid to induce tissue necrosis. Even though it has the advantage of preserving the normal anatomy with reduced pain and healing time, it has the disadvantage of persistence of the disease. This modality is under trial.[10]

Medical Treatment

Local application of 5-fluorouracil has been tried for the treatment of VIN.[11] Due to the high failure rate and local reaction, this has not gained acceptance. Imiquimod[12] is another drug tried for local use. The drug is an immune system modifier, which acts by producing interferons IFN- α and TNF-α, thus modifying macrophage function. Local skin reaction is an adverse effect.

14.3.7 Follow-up

In view of the high recurrence risk as well as malignant transformation, long-term follow-up is essential. Initial follow-up every 3-6 months should be advised for 4 years as the maximum recurrence occurs within this period. Later on yearly follow-up would suffice.

14.4 ULCERS OF THE VULVA

14.4.1 Herpes Genitalis

Genital herpes is the most common cause of genital ulceration in the developed world.[13] The causative organism in most cases is herpes simplex virus (HSV) type II. Type I usually causes infection in the mouth. Rarely type 1 too causes genital herpes. The infection is sexually transmitted. The virus is transmitted through the secretions from the ulcers. Infection can also occur through contact with a carrier of the disease. Risk factors for genital herpes infection include multiple sexual partners, sexual activity during adolescence, history of other STDs, relatively low educational status and a low socioeconomic status.[14]

Clinical Features

The first clinical episode of genital herpes can be:

1. Primary—in a person without prior HSV-1 or HSV-2 antibodies.
2. Non-primary—in a person with prior HSV-1 or HSV-2 antibody.

HSV infection is asymptomatic in a large proportion of women. Asymptomatic women also can spread the infection.

In symptomatic women, the typical presentation is bilaterally distributed crops of multiple small vesicles which break to form small shallow ulcers (Fig. 14.1). There can be moderate to severe local pain, dysuria, tender inguinal lymphadenopathy and systemic symptoms[15] like headache, muscle pain, fever, burning micturition and vaginal discharge.

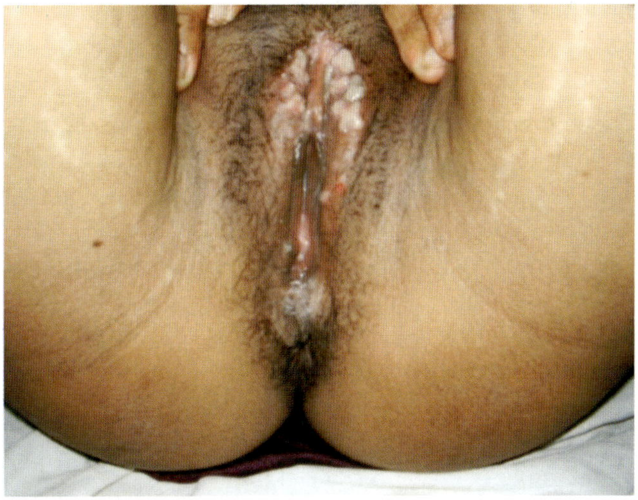

Fig. 14.1: Picture of vulva showing typical lesions of genital herpes infection. Multiple small vesicles are seen. Since several vesicles are seen it could be primary herpes

The primary infection is the most severe. Recurrences are milder and shorter in duration, and are due to a persistent chronic infection of sensory ganglia with a varying unpredictable degree of epithelial expression. Signs of recurrence differ from the primary in the smaller size of vesicles, closer grouping, lesser number of lesions and usual absence of constitutional symptoms.[16] Recurrences are more common (80%) with HSV type II infection than type I infection (50%). In the first year following the primary infection, about four recurrences usually occur. The triggering factors can be physical like local trauma, other sexually transmitted infections, sunlight or ultraviolet exposure, alcohol intake or psychological like stress or anxiety. The recurrences are preceded by warning symptoms like burning, tingling, numbness, pain in the back or buttock. There can be systemic symptoms like fever or malaise. Even after the lesions heal, pain and discomfort can persist as postherpetic neuralgia.

Pregnant women with active genital herpes infection are at risk of transmitting it to the newborn resulting in neonatal herpes infection.[17]

Management

Antiviral drugs are presently being used to reduce the severity, viral shedding, itching, average healing time and frequency of new lesion formation. The recommended regimen for primary episode includes acyclovir 400 mg 3 times a day or 200 mg 5 times a day for 7-10 days. Alternatively famciclovir can be given in a dose of 250 mg 3 times a day. Recurrent episodes can be treated with acyclovir in the same dose as mentioned earlier but only for 5 days. Nonsteroidal anti-inflammatory drugs can be given for symptomatic relief.

14.4.2 Syphilis

Syphilis is another sexually transmitted disease which cause genital ulcer. The disease is caused by the organism, *Treponema pallidum*. Even though, after the invention of penicillin the incidence drastically decreased, recently WHO has reported that there is an increase in the incidence of the disease.

A genital ulcer, the primary chancre, appears during the primary stage of the disease, at the site where the syphilis bacteria entered the body. The primary chancre is a painless regularly edged hard button like ulcer which is usually seen on the vulva, or on the cervix. The primary chancre appears about 21 days after the sexual contact and is highly infectious. Associated non-tender, rubbery, discrete lymph nodes are present bilaterally. As a rule the chancre heals in 3-8 weeks.[18]

Diagnosis

Diagnosis is by microscopic examination of fluid from the ulcer, taken with a swab. Serological tests will take 2-3 months to become positive. If tests are negative, serological tests should be repeated after 3 months.

Treatment

Penicillin is the drug of choice. It is important to ensure that the infection has cleared, by repeat testing. Screening for other STDs should also be done. Contacts should be traced and treated if indicated.

Prevention

Use of condom cannot absolutely prevent the transmission, as all the lesions cannot be covered by the condom. Even after complete treatment a person can contract the disease if there is a repeat exposure. Hence, women who are at the risk of STD should be on regular surveillance.

14.4.3 Lymphogranuloma Venereum

This sexually transmitted disease is caused by infection with *Chlamydia trachomatis*; serovars L I, L 2 and L 3.[19] The primary lesion is single painless evanescent erosion or ulcer or a herpetiform vesicle which appears 5-21 days after exposure. The lesions are more often hidden, since these are located in the fourchette or in the posterior vaginal wall. The infection spreads through lymphatics to the lymph nodes. Lymph node involvement manifests as unilateral, tender inguinal or femoral bubo after 10-30 days. These lymph nodes become fixed to the skin. In the final stage of disease progression, they become superlative with formation of abscesses, fistulas, strictures and sinus tracts.

Diagnosis

Diagnosis is by serological testing using compliment fixation. For identification of serovars, culture is necessary[19] which is often difficult and with poor sensitivity. PCR based tests have recently become available.

Treatment

Standard recommended treatment is doxycycline 100 mg orally twice a day for 21 days.[19]

14.4.4 Granuloma Inguinale

Granuloma inguinale (donovanosis) is a sexually transmitted infection caused by the bacterium, Calymmatobacterium granulomatis. The organism is seen as intracellular inclusion bodies called Donovan bodies. The disease is characterized by the presence of chronic indolent ulcers in the vulva and groin. Transmission can also occur through fecal route or by passage through an infected birth canal.

Clinical Features

The characteristic feature is multiple chronic progressive indolent ulcers which are seen in the labia minora, mons pubis, and the fourchette.[20] The ulcers are typically multiple, with a beefy red color. Four major clinical varieties are described.

1. Nodular
2. Ulcerovegetative
3. Hypertrophic
4. Cicatrical

Treatment

Prolonged treatment is necessary.[20] The recommended drug is doxycycline 100 mg orally twice daily for 3 weeks or until all lesions have completely healed. Follow-up is necessary as lesions can recur.

14.4.5 Behcet's Disease

Behcet's disease is a multisystem disease characterized by a combination of oral and genital ulcers and ocular inflammation. The condition is named after Turkish dermatologist who first described the symptom complex. It is thought to be immune mediated or thrombotic. Genital ulcers are seen in 60-80% of these patients. The ulcers are multiple and painful. These heal by scarring. The size of the ulcer is usually about 1-2 cm. These ulcers rarely erode deeper tissue and can result in urinary or fecal fistula formation.

Etiology

The etiology is unknown. A probable etiology proposed is altered immunity due to genetic predisposition. There is evidence of an association with the expression of some HLAs (B51, DR5, and DQw3) and a racial predilection for individuals of Asian or Middle Eastern descent.

Diagnosis

There is no specific test for diagnosis. The diagnosis is based on clinical findings following the international study group diagnostic guidelines[21] as given below.

Oral (*aphthous*) ulcers (any shape, size or number at least 3 times in any 12 months), along with 2 out of the next 4 "*hallmark*" symptoms:

1. *Genital ulcers* (including *anal* ulcers and spots in the genital region and swollen *testicles* or *epididymitis* in men).
2. *Skin lesions* (papulopustules, *folliculitis, erythema nodosum, acne* in postadolescents not on corticosteroids).
3. *Eye* inflammation (*iritis, uveitis*, retinal vasculitis, cells in the vitreous).
4. *Skin reaction* (papule >2 mm diameter 24-48 hours or more after needle-prick).

Treatment

Treatment is aimed at reducing the symptoms by controlling the immune system. Corticosteroids like Prednisolone at a dose of 1 mg/ kg/day can be given for severe disease. Topical hyaluronic acid has been found to reduce local inflammatory reaction.[22] Anti TNF agent, Etanercept[23] has been found to be useful in patients with skin and mucosal symptoms. Interferon α, azathioprine combination also has shown promise in treating genital and oral ulcers.

14.5 CONCLUSION

Vulvar preinvasive lesions that were earlier known by different names now come under the category of VIN. The incidence of preinvasive conditions of the vulva is on the increase especially among younger women due to an increase in HPV infection. Smoking is another important etiological factor. In older women the premalignant lesion recognized is lichen sclerosus. Most conditions present with symptoms of itching and pain. Women presenting with such symptoms should be properly evaluated. Since, VIN lesions are often multiple, representative biopsies after inspection with colposcope or after painting with 3-5% acetic acid is mandatory. The risk of malignancy being less, treatment is often conservative. Long-term follow-up is however essential to look for potential malignant transformation.

REFERENCES

1. Lynch B. Vulvar dystrophies and intraepithelial neoplasias. Dermatology Clin 1987;5:789-99.
2. Lynch PJ, Moyal-Barrocco M, Bogliatto F, Micheletti L, Scurry J. 2006 ISSVD classification of vulvar dermatoses: Pathologic subsets and their clinical correlates. Journal of Reproductive Medicine 2007;52(1):3-9.
3. Chan I, Oyama N, Neill SM, Wojnarowska F, Black MM, McGrath JA. Characterization of IgG autoantibodies to extracellular matrix protein 1 in lichen sclerosus. Clin Exp Dermatol 2004;29(5):499-504.

4. Bornstein J, Heifetz S, Kellner Y, Stolar Z, Abramovici H. Clobetasol dipropionate 0.05% versus testosterone propionate 2% topical application for severe vulvar lichen sclerosus. Am J Obstet Gynecol 1998;178(1 Pt 1):80-4.
5. Goolamali SK, Goolamali SI. "Lichen sclerosus". J Obstet Gynaecol 1997;17(1): 5-12.
6. American College of Obstetricians and Gynecologists. Diagnosis and management of vulvar skin disorders. National Guideline Clearinghouse. May, 2008.
7. Kagie MJ, Kenter GG, Fleuren GL,Trimbos JB. Vulvoscopy in benign and premalignant vulvar lesions: Results of seven years vulvoscopy clinic. J Gynecol Technol 1997;3:21-6.
8. Modesitt SC,Waters AB,Walton L.Vulvar intraepithelial neoplasia II:Occult cancer and the inpact of margin status on recurrence. Obstet Gynecol 1998;92:962-5.
9. Sideri M, Spinaci L, Spolti N, Schettino F. Evaluation of CO_2 laser excision or vaporisation for the treatment of vulvar intraepithelial neoplasia. Gynaecol Oncol 1999;75:277-81.
10 Baggish MS, Dorsey JH. Photodynamic therapy of vulval intraepithelial neoplasia. Cancer Res 2001;61:192-6.
11. Sillman FH, Sedlis A, Boyce JG. A review of lower genital intraepithelial neoplasia and the use of topical 5-fluorouracil. Obstet Gynecol Surv1985;40:190-20.
12. Beutner KR, Spruance SL, Houghham AJ, FoxTL, Owens ML, Douglas JM. Treatment of genital warts with an immune-response modifier (imiquimod). J Am Acad Dermatol 1998;38:230-9.
13. Mendel A. Genital herpes-how much of a problem. Lancet 1998;2351:16-8.
14. Conant MA, et al. Genital herpes an integrated approach to management. J Am Acad Dermatol 1996;35:601-5.
15. Pariera FA. Herpes simplex: Evolving concepts. J Am Acad Dermatol 1996;35:505-20.
16. Brown JJ, et al. An overview of STDs. Part I. J Am Dermatol 1999;41:511-29.
17. Brock Lehurst P, et al. Should acyclovir prophylaxis be used in late pregnancy in women with recurrent genital herpes infection? How to use a clinical decision analysis. Genitourin Med 1997;73:314-9.
18. Ndowa F, Dludlu S. Genital Ulcer –Adenopathy Syndrome. Kumar B, Gupta S, editors. Sexually Transmitted Infections. Ist edition. New Delhi: Elsevier 2005;493-50.
19. Willcox RR. Lymphogranuloma venereum. In Morton RS, Harris JRW. Eds. Recent advances in sexually Transmitted Diseases. Edinburgh: A Churchil Livingstonr 1975;188-93.
20. O'Farrell N. "Donovanosis". Sex Transm Infect 2002;78(6): 452-7.
21. International Study Group for Behcet's Disease. Criteria for diagnosis of Behcet's disease. Lancet 1990;335 (8697):1078-80.
22. Lee JH, Jung JY, Bang D. The efficacy of topical 0.2% hyaluronic acid gel on recurrent oral ulcers: Comparison between recurrent aphthous ulcers and the oral ulcers of Behcet's disease. J Eur Acad Dermatol Venereol 2008; 22(5): 590-5.
23. Melikoglu M, Fresko I, Mat C, et al. Short-term trial of etanercept in Behcet's disease: A double blind, placebo controlled study. J Rheumatol 2005;32(1):98-105.

15 Pelvic Inflammatory Disease

B Presannakumari

15.1 INTRODUCTION

Pelvic inflammatory disease (PID) is traditionally defined as infection of the upper genital tract; the uterus, fallopian tube and adjacent pelvic structures. The infection is usually an ascending infection from the vagina and endocervix, spreading to the endometrium, fallopian tubes, ovaries and the pelvic peritoneum. The most common organism involved is *C. trachomatis*, followed by *Gonococcus*. The disease involves a spectrum of inflammatory disorders of varying severity as well as different combinations of endometritis, salpingitis, tubo-ovarian abscess, pelvic peritonitis and generalized septicemia. PID has important health care implications as it affects younger women often leading to long-term sequelae in the form of infertility, ectopic pregnancies and chronic pelvic pain. However, the disease is often missed in clinical practice in spite of the fact that the incidence of the disease as well as its sequel is often preventable.

15.2 PUBLIC HEALTH IMPORTANCE

Cost of treating PID and its sequel will utilize significant health care resources. In UK, PID accounts for 1 in 60 visits to the general practitioner among women less than 45 years. In 1990, the total cost of treatment for chlamydial infection in the US was estimated to have exceeded $4 billion, $1,995 being the average cost per case of PID. In a large Indian study, an overall prevalence of 34% of reproductive tract infections was observed among women in the childbearing age group. Tubal damage appears to be the cause in 20-30% of the cases of female infertility. Occurrence of tubal infertility appears to be related to the number and severity of pelvic infections. The risk of ectopic pregnancy increases about 10 times following laparoscopically proven PID. Following a single attack of salpingitis, there is a 10% risk of infertility, which increases to 25% following a second and to 60% following subsequent episodes.[1]

PID is a disease of women of the childbearing age group. The exact incidence of the disease is not known, as asymptomatic and subclinical infections are common. Hospital statistics is not a surrogate of the incidence in the case of PID. The incidence is influenced by factors like age, sexual practice, method of contraception, etc. The use of barrier contraceptive significantly reduces the incidence of PID. By making the cervical mucus thick, hormonal contraceptives also reduce the incidence of PID. Sexual behavior and contraceptive practices vary among different regions of the world. Hence factors contributing to the prevalence of sexually transmitted diseases (STDs) and PID would also vary.

Chlamydial infection is the most common STD, world over. 10.3% of women under the age of 25 are found to be infected with *C. trachomatis*. The asymptomatic nature of chlamydial infections in women would mean that a vast majority may not seek medical attention and hence may go undiagnosed, resulting in serious sequelae. Some studies report high positivity (86%) for chlamydial antibodies in women with tubal infertility. 50% of all salpingitis and infertility in the UK are caused by chlamydial infection. Identification and treatment of chlamydial infection can reduce transmission of HIV. This could be because of the association between chlamydial infection and HIV viral shedding.

Though there was concern about the risk of PID associated with IUD use, recent reviews indicate that the risk of PID in modern IUD users is lower than was previously thought. However, the risk may be high in areas where gonorrhea and chlamydial infections are high. Actinomycosis is a rare infection associated with IUD use. PID attributed to the use of IUD is primarily confined to the first 3 weeks after insertion and is uncommon thereafter. A WHO study established that PID risk is temporally related to IUD insertion procedures. IUD use appears to be safe if inserted under aseptic precautions in women free from cervical infection. A Cochrane review suggests that there is no advantage in giving routine antibiotic prophylaxis[2] prior to IUD insertion.

Barrier methods and spermicidal creams offer protection against PID (60% reduction in the risk). A past history of PID is significant in that at least 25% of those women will go onto develop subsequent episodes.

The role of vaginal douching as a contributory factor in the development of PID is controversial. Pinworm infection in females can lead to PID, with the entire associated long-term sequelae. It is possible to predict the development of PID using a modified *Chlamydia* risk factor scoring system, with a view for educating and screening such women who secure a threshold score.

15.3 RISK FACTORS ASSOCIATED WITH PID (TABLE 15.1)

Cigarette smoking may result in generalized lowering of immunity which predisposes to PID. Substance abuse may contribute to PID by increasing "at risk" sexual behavior. While OCP is generally thought to reduce endometritis because of its effect on cervical mucus, it actually increases the chance of cervicitis by encouraging sex without using condoms. Termination of pregnancy is an iatrogenic cause of PID.

Table 15.1: Risk factors of PID

Young age at first intercourse
Lifetime number of sexual partners
Low socioeconomic status
Cigarette smoking, substance abuse
Oral contraceptive pill use
UCD insertion
Termination of pregnancy
Vaginal douching

15.4 MICROBIOLOGY (TABLE 15.2)

Previously, organisms causing PID were classified as gonococcal and non-gonococcal, with *C. trachomatis* titled

Table 15.2: Organisms involved in PID

Chlamydia trachomatis
Gonococcus
Mycoplasma genitale (?)
Peptostreptococcus/Peptococcus
Bacterial vaginosis causing organisms
Gardnerella vaginalis
Mobiluncus
Peptostreptococci
Mycoplasma—Mycoplasma hominis and *Ureaplasma urealyticum*
Aerobic vaginitis
E. coli
Group B streptococci
Enterococci
Other organisms
Mycobacterium tuberculosis
Actinomyces
Schistosoma sp

as the most prominent among non-gonococcal organisms. However, recent evidence suggests that *Chlamydia* itself is the commonest cause of PID world over especially among young women. This is attributed to the control of gonococcal PID as well as due to the improvements in the diagnosis of chlamydial infection. About 25-30% of infections are due to *C. trachomatis*. Ascending infection from the vagina in the presence of bacterial vaginosis, a condition characterized by a change in the vaginal ecology is another cause for PID. Normal vagina is colonized by lactobacilli which breakdown glycogen, keeping the pH acidic protecting it from invasion with pathogenic organisms. In bacterial vaginosis (BV), there will be a marked reduction of lactobacilli which is usually replaced by *Gardnerella vaginalis,* mobiluncus, peptostreptococci and *Mycoplasma—Mycoplasma hominis* and ureaplasma urealyticum. Aerobic vaginitis (AV) is caused by virulent aerobic bacteria like *Escherichia coli*, group-B streptococci and enterococci. Bacterial byproducts destroy the normal defence barriers of the cervical canal and lead to ascending infection of the upper genital tract.

The importance of chlamydial infection is that *chlamydia* being a slow growing organism can remain in the endosalpinx for months or years after initial colonization. Due to this insidious nature and mild or absent symptoms, treatment is often delayed or not initiated at all resulting in irreversible and severe damage to the fallopian tube. The important sequelae of chlamydial salpingitis (Table 15.3) are infertility, ectopic pregnancy and chronic pelvic pain. Damage caused by *Chlamydia* predisposes the genital tract for invasion by microorganisms from the vagina to extend upwards to the genital tract.

Chlamydia is an aerobic, gram-negative, obligate intracellular pathogen. They do not synthesize ATP, but depend on the host's energy sources. *Chlamydia trachomatis* has several serovariants, of which serovars A-C cause trachoma, and D-K cause conjunctivitis, urethritis, proctitis and cervicitis by infecting the columnar cells in the epithelium of the conjunctiva, urethra, rectum and cervix. They also infect the respiratory tract and can lead to pneumonia in the newborn.

The lifecycle of *Chlamydia* is completed in two phases- an infectious phase which is represented by the elementary body and a reproductive phase which is represented by the reticular body. *Chlamydia* infects non-ciliated cells and macrophages. Once inside the host cell, it has an incubation period of 7-21 days. Thereafter, it replicates every 3 hours. When the organism is intracellular it is not infectious and exists as reticulate body. The unique cell wall structure of *Chlamydia*, rich in lipopolysaccharides and cysteine, provides survival advantage by preventing phagocytosis. The infective invasive elementary bodies are released outside by rupture and destruction of the target cells. These elementary bodies enter other host cells by phagocytosis.

Table 15.3: Sequelae of chlamydial salpingitis

- Infertility
- Ectopic pregnancy
- Chronic pelvic pain

Neisseria gonorrhoeae are gram-negative, non-motile, kidney shaped intracellular diplococci. The primary site of infection of gonococcus in women is the cervix giving rise to a mucopurulent discharge. Spreading to the tubes it can lead to salpingitis by invading selectively, the ciliated secretory cells of the tubal mucosa, leading to ciliary sloughing and stasis. As the organism is intracellular it causes extensive destruction of the endosalpinx. Gonococcal infection is accompanied by an intense inflammatory reaction and activation of complement. There may be accumulation of inflammatory exudates and formation of tubo-ovarian abscesses. Subsequent fibrosis can result in tubal obstruction and infertility. The incidence of infertility may be as high as 20%.

15.5 PATHOGENESIS

PID results from spread of infection into the endocervical and endometrial cavity from the lower genital tract. The same organism simultaneously isolated from different ascending sites is proof of this. The upper genital tract is protected from invasion by microorganisms by the natural defence mechanisms, the most important of which is the cervical mucus plug which normally occludes the cervical canal. This barrier is disrupted during menstruation due to the flow of menstrual effluents predisposing to ascending infection. Instrumentation of cervical canal also may disrupt this barrier.

Infection of the endometrial cavity leads to endometritis; that of the tubes and ovaries results in salpingo-oophoritis and of the pelvic peritoneum leads to pelvic peritonitis. If not treated, the infection eventually spreads along the surfaces of abdominal viscera leading to periappendicitis, perihepatitis and perisplenitis. In early acute salpingitis, there is edema of the mucosa, submucosa and serosa. Fibrin deposits on the serosal surface of the tube bridges the abdominal and pelvic viscera forming flimsy adhesions which restrict tubal motility. These may later get organized with deposition of collagen to form permanent adhesions. The tubal ostia may be narrowed down, as a consequence of which the cavity gets filled with pus to form a pyosalpinx. Further, with pus exuding from the tubal ostium, the pelvic organs get densely adhered to form complex inflammatory masses. Tubo-ovarian abscess is a severe manifestation of PID. However, in up to 50% of women presenting with tubo-ovarian abscess, a preceding episode of PID may not be identified. Sometimes, there is ulceration of the ampullary mucosa which heals eventually. However, this may lead to agglutination of the plicae in the ampullary region and occlusion of the tubal folds leading to collection of clear fluid within the tubes forming a retort shaped mass-hydrosalpinx. Infection of the isthmus tends to cause more destruction than that of the ampullary region as the lumen is narrower here. Complete tubal obstruction may result from dense mucosal adhesions in this region.

Chlamydial and gonococcal infection damages the endocervical and tubal mucosa as a result of inflammatory reaction. This causes endogenous flora including organisms associated with BV or AV to ascend, and cause further infection. Presence of microbial flora in samples cultured from the fallopian tube indicates severe infection. While sexually transmitted infections like gonococcus or *Chlamydia* are isolated in early infection, isolation of endogenous organisms is associated with advanced disease. Tubo-ovarian abscesses usually harbor anaerobic organisms, Gonococci or *Chlamydia* rarely being isolated from them. Perihepatitis caused by *Chlamydia trachomatis* is known as Fitz Hugh-Curtis syndrome.

In acute salpingitis, there is dense polymorphonuclear infiltration of the mucosa, with inflammatory infiltrate present in the lumen. In chronic salpingitis, plasma cells, lymphocytes and histiocytes predominate.

15.5.1 Sequelae of Acute PID

With the advent of antibiotics, tubo-ovarian abscess, pyosalpinx, septicemia and death are very rare. Incompletely treated PID, especially chlamydial infection, due to its minimal symptoms and chronic nature, causes destruction of the endosalpinx leading to infertility, ectopic pregnancy or chronic pelvic pain. PID is one of the important causes for tubal factor infertility. A WHO study reported that the current chlamydial infection rate in infertile women is about 18-20 %. Infertility is becoming an emerging health problem in many countries of the world including India. The increase appears to be in fact due to the growing role played by *C. trachomatis*.[3]

Infertility in PID may be due to tubal block or peritubal adhesions leading to impaired ovum pick-up.

PID, especially chlamydial infection appears to be the reason for the increased incidence of ectopic pregnancy. Approximately 50% of ectopic pregnancies occur in fallopian tubes damaged by infection. Heterotopic pregnancy in IVF cycles are thought to be due to entrapment of embryo in the damaged fallopian tube.

Chronic pelvic pain can follow PID due to the formation of hydrosalpinx or pelvic adhesions. Rarely a tubo-ovarian abscess can persist in spite of antibiotic treatment resulting in chronic pelvic pain as well as recurrent attacks of acute PID.

15.6 CLINICAL FEATURES

15.6.1 Symptoms

Symptoms can vary from mild to severe depending upon the type of organism and host factors. It is to be noted that PID can exist without detectable symptoms. It has been found that more than half of the women with signs of PID[4] sequelae like tubal occlusion, hydrosalpinx or ectopic pregnancy often have no history of symptomatic PID suggesting that silent disease can lead to permanent tubal destruction.

Moreover, symptoms are neither specific nor exclusively diagnostic of PID. Women with PID commonly present with lower abdominal pain, pyrexia >38°C, deep dyspareunia, intermittent vaginal bleeding and/or abnormal vaginal discharge. Intermittent vaginal bleeding may take the form of postcoital bleeding or break-through bleeding while on pills. Just as it is important to rule out cervical neoplastic changes in women presenting with intermenstrual bleeding, it is mandatory to exclude cervicitis and endometritis as well. Women who develop perihepatitis (Fitz Hugh-Curtis syndrome) usually complain of right upper quadrant pain. In the presence of severe pelvic infection there can be associated nausea and vomiting, mimicking appendicitis.

15.6.2 Signs

There is a significant change in the clinical picture of PID over the years. This can be attributed to the decrease in the incidence of gonococcal and pyogenic infections and the effects of starting antibiotic early. Just like symptoms, signs can also vary depending upon the organism involved and the host factors. There have been wide disparities documented in the diagnosis of PID in women presenting with the same signs and symptoms. This infers that at least some cases of PID are undiagnosed. It should also be borne in mind that other conditions like ectopic pregnancy, endometriosis, ovarian cyst rupture, lower urinary tract infection and even acute appendicitis might present with similar history. It would be prudent to rule out ectopic pregnancy first, when a woman in the reproductive age group presents with lower abdominal pain. Bimanual pelvic examination may reveal tenderness in the fornices and cervical excitation pain due to peritoneal irritation and inflammation of the adnexal organs. In the presence of a tubo-ovarian abscess or pyosalpinx, a tender adnexal cystic swelling may be palpable. In the rare situation of peri-hepatitis there will be tenderness on palpation of the liver.

Chlamydial infection leads to PID in 20-40% of untreated women. However, the time-frame within which PID results from acute chlamydial infection is not clear.

15.6.3 Diagnosis (Table 15.4)

Table 15.4: 2006 center for disease control (CDC) and prevention criteria for the diagnosis of PID

Minimum criteria (1 or more)
• Lower abdominal tenderness
• Adnexal tenderness
• Tenderness with cervical motion
Additional criteria: Patients with PID should have 1 or more of the following:
• Signs of lower genital tract inflammation
• Oral temperature higher than 101°F
• Abnormal cervical and vaginal discharge
• Greatly increased numbers of white blood cells on saline microscopy of vaginal secretions
• Elevated erythrocyte sedimentation rate
• Elevated C-reactive protein level
• Laboratory documentation of cervical infection with *C. trachomatis* or *N. gonorrhoeae*
Elaborate criteria (additional findings include the following):
• Histopathologic evidence of endometritis at endometrial biopsy
• Thickened fluid-filled tubes with or without free pelvic fluid or a tubo-ovarian complex on transvaginal sonograms or images from other modalities
• Laparoscopic abnormalities that are consistent with PID

15.7 MANAGEMENT

15.7.1 Investigations

Investigations for pelvic inflammatory disease include:

1. **Pregnancy test:** To exclude the possibility of ectopic pregnancy.
2. **High vaginal swabs** should be taken for gram staining to rule out gonorrhea and anaerobic infections and intra-cervical swab for the diagnosis of *Chlamydia*. A positive result would favor a diagnosis of PID, though a negative result does not rule out PID entirely. PCR based tests have replaced cell culture for the definitive diagnosis of both symptomatic as well as asymptomatic chlamydial infection.
3. **Nonculture methods for the detection of *Chlamydia trachomatis*:** Nucleic acid amplification test or NAAT, is the most accurate of nonculture techniques. It amplifies and detects nucleic acid sequences that are unique to *C. trachomatis* and hence have a high sensitivity and specificity. These tests do not need viable micro-organisms. Some are sensitive enough to detect even a single nucleic acid sequence in the specimen.

   NAAT assays are of different types. This is based on the different technologies used. These include polymerase chain reaction (PCR), strand displacement amplification (SDA), transcription mediated amplification (TMA), Nucleic acid sequence based amplification (NASBA) and molecular beacon. Self-collected specimens can be used. These assays are automated and hence useful in screening programs.

   Disadvantages include high costs, reduced performance in the presence of inhibitors, and the need to freeze urine specimens to improve the test. Inhibitors include nitrates and crystals in urine. Other nonculture methods include enzyme linked immunoassays (EIA), DFA and nucleic acid hybridization techniques. Enzyme linked immunoassays use enzyme labeled antibodies against the membrane lipopolysaccharide of *Chlamydia*. However, false positives are very high due to cross reaction with other chlamydial species. EIAs are not as sensitive as culture methods.

   DFA involves direct visualization of chlamydial elementary bodies. It has a sensitivity of 80-90% and specificity of 99% compared to culture. However, it is not suitable for large specimens as it is very laborious.

   Nucleic acid hybridization techniques detect chlamydial RNA with a complimentary probe. The sensitivity is about 85% while the specificity is 99%.
4. **Indicators of infection** like raised CRP, raised ESR and increased WBC counts may be present.
5. **Ultrasound** might delineate thickened fluid filled fallopian tubes (Figs 15.1A and B) and free fluid in the pouch of Douglas. In the presence of tubo-ovarian abscess, a mixed echogenic mass can be located in the adnexa. Pyosalpinx will give rise to a cog-wheel appearance.

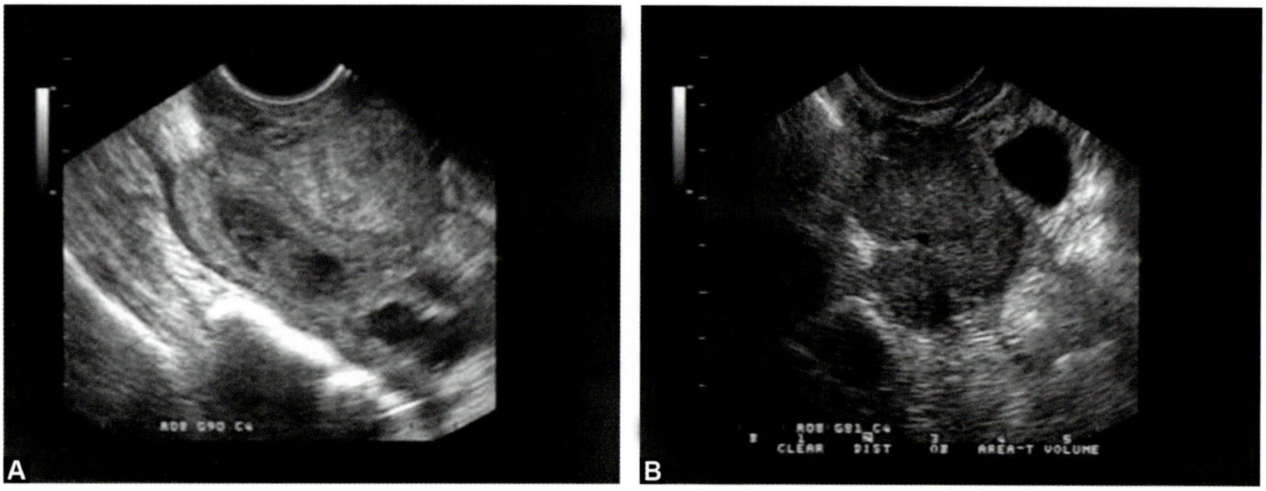

Figs 15.1A and B: TVS showing thickened fluid filled fallopian tube (A). Note the cog-wheel appearance of pyosalpinx in a patient with acute PID (B)

(Fig. 15.1) there will be increased free fluid in the peritoneal cavity. The hyperemia associated with acute inflammation can be demonstrated by power Doppler.[5] Tubo-ovarian abscess will appear as a heterogeneous complex mass in the adnexa.

6. The gold standard for the diagnosis of PID is visualization at laparoscopy (Figs 15.2 to 15.4). It offers the chance to diagnose PID as well as other causes for acute abdominal pain. Another advantage is confirmation of the diagnosis of PID and simultaneous treatment of the condition effectively by surgical interference when needed, supplemented with antibiotics, thus preventing complications and preserving fertility.

The appearance at laparoscopy varies depending on the pathology. Presence of swollen and inflamed tubes, inflammatory exudates and pus exuding from the tubal lumen or pyosalpinx can be visualized. Collection of samples from the tubal lumen for microbiological examination and sensitivity testing is of paramount importance. However, studies have shown that visual evidence of PID may not be present in about 23% of the patients who have PID. While some consider laparoscopy necessary in all cases of PID, it is not practical, or necessary to do laparoscopy for all patients. Moreover, laparoscopy may not be available in many of the clinical settings as emergency, is expensive and needs general anesthesia. However, laparoscopy has the advantage of draining the pus if there is a significant collection, as well as getting a sample of pus for culture. In situations where the diagnosis is in doubt or there is no response to treatment or where inflammatory pelvic masses including abscesses are suspected, laparoscopy should be done.

Indications for laparoscopy
- Doubt about diagnosis
- Absence of response to treatment
- Presence of pelvic abscess

7. **Endometrial biopsy:** Helps diagnosis by establishing the presence of inflammatory changes. However, curettage is not recommended as a means of diagnosing PID.

15.7.2 Treatment

The aim of treatment is to prevent serious acute complications of sepsis as well as to prevent the sequelae of PID; Empirical therapy should be started before culture result comes, as delay while waiting for culture result can lead to

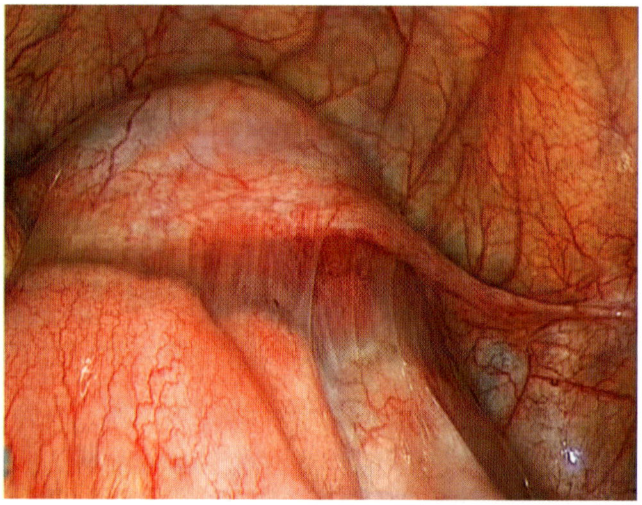

Fig. 15.2: Laparoscopic picture showing perihepatic adhesions (Fitz-Hugh-Curtis syndrome)

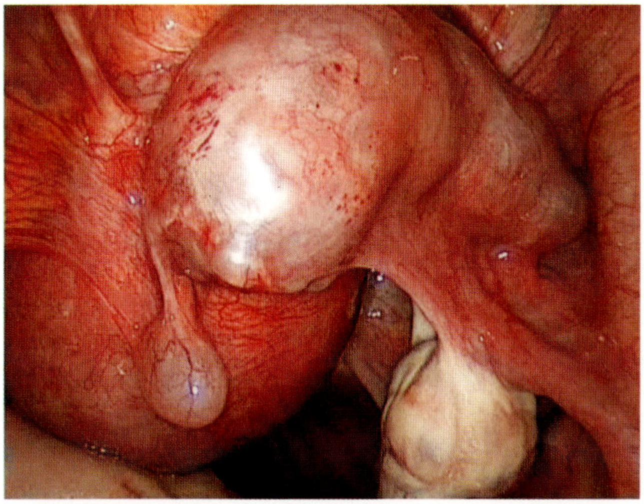

Fig. 15.3: Laparoscopic picture showing hydrosalpinx

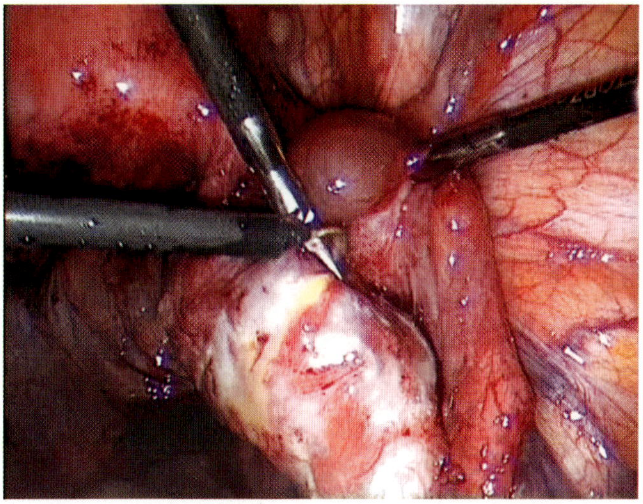

Fig. 15.4: Laparoscopic picture showing periovarian adhesions as sequelae of PID

acute complications of sepsis as well as sequelae of PID. The antibiotic started should cover common organisms which are involved in PID—*Chlamydia trachomatis*, *Neisseria gonorrhoeae*, anaerobic organisms, gram-negative and positive cocci, bacilli and *Mycoplasma*.

Medical Management

Outpatient antibiotic therapy is effective in both mild and moderately severe PID. In-patient treatment should be provided in the case of severe PID and in special circumstances. Patient should be advised to avoid intercourse till she and her partner are fully treated.

Since, the microbiological etiology of PID involves *Chlamydia, N. gonorrhoeae* and a variety of aerobes and anaerobes, treatment should include broad-spectrum agents.

On an outpatient basis, the following regimens have been recommended (Table 15.5).

Table 15.5: CDC recommended treatment regimens for outpatient therapy of acute PID

Regimen A
A single intramuscular injection of Ceftriaxone 250 mg/cefoxitin 2 g or Probenecid 1g orally in a single dose (or other parenteral third generation cephalosporin- cefotaxime), along with 100 mg of Doxycycline and 500 mg of Metronidazole, both given orally twice daily for 2 weeks.
Regimen B
A continuous 2 weeks treatment of 400 mg of oral Ofloxacin twice daily or Levofloxacin 500 mg orally once daily with or without 500 mg of Metronidazole twice daily. Ofloxacin as a single agent is found to be effective against both *C. trachomatis* and *N. gonorrhoeae.* Since, there is doubt about Ofloxacin's coverage of anaerobic organisms, Metronidazole is added.
Alternative oral regimens
Amoxicillin+Clavulanic acid along with Doxycycline is effective in obtaining clinical cure. Gastrointestinal side effect is a common problem encountered with this regimen. 1g Azithromycin given as a single dose is also found to be effective in acute PID.

After starting oral therapy, the patient should be re-evaluated within 48-72 hours. If the response is found to be poor, hospitalization (Table 15.6) and parenteral antibiotic administration is to be considered. Where available, Cefoxitin can replace Ceftriaxone, as it has been proven to be more effective in PID.

Table 15.6: Criteria for hospitalization in acute PID

- Presence of high fever, nausea and vomiting
- Presence of adnexal or pelvic masses
- Not responding to oral antibiotics
- Cannot tolerate oral regimen
- Other surgical conditions like appendicitis cannot be ruled out

It is better to hospitalize all adolescent patients since their future fertility is of concern due to non-compliance. In severe cases of pelvic inflammatory disease, the patient may be very sick. Supportive measures in the form of bedrest, hydration and adequate analgesia, may be necessary depending on severity of the symptoms. Inpatient treatment is also indicated in pregnancy, intolerance to oral therapy, and in the immunodeficient. Patients with adnexal masses should be given parenteral antibiotics (Table 15.7) as only parenteral antibiotics will give sufficient antibiotic levels to penetrate the abscess. Moreover, rupture of a tubo-ovarian abscess can lead to serious complications like septic shock which may need emergency resuscitation procedures. Intravenous therapy is maintained for 24 hours after the patient has become apyrexial and oral therapy is to be continued for the rest of the course.

Table 15.7: CDC recommended treatment regimens for inpatient therapy of acute pelvic inflammatory disease

Regimen A

Cefoxitin 2 g I.V 6th hourly/Cefotetan 2 g I.V 12th hourly plus Doxycycline, 100 mg I.V/orally 12th hourly to be continued for at least 24 hours after the patient shows relief in symptoms. It is followed by doxycycline 100 mg orally twice daily for 14 days. When tubo-ovarian abscess is present, clindamycin or metronidazole with doxycycline is preferred over doxycycline alone for its added anaerobic coverage. Ceftizoxime, Ceftriaxone, and cefotaxime can replace cefoxitin and cefotetan.

Regimen B

Clindamycin 900 mg I.V every 8 hours plus Gentamycin at a loading dose of 2 mg/kg body weight I.V/I.M followed by a maintenance dose of 1.5 mg/kg 8th hourly. This should be continued for 24 hours after relief of symptoms. It is to be followed with Doxycycline, 100 mg orally two times a day, or clindamycin 450 mg orally four times a day for 14 days. When tubo-ovarian abscess is present, clindamycin is preferred for continued therapy over doxycycline for the aforementioned reasons.

Alternative parenteral regimens

1. Ofloxacin 400 mg I.V every 12 hours, or levofloxacin 500 mg I.V once daily, with metronidazole 500 mg I.V every 8 hours.
2. Ampicillin/sulbactam 3 g I.V every 6 hours with doxycycline 100 mg i.v/oral every 12 hours. It is found to be effective in tubo-ovarian abscess as well as for anaerobes, *N. gonorrhoeae* and *C. trachomatis.*

In all cases of PID, patients should be made aware of the following:

- What treatment is being given and its possible adverse effects.
- That following treatment with the proper antibiotic in the proper dose and proper duration, fertility is usually maintained but there remains a risk of future infertility, chronic pelvic pain or ectopic pregnancy.
- Repeat episodes of PID are associated with an exponential increase in the risk of infertility.
- Future use of barrier contraception will significantly reduce the risk of PID.
- The need to screen her sexual contacts for infection, to prevent reinfection. The CDC recommends treatment of partners who have had sex with the patient during the preceding 60 days.
- Clinically more severe disease is associated with a greater risk of sequelae.
- The earlier the treatment is given, the lower the risk of future fertility problems.

15.7.3 Prevention of PID

Strategies for prevention of sexually transmitted diseases can in addition reduce the chances of occurrence of pelvic inflammatory disease as the two important organisms causing PID are gonococci and *Chlamydia* which are transmitted sexually. The clinician's important role is the primary prevention of PID which includes providing health education with emphasis on avoiding risky sexual behavior, encouraging the high-risk groups to undergo screening tests for PID as well as to teach the importance of treating the male sexual partners. Educating the adolescent group should be given more importance.

Secondary prevention in the form of screening for *Chlamydia* and treating while the organism is still confined to the cervical epithelium is important in preventing ascending infection. Those who have been screened and found positive should be treated with a single dose of azithromycin at a dose of 1 g as it will improve compliance. Screening should form one of the initial strategies in the evaluation of infertility.

Early diagnosis and therapy will reduce development of sequelae of PID.

15.7.4 Syndromic Approach to the Management of STDs

Since diagnosis of the specific STDs require laboratory facilities and clinical expertise which is lacking in developing countries, WHO has recommended a syndromic approach to the management of STD. The patients are categorized according to symptoms which include vaginal discharge, urethral discharge, genital ulceration, lower abdominal pain, etc. and a management protocol has been developed for each syndrome. For example, patients with vaginal discharge would be treated for fungal, trichomonilial as well as chlamydial infections. This type of management will improve patient compliance.

15.7.5 Surgical Management

With the advent of powerful antibiotics, surgical intervention is very rarely needed. Laparoscopy (Fig. 15.5) should be done whenever the diagnosis is in doubt as non-infective conditions like endometriosis can mimic PID. Whenever laparoscopy is done, pus should be collected from peritoneal cavity for culture. Abscess if any should be drained. Pelvic

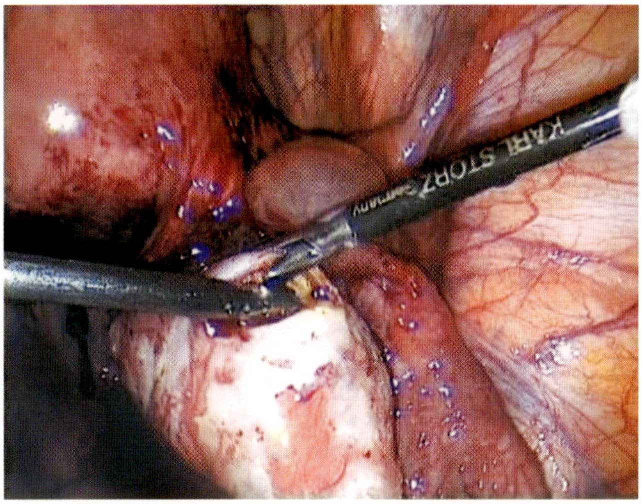

Fig. 15.5: Laparoscopic drainage of ovarian abscess

abscess can be drained by colpotomy. Prior to colpotomy, abscess cavity should be located by inserting a needle. Colpotomy can be proceeded with a knife along the track of the needle. Ultrasound is also helpful in locating pus.

Procedure of Colpotomy

With the patient in the lithotomy position, the posterior lip of the cervix is caught with volsellum. The vaginal mucosa is incised just below its reflection to the cervix. If there is doubt about the location of the pus, as previously mentioned, a needle aspiration will help. A small transverse incision is initially put and widened with artery forceps. Usually there will be several locules of pus which can be opened by inserting a finger. The pus should be sent for culture. Abscesses higher up in the abdomen which cannot be reached transvaginally, should be drained transabdominally. Ultrasound guided needle aspiration is less invasive than laparoscopy or laparotomy.

Women who develop recurrent attacks of acute PID, or who have persistent lower abdominal pain in the presence of an adnexal mass, not responding to antibiotic therapy needs surgical exploration. Unilateral mass can be treated by adnexectomy. When there is extensive adhesion, total abdominal hysterectomy with bilateral salpingo-oophorectomy should be preferred. The ideal time to perform definitive surgery is when the infection is quiescent which could be ascertained by estimating ESR and WBC count. The pelvic organs should be relatively non-tender. At laparotomy adhesions are commonly encountered. Flimsy adhesions can be released with fingers. Tubo-ovarian masses may be densely adherent to the cul-de-sac, uterus, lateral pelvic wall, etc. in which case there is risk of injury to ureters, sigmoid colon, rectum and small intestines. Dense fibrotic adhesions need sharp dissection. The ureter should be identified and traced to avoid injury. When extensive adhesions are anticipated during clinical examination by the presence of fixed adnexal masses, preoperative ureteric stenting should be done. When both adnexae have to be removed due to adhesions, hysterectomy might also be needed. But retaining the uterus should be thought of if the patient prefers to preserve the childbearing function as facilities for *in vitro* fertilization using donated eggs are available in the present setup. If total hysterectomy is done, vagina can be left open. It is ideal to keep a drain which can be removed postoperatively when drainage stops. In situations where inflammation is confined to one of the adnexa, unilateral adnexectomy can be the choice.

Management of Ruptured Pelvic Mass

Tubo-ovarian mass can rupture into the rectum, sigmoid colon or into the peritoneal cavity. Spontaneous rupture through the vagina is uncommon. Sometimes pus collection ruptures into the rectum, and the patient will have pus coming out through the anal opening. The infection will subside with antibiotics and does not need any additional surgical procedure. Posterior colpotomy in this situation is not necessary and may prove dangerous as it can cause rectovaginal fistula formation. When an abscess ruptures into the peritoneal cavity, septicemia and life-threatening septic shock can occur. Generalized peritonitis can result. On examination the abdomen will be distended, there will be rebound tenderness and the bowel sound will be sluggish or absent. Ultrasound will reveal presence of thick fluid in the peritoneal cavity.

Laparotomy should be done after achieving hemodynamic stability. Broad-spectrum antibiotics should be started and IV fluids should be administered under central venous pressure (CVP) monitoring. If there is significant distention of abdomen, bowel should be decompressed by inserting a nasogastric tube. Midline vertical incision is preferred for laparotomy. Pus should be drained and hysterectomy and bilateral salpingo-oophorectomy should be performed. For a young patient, unilateral salpingo-oophorectomy is the choice, but it should be kept in mind that there is a risk of recurrent abscess formation in the retained adnexa. At laparotomy if there are extensive adhesions with bowel loops involved, the pelvic structures will be obscured. The round ligament is a reliable landmark in such a situation. Bowel adhesions should be carefully separated as the risk of bowel injury is likely, due to the associated inflammation. If necessary, the surgeon's help should be sought. Oozing of blood from the dissected tissue will be difficult to control.

Postoperative Management

Septic shock, ileus, electrolyte and fluid imbalance are the complications which can occur. Adult respiratory distress syndrome is also a possibility due to septic shock. Subphrenic abscess can occur in the postoperative phase. If the general condition does not improve, a subphrenic abscess is to be looked for.

15.8 GENITAL TUBERCULOSIS

Female genital tuberculosis, a rare disease in developed countries is a frequent cause of chronic pelvic inflammatory disease and infertility in certain developing countries.[6]

About 1/3 of the world population is infected with the disease. This could be due to the poor management of treatment plans added to the lack of patient compliance. Development of multidrug resistant bacteria is a major public health problem.

15.8.1 Prevalence

The prevalence reported is 1-13% depending on the geographic area.[6]

15.8.2 Pathology and Pathogenesis

Mycobacterium tuberculosis hominis and *Mycobacterium tuberculosis bovis* are the usual types of bacteria involved. Atypical mycobacteria also are recently isolated. Genital tract tuberculosis is usually secondary to hematogenous dissemination during the time of active extragenital disease. The genital tract involvement can also be a part of gene-ralized military tuberculosis or may be a re-activation of a dormant disease in the fallopian tube. The initial infection probably begins in the fallopian tube and subsequently involves the endometrium, cervix, myometrium and ovary, vagina and vulva in decreasing frequency. The fallopian tubes are affected in about 90% whereas the endometrium is affected in 50% and the ovaries in 10-30%.[6-8]

The myometrium is involved microscopically, but involvement made out by imaging is uncommon. Tuberculous peritonitis may occur as a result of hematogenous dissemination from an active lesion in the neck, intestine or fallopian tube. Tuberculous peritonitis is seen associated with genital tuberculosis in about 50% of the cases.

The fallopian tube can become enlarged and form pyosalpinx. Tubo-ovarian abscess can also occur. Peritoneal adhesions are common and can involve bowel loops and abdominal wall. The fallopian tubes may be studded with miliary tubercles. Histopathological examination will reveal tubercle formation, multinucleated giant cells and epithelioid reaction with caseation.

Tuberculous peritonitis is of 3 types:

1. **The wet type**
   Plenty of straw colored fluid will accumulate in the peritoneal cavity. Tubercles will be seen studded over the visceral and parietal peritoneum.
2. **The fibrotic or the fixed type**
   In this type, there will be large omental masses, matted bowel loops and loculated ascites.
3. **The dry or plastic type**
   This type is characterized by caseous nodules, fibrous peritoneal reaction and dense adhesions.

15.8.3 Clinical Features

The disease usually affects women between the ages 20-40. Rarely adolescents and postmenopausal women are also affected. Genital tract tuberculosis is generally asymptomatic. The symptoms if present can be non-specific abdominal pain, vaginal discharge, infertility or menstrual irregularities including primary or secondary amenorrhea (Fig. 15.6). Rarely pelvic tuberculosis can present with menorrhagia or postmenopausal bleeding. Hence the diagnosis is sometimes incidental, while investigating for infertility or amenorrhea.[9]

In the presence of associated peritoneal tuberculosis, the presenting symptom will be distention of abdomen, loss of weight and loss of appetite, mimicking malignancy.

15.9 DIAGNOSIS

Genital tuberculosis is diagnosed by biopsy of cervical lesion, endometrial biopsy, or peritoneal biopsy. Isolating the bacilli is difficult. The diagnosis is usually based on histopathological features. In patients presenting with ascites, the diagnosis can be made by isolating the bacilli in ascetic fluid culture. However, the ascetic fluid cytology has a high false negative rate. CT scan of the abdomen can recognize thickened fallopian tubes, tubo-ovarian abcess and peritoneal thickening. Hysterosalpingography is better avoided due to the fear of dissemination of the infection. A peritoneal biopsy through minilaparotomy may help in diagnosis. Laparoscopy is not advisable as bowel perforation is likely due to adhesions. The diagnosis is usually made by histopathological examination of endometrial biopsy, which shows giant cells. Culturing the bacteria takes about 6 weeks. PCR done in endometrial biopsy specimen for microbacterial DNA is another method for the diagnosis which is reported to have 90% sensitivity.

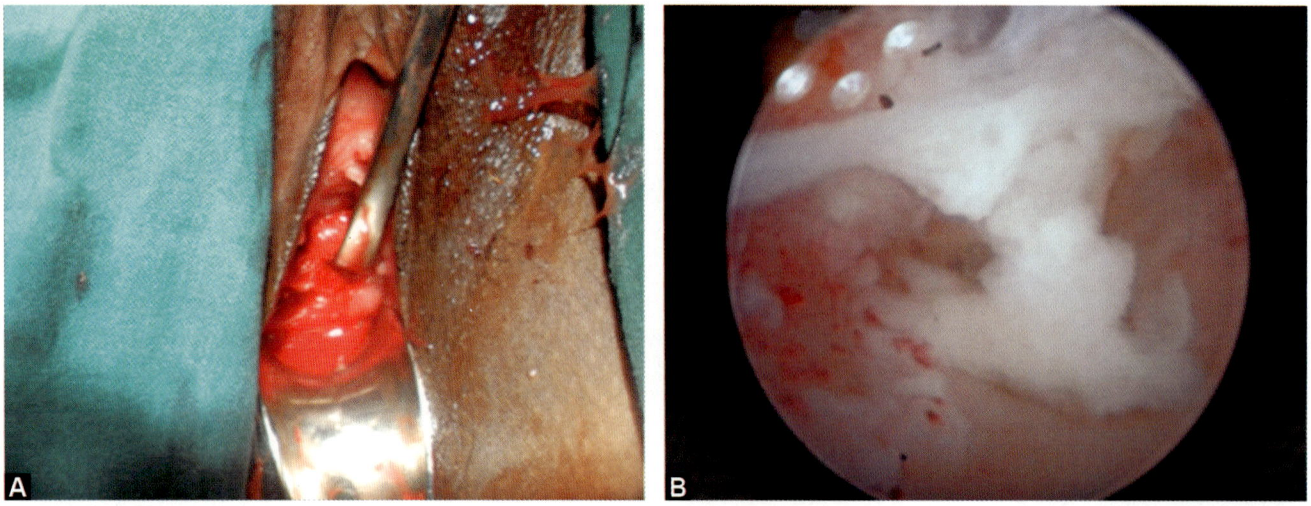

Figs 15.6A and B: Speculum examination (A) showing friable lesion in the cervix of 32-year-old lady who presented with secondary amenorrhea. Hysteroscopy picture of the same patient (B). The biopsy report was suggestive of tuberculosis

15.10 CONCLUSION

Pelvic inflammatory disease has important health implications as it affects the younger women in the reproductive age group. The important sequels of PID are infertility, chronic pelvic pain and increased incidence of ectopic pregnancy. The disease is often missed and not treated properly in spite of the fact that the sequelae are often preventable. There has been a shift in the organisms causing PID over the years. *Gonococcus*, which used to be the commonest organism involved, is much less at present especially in developed countries. As of now, chlamydial infection is reported to be the leading cause world over. Primary prevention of PID is through health education, emphasizing the importance of avoiding risky sexual behavior and promoting barrier contraception. Secondary prevention is by screening for *Chlamydia* and treating while the organism is still confined to the cervical epithelium. To improve compliance, a single dose regimen should be preferred. The aim of treatment of PID is to prevent serious acute complications of sepsis as well as to prevent long-term sequel. Empirical therapy should be started before getting culture report. This should cover most of the common organisms involved in PID. It is preferable to follow CDC guidelines in selecting the antibiotic as well as its dose and duration. Patients should be hospitalized whenever needed.

REFERENCES

1. Westrom. Human Reproduction 1999;14(8):1969-73.
2. Grimes DA, Schulz KF. Antibiotic prophylaxis for intrauterine contraceptive device insertion. Cochrane Database Syst Rev 2000;(2):CDOO1327.
3. WHO task force: Tubal infertility: Serologic relationship to past chlamydial and gonococcal infection. Sex Trans Dis 1995;29:71-7.
4. Sellors JW, Mahony JB, Chernesky MA, Rath DJ. Tubal factor infertility. An association with prior chlamydial infection and asymptomatic salpingitis. Fertil Steril 1988; 49:451-7.
5. Molander P, Sjöberg J, Paavonen J, Cacciatore B. Transvaginal power Doppler findings in laparoscopically proven acute pelvic inflammatory disease. Ultrasound Obstet Gynecol 2001;17:233-8.
6. Varma TR. Genital tuberculosis and subsequent fertility. Int J Gynecol Obstet 1991;35:1-11.
7. Sutherland AM. The changing pattern of tuberculosis of the female genital tract. A thirty-year survey. Arch Gynecol 1983;234:95-101.
8. Schaefer G. Female genital tuberculosis. Clin Obstet Gynecol 1976;19:223-39.
9. Figueroa-Damian R, Martinez-Velazco I, Villagrana-Zesati R, Arredondo-Garcia JL. Tuberculosis of the female reproductive tract:Effect on function. Int J Fertil Menopausal Stud 1996;41:430-6.

16 Infections of the Lower Genital Tract

B Presannakumari

Infections of the lower genital tract, which cause abnormal vaginal discharge, are a very common reason for gynecological consultation. Treatment of these diseases is thus important. Knowledge about the normal vaginal flora is important in understanding and treating vaginal infections.

16.1 NORMAL VAGINAL FLORA

Vagina is normally inhabited by bacteria of which the commonest is lactobacilli. Lactobacilli breakdown glycogen to lactic acid which maintain the vaginal pH acidic, creating an unfavorable environment for pathogens. A dynamic equilibrium exists between the vaginal epithelium, microorganisms which normally colonize the vagina the lactobacilli, local immune response and the vaginal pH.

16.2 MAINTENANCE OF VAGINAL pH

The normal pH of the vagina is 4.5. Normal pH is a critical determinant of good health in women. Estrogen increase epithelial glycogen. Lactobacilli metabolize glycogen to lactic acid and the pH is maintained acidic. Hence presence of lactobacilli protects against other bacterial infections. When the pH is alkaline, it alters the ecosystem causing epithelial desquamation. Low estrogenic states lower the glycogen and raise the pH. The pH is raised after menstruation and in the presence of seminal fluid which is alkaline.

Several other microorganisms are facultates in the vagina. These include diphtheroids, coagulase negative staphylococci, streptococci, *E. coli, Ureaplasma urealyticum and Mycoplasma hominis.* Anaerobic organisms are also present in low nonpathogenic concentrations. These include Peptostreptococci, Bacteroides, Fusobacterium, Mobilincus and Gardnerella.[1]

The normal vagina is moist because of physiological fluid which is formed of cervical mucus, vaginal transudate, uterine secretions and Bartholin's gland secretions. The physiological vaginal discharge is increased around the time of ovulation (ovulation cascade), in pregnancy, during COC use and at the time of sexual stimulation.

16.3 PATHOLOGICAL VAGINAL DISCHARGE

Vaginal discharge can be physiological or pathological. Physiological discharge should be differentiated from pathological, as misdiagnosis is common.

Abnormal vaginal discharge can be due to the following conditions:

1. Infections/inflammations of the lower genital tract
   a. Vaginitis
   b. Cervicitis
2. Foreign body in the vagina
   a. Forgotten tampon
   b. Pessary

3. Neoplasm
4. Fistulae
5. Allergic conditions
6. Upper genital tract infections

The common causes of vaginal discharge are:

1. Bacterial vaginosis
2. Trichomonas vaginitis
3. Candida vaginitis

16.3.1 Bacterial Vaginosis

Bacterial vaginosis is a polymicrobial alteration in the flora causing an increase in the vaginal pH, sometimes associated with a homogeneous vaginal discharge in the absence of demonstrable inflammatory response (Eschenbach et al 1988).

Etiology

The etiology is polymicrobial. The normal vaginal flora which is predominantly lactobacilli are replaced by

1. Gardnerella vaginalis
2. Bacteroides, Mobilincus, Prevotella
3. Mycoplasma hominis

Mobilincus produce trimethylamine which gives the smell of rotten fish. Production of succinate raises the vaginal pH. Absence of succinate and production of lactic acid blunt the chemotactic response of polymorphonuclear leukocytes and reduce their phagocytic ability. This explains absence of cellular inflammatory response.

Predisposing Factors

Increase in vaginal pH predispose to bacterial vaginosis. Hence, frequent douching can lead to reduction of lactobacilli and increase in pH. Smoking can suppress the immune system and facilitate the condition.

Symptoms

Since, there is no inflammation BV is asymptomatic in 50% of women. Symptomatic women may have a thin dark or dull grey vaginal discharge with a fishy odor, vaginal burning sensation and dyspareunia.

Apart from the presence vaginal discharge, the condition has gained importance due to the fact that it can predispose to the following conditions:

1. Pelvic inflammatory disease
2. Post cesarean endometritis
3. Postpartum endometritis
4. Posthysterectomy pelvic infection
5. Premature rupture of the membranes and chorio-amnionitis
6. Preterm labor.

Diagnosis

Certain characteristic features of the vaginal discharge lead to the diagnosis.

1. *Whiff test or amine test*—Addition of 10% KOH to a sample of vaginal discharge produces a fishy odor. The positive predictive value is 90% and specificity is 70%.
2. *Clue cells*—Examination of wet film will show vaginal epithelial cells studded with bacteria. Presence of clue cells is the most sensitive and specific criteria for the diagnosis of BV.
3. Vaginal pH > 4.5.
4. Gram staining and scoring systems based on the number of BV causing organisms compared to lactobacilli is an objective method. In the Nugent's Criteria,[2] a score of 0-10 is generated from combining three other scores. It is time consuming and requires trained staff but has high reliability.[3]
   - 0-3 is considered negative for BV
   - 4-6 is considered intermediate
   - 7+ is considered indicative of BV.

   At least 10-20 high power (1000 × oil immersion) fields are counted and an average determined.
5. DNA probe based tests to detect concentration of Gardnerella vaginalis is available but expensive.

   According to Amsel's criteria 3 of the following will lead to the diagnosis of BV.[8]
   - Homogeneous discharge
   - pH > 4.5
   - Amine test
   - Presence of clue cells.

Management

Bacterial vaginosis should be treated when a woman is symptomatic. Even if asymptomatic, BV should be treated in order to prevent the serious complications mentioned above, before pelvic surgery as well as in pregnancy. Metronidazole or clindamycin either orally or vaginally are effective treatment options.[7]

Metronidazole 500 mg twice daily for 7 days, while exhibiting poor activity against lactobacilli has excellent activity against BV causing organisms. Vaginal metronidazole 5 gm/day for 5 days also is effective. The cure rate reported is 75-84%.

Clindamycin ovule 2.5 gm containing 100 mg of clindamycin phosphate for 3 days has improved compliance compared to 7 days therapy.

Clindamycin cream single application (5 grams containing 100 mg clindamycin phosphate) administered intravaginally at anytime of the day has also been found to be effective.

Vaginal clindamycin scores over metronidazole due to better cure rate, better tolerability and less side effects.

In the 'syndromic management' recommended by WHO, a combination treatment of single dose tinidazole plus fluconazole is given to women who present with vaginal discharge.

"A woman presenting with vaginal discharge, who is at low risk for STIs and without symptoms indicative of upper reproductive tract infection may be given empirical treatment based on symptoms without taking swabs at first presentation.": WHO.[4]

Recurrent Bacterial Vaginosis

BV may recur at a rate of 15-30% within 3 months of treatment.

Predisposing factors are:

1. Douching
2. Smoking
3. IUD usage
4. Change of sexual partner

If BV occurs 3-4 times a year, the management includes the following:

- Give a clear explanation about bacterial vaginosis.
- Carefully go through their daily personal hygiene practices to identify the factors that may disrupt the normal balance of vaginal flora.
- Explain that although short course treatments often relieve symptoms, the imbalance in bacteria may persist, and that is why symptoms recur after treatment.
- A longer course of antibiotic such as metronidazole (500 mg) twice daily for up to seven days can be more effective in preventing or delaying recurrence.
- Additional use of lactic acid preparations may also be beneficial.
- Explore the impact on the patient's personal and sexual life and offer psychological support and psychosexual counseling when appropriate.
- If a woman with recurrent bacterial vaginosis has an intrauterine device *in situ,* alternative contraception could be discussed.

The role of probiotics in the management is controversial. A recent Cochrane review has not found beneficial effect, even though earlier reviews found it beneficial.[5,6]

16.3.2 Trichomonas Vaginitis

Trichomonas vaginitis is caused by Trichomonas vaginalis, a flagellate parasite. The infection is sexually transmitted. Transmission rate is very high. Female to male transmission is higher than male to female transmission. The organism can generate hydrogen which combines with oxygen to produce an anaerobic environment. The parasite exists in the trophozoite form. The organism has no cyst form, and can survive for up to 24 hours in urine, semen, or even water samples. It has an ability to persist on fomites with a moist surface for 1 to 2 hours. Often bacterial vaginosis will be seen in association.

Symptoms

Symptoms depend upon the severity of infection. Infection with a small inoculum can be asymptomatic. The typical symptom is the presence of profuse greenish yellow foul smelling vaginal discharge. Pruritus of the vulva may be present. Patchy erythema of the vagina and cervix (strawberry cervix) may rarely be seen.

Diagnosis

Microscopy of a wet film of the vaginal discharge will show motile organisms slightly larger than a neutrophil. The most sensitive laboratory method for the diagnosis is In Pouch TV culture, which has a sensitivity of 81%, whereas wet mount examination has a sensitivity of only 36% and Pap smear test has a sensitivity of 56%.[10] Absence of the organism in the smear does not exclude Trichomonas infection. Clue cells may be present due to the associated bacterial vaginosis. Whiff test may be positive. The vaginal pH will be > 5. Overnight culture has a sensitivity of 75-95% in diagnosing the presence of the organism. Since the infection is sexually transmitted, screening for other sexually transmitted infections should be done.

Treatment

Metronidazole is the drug of choice. It can be given as a single dose of 2 gm orally or as multiple dose of 500 mg twice daily for 7 days. Vaginal metronidazole is not effective in treating the infection. Those who do not respond can be treated with a repeat dose for 7 days. If still not responding a higher dose of 2 gm metronidazole for 5 days should be given. Tinidazole 5 gm daily for 5 days is an alternative treatment. The sexual partner should also be treated since they may be asymptomatic carriers.

16.3.3 Vulvovaginal Candidiasis (VVC)

VVC is common and affects women of all ages. About 75% of women will experience at least one episode of candidiasis in their lifetime. *Candida albicans* is the organism in 90% of the situations. Other species involved are *Candida glabrata* and *Candida tropicalis*.

Candida albicans exist in small numbers in the vagina, skin and the GI tract. Symptoms appear when the number of *Candida* exceeds the normal vaginal flora.

Predisposing Factors

Vulvovaginal candidiasis may follow a course of antibiotic taken for other reason. Pregnancy, diabetes mellitus, COC use and immunodeficiency states predispose to VVC.

Symptoms

The characteristic feature of VVC is curdy white discharge associated with itching of the vulva. There will be associated soreness, dyspareunia and painful micturition. The vulva will be reddish due to the inflammation.

Diagnosis

The characteristic vaginal discharge gives the clue to the diagnosis. Erythema and edema of the vulval skin will be present. The pH will be normal unlike in bacterial vaginosis. Microscopic examination will demonstrate mycelia and yeast forms of the fungus. Fungal culture is confirmatory but is not necessary as microscopic examination will give the diagnosis in 80% of the cases.

Treatment

The drug of choice is azole derivative. The dosages employed are the following:

- Clotrimazole vaginal suppository 100 mg once daily for 7 days.
- Clotrimazole vaginal suppository 100 mg twice daily for 3 days.
- Clotrimazole 500 mg vaginal tablet for single dose.
- Butoconazole 2% cream at a dose of 5 gm intravaginal as a single dose.
- Terconazole 0.4% cream intravaginal for 7 days.
- Terconazole 0.8% cream intravaginal for 3 days.

Oral fluconazole 150 mg as a single dose is as effective as vaginal clotrimazole. Since the symptoms can persist for 2-3 days after therapy, patients should be warned that further treatment is not necessary.

Chronic Vulvovaginal Candidiasis

Women who develop recurrent infection should be screened for predisposing factors.[9] Recurrent infection needs a longer course of antifungal agent. Fluconazole 150 mg daily for 3 days followed by 150 mg weekly for 6 months should be given. Topical treatment lasting for 10-14 days is also effective. Women who have severe irritation in the vagina can be treated with 1% hydrocortisone cream.

16.4 INFLAMMATORY VAGINITIS

This is characterized by profuse purulent vaginal discharge associated with vaginal burning and rarely pruritus. Vaginal erythema will be present. The condition is due to replacement of lactobacilli with gram-positive cocci usually streptococci. Treatment is with 2% clindamycin cream daily for 7 days. If relapse occurs in postmenopausal women, it is an indication to start hormone therapy.

16.5 ATROPHIC VAGINITIS

Atrophy of the vaginal epithelium in postmenopausal women due to estrogen deficiency can lead to bleeding. Treatment is by topical estrogen. Conjugated estrogen cream 1 gm intravaginally daily can be given for about 2 weeks.

16.6 CERVICITIS

Cervicitis could be endocervicitis or exocervicitis. The organisms responsible for these two entities are different. Exocervicitis is usually an association of vaginitis, the causative organism being the same. Endocervicitis is caused by *Neisseria gonorrhoea* and *Chlamydia trachomatis*. Examination will reveal mucopurulent discharge from the cervix. Improperly treated acute cervicitis can lead to chronic cervicitis. Chronic cervicitis is not a forerunner of malignancy of the cervix. Destruction of squamous epithelium of the exocervix results in its replacement with columnar epithelium. Mucous vaginal discharge can be a symptom of such an event. Management is by destroying the columnar epithelium by cryocautery, electrocautery or thermal cautery.

REFERENCES

1. Jaquiery A, Stylianopoulos A, Hogg G, Grover S. "Vulvovaginitis: Clinical features, aetiology, and microbiology of the genital tract". Arch Dis Child 1999;81(1):64-7.
2. Nugent RP, Krohn MA, Hillier SL. "Reliability of diagnosing bacterial vaginosis is improved by a standardized method of gram stain interpretation". J Clin Microbiol 1991;29(2):297-301.
3. Thomason JL, Gelbart SM, Anderson RJ, Walt AK, Osypowski PJ, Broekhuizen FF. "Statistical evaluation of diagnostic criteria for bacterial vaginosis". Am J Obstet Gynecol 1990;162(1):155-60.

4. Jacques Pépin, François Sobela, Nzambi Khonde, Thomas Agyarko-Poku, Soumaila Diakité, Sylvie Deslandes, Annie-Claude Labbé, Mohamed Sylla, Comfort Asamoah-Adu, and Eric Frost. The syndromic management of vaginal discharge using single dose treatments. A randomized controlled trial in West Africa. Bulletin of the World Health Organization 2006; 84(9):685-764.
5. Senok AC, Verstraelen H, Temmerman M, Botta GA. "Probiotics for the treatment of bacterial vaginosis". Cochrane Database Syst Rev 2009;4:CD006289.
6. Ogunsola FT. "The effects of antimicrobial therapy on bacterial vaginosis in non-pregnant women". Cochrane Database Syst Rev 2009;3:CD006055.
7. Joesoef MR, Schmid GP, Hillier SL. "Bacterial vaginosis: Review of treatment options and potential clinical indications for therapy". Clin Infect Dis 1999;28(1):S57-65.
8. Amsel R, Totten PA, Spiegel CA, Chen KC, Eschenbach D, Holmes KK. "Nonspecific vaginitis. Diagnostic criteria and microbial and epidemiologic associations". Am J Med 74 1983;(1):14-22. Brook I (2002).
9. Rodgers CA, Beardall AJ."Recurrent vulvovaginal candidiasis: why does it occur?". Int J STD AIDS 1999;10 (7): 435-9.
10. Ohlemeyer CL, Hornberger LL, Lynch DA, Swierkosz EM. "Diagnosis of Trichomonas vaginalis in adolescent females: In Pouch TV culture versus wet-mount microscopy". The Journal of adolescent health: Official publication of the Society for Adolescent Medicine 1998;22 (3):205-8.

17 Pelvic Organ Prolapse

B Presannakumari

17.1 INTRODUCTION

Pelvic organ prolapse is one of the most common reasons for hysterectomy in postmenopausal women. Some degree of prolapse occurs in 50% of parous women but only 20% of them are symptomatic. The exact prevalence is difficult to determine due to the differences in age, race, study population and examination techniques. In the Women's Health Initiative (WHI) study, incidence of uterine prolapse, cystocele and rectocele were reported to be 14.2%, 34.2% and 18.3% respectively in patients with intact uterus. The prevalence of cystocele and rectocele in women who had hysterectomy was 62.9% and 18.3% respectively.[1]

17.2 DEFINITION

The US National Institute of Health (NIH) in 2001 defined prolapse as the leading edge of any vaginal segment being less than 1 cm above the hymenal remnants. In 2002, the International Continence Society defined pelvic organ prolapse as the descent of one or more of the vaginal segments—the anterior, the posterior, and the apex of the vagina (cervix) or the vault (cuff) after hysterectomy.

A ***cystocele*** is a herniation of the urinary bladder through the anterior vaginal wall. Cystocele usually occurs when the pubovesicocervical fascia weakens in the middle or detaches from the lateral or superior connecting points.

A ***rectocele*** is a protrusion of the rectum into the vaginal lumen resulting from weakness in the muscular wall of the rectum and the Denonvillier's fascia.

An ***enterocele*** is a herniation of the peritoneum and small bowel which occurs downwards between the uterosacral ligaments.

Uterine prolapse is generally the result of lack of strength of cardinal and uterosacral ligaments leading to descent of the uterus towards the introitus.

Procidentia is descent of the uterus with complete eversion of the vagina.

The terms like cystocele, rectocele, and enterocele are now replaced by anterior compartment defects, posterior compartment defects and middle compartment defects respectively.

The reason is that these terms give an unrealistic certainty as to the visceral structures on the other side of the vaginal bulge especially in women who have undergone previous prolapse surgery. **Hence, pelvic organ prolapse is classified as anterior compartment, middle compartment and posterior compartment defects and a compartmental approach is adopted for treatment.**

It is important to understand the etiology, pathophysiology and risk factors associated with pelvic organ prolapse in order to prevent prolapse and also for the appropriate surgical correction.

17.3 ETIOLOGY

The etiology of prolapse is multifactorial. Over 90% of these patients are parous. Vaginal delivery is the most important factor causing prolapse. Instrumental delivery, delivery of a macrosomic infant and prolonged second stage of labor increases the chance of trauma of vaginal delivery. Obesity is another factor strongly associated with increased risk of vaginal prolapse. Genital atrophy and hypo-estrogenism play an important contributory role in the development of prolapse after menopause. Other factors implicated are chronic cough, constipation, previous hysterectomy and estrogen deficiency. Rarely the etiology may be congenital weakness of collagen as occuring in Ehlers-Danlos and Marfan syndrome or weakness of the muscle due to spina bifida.

17.3.1 Pathophysiology

The pelvic organs comprising the bladder, urethra, uterus, vagina and the rectum are supported and maintained in its normal position by the muscles of the pelvic floor and the pelvic fascia with its condensations, the pelvic ligaments.

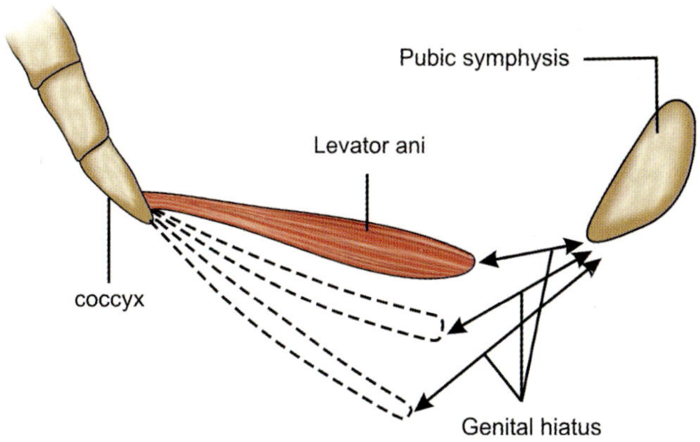

Fig. 17.1: Sagging of pelvic diaphragm causing widening of genital hiatus

Childbearing and aging predispose to damage of the muscular and fascial supports of the pelvic organs. Both childbearing and aging cause denervation of the pelvic floor muscles. This leads to sagging of the levators, widening of the levator hiatus and loss of support of pelvic viscera (Fig. 17.1). The endopelvic fascial support is also equally important in keeping the pelvic viscera in its normal position. This forms a network of supporting tissue which extends between the vagina and the pelvic sidewall.

Vaginal delivery causes discrete defects in this fascial network. The defects thus produced may be unilateral or bilateral, single or multiple, and may involve anterior, posterior or lateral vaginal walls. This can lead to stress urinary incontinence and genital prolapse. Childbirth and menopause cause changes in the collagen content of the endopelvic fascia causing weakness of the pelvic floor.

Collagen is the main component of the endopelvic fascia. Reduction in the quantity of collagen and increased turnover of collagen has been identified in women with prolapse. The remodeling of collagen due to hormonal changes following childbirth is one of the reasons for prolapse[2] uterus following delivery.

17.3.2 Anatomical Considerations

A thorough understanding of the pelvic anatomy is important in the diagnosis of pelvic support defects and most importantly in the surgical correction of these defects. Sagittal view of female pelvis showing the relation of pelvic viscera to endopelvic fascia is provided in Figure 17.2.

The anatomical supports of the pelvic organs were originally described by Victor Bonney. The uterus, vagina, bladder, urethra, rectum and anal canal are supported and kept in place by the pelvic floor. The pelvic floor comprises from below upwards the superficial and deep perineal

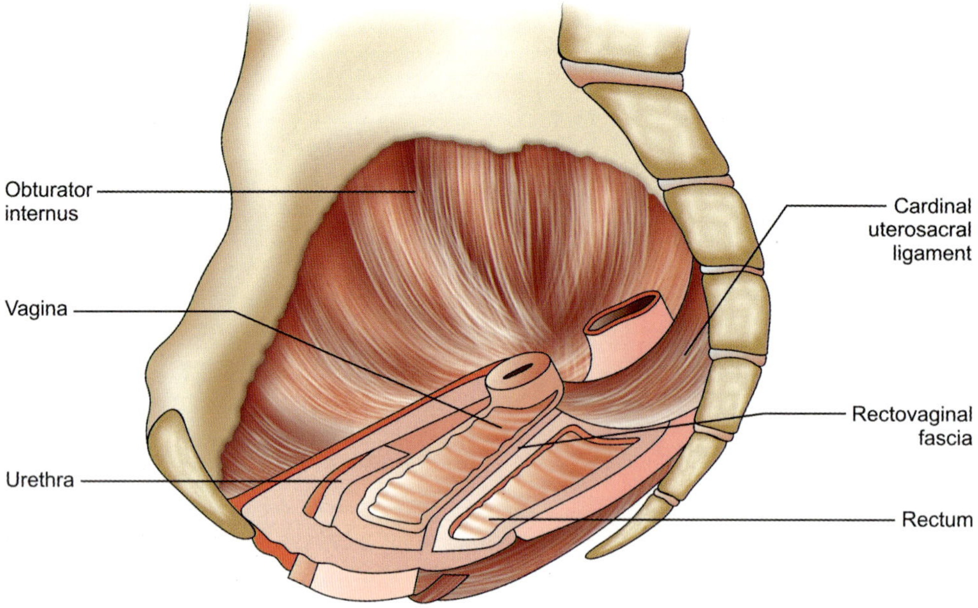

Fig. 17.2: Sagittal view of female pelvis showing relation of pelvic viscera to endopelvic fascia (redrawn from Skandalakis JE, et al (Eds). Hernia: Surgical anatomy and technique, 244-250)

muscles, the levator ani, the ligaments which are the condensations of pelvic cellular tissue, and the pelvic peritoneum. Posterolaterally are the obturator internus and the piriformis.

The levator ani is the most important muscle forming the pelvic diaphragm. It has two parts–the pubococcygeus and iliococcygeus. The muscle arises from the pelvic surface of the pubic bone and ischial spine. In between, it takes origin from the internal obturator fascia (arcus tendineus fascia pelvis).The anterior part of the pubococcygeus decussate around the vagina (pubovaginalis) and passes to the perineal body and anal canal. Anteriorly, the fibers are in relation to the urethra but are not attached to it. Posterior fibers join the raphe formed by the iliococcygeus. The deeper fibers of each side unite behind the anorectal junction (puborectalis). This slings the anorectal junction to the pubic bone. The iliococcygeus muscle proceeds downwards, medially and backwards and gets inserted on to the median raphe and to the last two pieces of the coccyx. The muscle is supplied by the anterior primary rami of S3 and S4. Both these muscles form the main support for the pelvic viscera and also act as sphincters for the rectum and vagina.

The muscles of the urogenital diaphragm, i.e. the sphincter urethrae and deep perineal muscles originate from ischial rami and are inserted on to the perineal body. They are supplied by the pudendal nerve. The muscles are covered inferiorly by the perineal membrane.

The endopelvic fascia is made of collagen, elastin and smooth muscle. It envelopes the pelvic structures, the uterus, vagina, bladder, urethra and rectum and attaches these to the walls of the pelvis with its condensations, the ligaments. This fascial sheath which lies anterior to and above the vagina is trapezoidal in shape with the narrow end located distally. It is known as vesicovaginal septum or the pubovesicocervical septum/fascia. It is attached distally to the pubic tubercles and the pubic arch. This fascial bridge is attached laterally to the arcus tendinus fascia pelvis. It forms the anterior vaginal support and suspends the bladder. Anterolateral detachment of this fascia results in anterior vaginal wall prolapse. The ATFP usually detaches from the ischial spine, but not from the pubis (Figs 17.3 and 17.4).

The endopelvic fascial sheath which lies in between the vagina and the rectum is also trapezoidal with the narrow end located distally. It supports the posterior vaginal wall and stabilizes the rectum. This fascial sheath is called the Denonvillier's fascia (described later).

Pelvic Ligaments

The ligaments are the condensations of the pelvic fascia in the upper part. They act as mooring for the cervix and upper part of the vagina. The following are the pelvic ligaments:

The cardinal ligament is the most important ligamentary support of the uterus. It extends from the lateral aspect of the cervix and upper vagina to the pelvic sidewall. It forms the base of the broad ligament. The ureter passes through a tunnel in the ligament.

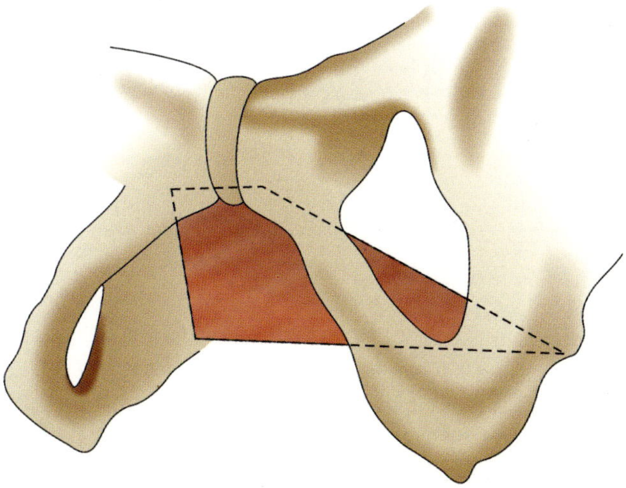

Fig. 17.3: Normal attachment of the anterior fibromuscular vaginal plane (redrawn from Berek and Novak's book of Gynaecology, 14th edition)

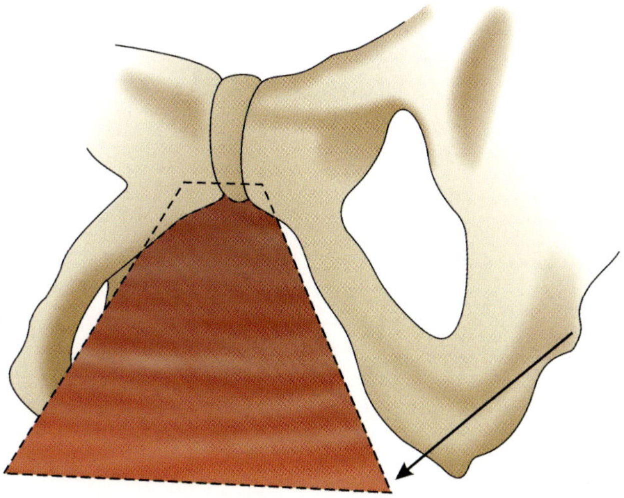

Fig. 17.4: Bilateral detachment of the anterior vaginal plane from the arcus tendineus (redrawn from Berek and Novak's book of Gynaecology, 14th edition)

The uterosacral ligament extends from the cervix and upper vagina to the sacrum. Near the cervix it inter digitates with the cardinal ligament fibers.

Posterior pubourethral ligament extends from the posteroinferior aspect of the symphysis pubis to the anterior aspect of the middle third of the urethra and on to the bladder. This ligament maintains the elevation of the bladder neck and prevents excess posterior displacement of the urethra. It is important in maintaining urinary continence.

Round ligament mainly consists of smooth muscle fibers and extends from the uterine cornua through the inguinal canal and ends at the labia majora. It does not have much of a supportive function but has some role in keeping the uterus in the anteverted position.

The rest of the endopelvic fascia envelopes the pelvic structures, the uterus, vagina, bladder, urethra and rectum and attaches these to the walls of the pelvis. It is made of collagen, elastin and smooth muscle.

The Supports of the Anterior Vaginal Wall

The pubovesicocervical fascia/septum: This is a trapezoid fascia which supports the anterior vagina. It extends from the vagina to the anterior and lateral walls of the pelvis. It is attached to the arcus tendineus fascia laterally from a point just posterior to the pubic ramus to a point just anterior to the ischial spine. This attachment supports the anterolateral vaginal wall. Its cephalad attachment is to the cardinal uterosacral ligament complex. Discrete defects in the fascial supports which are caused by vaginal delivery can end up in prolapse and stress urinary incontinence. This has been emphasized by Richardson in his important contributions.[3]

Anterior Compartment Defects

1. **Paravaginal defect** occurs when the pubovesicocervical fascia gets detached from its lateral attachment to the arcus tendineus fascia pelvis.
2. **Transverse (apical) defect** occurs when the fascia gets detached from its attachment to the pericervical ring. This results in descent of the apical vagina and uterus.
3. **Central defect** occurs when the defect is in the area immediately anterior to the vaginal mucosa in the center resulting in a midline defect (central cystocele).
4. **Descend of urethrovesical angle**—Loss of support of the urethrovesical angle results in the rotational descend of the bladder neck causing stress urinary incontinence.

The Supports of the Posterior Vaginal Wall

The posterior vaginal wall is supported by the Denonvillier's fascia which is the fibromuscular layer of the posterior vagina. Superiorly it fuses with the pericervical fascia and the fan shaped cardinal ligaments. This attachment from the cardinal-uterosacral ligament complex to the anterior rectal wall prevents enterocele formation. Thus, the upper part of the posterior vaginal wall is indirectly attached to the sacrum. Through the lateral attachment of the Denonvillier's fascia to the levator fascia, indirectly the vagina is laterally attached to the levator fascia. Caudally, the Denonvillier's fascia is attached to the perineal body. The pelvic floor muscle which is in a constant resting tone is another important support of the posterior vaginal wall. This serves to keep the genital hiatus closed. Contraction of puborectalis muscle pulls the rectum, vagina and bladder anteriorly.

When there is a tear in the Denonvillier's fascia, it results in posterior vaginal wall prolapse. The tear can be central, lateral, apical or caudal. The apical detachment results in enterocele. Central or caudal defects cause different types of rectocele or eversion of vagina.

Deficiency of the perineal body can occur, either due to tears sustained during vaginal delivery or attenuation due to menopausal atrophy.

17.3.3 Delancey's Three Levels of Support of the Vagina

Delancey (1992) suggested three levels of support of the vaginal wall. This concept is very important in the site specific repair of prolapse. Operations which do not take into account the normal attachments of the vagina[4] are likely to fail.

Level 1: Level 1 is the parametrium comprising the uterosacral and cardinal ligaments. Its main action is to support the cervix and the upper vagina by attaching to the pelvic side wall and the sacrum. Defective support at this level results in descent of the uterus. The detachment of the Denonvillier's fascia from its attachment to the uterosacral ligaments and pericervical ring can result in the descent of the upper posterior vaginal wall (enterocele).

Level 2: Level 2 is the attachment of the anterior and the posterior walls of the vagina to the pelvic side wall. The anterior attachment is to the fascia covering the obturator internus and levator ani—the arcus tendineus fascia and the posterior attachment is to the superior fascia of the levator ani. Defects at this level cause either a central or lateral anterior vaginal support defect (cystocele) or a posterior vaginal wall defect in the middle (rectocele). A lateral defect which extends to the urethrovesical junction can cause urinary stress incontinence.

Level 3: In the lower aspect, the endopelvic fascia fuses with the urethra and urogenital diaphragm and the pubis anteriorly. Laterally, it fuses with the levator ani fascia and posteriorly with the perineal body. Defects at this level cause urethrocele.

17.4 CLINICAL FEATURES

17.4.1 Symptoms

Urinary symptoms

- Stress incontinence
- Incomplete emptying or voiding difficulty
- Frequency of urination
- Positional changes in initiation of micturition
- Digital repositioning to initiate micturition
- Retention—A late complication which occurs when the prolapse is irreducible

Symptoms may not always correspond to the degree of prolapse. It can vary according to the site of defects. Eliciting the exact symptom is very important in planning surgical repair. *When eliciting the symptoms an effort should be made to pinpoint the site of defect; whether the symptoms are concerning the anterior, middle or posterior compartment.* The symptom which is common to all patients with prolapse is a feeling of mass coming down per vaginum. Patients may also complain of backache which is typically relieved by rest. Backache is caused due to stretching of nerves and it is usually more in mild degrees of prolapse than in severe degrees. A major degree of prolapse can interfere with sexual activity. Anterior compartment prolapse produces mainly urinary symptoms. Increased frequency can occur if the patient has a large cystocele with the urethrovesical angle well supported. In this situation, frequency is due to incomplete emptying. This is because when the patient strains, urine escapes into the cystocele and if the urethrovesical angle is well supported there will be kinking of the urethra and the cystocele will be at a lower level than the urethra causing incomplete emptying.

Posterior compartment defects mainly produce bowel symptoms which are as follows:

- Incomplete emptying of bowel
- Vaginal digital reposition for helping defecation
- Fecal urgency
- Incontinence of flatus or feces if the perineal body is deficient and there is decreased tone of the external anal sphincter

Unless the patient reduces the prolapse herself, she will not be able to empty the bladder. If the defect is in the urethrovesical junction there will be rotational descent of the bladder neck and the symptom can be stress urinary incontinence. When there is procidentia and the prolapse becomes irreducible it results in retention of urine with overflow incontinence. In long standing prolapse, the cervix and vagina may become ulcerated (Fig. 17.5) due to chronic congestion and may present as discharge per vaginum or bleeding per vaginum. In long standing prolapse of major degrees, there can be bilateral ureteric kinking leading to bilateral hydronephrosis and hydroureter which can lead to renal failure.

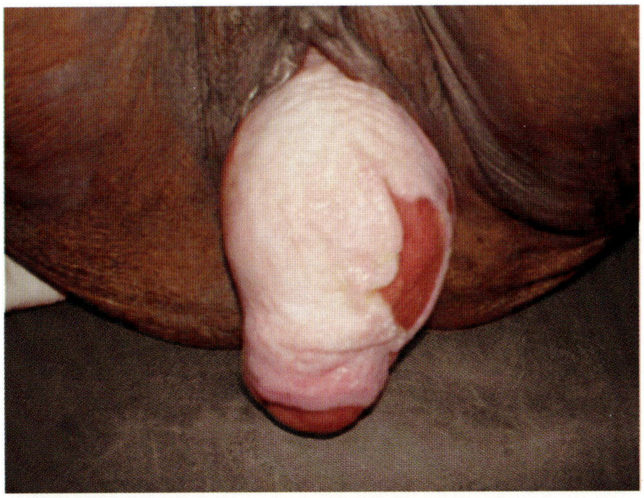

Fig. 17.5: Descent of the uterus with complete eversion of the vagina in a 70-year-old lady. Note the decubitus ulcer on the right side

17.4.2 Signs

Identification of the compartment and the site specific defect is important in planning surgical repair so that recurrence can be minimized. The patient should be examined at rest, while straining and also on traction. If the patient complains of stress incontinence she should be examined in full bladder to demonstrate incontinence while straining. *A site specific physical evaluation is essential*. When examining the patient, the site of pelvic defect should be correctly noted as the degree of defect in the anterior, middle and posterior compartment may not be uniform. A patient may have a large defect in the anterior compartment along with a small defect in the posterior compartment.

Prolapse of the lower anterior vaginal wall results in urethrocele. In most cases even with major degrees of prolapse the anterior vaginal wall in relation to the urethra will be spared.

Differentiating central cystocele from lateral cystocele—A defect in the central part of the pubovesicocervical fascia (the musculofascial wall of the anterior vagina) causing a central defect produces a ballooning type of defect of the upper anterior vaginal wall and the vaginal rugosity of the central aspect will be less or absent. The lateral sulci, which run along the anterolateral vaginal wall, will be preserved. A lateral defect (lateral cystocele) is demonstrated by keeping an open long curved artery forceps to retract the anterolateral aspect of the vagina. If the bulge disappears or becomes less prominent, the patient has a lateral defect. The lateral sulci also will be less prominent.

To demonstrate enterocele, the patient should be evaluated either in the dorsal position or in Sim's position. After reducing the prolapse and keeping the cervix in its normal position, i.e. at the level of the ischial spines, the Sim's speculum is inserted into the vagina and the posterior vaginal wall is retracted downwards and backwards as the patient strains. If the woman has anterior vaginal wall descent as well it may hinder proper visualization which can be overcome by retracting the anterior vaginal wall with the help of an anterior vaginal wall retractor. While the speculum is being withdrawn the site specific defect in the posterior vaginal wall can be made out. If there is a bulge in the upper one third, it is an enterocele and if there is a bulge in the middle one third, it is a rectocele and of course the deficient perineum can be demonstrated without the help of a speculum. As was mentioned earlier, abnormalities of the cervix and vagina should be made out and evaluated because there can be an ulcer in the vagina or a simultaneous malignancy of the cervix. After the local examination, a careful bimanual examination should be performed to exclude masses in the pelvis which may sometimes be the cause of prolapse and the levator ani tone should be assessed. In assessing the levator ani tone two fingers are kept in the vagina in the 4'o clock position and the thumb is placed at the outer aspect of the perineum. Meanwhile, the patient is asked to constrict the levator ani muscle as if she is stopping a stream of urine and the tone is assessed on the patient's left side. The same is repeated on the right side of the patient by keeping the vaginal fingers at the 8'o clock position. A rectal examination is also performed to assess the tone of the anal sphincter complex. The rectovaginal septum can be examined by a bi-digital examination.

The Q Tip Test

If the patient complains of stress incontinence or if the clinical examination findings suggest descent of the bladder neck as evidenced by a less prominent urethral sulcus, urethral hypermobility should be ascertained. This can be done by keeping a cotton tip in the urethra and asking the patient to strain. The angle between the axis of cotton tip and the horizontal is made out. If the angle is more than 30°, there is urethral hypermobility (Figs 17.6A and B).

When there is significant uterine prolapse, incontinence of urine should be excluded in the following manner. The bladder is filled with 300 ml sterile water after reducing the prolapse. The patient is asked to cough or strain. If there is leakage of urine the patient should have some form of incontinence and incontinence correction procedure is required. If it is neglected 30% of patients will have post operative urinary incontinence.

After examination, the degree of prolapse is classified.

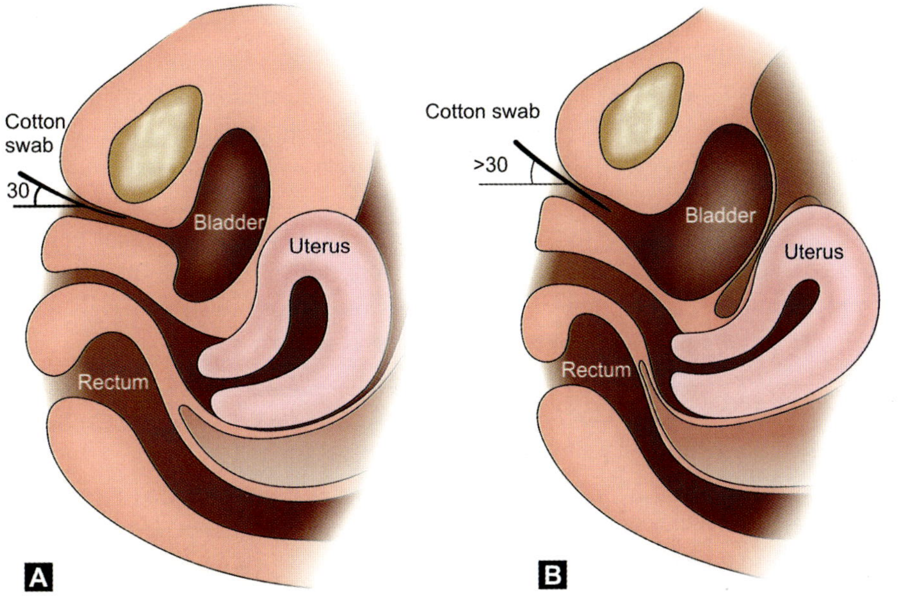

Figs 17.6A and B: Q tip test: (A) Normal angle of the cotton swab in the urethra with the horizontal (<30°). (B) Bladder neck descent resulting in >30° angle

17.4.3 Classification of Prolapse

There are 3 systems of classification of prolapse.

- Baden-Walker Halfway system
- ICS system using Pelvic Organ Prolapse Quantification (POPQ) system
- Revised New York classification (NYC) system (Baden, 1972; Bump,1976; Coti et al, 2000)

The classification system which has been in use since several years is the Baden and Walker classification which is as provided in Table 17.1.

Table 17.1: Baden and Walker classification

Grade I	Descent of any organ to the vaginal midplane
Grade II	Descent to the hymenal ring
Grade III	Descent to halfway through the introitus
Grade IV	Complete eversion

The NYC system preserves (Table 17.2) the Baden-Walker Halfway system and maybe converted to the POPQ.

Table 17.2: NYC system

Stage I	Descent of the uterus to any point in the vagina above the hymen
Stage II	Descent to the level of hymen
Stage III	Descent beyond the hymen
Stage IV	Complete eversion or procidentia

Pelvic Organ Prolapse Quantification (POPQ) System

Since the classification systems lacked reproducibility in the diagnostic evaluation of degree of pelvic organ prolapse in the various compartments and also in evaluating the outcome of various procedures for correction of pelvic organ prolapse, the International Continence Society standardized the terminology of pelvic organ prolapse. In 1993, an International Committee comprising of members of International Continence Society, American Urogynaecological Society and Society of Gynaec surgeons drafted the standardization document. This is the POPQ system (Fig. 17.7).

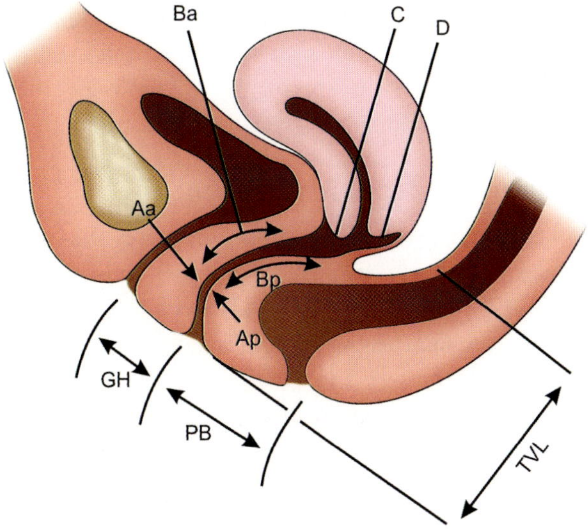

Fig. 17.7: Standardization of terminology for female pelvic organ prolapse (POPQ classification). Redrawn from Bump RC, Mattiason A, Bo K, et al. The standardization of terminology of female pelvic organ prolapse and pelvic floor dysfunction. Am J Obset Gynecol 1996; 175

In the POPQ system, anterior, midline and posterior compartments are separately evaluated for pelvic organ prolapse. Terms such as cystocele, rectocele and enterocele are replaced by corresponding segments of vaginal wall. Patient should be examined while straining and on traction.

The anterior compartment includes the anterior vaginal wall, the related pubovesicocervical fascia with the attached viscera—the bladder and urethra.

The middle compartment is composed of the uterus and the posterior fornix.

The posterior compartment is composed of the posterior vaginal wall with its posterior fibromuscular wall which is the Denonvilliers' fascia.

The defects are measured from a fixed point of reference which is taken as the hymen. The plane of the hymen is taken as 0. Six defined points from the hymen are taken as the reference points. The position of these points, if above the hymen is taken as negative and if below the hymen is taken as positive. The points are, two in the anterior compartment, two in the middle compartment and two in the posterior compartment.

Points in the Anterior Compartment

- **Aa** is a point 3 cm proximal to the hymen in the anterior vaginal wall. It will be -3 in a woman without prolapse and can range from -3 to +3 depending on the degree of prolapse.
- **Ba** is the most dependent position of the rest of the anterior vaginal wall. It will be in the same level as Aa (-3) in a woman without prolapse and can range from -3 in a woman without prolapse, to total vaginal length in the case of complete eversion of the vagina.

Points in the Middle Compartment

Cervix and posterior fornix comprise the middle compartment

- **Point C** refers to the tip of the cervix.
  C will be total vaginal length minus length of vaginal portion of the cervix in a lady with no prolapse.
- **Point D** denotes pouch of Douglas. It is equal to total vaginal length if there is no prolapse. It is omitted in the case of vault prolapse.

Difference between D and C gives the length of the vaginal portion of cervix. Points D and C are separately measured to differentiate between prolapse of uterus from an elongated cervix in which case also the external os will be seen at a lower level in the vagina.

Points in the Posterior Compartment

Posterior compartment also is measured similar to the anterior compartment making use of two points.

- **Ap** is 3 cm proximal to the hymen which will be -3 in a woman who has no prolapse and can range from -3 to +3
- **Bp** is the most dependent portion of the rest of the posterior vaginal wall. Bp can range from -3 in a woman without prolapse, to total vaginal length in a woman with procidentia.

The other measurements which are taken include:

- **Total vaginal length (TVL)** which is the total length of the vagina.
- **Genital hiatus (GH)** is measured from middle of the external urethral opening to the posterior hymenal ring. It will be 2 cm when there is no gaping of introitus and will be larger when the introitus is gaping.
- **Perineal body (PB)** is measured from fourchette to the middle of anal opening. If it is $>$ 2 cm there is no deficiency of perineal body.

Genital hiatus, perineal body and total vaginal length are measured after reducing the prolapse. All other measurements are taken with the prolapse in maximum protrusion.

Measurements can be recorded as a simple line of numbers (Fig. 17.8). For example, if there is no prolapse -3, -3, -7, -9, -3, -3, 9, 2, 2 for points Aa, Ba, C, D, Ap, Bp, TVL, GH, PB respectively.

There can be several different combinations of pelvic support defects. For example, a lady can have minimal

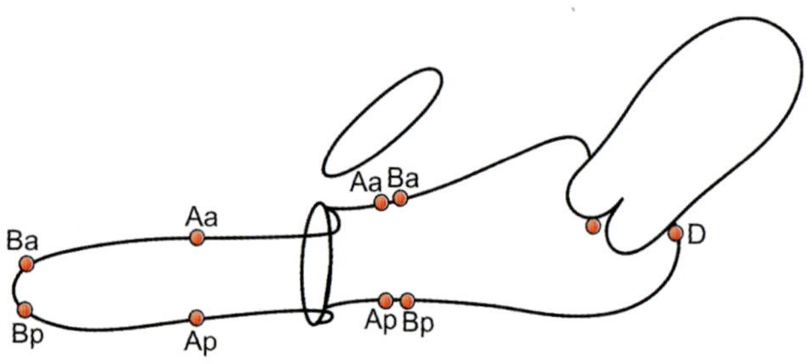

+3 Aa	+8 Ba	+8 C
4.5 GH	1.5 PB	8 TVL
+3 Ap	+8 Bp	—

−3 Aa	−3 Ba	−8 C
2 GH	3 PB	10 TVL
−3 Ap	−3 Bp	10 D

Fig. 17.8: Diagrammatic representation of measurements in post-hysterectomy vaginal eversion and normal support of the uterus (Left—complete vaginal vault eversion; Right—normal support of the uterus and cervix)

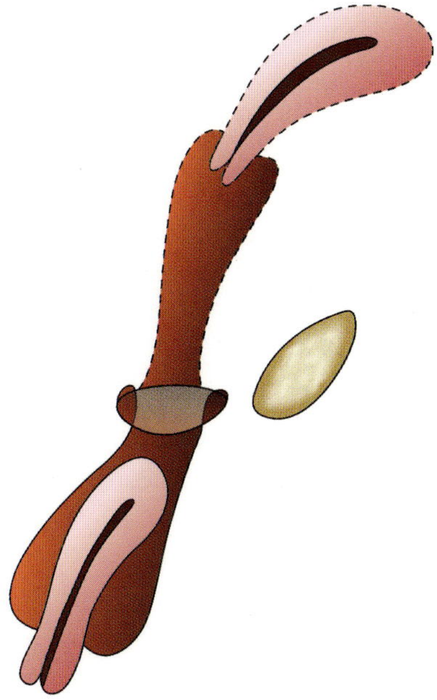

Fig. 17.9: Diagrammatic representation of procidentia. The normal position of the vagina and the uterus is shown in dotted line

descent of the uterus with a greater descent of the anterior vaginal wall and a lesser descent of the posterior vaginal wall. This can be precisely noted in a tandem method of report. This method of reporting several combinations cannot be used to compare when populations are being studied. So having completed quantitative description, an ordinal staging (Stage 0, 1, 2, 3, 4) has been given based on the most severe descent of the prolapse.

Stage 0—When there is no prolapse. Points Aa, Ap, Ba, Bp are all –3cm. Point D or C will be between –TVL cm and –(TVL –2) cm

Stage 1—The most distal portion of the prolapse is >1 cm above the hymen

Stage 2—The most distal portion of the prolapse is ≤ 1 cm above or below the level of the hymen

Stage 3—Most distal portion of the prolapse is >1 cm below the plane of the hymen but protrudes no further than 2 cm less than TVL.

Stage 4—Complete eversion of the total length of the lower genital tract (Fig. 17.9). The distal end protrudes to at least (TVL 2) cm. In most instances the leading edge will be the cervix or the vaginal vault.

17.5 PRETREATMENT EVALUATION

Prolapse by itself does not usually produce severe morbidity or mortality. Mortality can occur due to prolapse only if there is severe degree of long standing prolapse with renal failure. So before undertaking treatment decisions, several issues have to be kept in mind.

- Symptoms of the patient with respect to the three compartments of the pelvis.
- Objective examination to evaluate the specific defects in the three compartments.
- Diagnostic evaluation depending on patient's complaint.

Before deciding on the management option, patient's expectations and priorities should be discussed. The procedure selected should aim for the highest quality of life after surgery, at the same time keeping the lowest recurrence risk for the particular patient. Each patient's concerns and needs should be properly addressed.

17.5.1 Preoperative Investigations

Routine investigations for anesthesia and surgery as for any operative procedure must be performed.

Diagnostic imaging is not routinely performed, but in particular situations it may be necessary. When the uterus is not going to be removed, imaging of pelvic organs to exclude uterine and adnexal pathology is a must. Dynamic MRI is the investigation of choice for assessing enterocele.

Isotope defecography is useful in demonstrating rectocele.

Ultrasound imaging by transabdominal, endorectal, endovaginal, translabial or perineal routes is evolving as a diagnostic tool for detecting pelvic floor defects in prolapse. Endoanal ultrasound is helpful in diagnosing enterocele and anal sphincter defects. Transperineal 4D ultrasound is an efficient investigation to evaluate the levator ani muscle. MRI is a more accurate investigation in diagnosing the disorders of pelvic support as well as follow-up after surgery.

Urodynamic studies should be done in women with associated voiding problems or incontinence. If the patient is detected to have incontinence, an incontinence correction procedure should be planned along with prolapse repair.

17.6 MANAGEMENT OF PROLAPSE

Therapy should be decided based on

- Patient's general health
- Stage and type of pelvic organ prolapse
- The particular structural defect
- Presence or absence of stress urinary incontinence
- Need for preservation of coital function
- Desire for preservation of reproductive function
- Concomitant pelvic organ disease

17.6.1 Nonsurgical Therapies

There are several nonsurgical therapies which include

- Pelvic floor strengthening exercise
- Behavioral management
- Use of mechanical devices like pessary.

Pelvic floor muscle strengthening exercise may be advised for those women who desire childbearing and who develop prolapse after the first or second childbirth. It is useful in relieving stress urinary incontinence, but at present there is no evidence to suggest that it relieves prolapse. It may halt the progress of prolapse. Since it is not harmful, it may be advised.

Weight loss and avoiding weight lifting may be advised but there are no randomized controlled trials proving its efficacy.

Pessary Treatment

Pessary treatment is tried in the following situations:

- Women who develop mild or moderate degrees of prolapse following childbirth and who wish to conceive again. It is better to repair the prolapse after the completion of childbearing.
- Those who decline surgery.
- Those who are unfit for surgery.
- Pregnant women with prolapse uterus.
- Patients undergoing preoperative preparation for prolapse surgery.

Pessaries are not a permanent treatment for prolapse. However, symptoms can be relieved by pessary use temporarily. There are two types of pessaries. One is a ring pessary with support and the other a gel horn pessary which is a space fitting pessary. The ring pessary is the commonly used one and is particularly useful in treating stage I and II prolapse. In stages III and IV, prolapse, space fitting pessary is appropriate. According to a Cochrane review there is no evidence from randomized controlled trials upon which to base treatment of women with pelvic organ prolapse through the use of mechanical devices/pessaries. There is no consensus on the use of different types of device, the indications, nor the pattern of replacement and follow-up care.[5] The possible complications with the use of mechanical devices include vaginal discharge, malodor and ulceration of the vagina. Rarely, reduction of prolapse can lead to worsening of stress incontinence. If the vaginal ulcer caused by chronic irritation is neglected, it may lead to vesicovaginal fistula, urinary infection, bowel entrapment, all of which have been rarely described. Before advising pessary, lesions of the uterus, cervix and the vagina should be excluded. Pessary can be the option for very old patients and for those who are unfit for surgery due to medical problems.

Correction of Aggravating Factors

Reducing weight, quitting smoking, avoiding lifting of heavy weight, treating chronic cough and constipation etc should be considered before taking the patient for surgery.

Hormone Replacement Therapy (HRT)

Topical estrogen is useful in postmenopausal women to improve the quality of pelvic floor structures. But there is no evidence suggesting that it can cure prolapse.

17.6.2 Surgical Treatment

Is Hysterectomy Mandatory?

Vaginal hysterectomy with pelvic floor repair is the most commonly resorted procedure in women with pelvic organ prolapse who do not wish to conserve the uterus. Hysterectomy used to be done along with pelvic floor repair based on the following assumptions:

- The uterus causes prolapse to occur
- Removal of the uterus is necessary for the repair of prolapse
- Hysterectomy improves the chance of long-term success of repair

Recent research has indicated that hysterectomy is not always necessary for the successful surgical repair but may in fact cause further damage to the fascial support of the upper vagina (Mackenrodts-uterosacral complex) leading to a higher chance of recurrence. Repair using mesh after hysterectomy increases the chance of mesh erosion. Presently uterine suspension with either autologos material or artificial material like prolene mesh is being practiced without resorting to hysterectomy. Uterosacral ligament fixation, sacral uteropexy and sacrospinous colpopexy are being largely resorted to without hysterectomy.

The traditional surgical approach for uterine prolapse in elderly patients is vaginal hysterectomy with pelvic floor repair (*Ward Mayo's operation*). Attention should be given to the correction of the specific defect in each patient. As mentioned earlier, each patient can have different combinations of defects. Vaginal hysterectomy is performed initially for accessing the supporting structures. The most commonly resorted surgical technique is described below.

The anterior lip of the cervix is held with a Volsellum and two Allis forceps are placed on either side of the cervix. A third Allis forceps is placed below the external urethral meatus if the patient has urethrocele or below the urethrovesical junction if only a cystocele is present. The anterior vaginal wall is incised by an inverted T-shaped incision. The horizontal limb of the inverted T should be just below the bladder sulcus to avoid bladder injury. The vaginal wall is reflected from the bladder and the underlying fascia. The dissection should be carried till well below the external urethral meatus if the patient has urethrovesical angle descent also. Bleeding points should be coagulated. The attachment of the bladder to the cervix (vesicocervical ligament) is cut and the bladder is pushed up. The posterior lip of the cervix is now held with a Volsellum. The horizontal limb of the T incision is then carried around the cervix posteriorly, the pouch of Douglas opened and the uterus is brought forwards and delivered after cutting the uterovesical fold of peritoneum. Clamps are applied from below upwards. The first clamp is applied on the Mackenrodts' ligament and uterosacral ligament together. The second clamp is applied to the uterine vessels. The third clamp includes the round ligament, tube, broad ligament and the ovarian ligament. The ovaries should be inspected for abnormalities. In a postmenopausal patient, the ovaries can also be removed by clamping the round ligament initially and then the Infundibulopelvic ligament. If the patient has enterocele, it is corrected at this point. The enterocele peritoneal sac should be dissected and excised. The uterosacral ligaments are plicated in the midline. Peritoneal closure may be done with a single suture approximating the uterovesical fold of peritoneum anteriorly and pouch of Douglas peritoneum posteriorly. Traditional cystocele correction is done by plicating the pubovesicocervical fascia in the midline. Stanton SL reported a cure rate of 85% for prolapse and stress incontinence[6] following this procedure.

A lateral cystocele can also be corrected if the dissection is carried far laterally to reach the arcus tendineus fascia at the pelvic side wall. The pubovesicocervical fascia is reattached to the arcus tendineus fascia.

Women who have stress incontinence along with prolapse should undergo an incontinence correction procedure. Along with Ward Mayo's operation the procedure usually adopted is Kelly's plication. Plication sutures are applied at the region of bladder neck to reform the posterior urethrovesical angle. Redundant anterior vaginal wall is excised and the vagina is approximated preferably with sutures of polyglactin (no. 1 vicryl). It is ideal to put interrupted sutures to prevent shortening of the vaginal wall.

Posterior colpoperineorrhaphy: Two Allis forceps are placed at the lower end of labia minora and a third Allis forceps at the apex of the rectocele. A horizontal incision is put between the two Allis forceps and a vertical incision from the middle of this incision towards the third Allis forceps. The vagina is reflected from the perineal body below and the rectum above. The prerectal fascia (the Denonvilliers' fascia) is plicated in the midline to support the rectum. The levator ani muscles on either side are identified and caught with Allis forceps and plicated in the midline. This procedure is controversial as it can later lead to dyspareunia and also atrophy of the plicated part of the levator muscle. However, this step is advisable for patients who have widened genital hiatus. The redundant posterior vaginal wall is excised and the vaginal epithelium is sutured. Superficial perineal muscles are approximated. The skin of the perineum is closed and the vagina is packed for another 24 hours. An indwelling urinary catheter is kept for 3-4 days as the patient can have reflex retention of urine because of the pelvic floor repair.

Repair of Site Specific Defects

Repair of anterior compartment defect

Types of anatomical defects producing cystocele was first described by Raz[7] et al. Defective support of the anterior vagina can be caused due to a tear or weakness of the fibromuscular wall of the anterior vagina (pubovesicocervical fascia). The fascia may tear from its attachment to the arcus tendinous or from its attachment to the peri cervical ring. This can cause the following defects:

- central ballooning type of defect (central cystocele)
- descent of the bladder neck region
- lateral detachment (lateral cystocele)

The traditional anterior colporrhaphy of plicating the pubovesical fasia in the midline is presently replaced by a site specific repair. Following site specific repair, Walter et al[8] reported cure rates of 100% in a follow-up of one year.

In site specific repair, the exact site of pubovesicocervical fascial tear is identified by clinical examination as described earlier. The lateral tear producing a lateral defect and a central tear producing a central defect are repaired in different methods.

Repair of lateral cystocele

As lateral cystocele is the result of tearing of the musculofascial attachments of the vagina from the arcus tendinous fascia pelvis, the repair should be reattachment of the fascia to the arcus tendinous fascia. The arcus tendinous fascia can be approached transabdominally by dissecting through the cave of Retzius and going laterally to the pelvic side wall where the arcus tendinous fascia could be seen covering the obturator internus muscle.[9]

This can also be done through the vaginal route but with much difficulty.[10]

Repair of central cystocele

A central cystocele results from tearing of the pubovesical fascia in the midline which is usually repaired by plicating it. This can be performed along with Ward Mayo's operation after hysterectomy. It can also be done for cystocele repair where hysterectomy is not preferred.

When large central cystocele coexists with lateral defect the procedure of choice is to use a mesh to span the entire vesicovaginal space. The mesh has to be attached laterally to the white line. The procedure is usually done vaginally.

Prolapse of the bladder neck

Rotational descend of the bladder neck presenting with cystocele and stress incontinence may be corrected by Burch colposuspension which will be described later. It can also be repaired vaginally by Kelly's plication. The cure rates achieved is much better after Burch's colposuspension than Kelly's plication. An alternative procedure is inserting a tension free vaginal tape after correcting the anterior compartment defect.

Repair of middle compartment defect

Correction of uterine prolapse

When uterine conservation is not required, vaginal hysterectomy with pelvic floor repair is the treatment of choice. If the woman wants to retain her uterus there are several options:

1. **The Manchester Fothergill's repair**
   In this procedure, the vaginal portion of the cervix is amputated in order to reduce the total length of the cervix. The Mackenrodts' ligaments are cut and stitched to the front of the cervix by the Fothergill's stitch. For making the Fothergills stich a bite is taken from the Mackenrodts' ligament on one side and subsequently from the full thickness of the anterior lip of the cervix and then from the opposite Mackenrodts' ligament and tied. The external cervical os is reformed with the redundant vaginal wall. Simultaneously, cystocele, rectocele or enterocele if present are corrected. The disadvantage is the subsequent interference with fertility. If the patient conceives, there is risk of abortion and preterm labor as well as cervical dystocia. Because of all these disadvantages this procedure is at present rarely resorted to.
2. **Shirodkar's modified Manchester operation**
   For women who develop prolapse after childbirth and who desire to preserve childbearing function, this is one surgery of choice. In this procedure, a circular, incision is made around the cervix (at the cervicovaginal junction). When the posterior vaginal wall is separated from the cervix, the uterosacral ligaments can be identified. The ligament along with its peritoneal covering is isolated and brought to the anterior aspect through the lateral aspect of the cervix and sutured to the front of the cervix. The vagina is closed. Prolapse correction is better than what is achieved in Manchester Fothergill's operation and the advantage is that the cervix is preserved so that future fertility is not compromised. Along with this other compartment defects are also corrected.
3. **Sacrocervicopexy**
   Sacrocervicopexy is done transabdominally. It can be performed laparoscopically as well. In this procedure, the junction of the cervix and uterus is attached with the help of a mesh to the anterior longitudinal ligament over the first or second sacral vertebra. The mesh is then peritonised.
4. **Laparoscopic sacral colpopexy**
   Through a laparoscopic approach, the vagina can be fixed to the sacral promontory. In 363 patients operated laparoscopically, Rozet F et al[11] reported only 4% recurrence rate and a few complications including vaginal erosions, mesh infection and one bowel incarceration.
5. **McCall culdoplasty**
   To correct apical descent and for prophylaxis of future prolapse during vaginal hysterectomy, McCall in 1957 described a procedure in which the uterosacral ligaments are shortened and reattached to the vaginal cuff. Since the uterosacral ligaments are caught near the sacrum, it is advisable to perform cystoscopy to exclude ureteric obstruction.

   Cruishank and Kovac reported that modified McCall culdoplasty that reattaches the uterosacral ligament to the vault was most effective in preventing future apical defects.[12] During abdominal hysterectomy future enterocele can be prevented by an internal McCall suture. This is done by plicating the uterosacral ligaments.

Repair of enterocele

There can be 2 types of enterocele:

1. Traction enterocele where the upper posterior vaginal wall descends but bowel loops are not entering into the sac.
2. Pulsion enterocele where bowel loops enter into a sac formed by the peritoneum.

Enterocele can be treated by dissecting the enterocele peritoneal sac, excising it and approximating the uterosacral ligaments in the midline. Small defects when neglected at abdominal hysterectomy done for other conditions will later develop enterocele and vault prolapse. As a prophylaxis against vault prolapse uterosacral ligaments can be coapted after abdominal hysterectomy. Moschowitz procedure of inserting purse string sutures in the pouch of Douglas peritoneum for obliterating the pouch of Douglas is not recommended because of the risk of including the ureter while the sutures are taken in the pelvic peritoneum.

Repair of posterior compartment defects

If the patient has problems with defecation, it has to be properly evaluated before surgery. Posterior colpoperineorrhaphy is the traditional posterior compartment repair. Two Allis forceps are placed at the lower end of labia minora and a third allis forceps is placed at the apex of the rectocele or enterocele as the situation warrants. The vaginal wall is reflected from the underlying fascia and perineal body. The Denonvilliers' fascia is identified and plicated in the midline. The fascia can also be attached to the iliococcygeal muscle laterally. When hysterectomy is not performed, the fascia is attached to the cervix. If the patient has an enterocele also, the uterosacral ligaments are plicated after excising the peritoneal sac. Suture material can be PDS or vicryl. There is controversy about the traditional approximation of the levator ani muscles in the midline to reduce a widened genital hiatus. The opponents of this procedure claim that it is not anatomical and there will be postoperative dyspareunia. As a result of levator plication, the levator may go in for atrophy as mentioned earlier.

For a previous colporrhaphy failure, the use of a mesh is justified during the repair.

Perineal body

When the perineal body is also defective, it should be repaired along with colpoperineorrhaphy. The superficial muscles of the perineum and the bulbocavernosus are plicated in the midline and the skin closed. If the lower end of the Denonvilliers' fascia is found to be detached from the perineal body it should be reattached. As mentioned earlier, plicating the puborectalis to the midline is recently criticized. But if the urogenital hiatus is wide and the levator ani tone is poor then it has to be plicated or else there will be recurrence of prolapse. If the puborectalis muscles are plicated then one should make sure that two fingers can easily pass through the introitus to ensure that dyspareunia is unlikely following the procedure.

17.7 MANAGEMENT OF VAULT PROLAPSE

Before taking the patients for surgery, the precipitating factor should be evaluated and corrected. The exact defect must be identified. The patient may have an enterocele or descent of the vault or associated cystocele or rectocele. There can also be stress incontinence or bowel problems. The need for preserving the vaginal length for coital function should be evaluated. If the patient is sexually active, the procedure of choice is abdominal sacral colpopexy.

17.7.1 Procedure of Sacrocolpopexy

Sacrocolpopexy (Fig. 17.10) was first described by Falk HC who attached the vaginal vault directly to the sacrum. It was Lane FE[13,14] who used graft to suspend the vault to the sacral promontory. It is the procedure of choice for patients with apical vaginal prolapse and concomitant rectocele. In this procedure, the vault is suspended to the anterior longitudinal ligament of the first or second sacral vertebra. Loosely woven synthetic graft material, usually prolene is made use of for strengthening the vaginal wall. This graft will reinforce the posterior and anterior vaginal walls.

In patients with rectocele also, the mesh can be brought down and attached to the perineal body. Such a long mesh will support and suspend the perineal body to the sacrum thus correcting the posterior compartment defect (*Sacral colpoperineopexy*). Mesh erosion is a possible complication, the reported incidence ranging from 5- 40%. Mesh placed without opening the vagina results in fewer incidents of mesh erosion.

The procedure can be done through laparotomy or laparoscopy. After entering the abdomen, the vault is identified. This can be made easy by pushing the vagina from below with the help of an obturator introduced transvaginally. The peritoneum over the stretched vaginal vault free of bladder and rectum is identified and incised. The vault is then dissected from the bladder anteriorly and rectum posteriorly. The sigmoid colon is pushed cephalad and to the left side. Two separate mesh grafts are shaped like boat paddles, long enough to cover the anterior and posterior aspects of the vagina and to be fixed to the anterior aspect of the sacrum. The grafts are fixed to the anterior and posterior aspects of the vagina with interrupted sutures of 3 0 nylon.

The next step is identifying the anterior longitudinal ligament of the first or second vertebra. For this, the peritoneum over the sacrum is incised carefully to avoid injury to the presacral vessels. It is safer to cut the peritoneum slightly towards the right of the midline. The anterior longitudinal ligament is then identified. The two mesh grafts

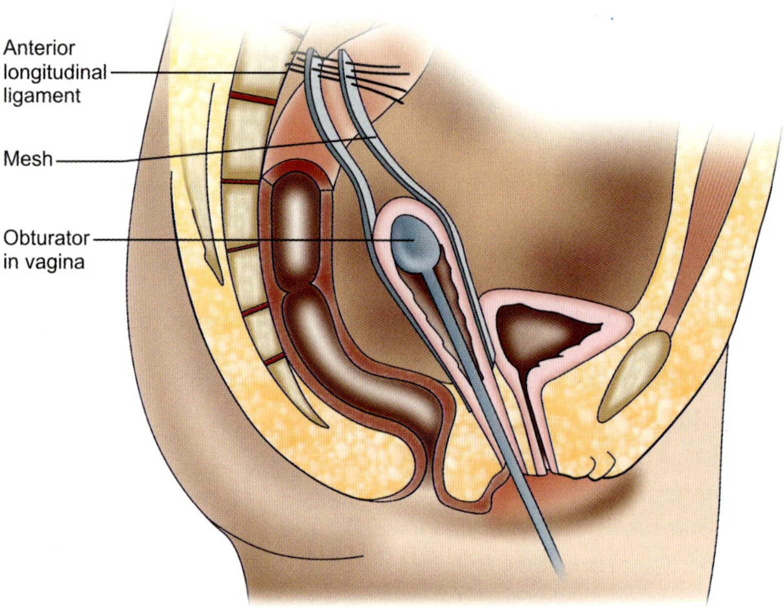

Fig. 17.10: Diagrammatic representation of the sagittal section of the pelvis showing sacral colpopexy. Note the obturator in the vagina and the mesh sutured to the anterior and posterior aspects of the vaginal vault, and the anterior longitudinal ligament

are approximated and brought to the sacral promontory. The mesh is trimmed in such a way that it can be stitched to the anterior longitudinal ligament of the first or second sacral vertebra without tension. Subsequently, the two ends of the mesh are sutured to the ligament using non absorbable sutures, preferably nylon. The entire graft should be covered with peritoneum dissected from the sacrum as well as from the redundant peritoneum dissected from the vault. This type of peritonisation will obliterate the posterior cul-de-sac to some extent.

During the dissection of the anterior longitudinal ligament, care has to be taken to prevent bleeding from the venous plexus and presacral artery. This procedure results in a better anatomical angle of the vagina compared to sacrospinous colpopexy. Abdominal sacrocolpopexy is associated with a lower rate of recurrent vault prolapse and dyspareunia than the vaginal sacrospinous colpopexy. One disadvantage reported is the post operative development of stress incontinence. In an excellent retrospective analysis evaluating long-term efficacy of sacral colpopexy for vaginal vault repair,[15] Le Franc et al reported that 27% patients had relapse of stress urinary incontinence.

It may be due to straightening of the anterior vaginal wall interfering with the sphincter mechanism of the urethra. Along with this procedure Burch colposuspension, mid urethral sling or a transvaginal perineorrhaphy may be performed as indicated.

17.7.2 Sacrospinous Colpopexy

In this procedure, the vaginal apex is fixed by non-absorbable or delayed absorbable sutures to the sacrospinous ligament (Fig. 17.11). There will be compression and thus closure of the vagina against pelvic floor muscles when there is an increase in the intra-abdominal pressure.[16] The ligament is approached transvaginally by dissecting through the rectovaginal space. The ischial spine is identified by palpating the pelvic sidewall. The prerectal fascia is pierced at the level of the ischial spine. There is significant risk of injury to the pudendal nerves and vessels and the inferior gluteal artery. The sacrospinous ligament is part of the coccygeus muscle. The coccygeus muscle can be felt, spanning medially from the ischial spine. To avoid injury to the pudendal vessel, the bite should be taken two finger breadths medial to the ischial spine (Fig. 17.11), through the sacrospinous ligament including part of the coccygeus muscle and the ligament is anchored to the vaginal vault. If the bite is taken above the level of the coccygeus muscle, there is a risk of injury to the sciatic plexus. It is usually done on the right side only, but may be performed on both sides. The bilateral suture has the disadvantage of producing a band of apical portion of the vagina across the rectum. The repair being extraperitoneal is comparatively safe. If done properly, it is a durable repair.

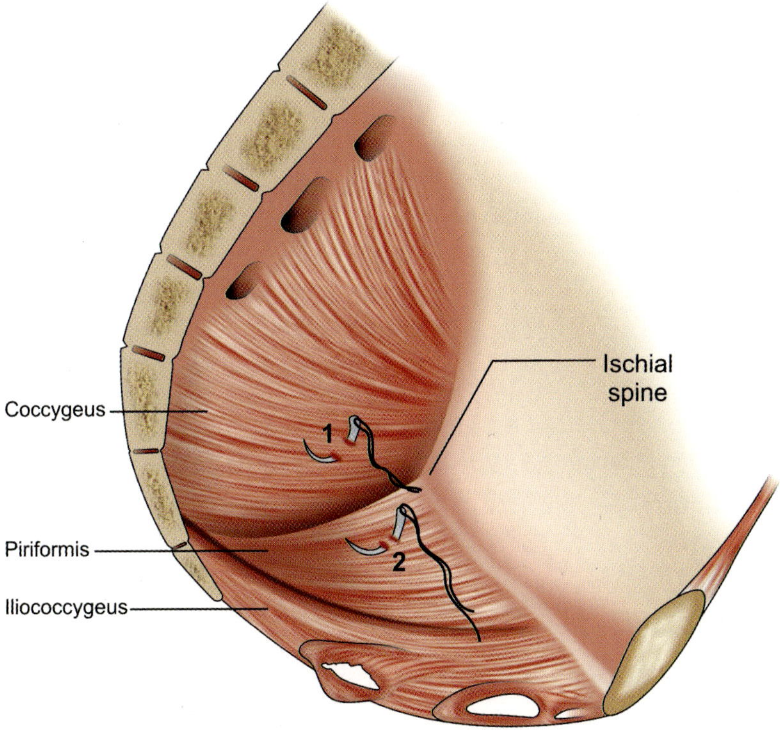

Fig. 17.11: Diagram showing location of suture placement in vaginal vault suspension—1. Site of suture placement for sacrospinous fixation. 2. Site of suture placement in iliococcygeal fixation

17.7.3 Iliococcygeal Fixation (Fig. 17.11)

This is yet another procedure for vault fixation, done through the vaginal route. The area is approached as in sacrospinous colpopexy through an incision in the posterior vaginal wall. The iliococcygeus muscle can be identified anterolaterally caudal to the ischial spine. Vaginal vault is fixed to the iliococcygeus using No.1 PDS sutures. This is an easier procedure compared to sacrospinous fixation and can be done bilaterally. A shorter length of the vagina is enough for the procedure. Risk of pudendal nerve and vessel injury is relatively low. Cure rates reported are comparable to sacrospinous fixation.

17.7.4 Uterosacral Ligament Suspension

Vaginal apex can also be suspended to the uterosacral ligaments. Through a transvaginal approach the uterosacral ligaments can be approached cephalad to the ischial spine. Up to three sutures can be taken from each ligament and anchored to the vaginal apex. The success rates reported are excellent but the serious complication which can occur is inclusion of the ureter. Hence, intraoperative checking of the patency of the ureter through cystoscope is recommen-ded. Since the ureter is lateral to the uterosacral ligament, including it in the sutures from the ligament is very unlikely.

17.7.5 Abdominal Uterosacral Suspension

Uterosacral ligament suspension can be performed through laparotomy or laparoscopy. The uterosacral ligament is identified and sutures of delayed absorbable or nonabsorbable material are placed on the uterosacral ligament and anchored to the anterior and posterior aspect of the vaginal cuff on the ipsilateral side. The procedure is repeated on the other side as well. Cystoscopy should be done after the procedure to check the patency of the ureter.

17.8 USE OF GRAFTS IN PROLAPSE SURGERY

There are no randomized controlled trials on the advantage or disadvantage of using grafts. Allograft, autografts, xenografts and synthetic materials have been tried in prolapse surgery. No ideal material is currently identified for reconstructive pelvic surgery. The most widely studied material is monofilament polypropylene mesh.

Mesh erosion is a significant complication of mesh use.

In situations where the fascia is very much attenuated the use of grafts may be considered to prevent prolapse recurrence. A Cochrane review suggested that the use of a polyglactin mesh at the time of repair may reduce the incidence of recurrence.[17] Success rates of 90% can be achieved in well selected patients.

The use of grafts should be considered in the following situations:

1. Previous failed repair
2. Elderly patients with atrophic tissues
3. Severe defects
4. Sacral colpopexy

Evidence supports the use of mesh in anterior vaginal wall prolapse surgery, abdominal sacral colpopexy, vaginal vault prolapse and posterior colporrhaphy[18] in recurrent rectocele.

17.9 LAPAROSCOPIC PROCEDURES

17.9.1 Laparoscopic Sacral Colpopexy

Sacral colpopexy was first done laparoscopically by Nezhat.[19] The procedure is identical to the open procedure except that it is done laparoscopically. The key anatomic landmarks to be considered while doing sacral colpopexy are the presacral artery and venous plexus which lie in front of the sacrum. Randomized controlled trials comparing laparoscopy and colposuspension showed similar subjective cure rates, but additional objective failure for laparoscopic procedure compared to traditional colposuspension.

17.9.2 Laparoscopic Cystocele Repair

Lateral cystocele can be repaired laparoscopically by dissecting through the cave of Retzius and going laterally. The obturator muscle and the arcus tendineus fascia are identified and the torn pubovesicocervical fascia is reattached to the arcus tendinous fascia as well as to the fascia overlying the obturator internus muscle. If the patient has stress incontinence as well, Burch colposuspension can also be performed laparoscopically.

17.10 VAGINAL OBLITERATIVE PROCEDURES

Procedures which obliterate the vagina are resorted to for patients who are very old and debilitated. The advantage is that it can be done as a simple procedure under local anesthesia. Intraoperative blood loss and morbidity are much less. Because the uterus is retained it is mandatory that uterine and cervical pathology should be excluded by an endometrial biopsy and a papanicolaou smear examination.

17.10.1 Le Fort Procedure

In this procedure, the cervix is pulled out with a Volsellum forceps and the vaginal mucosa is infiltrated with lignocaine and adrenaline. A rectangular area on the anterior vaginal wall is mapped. The proximal extent of the area should be at the bladder sulcus and the distal margin up to 4 cm away from the external urethral meatus. A mirror image of the same should be marked on the posterior vaginal wall. The vaginal mucosa over the marked area can be removed using sharp dissection. Hemostasis should be achieved. The cut edges of the anterior and posterior walls are stitched together with delayed absorbable sutures, e.g. polyglactin. Initially the vaginal edge near the cervix is sutured after reducing the prolapse. The sutures can be proceeded distally. This leaves an obliterated middle vagina and two tunnels on either side. Bladder-neck plication can also be combined to prevent the occurrence of stress urinary incontinence.

17.11 CONCLUSION

Pelvic organ prolapse is one of the common problems affecting about 50% of women in varying degrees. The incidence varies with the ethnicity and race. Etiology is multifactorial. Pelvic floor muscle weakness due to stretching and denervation caused by obstetric trauma and menopausal atrophy are the common causes. Understanding pelvic anatomy is basic to surgical repair. Surgical repair of prolapse is a challenge to the gynecologic surgeon due to the chances of recurrence. When eliciting history, an effort should be made to pinpoint the site of defect based on symptoms. On examination the site specific support defect should be identified and quantified. Conservative treatment like pelvic floor exercises and use of pessary when appropriate should be resorted to. Decision for surgery should be taken based on the physical fitness of the patient, the need for preserving the uterus as well as the need for preserving the coital function. The surgical approach should be individualized. Basis of success of surgery lies in the correction of site specific defect in the 3 compartments at the 3 levels. The use of mesh, the choice of mesh and abdominal approach to repair needs further evaluation.

REFERENCES

1. Swift SE. The distribution of pelvic organ support in a population of female subjects seen for routine gynecological health cases. Am J Obstet Gynecol 2000;183:277-85.

2. Delancey JO. Fascial and muscular abnormalities in women with urethral hypermobility and anterior vaginal wall prolapsed. Am J Obstet Gynaecol 2002;187(1):93-8.
3. Richardson AC, Iyon JB, Williams NL. A new look at pelvic relaxation, Am Obstet Gynecol 1976;126:568-72.
4. Delancey JO. Structural support of the urethra as it relates to stress urinary incontinence; the hammock hypothesis. Am J Obstet Gynecol 1994;170:1713-24.
5. Adams EJ, Thomson AJM, Maher C, Hagen S. Mechanical devices for pelvic organ prolapse in women. Cochrane Database of Systematic Reviews 2004, Issue 2. Art No CD004010. DOI: 10.1002/14651858.CD004010.
6. Stanton SL, Hilton P, Norton C, Cardozo L. Clinical and urodynamic effects of anterior colporrhaphy and vaginal hysterectomy for prolapse with and without incontinence. Br J Obstet Gynaecol 1982;89:459-63.
7. Raz S, Little NA, Jisa S, Sussman EM. Repair of severe anterior vaginal wall prolapse. J Urol 1991;146:988-92.
8. Walter S, Olesen KP, Hald T, et al. Urodynamic evaluation after vaginal repair and colposuspension. Br J Urol 1982; 54:377-80.
9. Shull BL, Baden WF. A six-year experience with paravaginal defect repair for stress urinary incontinence. Am J Obstet Gynecol 1989;160:1432-9.
10. Shull BL, Benn SJ, Kuehl TJ. Surgical management of prolapse of the anterior vaginal segment: an analysis of support defects, operative morbidity, and anatomic outcome. Am J Obstet Gynecol 1994;171:1429-36.
11. Rozet F, Mandrone E, Arroyo C, et al. Laparoscopic sacral colpopexy approach for genitourinary prolapse. Eur Urol 2005;47:230-6.
12. Cruishank SH, Kovac SR. Randomised comparison of three surgical methods used at the time of vaginal hysterectomy to prevent posterior enterocele. Am J Obstet Gynecol 1999; 180:859-65.
13. Lane FE. Repair of posthysterectomy vaginal vault prolapse. It is the procedure of choice for patients with apical vaginal prolapse and concomitant rectocele Obstet Gynecol. 1962; 20:72-7.
14. Maher C, Vasslerk, Glazener CMA, et al. Surgical management of pelvic organ prolapse in women. (Cochrane review) The Cochrane library, Chichester, Wiley, 2005.
15. Lefranc JP, Atallah D, Camatte S, Blondon J. Long-term follow-up of posthysterectomy vaginal vault prolapse abdominal repair: a report of 85 cases. J Am Coll Surg 2002; 195:352-8.
16. Randall CL, Nichols DS. Surgical treatment of vaginal inversion. Obstet Gynecol 1971;38:327-32.
17. Flood CG, Drutz HP, Waja L. Anterior colporrhaphy reinforced with Marlex mesh for the treatment of cystoceles. Int Urogynecol J Pelvic Floor Dysfunct 1998;9:200-04.
18. Birch C, Fynes MM. The role of synthetic and biological prostheses in reconstructive pelvic floor surgery. Curr Opin Obstet Gynecol 2002;14:527-35.
19. Nezhat CH, Nezhat F, Nezhat C. Laproscopic sacral colpopexy for vaginal vault prolapse Obstet Gynecol 1994; 84: 885-8.

18 Fistulae of the Lower Genital Tract

B Presannakumari

18.1 INTRODUCTION

The development of the genital tract, urinary tract and the lower gastrointestinal tract are closely related. This fact and the anatomic proximity of these structures predispose them to associated anomalies, injuries during surgery or radiation treatment as well as obstetric trauma. Hence fistulas can occur between urethra and vagina, urinary bladder and vagina, ureter and vagina, bladder and uterus or rectum and vagina.

18.2 VESICOVAGINAL FISTULA (VVF)

Continuous incontinence as a result of vesicovaginal fistula is one of the distressing symptoms a woman encounters. Obstetric vesicovaginal fistulas were very common in olden days. With improved antenatal and intrapartum care these fistulas are rare at present. Mariom Sims is considered the father of fistula repair as it was he who first successfully repaired obstetric vesicovaginal fistula after several attempts.

18.2.1 Etiology

VVF can be due to several causes:

1. Obstetric trauma
2. Surgery
3. Infection
4. Congenital
5. Malignancy
6. Treatment of malignancy

Obstetric fistulas are the commonest fistulas occurring in women. They occur due to injuries as a result of obstructed labor and traumatic delivery coupled with lack of medical care. Hence, obstetric fistulas occur in places where there is early childbearing, lack of obstetric care and poor nutrition.[1] They are preventable to a large extent by proper antenatal and intranatal care.

Obstetric fistulas result from pressure necrosis or due to incompletely repaired perineal or vaginal lacerations. The site of injury depends upon the level of obstruction. Obstetric injuries can involve multiple organs resulting in the occurrence of multiple fistulas. Scarring and reduced vascularity of tissues surrounding the fistula make them more susceptible to failure of surgical correction. Prolonged obstructed labor can result in cervical necrosis and vesicocervical fistula.

The major cause of VVF in developed countries is recognized as inadvertent bladder injury during gynecological surgery, predominantly abdominal hysterectomy

(85%). Advanced cervical cancer can extend to the vagina and bladder resulting in VVF. There is a 1% risk of development of urinary fistula among women who undergo radical surgery. Radiation treatment can also result in fistula formation.[2,3]

18.2.2 Classification

There is lack of agreement as to how VVF should be classified. Even though more than 20 classifications are reported in the literature, till now there is no standardized classification system which has been evaluated as to how it correlates with surgical outcome.

Earlier classifications are as follows:

1. Simple—small, non-radiation, single
2. Complex—medium, large size, resulting from radiation treatment, multiple, recurrent.

Depending on size

1. Small <2 cm
2. Medium 2-3 cm
3. Large 4-6 cm
4. Extensive >6 cm

The 2 most recent classification systems are as follows:

Waaldijk's Classification

Type I: Does not involve the urethral closing mechanism

Type IIAa: Involves the urethral closing mechanism, without (sub) total urethral involvement and without circumferential defect.

Type IIAb: Involves the urethral closing mechanism, without (sub) total urethral involvement and with circumferential defect.

Type IIBa: Involves the urethral closing mechanism, with (sub) total urethral involvement and without circumferential defect.

Type IIBb: Involves the urethral closing mechanism, with (sub) total urethral involvement and with circumferential defect.

Type III: Involves the ureter; other exceptional fistulas.

Source: Waaldijk K.1 Surgical classification of obstetric fistulas. Journal of Gynecology and Obstetrics, Volume 49, Number 2, May 1995; 161-163(3).

Classification by Goh

Type 1: Distal edge 3.5 cm from external urinary meatus.

Type 2: Distal edge 2.5-3.5 cm from external urinary meatus.

Type 3: Distal edge 1.5 to 2.5 cm from external urinary meatus.

Type 4: Distal edge 1.5 cm from external urinary meatus.

a. Size 1.5 cm in the largest diameter
b. Size, 1.5-3 cm in the largest diameter
c. Size 3 cm in the largest diameter.

- None or only mild fibrosis (around the fistula and/or vagina), and/or vaginal length 6 cm with normal capacity.
- Moderate or severe fibrosis (around the fistula and/or vagina), and/or reduced vaginal length and/or capacity.
- Special consideration, e.g. postradiation, ureteric involvement, circumferential fistula, or previous repair.

Source: Goh JT. A new classification for female genital tract fistula. Aust NZJ Obstet Gynecol 2004;44(6):502-4.

18.2.3 Clinical Features

Continuous leakage of urine is the main complaint. Those who have small fistula may complain of intermittent leakage and may be able to pass urine voluntarily. VVF should be suspected when a woman complaints of leakage of urine in the second postoperative week. In the case of obstetric fistula also the symptoms start after a few days when the tissues which had undergone necrosis breakdown. Abdominal pain, flank pain or distension in the postoperative period should raise the suspicion of urinary ascites or urinoma and needs evaluation. Hematuria, pyelonephritis and recurrent cystitis can occur as a result of VVF. The time interval between the injury and clinical manifestation depends upon the type of insult. Overlooked bladder laceration during pelvic surgery or bladder injury along with vaginal laceration during delivery presents with leakage within a few hours. Radiation induced fistulas which are due to avascular necrosis might present a few months to several years after radiation.

18.2.4 Diagnosis

Large fistulas can be diagnosed by speculum examination. Diagnosis of small fistula can be confirmed by filling the bladder with methylene blue after keeping a white gauze plug in the vagina. The patient should be re-examined after walking for a few minutes. If the plug is stained blue she has VVF. If the plug is stained with clear urine, she is presumed to have ureterovaginal fistula which also is a possibility after pelvic surgery. Cystoscopic examination should be done to rule out multiple fistulas and to assess the relation of the fistula to the ureteral opening, which is important in surgical correction. Cystoscopy is not possible in the presence of large fistula. In the instance of suspicion of concomitant ureteral fistula, intravenous pyeloureterogram should be done.

18.2.5 Management

VVF which occurs after hysterectomy for benign disease is a simple injury since the surrounding tissue is normal. Repair of such an injury carries high success rate. On the contrary, the fistula resulting from obstructed labor is due to a wider field injury so that the tissues around the fistula will exhibit dense scarring which makes surgical repair difficult.[4]

Conservative Management

Once a posthysterectomy fistula is diagnosed the patient should be managed by continuous bladder drainage. The fistula correction is better postponed to 3-4 months so that edema and inflammation around the fistula subsides. Small fistulas sometimes might close spontaneously during this time.

Timing of Surgery

Fistula repair gives best results if done after edema and inflammation subsides. Edema might subside by 6 weeks. However, by waiting for 3-4 months some fistulas heal spontaneously. Hence, it is better to wait for such a period.[5]

Basic Principles for Achieving Successful Repair[7]

1. Adequate mobilization of tissue so that approximation is achieved without tension.
2. Proper identification and excision of damaged parts.
3. Layer closure without tension.
4. The repair should be water tight at the time of closure.
5. Postoperative bladder drainage for 10-14 days.

Surgical Technique

The most appropriate method for the individual patient should be selected based on the following:
1. Lesion accessibility and mobility
2. Degree of scarring
3. Vaginal length
4. Site, size and number of fistula
5. Condition of the bladder and urethral sphincter

Historically, the surgical approach is based on the site of the fistula. Supratrigonal fistulas (fistulas above the interureteric ridge) were usually approached transabdominally. Infratrigonal fistulas (fistulas below the interureteric ridge) were better corrected transvaginally. Generally simple fistulas can be corrected by vaginal route and complex fistulas by abdominal route.

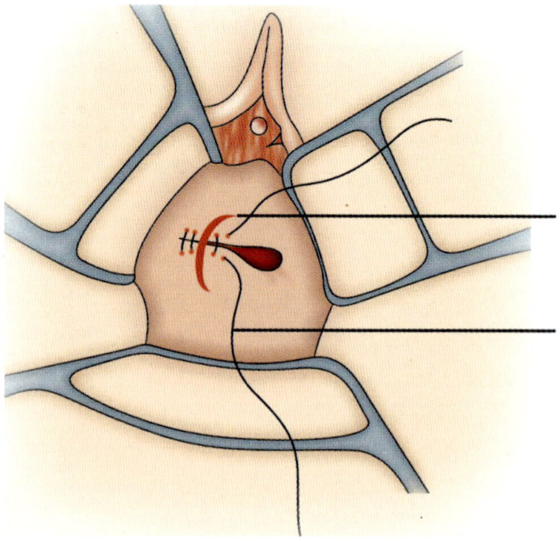

Fig. 18.1: Closure of simple vesicovaginal fistula

Vaginal method[8,9] (Fig. 18.1)

Adequate exposure is required. The fistula is circumscribed with a no15 blade and the vagina is separated from the bladder. The fibrous edges of the fistula are then excised and the vagina is adequately mobilized so that repair can be done without tension in the vagina as well as bladder wall. While mobilizing the bladder, if there is possible injury to the ureters, ureteric catheters should be inserted, if not done earlier. If the fistula is at the bladder neck or the urethra, a urethral catheter should be inserted before closing the fistula. The bladder is then closed with delayed absorbable suture, preferably 2 × 0 vicryl. Two layers of interrupted inverting sutures should be inserted. Methylene blue is introduced into the bladder to confirm water tight closure as well as to make sure another fistula is not overlooked. The catheter is strapped to the thigh so that there will not be drag on it. The vagina is then closed over the bladder with 0 vicryl.

Postoperative care

- The most important postoperative care is to keep the bladder decompressed by continuous bladder drainage for 7-14 days. Transurethral catheter should not be used if the fistula involves the lower trigone, bladder neck or urethra. A large suprapubic cather ensures unobstructed continuous drainage. Both transurethral and transabdominal catheters may be used simultaneously. The urethral catheter can removed on the 7th day. After confirming vesical integrity, the suprapubic catheter can be removed. Postradiation fistulas need longer postoperative bladder drainage.
- Acidification of urine with vitamin C, 500 mg three times a day diminishes risk of cystitis, mucous production and formation of bladder calculi.
- Postmenopausal patients may be given estrogen replacement for improving vascularity.

- Routine antibiotic is not mandatory. However, patient should be closely followed up for evidence of infection and antibiotic therapy promptly instituted if there is evidence of infection.
- Patient should avoid valsalva maneuvers. Stool softeners will avoid straining for stools.
- Since, the tissue is delicate it is better to avoid speculum examination and vaginal examination for 6-8 weeks postoperatively.

Routine excision of the fistula tract is not mandatory according to Raz.[6] The disadvantage of excising the fistula tract is increasing the size of the fistula as a result of excision of the scarred edges. The advantage of not excising the tract is increase in the strength of repair if the fibrous ring is not excised.

The advantages of transvaginal approach:

- Avoids laparotomy and cystotomy
- Only minimal blood loss
- Less postoperative discomfort
- Shorter hospital stay.

Contraindications to vaginal approach:

1. Poorly compliant bladder
2. Severe induration in the vaginal wall around the fistula
3. When the repair necessitates ureteral reimplantation due to the position of fistula or associated ureteral fistula
4. When the vagina is severely stenosed.

Abdominal methods

The abdominal methods are of 2 types:

1. **The bivalve technique:** In this method the bladder is incised down to the fistula starting from the dome. The margins of the fistula are dissected and a 2 layer closure of the vagina and bladder is carried out as in the vaginal method. This technique has the advantage of easy visualization and approach to the fistula. Also if the defect is near the trigone, the ureteral catheter can be conveniently introduced. In situations where tissue healing is expected to be impaired due to scarring, or poor blood supply, interposition of a tissue flap is easier with this method.
2. **Transvesical method**: In this method the fistula is approached transvesically, through an opening in the dome of the bladder.

The success of repairing postsurgical fistula is reported to be 91 and 96% for vaginal and abdominal route and also as congenital or aquired respectively.

Repair of Radiation Induced Fistula

Radiation induced fistulae are difficult to treat due to poor blood supply and fibrosis. As a routine tissue flaps are made use of to improve vascularity to the repaired area. Repair using flaps are reported to carry about 50% success rate. In patients who have distortion of anatomy, a vaginal approach with flaps can be tried as an initial procedure.

Repair Using Grafts

Recurrent fistulas, radiation induced fistulas and large fistulas are ideally repaired by inserting an interpositional vascular supply to prevent recurrence.

Advantages of using a graft

1. Covering minor defects in the suture line.
2. Bringing a fresh blood supply to the area of injured tissue.
3. Keeping the healing of the bladder and vaginal wall apart.

Martius flap[15]

In this procedure, a 5-6 cm long and 2-3 cm wide fat pad along the length of the labium majus is tunneled subcutaneously into the vagina to act as a flap. A myocutaneous flap of the bulbocavernosus muscle can also be made use of.

Urinary Diversion

When the repair is expected to fail or repeated failures occur, the alternative is urinary diversion. Radiation induced fistulas and multiple fistulas are the ones which need urinary diversion. In these situations there will be fibrosis and the consequent distortion of anatomy.

18.6 RECTOVAGINAL FISTULA (RVF)

Rectovaginal fistulas are abnormal communication between the rectum and vagina. Since, the symptom of rectovaginal fistula is incontinence of feces, it is very distressing and socially disabling as far as the affected individual is concerned. Surgical repair is a challenge to the surgeon.

18.6.1 Types of RVF (Table 18.1)

RVF can be classified as low, mid or high depending upon site of Fistula.

1. Congenital
2. Acquired
   a. Trauma
      i. Obstetric
      ii. Operative
   b. Infection
   c. Inflammatory bowel disease
   d. Radiation
   e. Carcinoma

Table 18.1: Types of RVF

Simple	*Complex*
• Lower or midvaginal • < 2.5 cm in diameter • Due to trauma or infection	• High vaginal fistula • >2.5 cm in diameter • Caused by inflammatory bowel disease, radiation, malignancy • Multiple failed attempts

Among the acquired causes obstetric trauma is the commonest, amounting to 88% of published series. Usually RVF results from a poorly sutured 4th degree perineal laceration or due to infection of the sutured laceration. Rectal or vaginal surgeries can result in RVF. This may be due to direct injury or postoperative infection. Penetrating injuries due to accidents can also result in RVF. Infections of the cul-de-sac if not properly treated can result in high fistula. Inflammatory bowel disease such as ulcerative colitis or Crohn's disease may lead to RVF. Malignancies of the cervix, endometrium and vagina as well as their radiation treatment can also be the cause.

18.6.2 Clinical Features

The symptom is involuntary passage of flatus and feces through the vagina. If the fistula is very small, the symptom will only be vaginal discharge which will be foul smelling. Symptoms like vaginal discharge, bleeding or rectal bleeding will be present depending on the underlying condition.

18.6.3 Diagnosis

History will often lead to the diagnosis. However, a thorough examination is very important to know the site, size and the underlying cause of the fistula. Multiple perineal fistulae suggest Crohn's disease. The fistula can be easily seen and felt on bimanual examination. Proctoscopy will help to locate small fistulas as well as to make out the health of the anal mucosa and the compliance of the rectum. Small fistula may be difficult to visualize. In such instances, methylene blue can be injected into the rectum after keeping a cotton swab in the vagina and retained for about 10-15 minutes. The fistula can be made out by looking for blue staining of the swab in the vagina. If the fistula is still not identified and the patient has symptoms, the possibility of a high RVF should be suspected. A barium enema should be performed to delineate the fistula and to make out the health of the colon and rectum. In obstetric fistula, the anal sphincter may be defective. Hence, the sphincter should be thoroughly evaluated. Endoanal ultrasound examination is a simple tool to assess the integrity of anal sphincter.[10] If the sphincter is found to be defective, it should be repaired. Otherwise patient satisfaction after repair will be affected due to the persistence of incontinence.

18.6.4 Management

Management depends upon the site, size, etiology and number of previous failed attempts and the presence of anal sphincter injury.

Timing of Surgery

The patient should be taken for surgery only after the inflammation or infection has subsided. This might need about 3-6 months. During this period some fistulas caused by trauma or infection might get closed. Waiting period is not necessary if the surrounding tissues are healthy. Fecal diversion is not necessary in all the fistulas but may be necessary before complex fistula repair.

Other than a simple obstetric rectovaginal fistula the surgery is better done by colorectal surgeon.

Surgical Correction of Obstetric Rectovaginal Fistula

The degree of continence should be assessed before surgery as it has been found that coexisting incontinence is present in about 40-50% of women who have obstetric RVF. A waiting period is advised to see that all inflammation has subsided. Transanal approach is usually preferred by colorectal surgeons. Gynecologists prefer transvaginal approach.

Transvaginal Approach

Preoperatively patients should receive mechanical preparation and prophylactic antibiotic.

In the transvaginal approach, the fistula is identified and a circular incision is made around the fistulous opening in the posterior vaginal wall. Infiltration with dilute adrenalin solution will help identify tissue plane and reduce bleeding. The fistulous tract is excised up to the rectum. The vaginal wall is mobilized from the underlying rectovaginal septum. A series of concentric purse string sutures are placed in the rectovaginal septum to occlude the fistulous opening. The levator muscle is then plicated in the midline so that intervening tissue is created between the rectum and the vagina. The vaginal wall is then closed.

Transperineal Approach (Fig. 18.2)

The type of fistula commonly encountered by the obstetrician is a low fistula which results from an incompletely

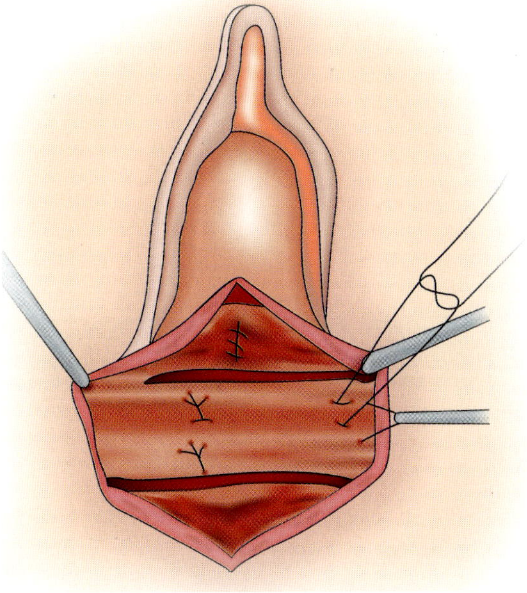

Fig. 18.2: Closure of low rectovaginal fistula. Perineoproctotomy and layered closure. An overlapping method of external sphincter approximation is seen

repaired 4th degree perineal laceration. Fistulotomy combined with perineoproctotomy followed by a layered closure is the preferred technique for patients who have associated sphincter defect also.[11-13,16] Preoperative mechanical preparation with enema should be done. Prophylactic antibiotic as usual should be given. The fistula is converted to a 4th degree tear by dividing the skin, sphincter and the perineal body. The fistulous tract is excised. The vaginal wall, the internal and external sphincter and the anal mucosa are identified and mobilized. The rectal mucosa is sutured with interrupted delayed absorbable sutures preferably vicryl. A second layer of sutures are inserted to invert the first layer of sutures so as to withstand the pressure in the rectum. The internal sphincter is then sutured over the mucosa. The external sphincter is identified and mobilized up to the ischiorectal fossa. An overlapping sphincteroplasty is then performed with horizontal mattress sutures. The perineal body is then reconstructed. The success rate reported is 85-100%.

18.6.5 Radiation Induced Fistula

Radiation induced fistulae are difficult to treat due to radiation damage to the surrounding tissues. Fistula can occur in such patients as a result of recurrence of malignancy also. Hence, it is important to exclude malignancy by imaging and biopsy from the site.

The compliance of the rectum should be assessed prior to the surgery. Fecal diversion either before or during the surgery may be necessary.

Transperineal approaches are preferred due to the less radiation effects in the vagina compared to the rectum.[14] The method is similar to that of obstetric fistula repair. For better healing, healthy vascular non-irradiated tissue can be interposed between the rectum and vagina. The gracilis muscle or the sartorius can be used for the purpose. The gracilis muscle may be preferred as harvesting the muscle will not cause any difficulty in ambulation. The Martius technique of incorporating the subcutaneous tissue and the bulbocavernosus muscle can also be preferred. Even when tissue interposition is resorted to, fecal diversion either before or in conjunction with the repair should be done.

REFERENCES

1. Kelly J, Kwast BE. Epidemiologic study of vesicovaginal fistulas in Ethiopia. Int Urogynecol J 1993;4:278-81.
2. Elkins TE, Drescher C, Martey JO, Fort D. Vesicovaginal fistula revisited. Obstet Gynecol 1988;72:307-12.
3. Lee RA, Symmonds RE, Williams TJ. Current status of genitourinary fistula. Obstet Gynecol 1988;72:313-15.
4. Wall LL, Karshima J, Kirschner C, Arrowsmith SD. The obstetric vesicovaginal fistula: Characteristics of 899 patients from Jos, Nigeria. Am J Obstet Gynecol 2004;190:1011-9.
5. Waaldijk K. The immediate surgical management of fresh obstetric fistulas with catheter and/or early closure. Int J Gynecol Obstet 1994;45(1):11-6.
6. Raz S. Female urology. Philadelphia, Pa: WB Saunders 1893;373-7.
7. Kelly J. Obstetric fistulae. Contemp Rev Obstet Gynaecol 1995;7:56-9.
8. Sims JM. On the treatment of vesicovaginal fistula. Am J Med Sci 1852;23:59-82.
9. Kelly J. Repair of obstetrical fistula: Obstet Gynaecol 2002; 4:205-11.
10. Yee LF, Birnbaum EH, Read TE, et al. Use of endoanal ultrasound in patients with rectovaginal fistulas. Dis Colon Rectum 1999;42:1057-64.
11. Russell TR, Gallagher DM. Low rectovaginal fistulas: Approach and treatment. M J Surg 1977;134:13-8.
12. Given FT Jr. Rectovaginal fistula. A review of 20 years experience in a community hospital. Am J Obstet Gynecol 1970;108:41-6.
13. Hibbard LT. Surgical management of rectovaginal fistulas and complete perineal tears. Am J Obstet Gynecol 1978; 130:139-41.
14. WP, Senagore AJ, Schiesel EC. Operative repair of ano-vaginal and rectovaginal fistulas. Dis Colon Rectum 1995; 38:4-6.
15. Martius J. Operations for urinary incontinence. In: McCall M, Bolten KA, editors. Operative gynecology. Boston: Little, Brown 1956;318-27.
16. Wise WE, Aguilar PS, Padmanabhan A, et al. Surgical treatment of low rectal vaginal fistulas. Dis Colon Rectum 1991;34:271-4.

19 Carcinoma of the Ovary

B Presannakumari

19.1 INTRODUCTION

Ovarian carcinoma poses a great challenge to the practitioner as most women present late in the course of the disease. It has the highest mortality rate among all the gynecological malignancies and accounts for 3% of all malignancies, 31% of female genital tract cancers and 6% of deaths from cancer in women. A woman's lifetime risk of ovarian cancer is 1-1.5%; one out of every 70 woman is at risk of developing ovarian cancer. The incidence of ovarian malignancy increases with age. As per SEER data base, 2001-2005, the incidence is 1.3% under age 20, 3.4% between 20-34 years, 7.9% between 35 and 44, 19% between 45 and 54, 21.8% between 55 and 64 and 20% between 65 and 74 with a median age of diagnosis at 63 years. However, a recent report shows that the peak incidence is in the eighth decade with 57/100,000 in the 70-74 year age group.[1]

19.2 ETIOLOGY AND RISK FACTORS

The molecular events related to ovarian malignancy are not yet fully understood. Since epithelial ovarian tumors are frequently associated with nulliparity, early menarche and late menopause, incessant ovulation is thought to be an etiological factor. Other risk factors (Table 19.1) that were identified are family history and increasing age. About 10% of cancers are attributed to familial predisposition. Women who have mutations of BRCA1 and BRCA2 genes carry the greatest genetic risk of ovarian cancer, particularly non-mucinous. For BRCA1 (chromosome 17) carriers, the

Table 19.1: Risk factors for ovarian malignancy

Risk factors
Nulliparity
Early menarche
Late menopause
Increasing age
Family history
• BRCA 1 carrier-25-40%
• BRCA 2 carrier-15-25%
• Hereditary colorectal cancer syndrome (HNPCC mutation carrier)—10-12%

lifetime risk is estimated to be 25-40%. Those who have BRCA2 (chromosome 13) have a lifetime risk of 15-25%. These mutations are inherited in an autosomal dominant mode. These women develop malignancy at an earlier age than women who do not have familial predisposition. Women who have hereditary non-polyposis colorectal cancer (HNPCC) syndrome also are at an increased risk for ovarian malignancy. HNPCC mutations which involve the repair genes hMLH1 and hMSH II account for about 10-12% of hereditary ovarian cancer. Many studies have addressed the issue of increased risk of ovarian cancer in women undergoing ovulation induction, but are inconclusive.

19.3 PATHOLOGY

As the ovaries develop from the following three types of cells, ovarian tumors are mainly of three different types.

1. Coelomic epithelium of the genital ridge—Epithelial ovarian tumors
2. Germ cells which migrate from the yolk sac—Germ cell tumors. Since the germ cells are totipotent, different histological varieties of tumors can occur.
3. Mesenchyme of the genital ridge—Sex cord stromal tumors

The ovary is a common site for secondary deposits from the colon, stomach, breast as well as other pelvic malignancies.

Ovarian tumors are classified by WHO (1999) based on the histology into 46 different types of epithelial tumors, 24 sex cord stromal tumors, 29 germ cell tumors and 13 other categories.

This classification is approved by FIGO and allows comparisons of prognosis in treatment trials. Many of the histological types are very rare. The biological behavior of different tumors varies. Within the same histological type, the biological behavior can differ based on the degree of differentiation of the cells. Hence, meticulous assessment of histology of every ovarian tumor is important.

19.4 WHO HISTOLOGICAL CLASSIFICATION OF TUMORS OF OVARY (2003)

1. Surface epithelial tumors

a. Serous tumors
   - i. Malignant
     - Adenocarcinoma
     - Surface papillary adenocarcinoma
     - Adenocarcinofibroma
   - ii. Borderline
     1. Papillary cystic tumor
     2. Surface papillary tumor
     3. Adenofibroma and cystadenofibroma
   - iii. Benign
     1. Cystadenoma
     2. Papillary cystadenoma
     3. Surface papilloma
     4. Adenofibroma and cystadenofibroma

b. Mucinous tumors
   - i. Malignant
     1. Adenocarcinoma
     2. Adenocarcinofibroma
   - ii. Borderline
     1. Intestinal type
     2. Endocervical like
   - iii. Benign
     1. Cystadenoma
     2. Adenofibroma and cystadenofibroma
     3. Mucinous cystic tumors with mural nodules
     4. Mucinous cystic tumors with pseudomyxoma peritonei

c. Endometrioid tumors including variants with squamous differentiation
   - i. Malignant
     1. Adenocarcinoma not otherwise specified
     2. Adenocarcinofibroma [malignant adenofibroma]
     3. Carcinosarcoma
     4. Adenosarcoma
     5. Endometrial stromal sarcoma (low grade)
     6. Undifferentiated ovarian sarcoma
   - ii. Borderline
     1. Cystic tumor
     2. Adenofibroma and cystadenofibroma
   - iii. Benign
     1. Cystadenoma
     2. Adenofibroma and cystadenofibroma

d. Clear cell tumors
   - i. Malignant

1. Adenocarcinoma
2. Adenocarcinofibroma (malignant adeno-fibroma)

ii. Borderline
1. Cystic tumor
2. Adenofibroma and cystadenofibroma

iii. Benign
1. Cystadenoma
2. Adenofibroma and cystadenofibroma

e. Transitional cell tumors
i. Malignant
1. Transitional cell carcinoma (non-Brenner type)
2. Malignant Brenner tumor

ii. Borderline
1. Borderline Brenner tumor
2. Proliferating variant

iii. Benign
1. Brenner tumor
2. Metaplastic variant

f. Squamous cell tumors
i. Squamous cell carcinoma
ii. Epidermoid cyst

g. Mixed epithelial tumors (specify components)
i. Malignant
ii. Borderline
iii. Benign

h. Undifferentiated and unclassified tumors

2. Sex-cord stromal tumors

a. Granulosa stromal cell tumors

b. Granulosa cell tumor group
i. Adult
ii. Juvenile

c. Thecoma-fibroma group
i. Thecoma not otherwise specified
1. Typical
2. Luteinized

ii. Fibroma
iii. Cellular fibroma
iv. Fibrosarcoma
v. Stromal tumor with minor sex cord elements
vi. Sclerosing stromal tumor
vii. Signet ring stromal tumor
viii. Unclassified

d. Sertoli-stromal cell tumors
i. Sertoli Leydig cell tumor group
1. Well differentiated
2. Of intermediate differentiation
3. Poorly differentiated
4. Retiform

ii. Sertoli cell tumors
iii. Stromal Leydig cell tumors
iv. Sex cord stromal tumor of mixed or unclassified type
1. Sex-cord stromal tumors with annular tubules
2. Gynandroblastoma

v. Leydig cell tumor group
1. Hilus cell tumor
2. Leydig cell tumor

a. NOS (Not otherwise specified)
b. Non-hilar type

vi. Steroid cell tumors
1. Stromal luteoma
2. Steroid cell tumor

a. NOS
b. Well differentiated
c. Malignant

19.5 EPITHELIAL TUMORS

Epithelial ovarian tumors comprise 90% of ovarian malignancies. They develop from the invagination of the epithelium covering the ovary. The coelomic epithelium has the ability to develop into many different types (Table 19.2) of Mullerian (fallopian tube epithelium-serous tumors, endometrium-endometrioid and endocervical-mucinous) and non-mullerian epithelium (intestinal epithelium-mucinous tumor of intestinal type) and transitional epithelium (Brenner tumor).

Table 19.2: Epithelial tumors

Mullerian
• Fallopian tube epithelium—serous tumors
• Endometrium—endometrioid
• Endocervical—mucinous
Non-mullerian
• Intestinal epithelium-mucinous tumor of intestinal type
Transitional epithelium
• Brenner tumor

19.5.1 Screening

Ovarian cancer is the fourth most common cancer among women, but is the most lethal malignancy. At the time of diagnosis 70% will be having stage III disease as the disease is asymptomatic till late stage. Hence, there is a need for a screening method to detect early stage disease. If the disease is diagnosed early, i.e. when it is confined to the ovary, the 5-year survival is good. Five-year survival rate for early stage disease is 90% and for advanced disease it drops to 30%.

Unlike cancer of the cervix, ovaries cannot be easily approached for screening and early ovarian cancer is asymptomatic. There is no pre-invasive stage or latent phase. So far there is no ideal screening method. But of late, with improvement in ultrasound and development of tumor markers, the sensitivity and specificity of screening strategies of ovarian cancer have improved.

Two large randomized trials, one in the UK and the other in US are being undertaken to study the sensitivity and specificity of screening methods in detecting ovarian malignancy among postmenopausal women, the results of which are awaited. The former is the United Kingdom Collaborative Trial of Ovarian Cancer Screening- UK CTO CS trial. In this trial, initially CA-125 screening is done on the basis of which volunteers are categorized into low risk, intermediate risk and elevated risk groups. Low risk group will undergo annual CA-125, intermediate group will have CA-125 repeated and elevated risk group will be taken for TVS and if TVS is also abnormal, surgery is advised. The latter is the NIH PLCO (Prostate, Lung, Colorectal and Ovarian cancer) Study in which the presence of malignancy is assessed by clinical examination, ultrasound and CA-125. The results of these two studies will come out with the feasibility of screening general population for ovarian malignancy.

The strategies presently available for ovarian cancer screening will not fulfill the WHO criteria of an ideal screening test. However, it is worth going into the status of various screening strategies available at present.

Vaginal Examination

Vaginal examination is not dependable for the early diagnosis of ovarian malignancy. Due to the lack of sensitivity, vaginal examination alone cannot be used as a first line screening method among asymptomatic women.

Tumor Markers

Tumor markers are substances produced in the body, either elaborated by the cancer cells or by normal cells in response to the presence of malignant cells. These markers can be used to screen for malignancy, to predict the malignant nature of an existing neoplasm, to assess the response to treatment as well as for detecting recurrence of the disease while on follow-up. They can be tumor antigens, enzymes, hormones, oncogenes or other substances.

Unfortunately, no single test or combination of tests developed is sensitive or specific enough for detecting the presence of ovarian malignancy.[2]

Tumor markers of epithelial tumors (Table 19.3)

Table 19.3: Tumor markers of epithelial ovarian malignancy

- CA 125
- Carcino embryonic antigen (CEA)
- CA 19-9
- Tumor associated trypsin inhibitor (TATI)
- Cancer associated serum antigen (CASA)

1. **CA (Cancer antigen) 125:** The most extensively investigated tumor marker for epithelial tumor is CA 125. It is a glycoprotein, the blood level of which is elevated in 80% of non-mucinous epithelial ovarian cancers. In stage I disease it is elevated only in 50% of the patients. It is insensitive in mucinous and germ cell tumors. But since serous epithelial malignancies are highly aggressive and germ cell tumors have comparatively good prognosis, it is worthwhile to use CA 125 level as a screening test for ovarian malignancy. Levels below 35 IU/ml are considered normal. It can be elevated in non-ovarian malignancies, e.g. endometrial cancer, several benign as well as inflammatory conditions like endometriosis, PID, pancreatitis, pericarditis, colitis, diverticulitis, peritonitis, pleuritis and SLE. Serial estimation is mandatory and rising titers signify malignancy. In benign conditions it almost maintains the same level. The specificity is more in post menopausal women than in pre-menopausal women. If the levels are found to be high, it can be used for the follow-up of patients while on treatment and also to detect recurrence. In patients who respond to treatment, the CA 125 levels return to normal in 3 months time. Elevated CA 125 level alone should not be an indication to treat patients with chemotherapy, when there is a clinical situation giving the impression of an inoperable ovarian malignancy. Conditions like peritoneal tuberculosis can mimic ovarian malignancy on clinical examination. Malignancy should always be confirmed by histopathology before administering chemotherapy.
2. **Carcinoembryonic antigen (CEA):** CEA is a complex glycoprotein found in the plasma membrane of tumor cells. It is found to be elevated in the blood of patients with mucinous tumors of the ovary. This is also not a specific tumor marker for ovarian mucinous tumors. It is elevated in cancer of the breast, lung, pancreas, stomach and in benign conditions like cirrhosis, inflammatory bowel disease, chronic bowel disease and pancreatitis. Levels are tested in sera.

3. **CA 19-9:** This is also a marker for mucinous tumors. Like CEA it is elevated in malignancies of the stomach, colon and pancreas also.
4. **Tumor associated trypsin inhibitor (TATI):** Tumor associated trypsin inhibitor is a protease inhibitor elevated in mucinous tumors.
5. **Cancer associated serum antigen (CASA):** Cancer associated serum antigen is another marker for ovarian malignancy. However, it is elevated in other malignancies like prostate, breast, colon, etc. The optimal cut off level is 8 U/ml. It also has an independent prognostic value for survival.

Since, CA 125 is elevated mainly in non-mucinous epithelial ovarian cancers, a combination of markers which include markers for other types of ovarian malignancy has been suggested. CA 72-4, M-CSF, OVXI, LPA, prostacin, osteopontin, inhibin and kallikrein have given promising results.

Proteomics

A recently evolved screening method is analysis of serum proteins by surface enhanced laser desorption ionization time of flight (SELDI-TOF) mass spectrometry. This is based on the principle that malignant tissue produces abnormal proteins which can be analyzed in serum. The proteins in the serum can be separated according to their molecular weight. Based on the pattern of different proteins, women who have malignancy could be sorted out. Preliminary data by Petricon[3] and colleagues on proteomics reported sensitivity of 100% and specificity of 95% in identifying patients who had ovarian cancer. This method is under investigation.

Ultrasound

Ultrasound, especially TVS has evolved as a powerful tool for the evaluation of pelvic organs. TVS helps to detect even small adnexal masses. It has high sensitivity in predicting malignancy. Nagell and colleagues[4] screened 25327 women from 1987 to 2005 with annual USS and reported detection at an earlier stage of the disease and decreased mortality. Due to the high sensitivity of TVS in detecting adnexal masses, unnecessary surgical intervention is a disadvantage. Ovarian masses with septations >3 mm in thickness, mural nodules, presence of solid components within the mass and papillary projections are suggestive of malignancy. A morphologic index[5] based on ultrasound features has been developed, which has a positive predictive value of 45%. Benign lesions like endometriomas and hemorrhagic cysts may simulate malignancy, but Doppler ultrasound helps in predicting malignancy in ovarian tumor by studying the pulsatility index (PI) and resistive index (RI) of the vessels in the ovarian mass. Malignant tissue will have new vessels formed with thin walls and hence have low resistance flow. An RI <0.4 and PI <1 predicts malignancy. Scoring systems based on morphological index to calculate the risk of malignancy in an ovarian cyst has been proposed by several authors, of which the one published by Gramberg et al is the generally followed one. The specificity and the positive predictive value has been found to increase from 82 to 97% and 63 to 97% respectively by adding color Doppler to gray-scale morphologic information (Figs 19.1A and B). A large meta-analysis comparing morphologic assessment, Doppler ultrasound, color Doppler flow imaging, and combined techniques for characterization of adnexal masses using summary receiver operator curves found the best diagnostic

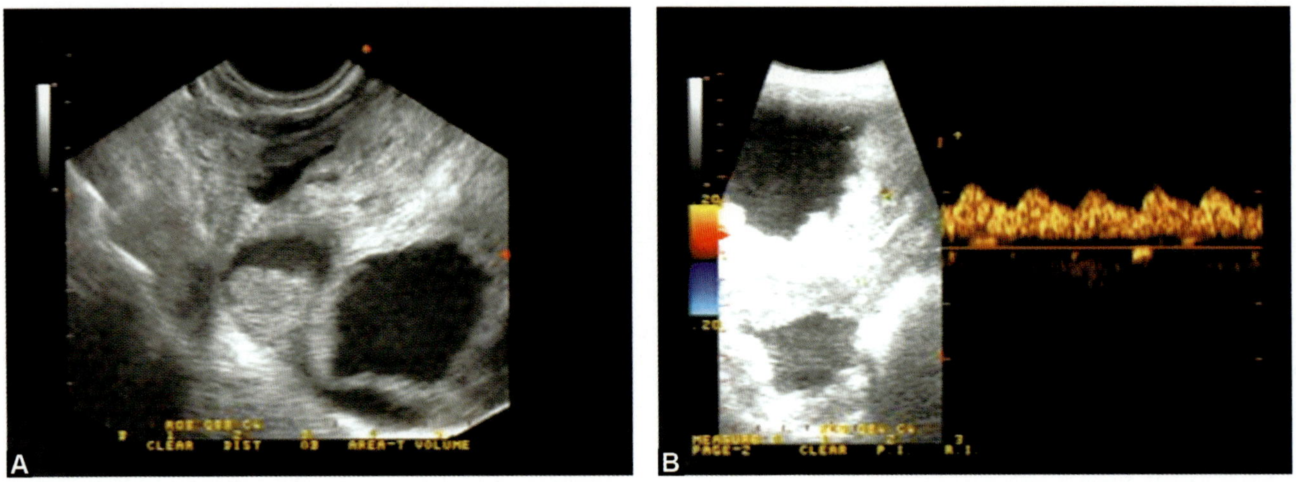

Figs 19.1A and B: TVS showing solid areas and cystic spaces with thick wall suggestive of malignancy in an 8 cm ovarian tumor (A), which was not clinically suspected to be malignant. Spectral Doppler picture showing increased vascularity with high diastolic flow (B)

> **Ultrasound features of malignancy (Gramberg et al)**
> - Presence of solid areas
> - Thick septa >3 mm
> - Increased vascularity
> - Blood vessels with RI<0.4, PI<1
> - Confluence of vessels

performance for combined techniques[6] (0.92), followed in decreasing order by morphologic assessment alone (0.85), Doppler indices (0.82), and color Doppler flow (0.73). Histologic subtypes cannot be accurately differentiated by ultrasound features.

Multimodal Screening

To improve the positive predictive value, it is better to do CA 125 as a first line test and USS if CA 125 is abnormal. The sensitivity of USS is greater than that of CA 125, but CA 125 is done first to decrease the number of TVS, which involves expense and discomfort. However, the sensitivity of the combined test is comparable to those utilizing Doppler ultrasound along with morphological scoring.

Risk of Malignancy Index (RMI)

RMI gives an estimate of the risk of Ovarian Ca for women with adnexal masses.The RMI is calculated using ultrasound findings (U), menopausal status (M) and CA125 value (serum levels >35 U/ml abnormal).

Risk	*RMI*	*Risk of cancer*
Low	<25	<3
Moderate	25-250	20
High	> 250	75

RMI = U x M x CA125

Ultrasound findings are scored with one point for each of the following:

- Multilocular cyst
- Evidence of solid areas
- Evidence of metastases
- Presence of ascites
- Bilateral lesions

U = 0 (ultrasound score of 0)
U = 1 (ultrasound score of 1)
U = 3 (ultrasound score of 2 - 5)

Menopausal status is scored as follows:
Postmenopausal status is graded M = 3,
Pre-menopausal status is graded M = 1

Who should be screened?

Recommendations for screening

Screening general population lacks specificity. But high risk population screening will give better positive predictive value. Currently, there is no scientific evidence for screening with good efficacy among low risk or average risk women. At present screening is not recommended for general population of women with or without a family history of sporadic ovarian cancer. To improve the sensitivity of the screening test, it is important to screen high risk population where the prevalence is high compared to the general population. When the lifetime risk of ovarian cancer is only 1-1.5% in the general population, it is 12% in women with genetic predisposition. For high risk women and those with genetic mutations, screening is recommended which should include annual rectovaginal examination, CA 125 and TVS. Twice a year screening has also been recommended from 35 years.

However, as of today, there is no evidence that screening reduces the mortality from ovarian cancer.

Inclusion criteria as high risk

- Two first degree relatives with ovarian cancer
- One ovarian cancer and one breast cancer, in first degree relative occurring at <50 years of age
- One ovarian cancer and two breast cancer, occurring at <60 years of age
- One ovarian cancer and 3 colorectal cancer, one <50 years of age
- Known mutations of BRCA I/BRCA II or HNPCC genes.

Spread of ovarian cancer

Primary spread is to the opposite ovary through the uterus. Peritoneal (trans-coelomic) spread is the most common route of spread. As the ovary is covered with a single layer of surface epithelium, tumor cells exfoliate from the surface and spread by the peritoneal fluid circulation effected by local peristalsis and respiratory movements. The peritoneal fluid normally circulates in a clock-wise manner from the right paracolic gutter to the right side of the diaphragm, crossing the midline and circulating through the left paracolic gutter to the left side of the pelvis. Peritoneal deposits appear as metastatic plaques of varying sizes. It is more in the peritoneal reflections. The omentum will be diffusely infiltrated and large deposits can occur in the omentum—omental caking.

Lymphatic metastases occur in ovarian cancer but are not given much importance. Maximum drainage is into the retroperitoneum, i.e. to the para-aortic group of nodes along the ovarian vessels. Along the uterine vessels lymphatics drain to the internal iliac, obturator and external iliac nodes. Along the round ligament, lymphatics can reach the inguinal group of nodes. Hence, occasionally ovarian cancer deposits can occur in the groin.

Distant metastasis is rare. The common sites of distant spread are the liver, lungs, pleura, adrenal glands and spleen. Bone and brain metastases are very rare.

19.5.2 Clinical Presentation of Epithelial Ovarian Tumor

Epithelial ovarian tumors can occur in any age group but the maximum incidence is in the 6th to 8th decade. Borderline tumor usually occurs in the younger age group, but the disease can occur at any age.

Symptoms and Signs

It is unfortunate that ovarian malignancies are asymptomatic till an advanced stage. Symptoms are often vague, like feeling of fullness, bloating sensation and vague pain abdomen. Loss of weight and loss of appetite occurs when the tumor grows to a large size. The symptoms for which women usually seek medical advice, are distension of abdomen, loss of weight and loss of appetite. Tumor impacted in the pelvis can cause constipation or tenesmus. Acute abdominal pain is not the usual presentation of malignant ovarian tumor. But rarely malignant ovarian tumors can present as acute abdomen when it undergoes torsion, infection or hemorrhage.

Postmenopausal women with large epithelial ovarian tumor can present with irregular vaginal bleeding due to the tumor stimulating the surrounding ovarian tissue to produce hormones (misfit tumor). Rarely, the symptom can be frequency of micturition.

When a woman presents with ascites and mass abdomen, an effort should be made to elicit symptoms suggestive of primary malignancy of the breast, gastrointestinal tract or urinary tract as the ascites and mass may be due to secondary deposit in the ovary. Hence, a history of hematuria, malena, vomiting, nipple discharge or lump in the breast should be elicited.

Women presenting with advanced disease would be emaciated and on examination the abdomen will be distended and a hard fixed mass will be palpable in the hypogastrium. Deposits in the porta hepatis and the root of mesentery may be palpable in the upper abdomen. Bimanual examination can make out deposits in the pouch of Douglas and hard fixed mass inseparable from the uterus can be appreciated. Pouch of Douglas deposits can be better appreciated by rectal examination. Rarely, the tumor can grow in between rectum and vagina, in which case rectal examination will help differentiate it from retroperitoneal tumors. When a woman presents with symptoms like bloating, vague abdominal pain, etc. bimanual examination should be performed, lest a malignant ovarian tumor which is limited to the pelvis be missed. In the presence of a mobile tumor without ascites and secondary deposits, imaging by ultrasound/CT and tumor markers will help differentiate between malignant and benign mass.

19.5.3 Management of Epithelial Ovarian Tumor

The primary mode of treatment of malignant ovarian tumor is surgical. The disease is staged surgically following systematic exploratory laparotomy. Management of epithelial ovarian tumor is different from germ cell tumors. Malignancy can be predicted in ovarian tumors from the history, clinical features, ultrasound appearance supplemented with Doppler and tumor markers. The final confirmation is by histopathology. Histopathological diagnosis can be made before surgery from cytology of ascitic fluid or by ultrasound-guided needle aspiration biopsy.

Preoperative Evaluation

Before surgical exploration, patients should have complete blood count, liver function tests and chest X-ray. The usual imaging is by ultrasound and Doppler. If clinically indicated, CT or MRI may have to be done to assess operability, extent of invasion and to exclude primary site elsewhere when a pelvic mass is suspected to be a secondary deposit. Multi detector CT is highly accurate in detecting tumor implants larger than 1 cm. Implants measuring <1 cm are difficult to detect. MRI is slightly more accurate than CT in detecting nodal metastases. When the nodes are not enlarged but harbor tumor cells, CT and MRI cannot detect the disease. Positron emission tomography (PET) is evolving as an imaging modality. PET can detect lesions more than 0.5 cm in diameter. Tumor markers should be done as appropriate. Tumor markers help predict malignancy. If the marker is positive, it will help in assessing response to treatment and will be a surrogate marker for recurrence.

If a patient has symptoms suspicious of colon cancer, a barium enema should be done. Patients with hematemesis, dysphagia or vomiting should have esophago-gastroscopy. Breast examination should be routine because occasionally the primary in the breast may be small, in the presence of large secondary deposits in the ovary with ascites. Postmenopausal women who have vaginal bleeding should have endometrial and endocervical evaluation to exclude concomitant endometrial malignancy.

Differential Diagnosis

Inflammatory conditions like pelvic or peritoneal tuberculosis can mimic ovarian malignancy due to the associated loss of weight, loss of appetite and ascites. Endometriosis produces bilateral adnexal masses with fixity and nodules in the pouch of Douglas. Ultrasound helps to diagnose endometriotic cysts by the typical appearance. It should be kept in mind that clear cell carcinoma can occur in endometriotic cysts. Subserous pedunculated uterine fibroids can simulate solid ovarian tumors. Other neoplastic conditions like colon cancer and retroperitoneal tumors also can mimic ovarian malignancy. Clinical examination, ultrasound and if necessary CT/MRI would prove beneficial in these situations. A pelvic kidney which is a very rare occurrence should be excluded when a firm mass is palpable in the pelvis in close proximity to the pelvic side wall. Kidney can be easily spotted out by ultrasound. Usually it will be the opposite side kidney that is seen in the pelvis. Hence the absence of kidneys in the normal position has to be confirmed.

Surgical Management

Ovarian tumor is staged surgically (Table 19.4). Surgical staging by FIGO was introduced in 1964 and revised in 1985.

The histological grade determined by pattern of differentiation, extent of cellular atypia and proportion of undifferentiated cells are not given much importance these days because studies have shown poor reproducibility and interobserver variation. Further the value of grading in prognosis has not been conclusively established.

Table 19.4: Carcinoma of the ovary: FIGO Staging (with permission from FIGO)

FIGO	*Characteristics*	*TNM*
	Primary ovarian tumors cannot be assessed	TX
0	No evidence of primary tumor	T0
I	Tumor confined to ovaries	T1
	Tumor limited to one ovary, capsule intact	T1a
IA	No tumor on ovarian surface	
	No malignant cells in the ascites or peritoneal washings	
	Tumor limited to both ovaries, capsules intact	T1b
IB	No tumor on ovarian surface	
	No malignant cells in the ascites or peritoneal washings	
IC	Tumor limited to one or both ovaries, with any of the following:	
	Capsule ruptured, tumor on ovarian surface, positive malignant cells in the ascites or positive peritoneal washings	T1c
II	Tumor involves one or both ovaries with pelvic extension	T2
IIA	Extension and/or implants in uterus and/ or tubes	T2a
	No malignant cells in the ascites or peritoneal washings	
IIB	Extension to other pelvic organ	T2b
	No malignant cells in the ascites or peritoneal washings	
IIC	IIA/B with positive malignant cells in the ascites or positive peritoneal washings	T2c
III	Tumor involves one or both ovaries with microscopically confirmed peritoneal metastasis outside the pelvis and/or regional lymph node metastasis	T3 N1
IIIA	Microscopic peritoneal metastasis beyond the pelvis	T3a
IIIB	Macroscopic peritoneal metastasis beyond the pelvis 2 cm or less in greatest dimension	T3b
IIIC	Peritoneal metastasis beyond pelvis more than 2 cm in greatest dimension and/or regional lymph node metastasis	T3c N1
IV	Distant metastasis beyond the peritoneal cavity	M1

Note: Liver capsule metastasis is T3/Stage III, liver parenchymal metastasis M1/Stage IV. Pleural effusion must have positive cytology

Management of Patients in the Reproductive Age Group with a Suspicion of Ovarian Cancer

When a young woman in the reproductive age group presents with pelvic mass, surgical decision making is of crucial importance. For a benign tumor, conservative surgery is the rule and for malignant tumor, the definitive treatment involves removal of uterus and both ovaries. Judging whether the tumor is malignant or benign frequently becomes a difficult task before surgery. Clinical assessment supplemented with imaging and tumor markers help to a great extent in deciding whether the mass is benign or malignant. The following factors point in favor of malignancy:

1. Rapid progression of symptoms with loss of weight and loss of appetite
2. Presence of bilateral tumor

3. Tumor fixation and nodularity of the pouch of Douglas
4. Presence of ascites (benign tumors like fibromas can be associated with ascites—Meig's syndrome)
5. Ultrasound appearance of thick septa, solid areas and vascularity with RI<0.4 and PI< 1.
6. CT/MRI finding of metastatic nodule
7. Elevated tumor markers

Laparoscopic evaluation gives an opportunity for assessment of the nature of the tumor, whenever clinical examination and investigations are not conclusive of malignancy, but suspicious. If at laparoscopy, the tumor appears to be malignant, laparotomy should be performed. When the suspicion of malignancy is strong, laparotomy should be resorted to without performing laparoscopy. Laparotomy should be done only with frozen section facility. Laparoscopic management of early stage ovarian malignancy is controversial. There are only very few trials and a Cochrane review has not found evidence to support laparoscopic management of ovarian tumor if malignancy is predicted.[7]

Management of Early Stage Ovarian Cancer

Only about 25% of ovarian cancers are diagnosed in stage I. The primary mode of treatment of ovarian malignancy is surgery. The aim of surgical treatment is to remove as much malignant tissue as possible. If residual tissue is present, its size and extent should be delineated. Staging laparotomy is the most important part of management. Hence, comprehensive surgical staging should be done for all patients. Even if macroscopic spread is not made out, microscopic spread can be present which needs to be treated postoperatively for better survival.

For staging laparotomy, a vertical midline incision, which should extent well above the umbilicus should be preferred. For a small tumor confined to the pelvis, a transverse Cherney or Maylard incision may be chosen. If ascites is present, it is collected for cytological study. If there is no ascites, the peritoneal cavity should be washed with 200 ml saline and sample collected from subdiaphragmatic area, paracolic gutters and pouch of Douglas. The entire peritoneal cavity is inspected and palpated systematically in a caecocephalad manner to delineate the extent of the disease. The primary tumor should be inspected for capsule rupture or tumor excrescence on the surface (Fig. 19.2). If the appearance of the tumor is suggestive of Krukenberg tumor, probable primary sites like stomach, colon or pancreas should be kept in mind and these structures palpated in order to exclude primary. If macroscopic disease is not seen in the upper abdomen, the diaphragm should be scraped and smear taken for cytology, to exclude microscopic disease in these sanctuary areas.

Total hysterectomy with bilateral salpingo-oophorectomy and infracolic omentectomy should be performed (Figs 19.3 and 19.4). Even if on gross examination the tumor appears to be confined to the ovary, peritoneal biopsy from the paracolic gutters, cul-de-sac, uterovesical fold and subdiaphragmatic area should be taken to exclude microscopic deposits.

The para-aortic and pelvic lymph nodes should be removed for histological examination as they are the primary areas of drainage. Removal of omentum, lymph nodes and peritoneal biopsy allows accurate staging of early disease and optimal debulking if disease is advanced. Surgical staging including peritoneal biopsy detects occult stage III disease.[8] Lymphadenectomy is reported to improve survival in women with early stage ovarian cancer.

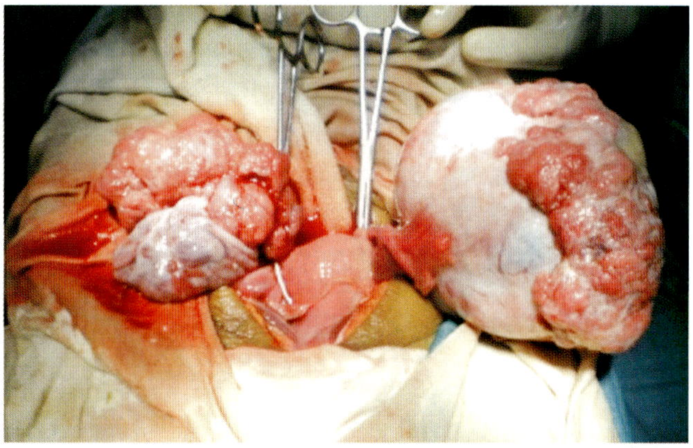

Fig. 19.2: Bilateral papillary serous cystadenocarcinoma. Note the papillary excrescences on the surface

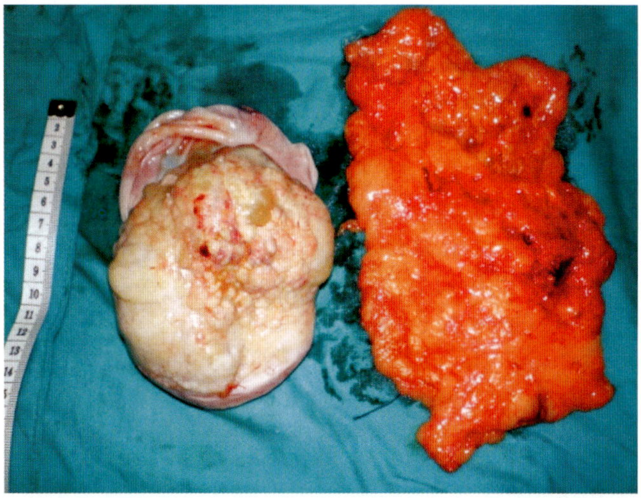

Fig. 19.3: Solid ovarian tumor and omentectomy specimen of a 50-year-old lady who had total hysterectomy with BSO. Pathology revealed clear cell carcinoma. There was no evidence of disease outside the ovary. Postoperatively the patient was administered chemotherapy based on the pathology report

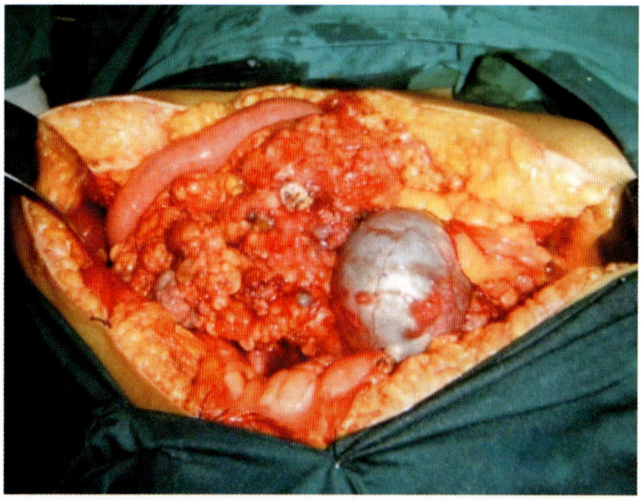

Fig. 19.4: Papillary serous cystadenocarcinoma. Note the multiple secondary deposits on the omentum

Role of Conservative Surgery in Early Stage Epithelial Ovarian Cancer

Epithelial ovarian cancers can occur in younger age group also. The stage at which the tumor is confined to the ovary and hence is curable by ovariotomy is very limited in the biological time-table of the tumor. If the patient is fortunate enough the tumor will be detected in this stage when conservative surgery is possible. Unilateral well-differentiated well-encapsulated tumor without ascites (Stage IA) diagnosed after proper staging can be treated conservatively by unilateral ovariotomy, if the woman is particular to preserve the childbearing function, after getting an informed consent. After completion of family, re-laparotomy and total hysterectomy with removal of the remaining ovary should be undertaken. Oncologic outcome for conservatively treated early stage disease has been found to be as good as for those women treated with TH with BSO.[9]

In the event of an unexpected finding of malignancy in an ovariotomy specimen, the patient should have re-laparotomy and proper staging of the disease before taking a decision to restrict ovariotomy as management. It has been reported that when a proper surgical staging (revision staging) is done following an inadequate staging, the disease has been found to be upstaged in 22% of patients. If the initial findings favor adjuvant treatment based on risk factors, immediate re-staging need not be done. Completion surgery may be done at the end of adjuvant chemotherapy.

Adjuvant Therapy for Early Stage Disease

After staging laparotomy and definitive surgery, adjuvant chemotherapy is not required for patients who had stage Ia or Ib with intact capsule, no excrescences, negative peritoneal biopsy and washings and the histopathology is non-clear cell type.

If the histology is clear cell type or grade 3 non-clear cell type or the disease is stage Ic or above (positive peritoneal washing or omentum positive), the patient should be given postoperative chemotherapy (Table 19.5). Two major studies addressed the issue of survival benefit following adjuvant chemotherapy after surgery for early stage ovarian cancer, the EORTC trial and the British Medical Research Council trial. Survival for the chemotherapy arm was 82% vs 74% for the non-chemotherapy arm.[10] The standard approach is to give a combination of Carboplatin and Paclitaxel. Carboplatin is preferred over Cisplatin due to its lower side effect profile.

Table 19.5: Indications for adjuvant therapy for early stage disease

Histology
• Clear cell type
• Non-clear cell but grade 3
Positive peritoneal washing
Omentum positive
Capsule involvement
Tumor rupture during surgery

GOG 157 trial addressed the issue of the number of chemotherapeutic regime for adjuvant treatment. 321 women who had surgery for stage 1A- stage II ovarian cancer were randomized to 3 or 6 cycles of Carboplatin and Paclitaxel. The decrease in recurrence in the 6 cycle arm was 27% vs 19% in the 3 cycle arm. Hence, the standard is to give 6 cycles of chemotherapy.

Presently radiotherapy is not routinely resorted to for the treatment of residual disease. Since the entire peritoneal cavity is at risk of tumor spread, radiation needs to be given to the whole abdomen. Radiation dose adequate enough to destroy the tumor cannot be given for fear of damaging the intestine, kidneys and the liver.

Management of Advanced Disease

The primary aim of treatment is an aggressive removal of as much of the tumor as possible so that the least amount of tumor tissue is left behind. The 5-year cure rate depends on the volume of tumor tissue left behind rather than the stage of the disease. Optimal cytoreduction was previously defined as < 2 cm residual tumor. Later <1 cm residual tissue was defined as optimal cytoreduction because improved survival was reported in patients with a <1 cm residual tumor compared to < 2 cm size[11] The recently completed trials by GOG 52, 158 and 172 has defined complete removal of gross residual disease as the treatment option conferring survival benefit. It is preferable to undertake optimal cytoreduction in dedicated centers having experienced hands. The smaller the tumor volume, the more effective will be the chemotherapy. By debulking, the improved survival benefit is because of the following facts.

1. Large volume tumors are poorly vascularized so that chemotherapeutic agents will not reach deep into the tumor tissue leading to suboptimal response whereas chemotherapeutic agents reach small volume tumors better.
2. Debulking removes resistant clones of cells.
3. Large volume tumor will have more cells in the resting phase (G0 phase) which are resistant to chemotherapy. As tumor volume is reduced a greater proportion of cells will be transitioned to the growth phase of the cycle making them more susceptible to chemotherapy.

Patients with massive ascites can develop hemodynamic instability while decompression during surgery. If there are bowel adhesions, the same should be released. If the pelvic structures cannot be delineated, the tumor along with the uterus, tubes and ovaries and the pelvic peritoneum are separated from the retroperitoneum, rectosigmoid, bladder and urethra through a retroperitoneal approach and the whole tumor is removed en-mass. Cytoreductive surgery in the presence of extensive disease in the diaphragm, liver parenchyma, lesser omentum or portahepatis is difficult. However, removal of the supracolic omentum as well as resection of diaphragmatic secondaries is being practiced in dedicated centers.

Role of Bowel Resection as Part of Debulking

In the event of the mass invading into the wall of the rectosigmoid, the rectosigmoid can be removed with the tumor in a posterior exenteration. A colostomy is inevitable in this situation. Depending on the area of involvement, a partial resection and end to end anastomosis may be performed. Anastomotic leak and its sequelae are the major postoperative problems.

Diaphragmatic Secondaries

Secondaries in the diaphragm can be resected as a part of debulking. There is evidence that peeling of diaphragmatic peritoneum, partial thickness diaphragm resection or excision of nodules from the surface of diaphragm improved 5-year survival rate from 15 to 53% compared to those who did not have diaphragmatic surgery.[13]

Role of Lymphadenectomy in Advanced Stage Ovarian Malignancy

Removal of obviously involved lymph nodes in patients during cytoreduction for advanced ovarian malignancy is justifiable as it improves survival by debulking the tumor tissue.[24]

Role of Neoadjuvant Chemotherapy in the Initial Treatment of Advanced Disease

A Cochrane review has found that neoadjuvant chemotherapy prior to debulking surgery for advanced epithelial ovarian cancer is not superior to conventional debulking surgery followed by platinum based chemotherapy.[14] Two prospective randomized controlled trials are evaluating the role of neoadjuvant chemotherapy prior to debulking-CHORUS 2003 and EORTC 55971. However, patients who have clinically inoperable tumor can be treated with chemotherapy after cytological confirmation.

Adjuvant Therapy after Surgery for Advanced Ovarian Cancer

The standard therapy after primary surgery for advanced ovarian cancer is 6 cycles of Carboplatin and Paclitaxel. 80% will respond and 60% will achieve complete clinical remission with this regime. But majority of them will go for recurrence later on.

FIGO recommends the following regimes:

- Paclitaxel 175 mg/m^2 over 3 hours and Carboplatin AUC 6 over 1 hour
- Docetaxel 75 mg/m^2 over 1 hour and Carboplatin AUC 5 over 1 hour.

The dose of Carboplatin is based on Calvert's formula using Creatinine clearance calculated by Cocroft formula-(140- age) × weight in kg × .85/serum creatinine × 72. (AUC-Area under the curve).

The following regimes may also be considered:

- Paclitaxel 135 mg/m^2 over 24 hours, cisplatin 75 mg/m^2 over 6 hours
- Paclitaxel 175 mg/m^2 over 3 hours and cisplatin 75 mg/m^2 over 6 hours.

Role of Intraperitoneal (IP) Chemotherapy

To reduce recurrence, the role of intraperitoneal Cisplatin as frontline primary adjuvant therapy was studied in trials. In GOG 172 study, IV Cisplatin and Paclitaxel were compared with intraperitoneal Cisplatin (100 mg/m^2) on day 2 and Paclitaxel 135 mg/m^2 IV over 24 hours on day 1 and Paclitaxel 60 mg/m^2 intraperitoneally on day 8. Six such cycles are given every 21 days. There was a 25% reduction in the risk of death in the intraperitoneal group. A Cochrane meta-analysis found an increase in overall survival and progression free survival in advanced ovarian cancer in the IP group. The results of this provide the most reliable estimates of the relative survival benefits of IP over IV therapy and should be used as part of decision-making process. However, the potential for catheter related complications, the discomfort of abdominal distension and toxicity needs to be considered when deciding on the most appropriate treatment for each individual woman. Opinion about the optimal dose, timing and mechanism of administration needs to be addressed in the next phase of clinical trials.[15]

Role of Secondary Cytoreduction

Secondary cytoreduction is an attempt at cytoreductive surgery if secondaries develop following completion of first line chemotherapy. The decision for cytoreductive surgery in patients who develop recurrence is based on the period of disease free survival and the number of recurrence sites. Patients who had disease free interval longer than 30 months and single site recurrence will benefit from secondary cytoreduction by the removal of all macroscopic disease.

Inoperable Tumors

Operability of the tumor is assessed by clinical examination supplemented with imaging. The tumor is considered inoperable in the following situations.

1. Presence of extensive upper abdominal secondaries (Nodes in the portahepatis, base of small bowel mesentery and lesser sac)
2. Perisplenic and diaphragmatic involvement
3. Liver parenchymal and pulmonary metastasis
4. Poor general condition

Management of Inoperable Tumor

Histopathological diagnosis of malignancy is a must before planning treatment. Clinically inoperable tumors should have ultrasound-guided needle biopsy to confirm malignancy. If the needle biopsy is negative, laparotomy and biopsy is warranted. Neo-adjuvant chemotherapy is given for these patients followed by interval debulking surgery (see in next column). 3-6 courses of chemotherapy are given and the operability reassessed. If needed, imaging studies with CT/MRI should be done. Pleural effusion *per se* is not a contraindication for primary cytoreductive surgery. About 60-80% patients can be optimally debulked by neo-adjuvant chemotherapy followed by debulking.[16]

Interval Debulking Surgery (IDS)

When primary cytoreduction is considered suboptimal, an attempt at cytoreduction can be tried after three cycles of systemic chemotherapy. This interval debulking reduces the dose of chemotherapeutic agents used so that cost of treatment and side effects are reduced. Patients who could not undergo primary cytoreduction due to poor physical fitness can also be considered for debulking after a few courses of chemotherapy.

An EORTC trial was conducted on 319 patients who had suboptimal initial debulking. After 3 courses of chemotherapy, patients were randomly assigned to interval debulking followed by chemotherapy vs continued chemotherapy. There was a reduction in death of 33% at 2 years follow-up in the group who had interval debulking. In a Cochrane review of 3 RCTs no conclusive evidence was found to determine whether IDS between cycles of chemotherapy would improve or decrease the survival rates of women with advanced ovarian cancer, compared with conventional treatment of primary surgery followed by adjuvant chemotherapy.[17] However, in situations where the primary surgery was not performed by gynecologic oncologists or was less extensive, IDS appeared to yield benefit.

19.5.4 Prognostic Factors

The overall 5-year survival reported is 48.4%. Stage of the disease at presentation is the most important prognostic factor. Stage Ia has a survival of 89.9% and for stage IV it drops to 16.8%.[18]

The prognosis of patients with epithelial ovarian tumor is affected by the following factors.

1. Stage at diagnosis
2. Histological subtype
3. Grading
4. Volume of the residual disease

Early detection has a significant effect on survival. Clear cell tumors are very aggressive compared to other types of epithelial tumors. Tumor grade is an independent prognostic factor, with well differentiated tumors carrying good prognosis. Because of the poor outcome with chemotherapy in patients with large volume tumor, the initial management of advanced disease patients should be by primary optimal cytoreduction.

19.5.5 Post-treatment Follow-up

Even patients, who have excellent initial response to treatment, might relapse. Early diagnosis and management of recurrence after progression free interval gives the best results. The objectives of a proper follow-up are:

Flow chart 19.1: Management algorithm for epithelial ovarian cancer

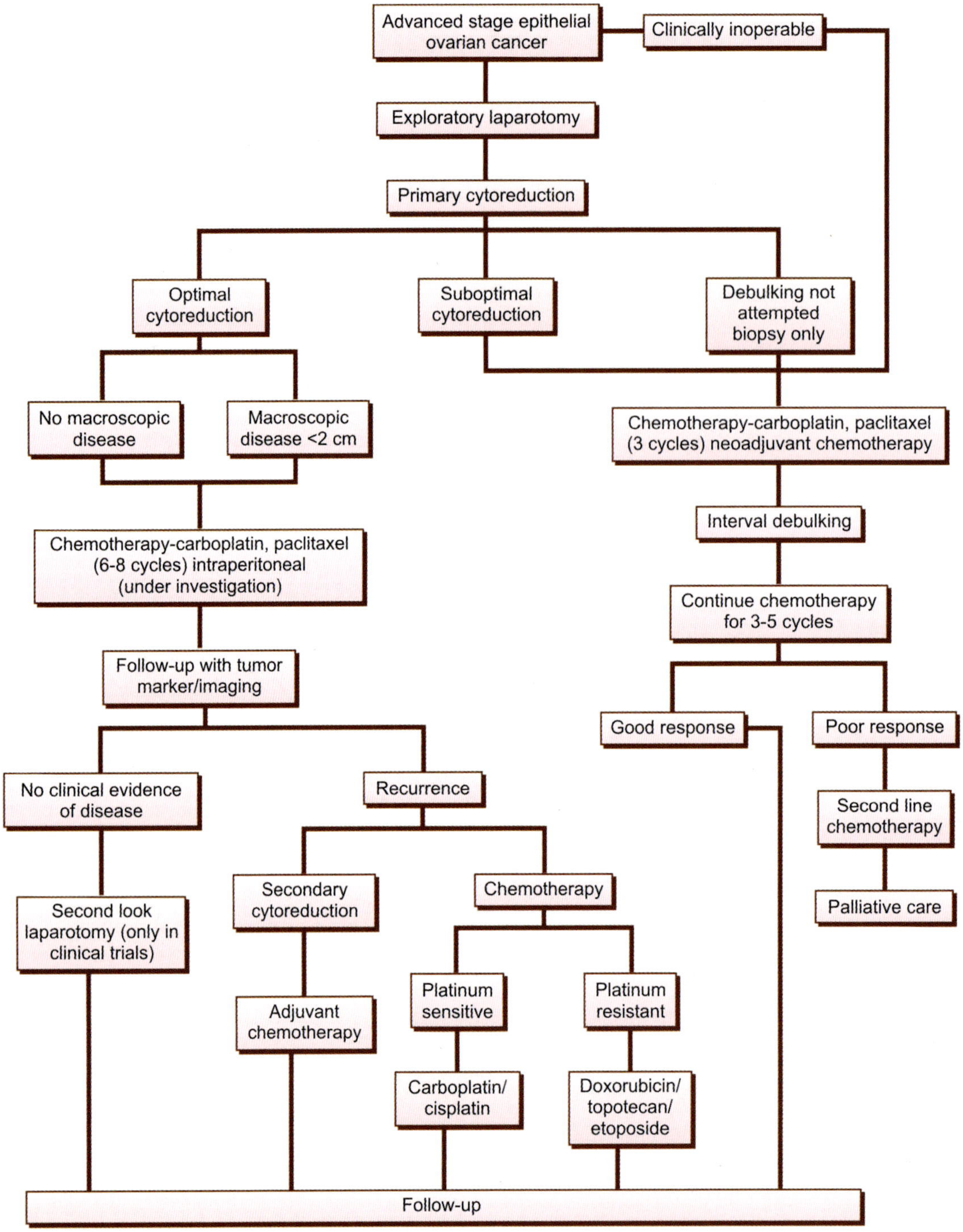

- Immediate response to treatment can be assessed
- Early recognition and management of complications of treatment
- Assessment of efficacy of treatment modalities

During the first year the patients should be seen every 3 months. In the subsequent years the interval can be gradually increased to every 4-6 months and then annually after the fifth year. During follow-up visits, a detailed history should be taken and a complete physical examination which should include pelvic and rectal examination must be performed. Women, who have elevated CA 125 preoperatively, can be followed up with CA 125. CT or MR imaging of the abdomen and pelvis may have to be done if there is clinical suspicion of recurrence. Chest CT need not be performed routinely. If the tumor markers are elevated and no lesion is detected in the abdomen and pelvis, CT chest should be performed.

During follow-up, even if the CA 125 level is in the normal range but is more than the previous value there is a significant risk of recurrence and imaging is indicated. Recurrent tumor is usually seen as pelvic masses, peritoneal tumor implants, ascites or as lymphadenopathy. Occasionally recurrence can be pleural or parenchymal disease of the lung or liver.

The different terms used to describe disease after the initial treatment are:

1. *Persistent disease*: After the tumor has partially responded to initial therapy, there is an immediate elevation of CA 125 or clinical evidence of disease.
2. *Chemotherapy resistant disease*: Tumor recurrence detected within 6 months of completion of initial treatment.
3. *Refractory tumor*: Tumors that progress during initial therapy
4. *Recurrent ovarian cancer*: Tumor recurrence after complete initial response (a disease free interval of at least 6 months) to first line therapy.

Management of Recurrent Disease

Recurrent disease is tumor recurrence after a complete initial response to first line therapy, a negative second-look surgery (if performed) and a disease free interval >6 months. The management depends upon tumor bulk, location, number and the general fitness of the patient. Treatment can be surgical (secondary debulking) or medical. Resectability of the tumor should be assessed before deciding on surgical intervention. Survival rate reported after secondary cytoreduction varies from 17-62%. Unnecessary surgery should be avoided by proper preoperative assessment with imaging studies. MR imaging is found to have better sensitivity, specificity, accuracy and positive predictive value compared to CA 125 estimation and physical examination. FDG-PET is also used in advanced centers for preoperative evaluation. The sensitivity of PET is found to be superior to MR imaging. PET is usually used in patients who have increased CA 125 and no definite deposit detected in CT or MRI. Preoperative imaging should confirm absence of tumor elsewhere.

Recurrence usually occurs in the pelvis. There are two types of pelvic recurrence.

1. Central recurrence
2. Pelvic side wall recurrence

The size of the central mass is not a factor which decides operability, but extension to pelvic side wall denotes inoperability. MR imaging helps to make out inoperability by identifying the fat plane between the tumor and the pelvic side wall. Fat plane of at least 3 mm in thickness is necessary for resectability. Tumor invasion to bladder or rectum is not a contraindication for surgery provided the patient is willing for exenteration and is fit for such a procedure. Anterior exenteration which necessitates the removal of lower urinary tract requires a urinary diversion procedure and posterior exenteration necessitates colostomy. As in primary debulking, tumor in the gastrohepatic ligament, gallbladder fossa, portahepatis, root of the mesentery, etc. precludes surgical intervention. Platinum sensitive patients with recurrence can be given platinum-taxol combination itself. Recurrence rates of 15-20% were reported. For platinum resistant patients, the agents used are topotecan, docetaxel, liposomal doxorubicin, gemcitabine and etoposide. The Ovarian Cancer Guideline Panel of the NCCN broadened the list by adding anastrazole, bivacizumab, irinotecan, ifosfamide and letrozole. Tamoxifen also has been evaluated in the treatment of relapsed ovarian tumor. According to a Cochrane review, there is some evidence from observational studies that tamoxifen may induce response in a modest proportion of women with relapsed ovarian cancer, whose tumor is positive for estrogen receptor.[19]

Tumor involvement of bowel, radiation fibrosis and adhesions are the causes of intestinal obstruction. Acute obstruction necessitates surgical interference and subacute obstruction can be managed by conservative measures. Large bowel obstruction is a contraindication for cytoreduction. Palliative chemotherapy should be preferred in such a situation.

19.5.6 Prevention of Ovarian Cancer

Prevention should identify those at high risk for the disease. Risk factors associated with increased incidence of epithelial ovarian cancer are:

1. Advanced age
2. Previous history of breast, endometrial or ovarian cancer
3. Family history of ovarian cancer
4. Persons who have been identified to have BRCA I and II mutations
5. Lynch II syndrome (hereditary non-polyposis colorectal cancer syndrome)

A large volume of data indicates that oral contraceptive pill use for 5 years reduce the risk of ovarian cancer by 50%. Studies have demonstrated that the protective effect lasts for 10-20 years after discontinuation of OCP use. Even the low dose pills have protective effect against ovarian cancer. Tubal ligation reduces the incidence of ovarian cancer to over one-half.

Prophylactic oophorectomy in carriers of BRCA I and II and HNPCC mutation has been shown to reduce ovarian, fallopian tube and breast cancer. Oophorectomy should be done at the age of 35-40 years since the risk of BRCA associated cancer risk has been seen to dramatically increase during this period. For those who are not willing for oophorectomy, oral contraceptives are to be advised. These women should have yearly rectovaginal examination, TVS, mammogram and CA 125 estimation. Even after oophorectomy, these women should be followed up for primary peritoneal cancer by annual clinical examination including rectovaginal examination. GOG is presently studying the effect of Fenrelinide as a chemopreventive agent in those with genetic risk of ovarian cancer, the results of which are awaited.

19.5.7 Future Prospects

Immunological methods targeted at cancer cells alone hold promise due to the absence of side effects and unwanted damage to normal tissues. One such drug under trial is Bevacizumab. This is a recombinant antibody to VEGF. It has been found to improve survival in colorectal, lung, breast and renal cancers. It is incorporated as frontline adjuvant treatment with carboplatin and paclitaxel in the ongoing GOG 218 trial. One important problem with this drug is the incidence of bowel perforation especially in patients who have bowel involvement, prior radiation exposure or recent surgery. CA 125 monoclonal antibody is also being used alone and in combination with chemotherapeutic agents. Intraperitoneal immunotherapy with interferon for minimal residual disease has shown response rate similar to that of cytotoxic agents.

19.6 NON-EPITHELIAL OVARIAN TUMOR

Non-epithelial ovarian tumors include:

1. Germ cell tumors
2. Sex cord stromal tumors
3. Metastatic carcinomas
4. Sarcomas, lipoid cell tumors, etc.

19.6.1 Germ Cell Tumors

Germ cell tumors comprise 3-5% of ovarian malignancies. These tumors occur in children and adolescents. 67-87% of ovarian tumors in children and adolescents are germ cell tumors. They range from benign cystic teratoma to very aggressive embryonal carcinoma. Since they originate from primitive germ cells these tumors have the capacity for multipotent differentiation. Thus, any cell type may predominate in teratomas. The tumor with predominant thyroid tissue is called struma ovarii. As in epithelial ovarian tumor a comprehensive surgical staging is mandatory for germ cell tumor also. Since these tumors are typically seen in girls and young women, ovarian conservation is necessary.

Characteristic features of ovarian germ cell tumor

- Peak incidence in young women and adolescent girls
- Usually unilateral
- Usually detected in earlier stages
- Tumor markers are α fetoprotein, hCG and LDH
- Excellent chemosensitivity
- Highly curable by cytoreductive surgery followed by chemotherapy
- BEP is the preferred chemotherapeutic regime
- Within the same tumor there can be different malignant types or a mixture of benign and malignant types

Germ cell tumors bear certain characteristic features which are different from epithelial tumors. One particular feature is that there can be different malignant types in a single tumor or a mixture of benign and malignant tumors. Understanding this is important during histopathological examination since management depends upon the most malignant portion of the tumor. Presence of tumor markers like AFP and β-hCG are characteristic features of germ cell tumors. Before the advent of chemotherapeutic agents, surgical management carried very poor prognosis for the malignant tumors. With the introduction of chemotherapeutic agents especially cisplatin and carboplatin, germ cell tumors happen to carry very good prognosis. This has led to conservative surgery followed by chemotherapy, even in advanced stages.

19.6.2 Classification

WHO Histologic typing of ovarian germ cell tumors is provided in Table 19.6.

In a review of forty-one patients with malignant ovarian germ cell tumors twenty-three (56%) were dysgerminomas, eight (19.5%) mixed germ cell tumors, three (7.3%) yolk sac tumors, three (7.3%) immature teratomas, two (4.8%) squamous cell carcinoma arising from a mature teratoma, one (2.4%) was embryonal carcinoma and one choriocarcinoma.[20]

Tumor markers (Table 19.7).

Table 19.6: WHO histologic typing of ovarian germ cell tumors

Primitive germ cell tumor
- Dysgerminoma
- Yolk sac tumor
- Embryonal carcinoma
- Polyembryoma
- Non-gestational choriocarcinoma
- Mixed germ cell tumor

Biphasic/triphasic teratoma
- Immature teratoma
- Mature teratoma
  - Solid
  - Cystic
  - Dermoid cyst
  - Fetiform teratoma (homunculus)

Monodermal teratoma
- Thyroid tumor
  - Struma ovarii
  - Benign
  - Malignant
- Carcinoid
- Neuroectodermal carcinoma
- Melanocytic sarcoma
- Sebaceous tumor
- Pituitary type tumor
- Others

Adapted from Tavassoll FA, Devllee P, eds. World Health Organisation classification of tumors. Pathology and Genetics of Tumors of the Breast and Female Organs. Lyon: IARC Press, 2003

Table 19.7: Markers of germ cell tumor

EST	*AFP*
Dysgerminoma	LDH, AFP (if EST elements are present), β-hCG (if choriocarcinoma elements are present), PLAP
Embryonal carcinoma	AFP (if EST elements are present), β-hCG (if choriocarcinoma elements are present)
Immature teratoma	AFP (if EST elements are present)
Choriocarcinoma	hCG

The presence of tumor markers, AFP or β-hCG confirms germ cell tumors. AFP is the tumor marker for endodermal sinus tumor (EST). In pure dysgerminoma and embryonal carcinoma, β-hCG and AFP are negative. There can be a mixture of dysgerminoma and endodermal sinus tumor in which case AFP may be positive.

Placental alkaline phosphatase (PLAP) and Lactate dehydrogenase (LDH) will be positive in most patients with dysgerminoma. They can be used for monitoring, if they are initially positive. Both β-hCG and AFP can be positive in embryonal cell carcinoma. Choriocarcinoma (non-gestational) arising from extraembryonic cells secrete hCG. Immature teratoma, do not usually produce tumor markers. But if EST elements are present AFP will be positive.

19.6.3 Dysgerminoma

Dysgerminomas are the most common malignant germ cell tumors. They are usually seen in the 2nd-3rd decades of life. Most patients present with mass abdomen or pain abdomen. Even though fast growing, the disease usually presents in the early stage. It is bilateral in 10-15% of cases.

On gross examination, the tumor has a bosselated appearance and the cut surface is spongy and grayish-brown in color. Microscopically, the tumor is characterized by large round ovoid cells with abundant clear cytoplasm and large nuclei with prominent nucleoli (Fig. 19.5). There will be lymphocytic infiltration and presence of multinucleated giant cells. Extensive areas of necrosis are also seen mimicking tuberculosis.

Clinical examination reveals a large lobulated solid mass. Ultrasound appearance will be of a large echogenic multi-lobulated mass with prominent fibrovascular septa. Placental alkaline phosphatase (PLAP) and lactate dehydrogenase (LDH) will be positive in most of the patients. Rarely, β-hCG may be positive. AFP may be positive in the presence of associated endodermal sinus tumor elements which is rare. Dysgerminomas can occur in dysgenetic gonads; hence if pre-menarchal girls present with dysgerminoma, karyotyping is mandatory. If the karyotype shows Y chromosome, removal of the other gonad even if it is a streak is essential. Incidence

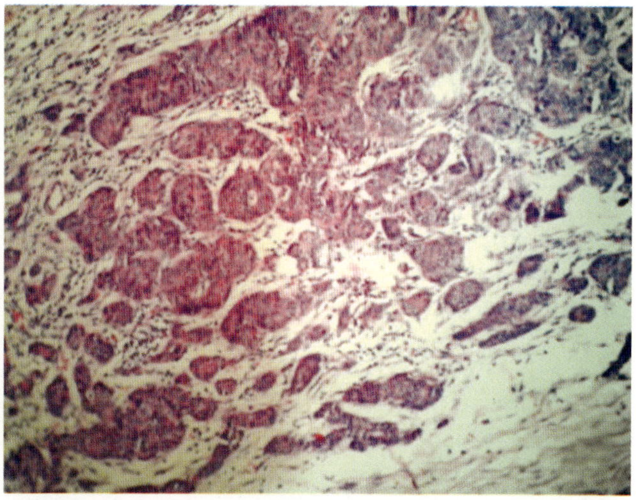

Fig. 19.5: Microscopic appearance of dysgerminoma. Note cells showing clear cytoplasm and fibrous septa rich in lymphocytes

of dysgerminoma is also high in women, who develop secondary amenorrhea, who are chromosomal mosaics carrying Y chromosome component. Hence, karyotyping is also indicated for those presenting with secondary amenorrhea and high gonadotropin levels to find out individuals with Y chromosome (usually mosaics).

Management (Fig. 19.7)

Since this tumor occurs in the 2nd and 3rd decades, fertility sparing surgery is most often necessary. Laparotomy and comprehensive surgical staging should be done as in epithelial ovarian tumor. Staging procedure is same as in epithelial tumors. In the presence of a unilateral tumor, every effort should be made to exclude extraovarian disease. Transperitoneal spread can also occur. The common mode of spread is through lymphatics. Since lymphatic spread is more common than in epithelial tumors, lymphadenectomy which might influence adjuvant therapy should be part of staging. For those patients whose tumor is confined to the ovary (Stage IA), unilateral ovariotomy (Fig. 19.6) and ipsilateral pelvic and para-aortic lymphadenectomy will suffice as treatment. If there is no evidence of extraovarian disease (Stage IA, lymph nodes are also negative) the patient can be observed without adjuvant chemotherapy. Chemotherapy, which has side effects as well as complications, can thus be avoided in patients who do not require it. For all other stages, postoperative chemotherapy with bleomycin, etoposide and cisplatin/carboplatin (BEP) is advised (Table 19.8). Even though these tumors are radiosensitive, radiation is not advised in view of the possible damage to the retained ovary. Combination chemotherapy has long-term side effects like development of second malignancies and premature menopause. The incidence of development of leukemia is reported as 4.7% in one follow-up study.[21]

Table 19.8: Combination chemotherapy for ovarian germ cell tumors

BEP regimen
Bleomycin: 15 units/m^2/week IV × 3 weeks
Etoposide: 100 mg/m^2/day IV × 5 days every 3 weeks
Cisplatin: 20 mg/m^2/day IV × 5 days or 100 mg/m^2/day × 1 day every 3 weeks
VBP regimen
Vinblastine: 0.15 mg/kg IV, days 1 and 2 every 3 weeks
Bleomycin: 15 units/m^2/week IV × 5; then on day 1 of course 4
Cisplatin: 100 mg/m^2 IV on day 1 every 3 weeks
VAC regimen
Vincristine: 1-1.5 mg/m^2 IV on day 1 every 4 weeks
Actinomycin D: 0.5 mg/day IV × 5 days every 4 weeks
Cyclophosphamide: 150 mg/m^2/day IV × 5 days every 4 weeks
POMB-ACE regimen
Cisplatin, Vincristine, Methotrexate, Bleomycin, Actinomycin D, Cyclophosphamide, Etoposide

Side effects of chemotherapy

- Gastrointestinal symptoms
- Bone marrow suppression
- Premature menopause
- Secondary malignancy

Since these tumors do not have consistent and reliable tumor markers, follow-up is by clinical examination supplemented by imaging using CT/MRI. The patients are to be followed every 1-2 months in the first year, every 2 months in the second year, every 3 months in the third year,

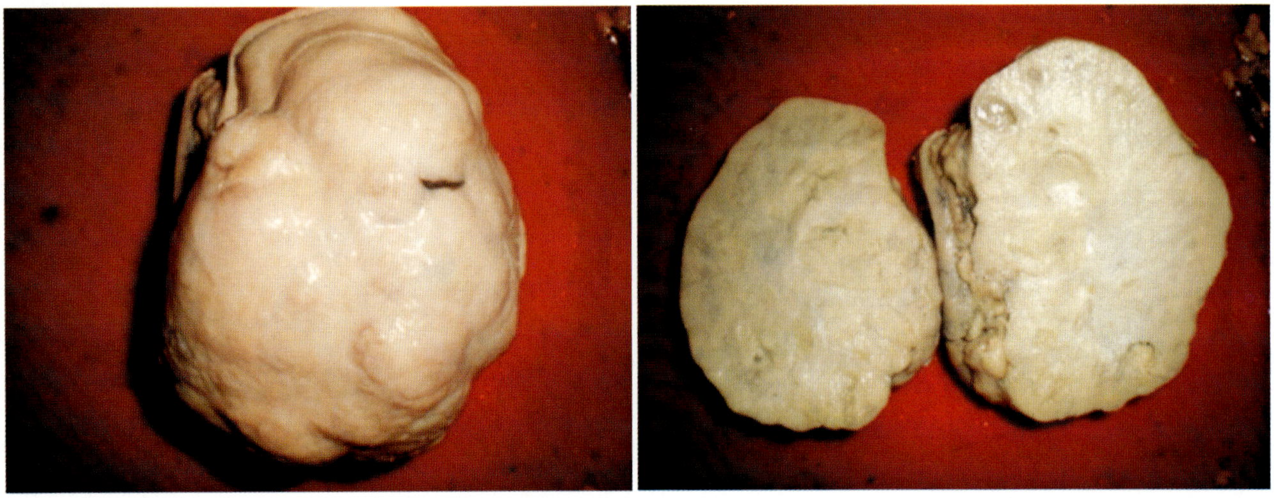

Fig. 19.6: Ovariotomy specimen (gross and cut-section) showing solid ovarian tumor measuring 20 cm of a 23-year-old unmarried lady. Note the bosselated appearance typical of dysgerminoma. Her LDH level was 3829 IU/L and β-hCG 293 IU/L. She was administered chemotherapy (BEP) as peritoneal washings were positive for malignant cells even though para-aortic nodes were negative

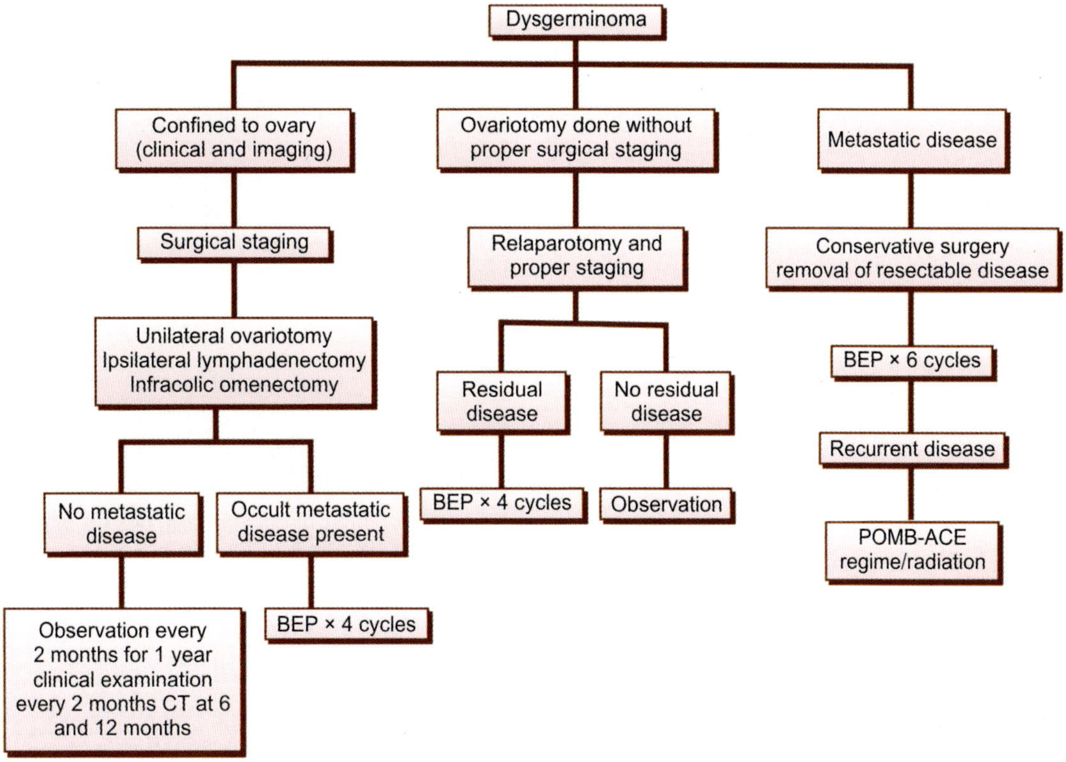

Fig. 19.7: Management algorithm for dysgerminoma

every 4 months in the fourth year, twice annually in the fifth year and once a year subsequently.

The cure rate for Stage IA tumors is as high as 95%. Even for advanced disease, cure rate as high as 85-90% can be expected with the advent of modern chemotherapeutic agents.[22]

19.6.4 Immature Teratoma

Immature teratoma is the second most common malignant germ cell tumor which also usually occurs in children and young adults. Occasionally it occurs in combination with other germ cell tumors. Rarely, postmenopausal women are affected. The tumor has a predominantly solid appearance except when it occurs in a cystic teratoma in which case the solid part can be identified in the cystic teratoma (Fig. 19.8). The presence of immature elements determines the aggressiveness of the tumor. Hence, based on the proportion of immature elements, three grades are recognized (I, II and III). In grade I, <1 low power field contains immature neural elements. In grade II, 1-3 low power fields contain immature elements and in grade III, >3 low power fields contain these elements. Prognosis is poor in the presence of higher grade lesions. Malignant change, very rarely (0.5%), occurs in cystic teratoma which is usually squamous cell carcinoma but rarely sarcoma. In very few cases, the immature teratomas elaborate steroid hormones in which case the patient can present with precocious puberty. Production of corticosteroids can cause osteoporosis and bone fracture.

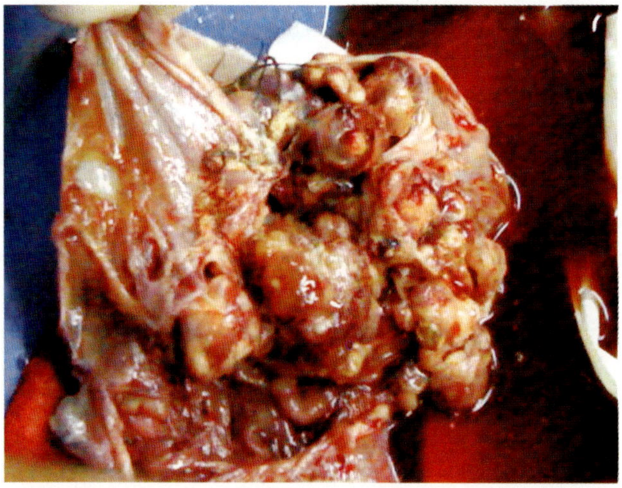

Fig. 19.8: Cut-open specimen of immature teratoma of a 30-year-old lady who presented with mass abdomen. She had a large mass measuring 30 cm arising from right ovary. Ultrasound features were suggestive of malignancy with tumor markers negative. Since she had completed family, total hysterectomy with BSO was done. Postoperatively chemotherapy was administered since the tumor was grade III

Tumor markers are usually negative. However, in mixed tumors, depending upon the other germ cell element present, AFP or β-hCG may be positive.

Management in young women and children involve proper surgical staging and unilateral oophorectomy. For older women, total hysterectomy with bilateral salpingo-oophorectomy should be preferred. Since these tumors respond to chemotherapy better than epithelial tumors, multiple peritoneal secondaries need not be resected. Stage IA grade I tumor does not need adjuvant chemotherapy, but stage IA grade II-III should be given adjuvant chemotherapy for which BEP regime is preferred. Patients with malignant squamous elements have poor prognosis.

Survival of Stage I, grade I patients is 100%, but for stage III it is only 50%.

19.6.5 Endodermal Sinus Tumor (EST)

Endodermal sinus tumor is the most malignant ovarian germ cell tumor, usually seen in children and adolescents as other germ cell tumors. Since the tumor originates from yolk sac, it is otherwise called yolk sac tumor. EST can occur in association with other types of germ cell tumors. In a retrospective analysis of 47 patients with yolk sac tumors, 22 were pure EST and 25 EST with components of other malignant ovarian germ cell tumors (9 EST with mature teratoma, 5 EST with immature teratoma, 7 EST with dysgerminoma, 2 EST with immature teratoma and embryonal cell carcinoma, 1 embryonal carcinoma with EST component and 1 polyembryoma with EST component).[23]

The usual presentation is with mass abdomen, but can also present as acute abdomen due to rupture, hemorrhage or necrosis and rarely as fever. The tumor grossly appears as a solid friable mass with areas of hemorrhage and necrosis. They are usually unilateral, but rarely bilateral (5%). Consistency varies from soft to firm. Cut surface is reddish in color. Cystic areas can be seen if there is degeneration. Microscopic appearance is characterized by the presence of Schiller Duval bodies (Fig. 19.9). These are cystic spaces lined by flattened endothelium in the center of which glomerulus like vascular core is present.

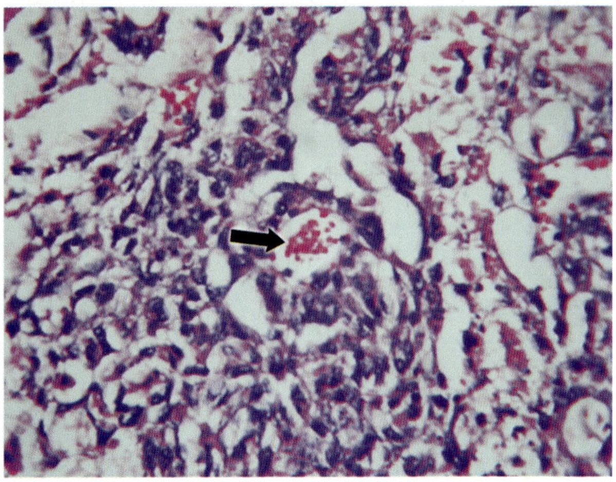

Fig. 19.9: Microscopic picture of endodermal sinus tumor showing Schiller Duval body—central vessel and surrounding endoderm (arrow)

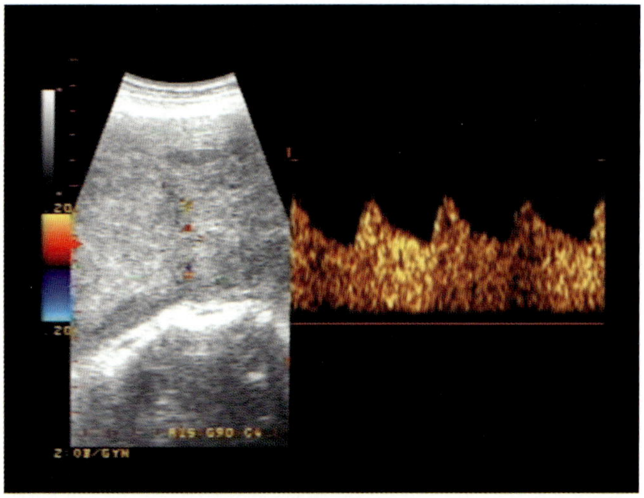

Fig. 19.10: Triplex ultrasound scan picture of endodermal sinus tumor. Note the low resistance flow characteristic of malignancy. The patient was an adolescent girl who presented with pain abdomen and fever

The usual association is with dysgerminoma. AFP is the tumor marker which will be elevated in serum and there is good correlation between the serum level and extent of disease. Hence, it is a useful marker for monitoring response to treatment. AFP can be demonstrated in the tumor by immunohistochemistry. On performing tumor marker estimation for pre-menarchal girls and young adults with clinically suspected malignant ovarian tumor, presence of AFP strongly suggests endodermal sinus tumor. On immunohistochemistry PAS will be positive. On imaging, the tumor appears as a predominantly echogenic mass with/without cystic spaces (Fig. 19.10). There will not be fibrous septa as in dysgerminoma.

Management is exploratory laparotomy, surgical staging and unilateral ovariotomy as the tumor is almost always unilateral. Hysterectomy and contralateral oophorectomy need not be done as it does not alter outcome, even if the patient does not want to conserve the childbearing function. If the tumor appears obviously confined to the ovary, thorough surgical staging by peritoneal biopsy need not be done when EST is confirmed at laparotomy, as all patients need postoperative chemotherapy unlike dysgerminoma. The preferred chemotherapy is the BEP regime. GOG protocol has used 3-4 treatment cycles every 4 weeks. It is preferable that the patient gets two more courses of chemotherapy after AFP becomes negative. Those who do not respond to treatment as documented by persistently high AFP levels can be given POMB-ACE regime.

Survival for stage I and II EST is reported to be 60-100%, but for those with stage III and IV it is less favorable at 50-75%.

19.6.6 Embryonal Carcinoma

Embryonal carcinoma is a highly malignant germ cell tumor. It usually occurs in children and young adults, the median age being 14 years. It usually occurs in combination with yolk sac tumor. They may elaborate estrogens and hence the patients can present with precocious puberty. Primary lesions are large, usually unilateral but may be rarely bilateral. On gross examination, it appears as a solid, necrotic, hemorrhagic lesion. AFP and hCG may be positive. Management is similar to endodermal sinus tumor. Survival for embryonal carcinoma is slightly more than EST.

19.6.7 Choriocarcinoma

Primary choriocarcinoma of the ovary is an extremely rare tumor. Histologically, it is same as gestational choriocarcinoma. hCG is the tumor marker and is useful in diagnosis and follow-up. Due to the high hCG, precocious puberty can occur. MAC (Methotrexate, Actinomycin, Cisplatin) regime is preferred over BEP.

19.6.8 Polyembryoma

Polyembryoma is formed of all three embryonal components. They are usually seen in pre-menarchal girls and usually presents as precocious puberty. AFP and hCG may be elevated.

19.6.9 Ovarian Lymphoma

Primary lymphoma of the ovary is rare, but usually ovarian lymphomas are a part of systemic disease. Hence if ovarian lymphoma is encountered, systemic disease should be searched for. Diagnosis is made by fine-needle biopsy. Ovarian lymphoma can occur as a part of Burkitts' lymphoma. Management is chemotherapy depending upon the histologic subtypes.

19.6.10 Sex-cord Stromal Tumors

These tumors develop from the gonadal stroma and accounts for 5-10% of all gonadal neoplasms. Classification of sex cord tumors is provided in Table 19.9.

Table 19.9: Classification of sex-cord tumors

1. Granulosa cell tumor
2. Theca cell tumor
3. Thecoma
4. Fibroma
5. Sertoli-Leydig cell tumor
6. Sex-cord tumors with annular tubules
7. Lipoid cell tumor
8. Gynandroblastoma

Etiology

About 30% of patients with sex-cord stromal tumors have associated Peutz-Jeghers' syndrome; an autosomal dominant disorder characterized by multiple hamartomatous gastrointestinal polyps and an increased risk of various neoplasms and pigmented macules over the lips and buccal mucosa. Fibromas are associated with Meigs' syndrome. They are thought to develop from mesenchyme of the genital ridge.

Granulosa Cell Tumor

Granulosa cell tumors account for 3-5% of all ovarian neoplasms and 70% of sex cord stromal tumors. The adult type occurs in postmenopausal women (Figs 19.11A and B) and the juvenile type occurs in children and young adults. They are benign or less aggressive malignant lesions. Due to the estrogen produced by the stromal tumors, premenarchal girls may present with iso-sexual precocious puberty. When it occurs in postmenopausal women, the symptom can be irregular bleeding due to endometrial hyperplasia. Rarely, coexisting endometrial carcinoma may also occur. Testosterone is also rarely elaborated by these tumors in which case the patient may present with virilization (Figs 19.12A to C). Serum inhibin is a useful marker of the tumor. Intra-abdominal bleeding due to rupture of tumor can also be a presenting symptom.

Grossly, the tumor appears to be a mixture of solid and cystic components with areas of hemorrhage. The histology can vary between microfollicular, macrofollicular, trabecular and insular. The microfollicular pattern is characterized by Call-exner bodies (Fig. 19.13) which are the most common histologic subtype. Call-exner bodies are formed by rings of granulosa cells surrounding eosinophilic body.

Management depends upon the age of the patient and the stage of the disease. When child bearing is desired, unilateral salpingo-oophorectomy is the preferred treatment after proper staging laparotomy. In peri-menopausal and postmenopausal women, total hysterectomy and bilateral salpingo-oophorectomy is preferred.

The tumor has a tendency for late relapse, but there is no role for adjuvant chemotherapy after surgery for preventing this relapse. But residual disease following surgery and late recurrence can be managed by chemotherapy.

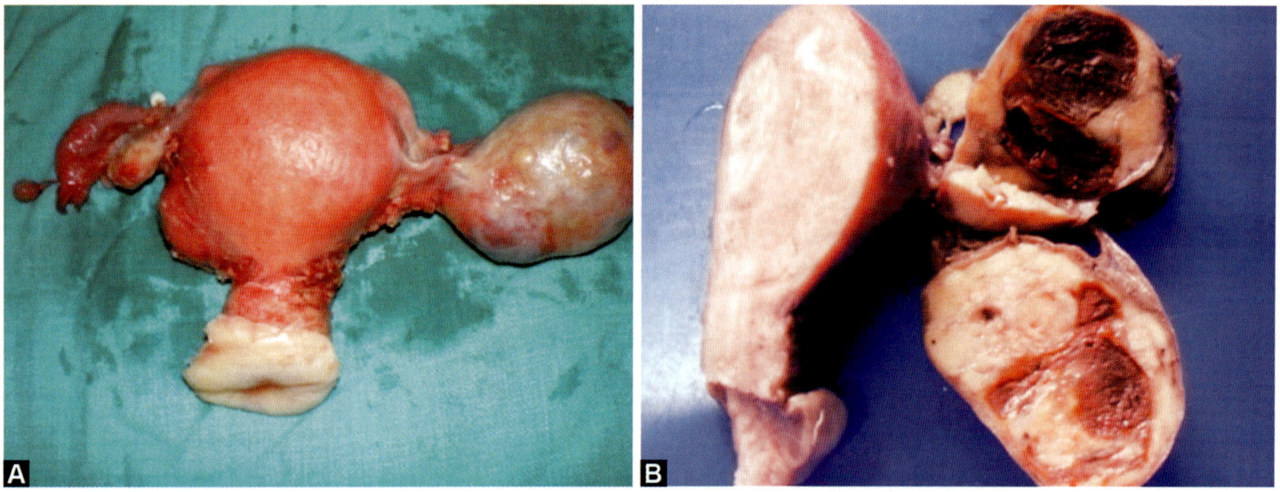

Figs 19.11A and B: Total hysterectomy with BSO specimen (A) showing unilateral solid ovarian tumor. The patient was a postmenopausal lady who presented with vaginal bleeding. Pathological examination revealed granulosa cell tumor. Cut section (B) shows areas of hemorrhage and necrosis

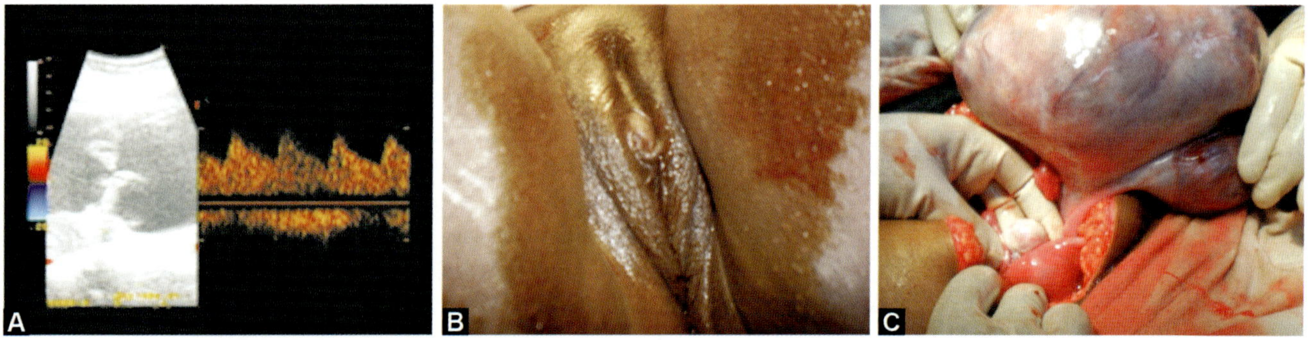

Figs 19.12A to C: TAS showing solid and cystic mass with increased diastolic flow in Doppler (A) in a 23-year-old nulliparous lady who presented with history of irregular vaginal bleeding, hirsutism and voice change. Clinical examination revealed clitoromegaly (B). Laparotomy picture (C) of the same lady showing large unilateral well encapsulated mass. Pathological examination revealed granulosa cell tumor. Rarely granulosa cell tumor elaborates androgen

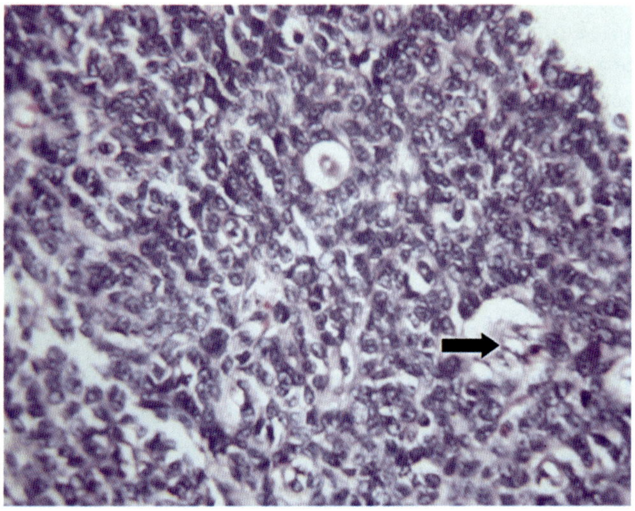

Fig. 19.13: Microscopic picture of granulosa cell tumor showing Call-Exner body (arrow)

Sertoli-Leydig Cell Tumor

These tumors are usually seen in the second and third decades of life. Usually, they are of low grade malignant potential, but rarely aggressive tumors may be encountered. The malignant potential depends upon nuclear atypia and the number of mitotic figures. Since these tumors typically produce androgen, testosterone is a marker. Hence defeminization followed by virilization is the usual presentation. Rarely, they may elaborate estrogen. These tumors are usually unilateral, but may be very rarely bilateral (<1%). The microscopic picture is similar to the histology of testis in well-differentiated tumors—tubules composed of Sertoli cells surrounded by stroma filled with Leydig cells. One characteristic feature is the presence of Reinke's crystals which are eosinophilic rod shaped structures seen inside Leydig cells.

Management is unilateral salpingo-oophorectomy in younger patients and hysterectomy with bilateral salpingo-oophorectomy in older women. Prognosis is good and recurrences are very rare with 5-year survival rate of 70-90%.

Thecoma

Thecomas are formed exclusively of theca cells. Grossly, they are solid tumors and the cut section is yellow-orange in color. It can vary in size from small tumors which may escape clinical examination to large ones measuring 5-10 cm. They are similar to fibromas, but secrete estrogen. Thecomas are usually benign or have low grade malignant potential.

Management is surgical and 5-year survival is nearly 100%.

Fibroma

Fibromas are benign tumors composed of fibrous connective tissue. Presence of ascites and pleural effusion associated with fibroma is Meigs' syndrome. Its malignant counterpart is fibrosarcoma. In the presence of associated thecomatous areas, the tumor is called fibrothecoma.

Sarcoma

Sarcoma of the ovary is a very rare tumor occurring in post menopausal women. There are different subtypes of sarcoma. Management is optimal cytoreduction followed by platinum based chemotherapy.

19.7 BORDERLINE TUMORS OF THE OVARY

19.7.1 Definition

Epithelial cancers of low malignant potential are called borderline tumors. According to WHO, borderline ovarian tumors are characterized by lack of stromal invasion, budding multilayered epithelium, mitotic activity and nuclear atypia.

19.7.2 Incidence

The incidence reported is 2.5/1 lakh woman years. Ovarian tumors exhibiting 2 or more of the above features involving 10% or more of the tumor may be classified as borderline. They are usually seen in younger patients, about 10 years younger than women with frank malignancy and constitute nearly 15% of all epithelial ovarian cancers. Because of their indolent nature, they are usually diagnosed in stage I (75%).

19.7.3 Risk Factors

The risk factors are not clearly known. Multiparity and lactation are reported to reduce the incidence. Association with any genetic factors has not been established.

19.7.4 Pathology

They show intracystic and exophytic papillary growth pattern. Since they are epithelial tumors, the histological types are serous, mucinous, clear cell, endometroid and Brenner types. The most commonly encountered histological type is the serous, followed by mucinous. The mucinous types can be either intestinal type or the endocervical type; the intestinal type being more common. The recurrence rate is less for mucinous tumors. Advanced tumors are associated with pseudomyxoma peritonei.

Histologically, they are characterized by epithelial multilayering with not more than 4 mitosis/10 HPF. The cells show mild nuclear atypia and increased nucleo-cytoplasmic ratio but without destructive stromal invasion.

19.7.5 Clinical Features

Clinical features are same as epithelial ovarian cancers except for the gradual growth. Abdominal discomfort, pain, distension and mass abdomen may be complained of. It is difficult to diagnose as it remains asymptomatic.

19.7.6 Diagnosis

Tumor markers may be elevated but cannot be used to differentiate between borderline tumors and frankly malignant tumors. CA-125 may be elevated in serous types and CA19-9 may be elevated in mucinous types. Ultrasound appearance of mural nodules is characteristic of these types of tumors. But Doppler studies alone cannot differentiate malignant tumors from borderline tumors as RI and PI are decreased even in borderline tumors. MRI and CT can be used to delineate the extent of the disease before surgery. The diagnosis can be confirmed only by histopathology.

19.7.7 Treatment

At laparotomy, FIGO staging is used for these tumors also. Extensive peritoneal deposits may be encountered. These peritoneal implants can be of invasive or noninvasive type. Invasive implants invade the underlying peritoneum and will show mild to moderate cytological atypia. Noninvasive implants lack invasion and will show only minimal or mild cytological atypia and lack mitosis. Noninvasive implants occur more commonly and are associated with better overall survival (95.3% vs 22%). Since these tumors occur in younger patients, ovarian conservation is a dilemma. Unless extensive sections are studied, frank invasion cannot be ruled out. Hence, total hysterectomy and bilateral salpingo-oophorectomy should be recommended for women who have completed their family. For those who have not completed their family, conservative surgery can be resorted to. Since women undergoing cystectomy are more likely to have recurrence compared to those undergoing oophorectomy (75% vs 24%), oophorectomy should be preferred when conservative surgery is needed. It is ideal to do the definitive surgery after completing family.

19.7.8 Prognosis

Prognosis depends on
- Age at diagnosis
- DNA ploidy
- Presence of invasive implants
- Stage of the disease
- Histological type

10-year survival after optimal cytoreduction is excellent (95%). If cytoreduction is optimal, i.e. without any macroscopic residual disease and the implants do not show invasion, adjuvant chemotherapy is not needed. However, the patient should be observed periodically. If residual invasive disease is present, chemotherapy is indicated. Those who had unilateral ovariotomy should have periodic transvaginal ultrasonogram at least once a year. Women who are young at diagnosis and with serous histology carry a more favorable prognosis. Those who develop recurrence can be managed by repeat surgery and chemotherapy.

Recurrences usually occur within 6 years of initial surgery. Very late recurrences have also been reported. Whether this represents recurrence or another primary is disputable. Since late recurrence is common, patients should be followed up albeit at less frequent intervals.

19.8 METASTATIC TUMORS OF THE OVARY (FIGS 19.14A TO C)

About 5% of the ovarian tumors are metastatic from other organs. The frequent sites are uterus, fallopian tube, breast and the gastrointestinal tract. The mode of spread is hematogenous, lymphatic, transcoelomic or by surface implantation.

Krukenberg tumors of the ovary are metastatic tumors from stomach, colon, breast or biliary tract. They are typically bilateral solid tumors which preserve the shape of the ovary. In most of the situations, the patient presents with ascites and ovarian masses and the primary tumor will be insignificant. Hence, it is important to take a proper history when bilateral solid ovarian tumors are encountered. Primary in the stomach may be undetectable on clinical examination but could be diagnosed by endoscopy.

Melanoma, carcinoid tumor, lymphoma and leukemia can all metastasize to the ovary.

19.9 CONCLUSION

Even though ovarian cancer ranks as the 4th common genital tract malignancy, it is a leading cause of death due to malignancy among women. The reason is absence of a premalignant stage or effective screening strategy as well as failure to diagnose early stage disease. As of now there is no effective population screening strategy for ovarian cancer detection unlike cervical cancer. Ultrasound has come up as an effective tool for the diagnosis of ovarian malignancy. Those who are at high risk for ovarian cancer (BRCA and HNPCC mutation carriers) should be advised screening with TVS and CA 125 level. Most of the women affected belong to the 6th-8th decade of life. However, rarely young women are affected. About 90% of ovarian malignancies are epithelial in origin. When the ovary is involved with malignancy, the entire peritoneal viscera are at the risk of tumor spread and the disease is usually

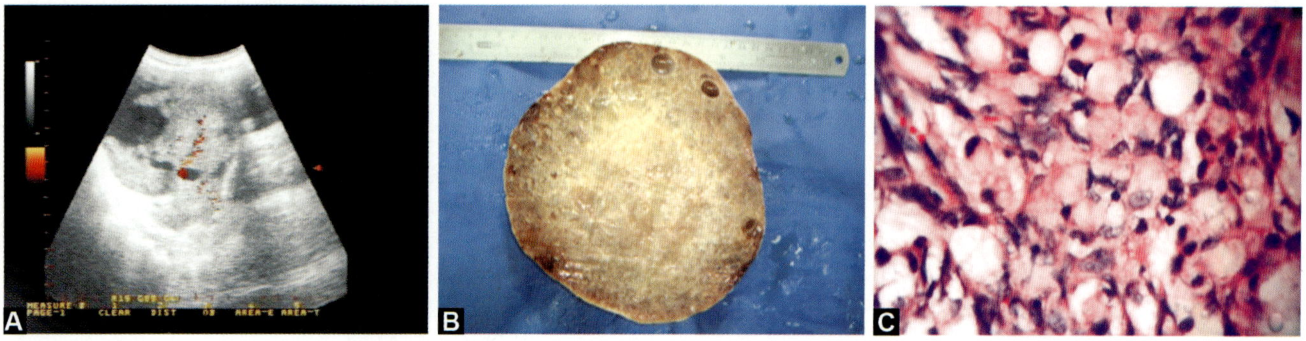

Figs 19.14A to C: Ultrasound picture, section and microscopy of Krukenberg's tumor of the ovary in a 39-year-old lady. The primary was in the stomach. Note the predominantly solid appearance and the cystic spaces seen in the ultrasound picture and the cut section of the tumor. This appearance is typical of Krukenberg's tumor

diagnosed in stage III. With the discovery of platinum based chemotherapeutic agents and taxanes, the 5-year cure rate of ovarian malignancy has improved significantly. As the survival depends upon the volume of residual disease, systematic exploratory laparotomy, delineation of extent of disease and optimal cytoreduction should be given prime importance. Surgery of advanced disease should be undertaken by experienced team in dedicated centers. Residual disease should not be missed and even for microscopic residual disease adjuvant chemotherapy with Cisplatin-Taxol combination should be employed. Borderline ovarian malignancies have been understood as a separate entity occurring in younger women with better survival after conservative surgery and delayed recurrence. When adolescents and young adults present with ovarian tumor, possibility of a germ cell tumor should be kept in mind. Even for stage III GCTs conservative surgery followed by chemotherapy with BEP regime should be the choice for those who have not completed childbearing. GCTs are usually unilateral but can rarely be bilateral. Even if bilateral, if normal ovarian tissue can be identified, resection of the tumor leaving normal ovarian tissue followed by chemotherapy can be advised. If GCTs occur in girls who have not attained menarche, karyotyping should be done to look for Y chromosome or segments, as they may be XY females or mosaics, who need gonadectomy. In future with the evolution of more sensitive and specific tumor markers which can be employed in the screening of the general population like proteomics and with the development of immunotherapeutic agents targeted specifically to the tumor tissue, early detection as well as cure rates of ovarian cancer would definitely be better.

19.10 CASE SCENARIOS

Case Scenario 1 (Fig. 19.15A to D)

M/s M, a 45-year-old lady presented with complaints of watery discharge per vaginum of 6 months duration. She

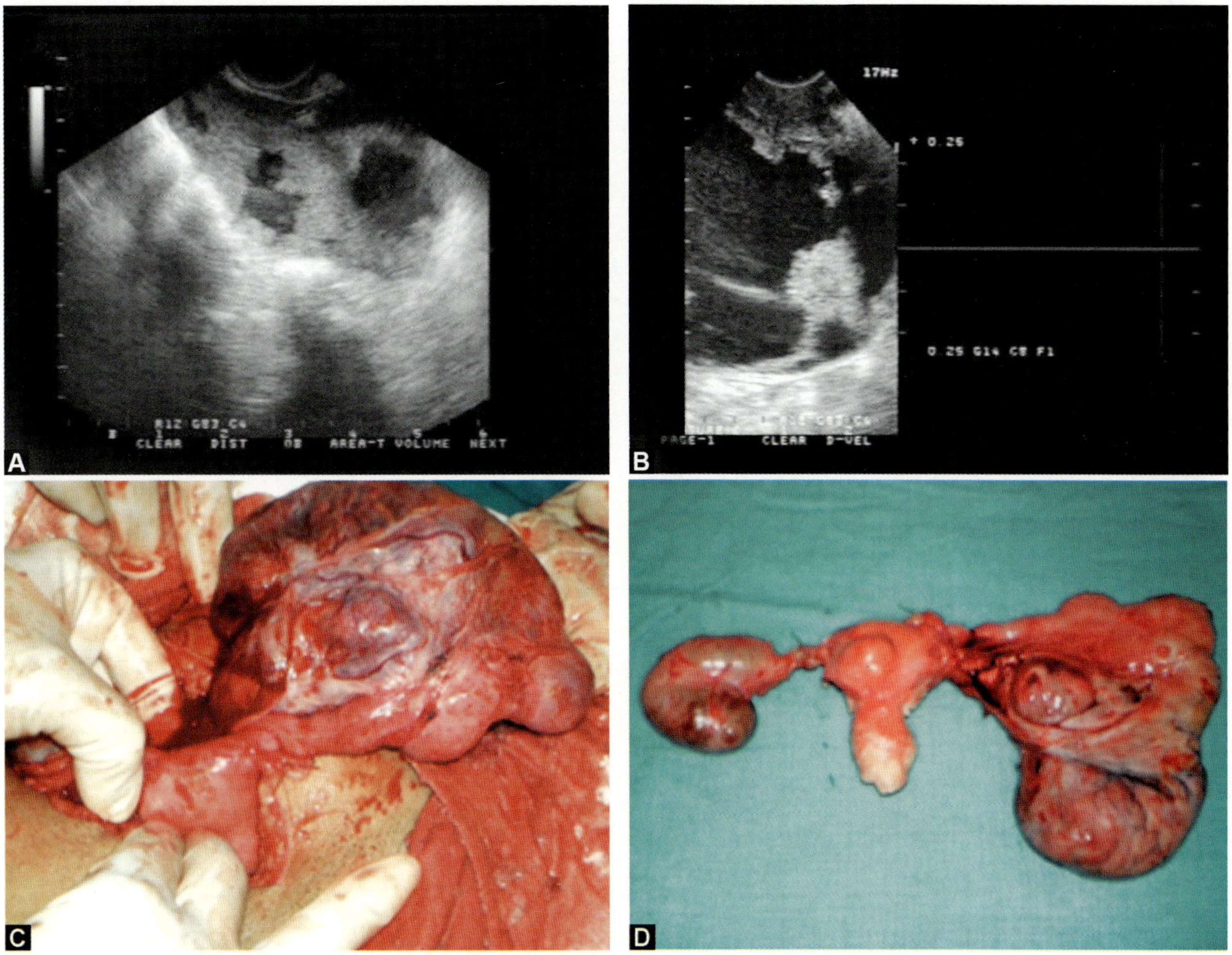

Figs 19.15A to D: TVS showing the whole of the adnexal mass (A), TVS of the distended part of the mass (B), Laparotomy picture showing the uterus, and the enlarged fallopian tube (C), and the operated specimen showing uterus, fallopian tube with the growth (D)

attained menopause 1 year back. She is a para 1 who had normal vaginal delivery 13 years back. No history of bleeding per vaginum. No history of loss of weight or loss of appetite.

On examination, her general condition was satisfactory. Nothing abnormal was seen on general examination. There was no mass palpable in the abdomen and no free fluid was elicited. On speculum examination, cervix and vagina appeared normal. Bimanual examination revealed atrophic uterus and a cystic mass about the size of a lemon was felt through the right fornix.

TVS- uterus was normal in size. The endometrium measured 4 mm. Right adnexal mass of 6 cm × 5 cm with cystic and solid elements was seen. Doppler showed low resistance flow with RI 0.41 and PI 0.94. Right ovary could not be separately made out.

What could be the most probable diagnosis? What are the other diagnostic probabilities?

Considering the history of watery vaginal discharge and adnexal mass with solid areas showing increased vascularity and low resistance flow, the possibilities are:

1. Fallopian tube malignancy
2. Ovarian malignancy
3. Degenerated subserous pedunculated fibroid
4. Malignant growth from bowel.

Considering the symptom of watery vaginal discharge and the presence of a complex adnexal mass on TVS, a provisional diagnosis of fallopian tube malignancy was made. CA 125 estimation was done, which was reported as 106 IU/ml Exploratory laparotomy was done. Laparotomy findings were as follows:

There was no ascites. Uterus was normal in size. Both ovaries were normal. Left fallopian tube was found to be distended with blood. No tumor was palpable in the left tube. The right tube was found to be enlarged to form a cystic tumor of about 6 cm in size. Peritoneal washing was done with about 200 ml saline and was collected for cytology. The entire peritoneal surface was palpated for secondary deposits. There was no evidence of secondaries macroscopically. Total hysterectomy bilateral salpingo-oophorectomy and Infracolic omentectomy was done. The specimen was sent for pathology. The pathology report was adenocarcinoma fallopian tube Grade III, involving the distal half, with infiltration to the muscular layer. The omentum and peritoneal washing were negative for malignancy. The patient was treated with adjuvant chemotherapy as the tumor was of Grade III.

Fallopian tube carcinoma usually occurs in the fifth and sixth decade of life. BRCAI and BRCA2 mutation carriers are at increased risk for fallopian tube malignancies also. Hence prophylactic ovariotomy in BRCA gene mutation carriers should include removal of both fallopian tubes also. The usual symptom is watery vaginal discharge. Bleeding per vaginum can also be complained of. A pelvic mass may be present. Patients with advanced disease will present with ascites. Staging and management are the same as epithelial ovarian carcinoma. The disease is usually diagnosed at an earlier stage than epithelial ovarian carcinoma due to the symptoms of vaginal discharge or bleeding.

Case Scenario 2

Thirty-one year old M/s N presented with abdominal pain, vomiting, loss of weight and loss of appetite of 3 months duration. She was married for 10 years and has one 4-year-old child. Her periods were regular. She had no bowel or bladder symptoms. On examination her general condition was good. She had a cystic mass about 10 × 15 cm in size occupying the hypogastrium. There was no free fluid on clinical examination. No other mass was palpable. Local examination revealed normal cervix and vagina. Bimanual examination showed a cystic mass filling the pouch of Douglas. Uterus could be made out separately. There was no nodularity in the pouch of Douglas. Ultrasound examination showed large multiloculated cystic mass in the pelvis with thick septations, possibly arising from the left ovary. Doppler showed increased vascularity with low resistance flow. Another mass of 8 cm size which was predominantly solid was noted in the right fornix. There was no ascites.

What is the most probable diagnosis?

The most probable diagnosis is malignant ovarian tumor because of the history of short duration, ultrasound showing bilateral tumors, thick septations and increased vascularity.

What is the role of tumor markers in this clinical situation?

Tumor markers for epithelial as well as germ cell tumors should be done. If markers for GCTs are positive conservative surgery should be planned as the patient is young and has not completed family. Since the tumor is multiloculated and bilateral, epithelial ovarian tumor is the most probable diagnosis. If any marker of epithelial ovarian tumor is positive, it can be made use of in the follow-up of the patient after surgery.

Her tumor markers were as follows:

- CA 125-387.4 IU/ml
- CEA-1.4 ng/ml
- aFetoprotein and β-hCG were normal.

How should the results be interpreted? How should the patient be counseled?

Epithelial ovarian tumor is likely.

She should be counseled that she might need total hysterectomy and bilateral salpingo-oophorectomy, even though she is young and has only one child. Even if the uterus looks normal might contain involved lymphatics.

Exploratory laparotomy was done through a midline vertical incision. Peritoneal cavity contained about 150 ml of straw colored ascitic fluid. Peritoneal washing was taken for cytological examination. The uterus was normal in size. The left ovary was replaced by a large multiloculated cystic tumor with solid elements. Right ovary showed another tumor which was predominantly solid with cystic areas. The entire peritoneal cavity and viscera were inspected systematically and palpated for evidence of secondaries. There were no macroscopic secondary deposits. Peritoneal biopsies were taken from the paracolic gutter, uterovesical fold of peritoneum and the under surface of the diaphragm. TAH with BSO and infracolic omentectomy was done.

The postoperative period was uneventful.

The pathology report was papillary serous cystadenocarcinoma Grade I with intact capsule and omentum, peritoneal biopsy and washings were negative for malignancy.

What postoperative treatment should be advised?

Since a proper staging laparotomy was done and since there is no residual disease (stage I b) she needs only follow-up. CA 125 level should be done at each visit since it was previously found to be elevated.

If the level has become 20 IU/ml at 4 months post surgery and after 1 year it shows mild elevation to 37 IU/ml, what should be done?

Even though the level is in the upper limit of normal, since there is a rise in titer, recurrence should be suspected. If clinical examination is negative CT/MRI should be done to find out recurrent disease. Even if CT/MRI is negative, PET scan should be done if available to detect the recurrence early.

Case Scenario 3

Sixty-two year old M/s K presented with loss of weight and loss of appetite of 3 months duration. She was a multiparous lady who attained menopause 18 years back. She did not give history suggestive of any gastrointestinal or urinary problem. On examination she was emaciated. She had enlarged left supraclavicular lymph nodes. Her abdomen was distended. Ascites was present. Multiple masses were palpated all over the abdomen. Local examination of vulva was unremarkable. Cervix and vagina looked normal. Bimanual examination revealed multiple nodules in the pouch of Douglas. Uterus exact size could not be made out and there was no definite adnexal mass.

What are the diagnostic probabilities?

She may be having malignancy with multiple secondary deposits. The primary is difficult to spot out, as symptoms as well as signs are not giving a clue about the site.

Tuberculosis of the abdomen is another possibility.

How to proceed?

Ultrasound of the abdomen is the primary imaging modality. Ultrasound revealed mild ascites and multiple mixed echogenic masses in the abdomen. Multiple masses were also seen in the pelvis. Uterus was atrophic and appeared normal. The ovaries could not be made out.

Could she be having malignant ovarian tumor?

Malignant ovarian tumor is a possibility, as it is common and she has no symptoms suggesting malignancy of other systems.

How to arrive at a diagnosis of malignancy before doing laparotomy?

Aspiration of peritoneal fluid and cytological examination.

What about tumor markers?

Tumor markers like CA 125 and CEA can be elevated in non-mucinous or mucinous tumors of the ovary. However, it can be elevated not only in ovarian tumors but in other tumors also.

Her cytology showed adenocarcinoma cells. Tumor markers, CA125: 160IU/ml; CEA: 1885 ng/ml. How will you manage the case?

Since operability is doubtful as she is clinically suspected to have upper abdominal masses, she needs CT imaging to exclude deposits in the lesser sac and porta hepatis, the presence of which is a contraindication for primary surgery.

CT was taken (Fig 19.16) which showed enlarged para-aortic nodes and deposits in the lesser sac.

As a part of metastatic work-up lung CT was taken which showed multiple parenchymatous deposits (Fig 19.17).

Since this lady had stage IV disease, she should be considered inoperable and can be given only palliative chemotherapy. Hence, she was started on chemotherapy with Cisplatin and Paclitaxel. She should be evaluated after 6 courses of chemotherapy.

After 3 courses of chemotherapy, the mass was found to be progressing. What is the next step in management?

The tumor is platinum refractory. She should be started on second line chemotherapy. She was given Gemcitabin. The

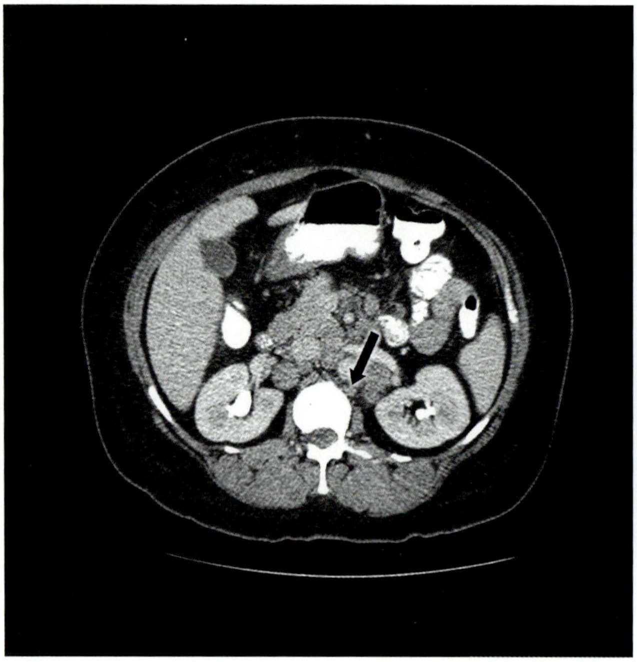

Fig. 19.16: CT picture showing malignant deposits in the lesser sac (arrow)

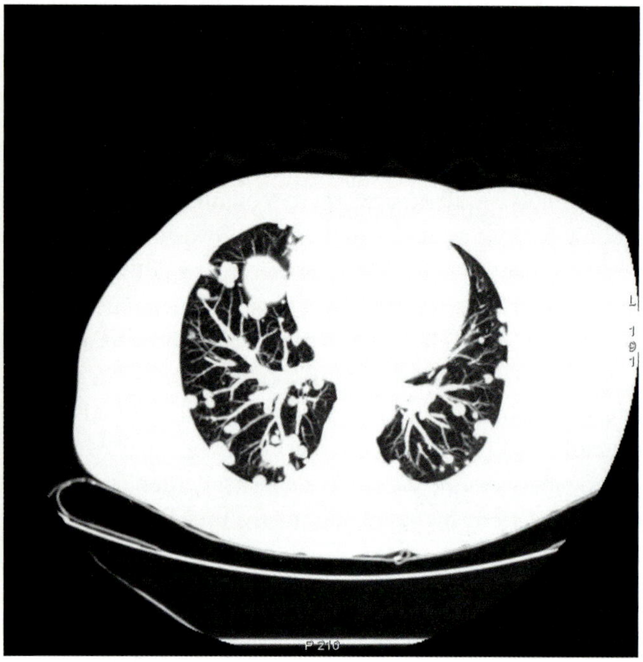

Fig. 19.17: CT lung showing multiple deposits

patient became symptomatically better after administration of Gemcitabin.

REFERENCES

1. Nishan Chobanian, et al. Ovarian cancer. Surg Clin N Am 88 2008;285-99.
2. Sterling D, et al. Screening for familial ovarian cancer: failure of current protocols to detect ovarian cancer at an early stage according to The International Federation of Obstetrics and Gynaecology System. J Clin Oncol 2005;23(24):5588.
3. Petricon EF, et al. Use of proteiomic patterns in serum to identify ovarian cancer. Lancet 2002;359:572-7.
4. Nagell TR, et al. Ovarian cancer screening with annual transvaginal sonography: Finding of 25000 women screened. Cancer 2007;109(9):1887-96.
5. DePriest PD, Shenson D, Fried A, et al. A morphology index based on Sonographic findings in ovarian cancer. Gynecol Oncol 1993;51:7-11.
6. Kinkel K, Hricak H, Ying Lu, et al. US characterization of ovarian masses: a meta-analysis. Radiology 2000;217:803-11.
7. Medeiros LRF, Rosa DD, Bozzetti MC, Rosa MINES, Edelweiss MI, Stein AT, Zelmanowicz A, Ethur AB, Zanini RR. Laparoscopy versus laparotomy for FIGO Stage I ovarian cancer. Cochrane Database of Systematic Reviews 2008; Issue 4. Art. No.: CD005344. DOI: 10.1002/14651858. CD005344. pub2.
8. Young RC, et al. Staging laparotomy in early ovarian carcinoma JAMA 1983;250:3072-6.
9. Maltaris T, et al. Reproduction beyond cancer: A message of hope for young women. Gynaecol Oncol 2006;103:1109-21.
10. Bolis G, et al. Adjuvant treatment for early epithelial ovarian cancer: Results of two randomized clinical trials comparing Cisplatin to no further treatment or chromic treatment-GIGOG. Ann Oncol 1995;6:887-93.
11. Bristow RE, et al. Survival effect of maximal cytoreductive surgery for advanced ovarian carcinoma during the platinum era: A meta analysis. J Clin Oncol 2002;20:1248-59.
12. Michel G, et al. Extensive cyto reductive surgery in advanced ovarian cancer. Eur J Gynec Oncol 1997;18:9-15.
13. Montz FJ, Schlaerth J, Berek JS. Resection of diaphragmatic peritoneum and colon: Role in cytoreductive surgery for ovarian carcinoma. Gynaecol Oncol 1989;35:338-40.
14. Morrison J, Swanton A, Collins S, Kehoe S. Chemotherapy vs. surgery in initial treatment advanced ovarian epithelial cancer. Cochrane Database of Systematic Review 2007, Issue 4 Art No. CD005343.DOI:10.1002/146518 58.CD005343.
15. Jaaback K, Johnson N. Intraperitoneal chemotherapy for the initial management of primary epithelial ovarian cancer. Cochrane Database of Systematic Reviews 2006, Issue 1. Art. No.: CD005340. DOI: 10.1002/14651858. CD005340. pub2.
16. Mezzo F, et al. Neoadjuvant chemotherapy followed by surgery in patients with primarily unresectable advanced stage ovarian cancer. Gynecol oncol 2003;90:103-69.
17. Tangjitgamol S, Manusirivithaya S, Laopaiboon M, Lumbiganon P. Interval debulking surgery for advanced

epithelial ovarian cancer. Cochrane Database of Systematic Reviews 2009, Issue 2. Art. No.: CD006014. DOI: 10.1002/14651858.CD006014.pub4.
18. Heintz APM, Odicino F, Maisonneuve P, Carcinoma of the ovary. J Epidemiol Biostat 2001;6:108-38.
19. Williams C, Simera I. Tamoxifen for relapse of ovarian cancer. Cochrane Database of Systematic Reviews 2001, Issue 1. Art. No.: CD001034. DOI: 10.1002/14651858.CD001034.
20. Topuz S, Iyibozkurt AC, Akhan SE, Keskin N, Yavuz E, Salihoglu Y, Bengisu E, Berkman S. Malignant germ cell tumors of the ovary: A review of 41 cases and risk factors for recurrence. Eur J Gynaecol Oncol 2008;29(6):635-7.
21. Pederson, Bjugard J, et al. Increased risk of myelodysplasia and leukemia after etoposide, cisplatin and bleomycin for germ-cell tumor. Lancet 1991 Aug 10;338(8763):359-63.
22. William SD, Blessing JA, Hatck KD, et al. Chemotherapy of advanced dysgerminoma: Trials of the Gynecologic Oncologic Group. J Clin Oncol 1991;9(11):1955-91.
23. Akihiro Nawa, Naoko Obata, Fumitaka Kikkawa, Michiyasu Kawai, Tetsuo Nagasaka, Setsuko Goto, Katsuhiko Nishimori, PhD, d and Nobuo Nakashima. Prognostic factors of patients with yolk sac tumors of the ovary. Am J Obstet Gynecol 2001;184(6):1182-88.
24. Giovanni D, et al. Am J Obs gynaec 2006;195:1268-9.

20 Malignancies of the Uterine Corpus

B Presannakumari

20.1 INTRODUCTION

Endometrial cancer is the most common malignancy of the uterine corpus. Worldwide, cancer of the endometrium ranks the third most common genital malignancy after cancers of the cervix and ovary. The estimated total number of new cases of cancer of the corpus uteri is 142,000 per year worldwide which constitutes 3.7% of cancers in women.

Reported global cancer statistics show the incidence of endometrial carcinoma to be the highest in North America, followed by Europe and temperate South America. The increased prevalence of the disease in the United States relative to other gynecologic cancers is influenced by the earlier diagnosis and decreasing incidence of cervical cancer, prolonged life expectancy, and dietary factors (perhaps related to increased obesity). The incidence is low in southern and eastern Asia, as well as in most of Africa.

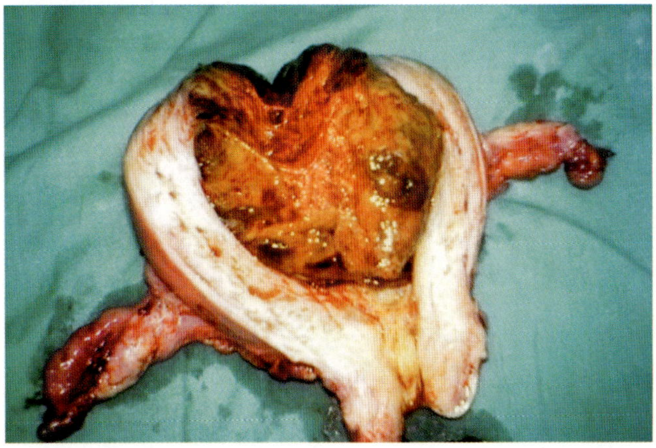

Unopposed estrogen should never be used as HRT to treat women who have not had hysterectomy. It increases the risk of endometrial cancer 4-8 times.

20.2 TYPES OF ENDOMETRIAL CARCINOMA

There appears to be two different types of endometrial cancer affecting two different age groups.

Type I—Estrogen dependent
- occurs in women exposed to unopposed estrogen
- is better differentiated
- carries a good prognosis
- is mucinous and secretory in type

Type II—Nonestrogen dependent
- occurs in older women
- no associated endometrial hyperplasia
- is less differentiated
- carries a poor prognosis

20.3 ETIOLOGY

The precise etiology of endometrial carcinoma is not known, but several factors are known to influence its development. Factors that increase the risk of developing endometrial cancer include:

a. **Prolonged unopposed estrogen:** This is probably one of the greatest risk factors especially in women with PCOS and chronic anovulation. This risk can be decreased by giving progestagens for at least 10 days a month, starting from the adolescent years to prevent endometrial hyperplasia.

   Premenopausal women with endometrial cancer usually have a history of chronic anovulation. They have a pre-malignant state of endometrial hyperplasia and develop type 1 cancer. Hence, all women presenting with chronic anovulation should undergo endometrial evaluation to exclude endometrial cancer/hyperplasia.

   Women under the age of 40, who develop endometrial cancer, are those who have PCOS. Carriers of mismatch repair gene defects also develop the disease at a younger age.

Relation between Endometrial Hyperplasia and Endometrial Cancer

Endometrial hyperplasia represents a spectrum of morphological and biological alterations in the endometrial glands and stroma ranging from simple hyperplasia without atypia through complex hyperplasia without atypia, simple hyperplasia with atypia, to complex hyperplasia with atypia. The risk of progression to endometrial cancer ranges from 1, 3, 8 to 29% respectively.

b. **Nulliparous women** have 2-3 times the risk as parous women.

c. **Late menopause** after the age of 52 has a relative risk of 2.4 for the development of endometrial cancer.

d. **Early menarche** also poses an increased risk.

e. **Obesity:** Women who weigh greater than 50 lbs over the expected weight for their height have a relative risk of 10 for the development of endometrial cancer. This is due to the excess estrone production as a result of peripheral conversion of adrenal-derived androstenedione. A BMI >30 triples the risk of developing endometrial cancer.

f. **Physical inactivity, high calorie intake, and high serum glucose** are BMI independent risk factors. It has been demonstrated that a diet high in animal fats and low in fruits and vegetables can increase the risk for endometrial cancer. A substantial chunk of endometrial cancers can be avoided by maintaining normal weight with a regular exercise schedule and dietary adjustments.

g. **Diabetes mellitus** increases the risk 1.3 to 2.8 times.

The role of tamoxifen in causing endometrial carcinoma is controversial. Tamoxifen was believed to be a risk factor for endometrial cancer. There were reports that the use of Tamoxifen increases the risk of endometrial cancer 3-6 fold. However, according to the SEER database, risk of endometrial cancer does not appear to be increased by taking tamoxifen. But carcinosarcomas have been found to be increased among long-term users of tamoxifen.

20.4 GENETICS OF ENDOMETRIAL CANCER

Hereditary Nonpolyposis Colon Cancer (HNPCC) results from germ line mutations in DNA mismatch repair genes (Froggatt et al 1996). These individuals are at increased risk for malignancies in the colon, endometrium, ovary, biliary tract, stomach, small intestine and renal tract. The risk for development of endometrial cancer is 46%. The majority of the mismatch repair gene defects involve the genes MLH1, MSH2 and MSH6. Defects in PMS1 and PMS2 being less common (Papadopoulos and Lindblom 1997). Family history will help to identify women carrying these mutations. If a woman is found to be at high risk, there may be a role for prophylactic hysterectomy and salpingo oophorectomy.

Mutations in BRCA1 or BRCA2 genes have been shown to contribute to increased risk of breast and ovarian cancers. However, it is unclear whether these mutations are also associated with increased risk of endometrial cancer as studies have produced inconsistent findings. A recent study by Beiner et al suggested that BRCA mutations are not directly associated with increased risk of endometrial cancer.

5-10% of endometrial carcinomas have a familial predisposition. Mutations of DNA mismatch repair genes which cause HNPCC, predispose to endometrial and ovarian carcinoma. The risk of development of endometrial cancer is 46%. It is not conclusive whether mutations of BRCA I and II predispose to development of endometrial cancer.

Table 20.1: WHO histological classification of endometrial carcinoma

Endometrioid adenocarcinoma	With squamous differentiation Villoglandular Secretory With ciliated cells
Other adenocarcinomas	Mucinous adenocarcinoma Serous adenocarcinoma Clear-cell adenocarcinoma Mixed adenocarcinoma Squamous-cell carcinoma Transitional-cell carcinoma Small-cell carcinoma Undifferentiated carcinoma

20.5 PATHOLOGY

20.5.1 WHO Histological Classification of Endometrial Carcinoma (Table 20.1)

Endometrioid adenocarcinoma is composed of glands that resemble normal endometrial glands. In poorly differentiated adenocarcinomas there will be more solid areas, less glandular formation and more cytological atypia. The well differentiated lesions (Fig. 20.1) may be difficult to differentiate from atypical hyperplasia.

According to FIGO (1989) tumors are grouped into three grades:

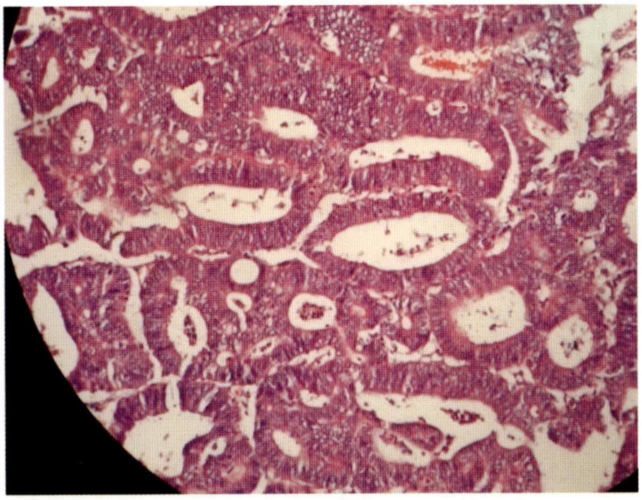

Fig. 20.1: Well-differentiated adenocarcinoma endometrium. The glands are arranged in back-to-back appearance with no intervening stroma

Grade 1: <5% of tumor shows solid growth pattern

Grade 2: 6-50% of tumor cells show a solid growth pattern

Grade 3: >50% of tumor cells show a solid growth pattern

Nuclear atypia that is inappropriate for the architectural grade increases tumor grade by 1. Adenocarcinomas with squamous differentiation are graded according to the nuclear grade of the glandular component.

15-25% of endometrioid carcinomas have areas of squamous differentiation. In the past, tumors with benign appearing squamous areas were called adenoacanthomas and tumors with malignant looking areas were called adenosquamous carcinomas. The degree of differentiation of squamous component parallels that of glandular component and the behavior of the tumor is largely dependent on the glandular component.[1] This has led to the new term 'endometrial carcinoma with squamous differentiation' to replace the previous two designations 'adenoacanthomas' and 'adenosquamous carcinomas'.

20.5.2 Other Adenocarcinomas

Mucinous Carcinomas

About 5% of endometrial carcinomas have cells composed of intracytoplasmic mucin. They have well differentiated glandular architecture and resemble endocervical adenocarcinoma. Positive perinuclear immunohistochemical staining with Vimentin suggests an endometrial origin.

> Endometrioid adenocarcinomas have the best prognosis. Areas of squamous differentiation make the prognosis worse.
>
> Clear cell adenocarcinoma has the worst prognosis followed closely by papillary serous carcinomas.

Papillary Serous Carcinoma

About 3-5% of endometrial carcinomas are papillary serous. They resemble serous carcinomas of the ovary. They are composed of highly atypical cells and are considered high grade lesions. They are sometimes seen mixed with other histological patterns. Papillary serous carcinoma is associated with involvement of the lymph vascular space and shows deep myometrial invasion. Though they are confined to the endometrium, they have a propensity for intraabdominal spread.

A preoperative diagnosis of papillary serous carcinoma warrants para-aortic sampling, even if the tumor is seen not to involve the myometrium. In a report of 50 surgically staged patients with papillary serous carcinomas, extrauterine spread was found in 72%.[2]

Clear Cell Carcinomas

5% of endometrial carcinomas are of the clear cell type. They have a mixed histological pattern including papillary, tubulocystic glandular and solid types. The cells have highly atypical nuclei and abundant clear/eosinophilic cytoplasm. They often have a hobnail appearance. This is a very aggressive endometrial cancer and prognosis is worse than papillary serous carcinoma.

Squamous Carcinoma

Squamous carcinomas of the endometrium are rare. They are often seen associated with cervical stenosis, chronic inflammation and pyometra. Their prognosis is poor and 5 year survival in stage 1 disease is only 36%.

20.5.3 Simultaneous Tumors of Endometrium and Ovary (Synchronous Tumors)

The reported incidence of synchronous tumor is 1.4-3.8%. Usually, both endometrial and ovarian tumors are well differentiated and have excellent prognosis. These types of tumors occur in premenopausal women. The ovarian tumor is diagnosed at an earlier stage due to the simultaneously occurring uterine tumor which is symptomatic.

20.6 CLINICAL FEATURES

20.6.1 Symptoms

Endometrial carcinoma is predominantly a disease of the elderly. 75% of the cases occur in women older than 50 years of age. In the vast majority (90%), the presenting symptom is abnormal vaginal bleeding, usually after menopause. In the remaining, the symptoms could be discharge per vaginum or pain. In less than 5% of women having endometrial cancer, the disease may be asymptomatic and is diagnosed due to the fortuitous finding of thickened endometrium observed on an ultrasound scan performed for some other purpose. In some, absence of bleeding may be because of cervical stenosis. These women are likely to develop pyometra and their presenting symptom may be pelvic pain. Later on, these patients present with purulent discharge per vaginum. Sometimes the endometrial cancer may be found in a uterus removed for some other reason. Rarely, a pap test may be positive due to spillage of malignant cells from the endometrium through the cervical canal.

Premenopausal women with endometrial cancer usually present with endometrial bleeding which may be menometrorrhagia. Patients having PCOD and chronic anovulation may present with infrequent and profuse periods. So, all women with chronic anovulation should have periodic endometrial evaluation and an abnormally thick endometrium should be sampled in order to exclude endometrial cancer.

Atrophic vaginitis and malignant growths of the vagina and cervix can also present with postmenopausal bleeding.

Among patients who present with postmenopausal bleeding, only 10% are due to endometrial carcinoma. Another 10% will have some pathology in the endometrium other than malignancy (Gredmark et al 1995). Endometrial atrophy is the most common endometrial finding in postmenopausal bleeding accounting for 60-80% of such bleeding. Refer Table 20.2. Endometrial polyp accounts for 2-12% of cases of postmenopausal bleeding. The thickness of the endometrial stripe, as measured by ultrasound, has been advocated as a factor in determining the need for dilatation and curettage. Although considerable overlap exists in the endometrial thickness and appearance between the various benign and malignant histologic types several reports suggest that the presence of a thin stripe is usually associated with atrophic endometrium and may indicate that a histologic diagnosis is not necessary.

In 1991, Granberg et al reported that if a cut off value of 5mm was used to define the thickness of the normal endometrial stripe in symptomatic postmenopausal patients approximately 70% of patients with vaginal bleeding could have avoided curettage. In 1995, a multicentric study reported by Karlsson et al revealed that dilatation and curettage found cancer in 2 out of 88 patients with a 5 mm stripe, whereas cancer was detected in none of the 518 women with a stripe ≤ 4 mm; hence a 4 mm cutoff may be more prudent. Women on estrogen replacement therapy typically have endometrial stripe thickness measuring up to 8-10 mm.[7]

Postmenopausal bleeding and discharge per-vaginum are the most common complaints of patients with endometrial cancer. Even though endometrial cancer is the most common malignancy causing postmenopausal bleeding, causes in the vagina and cervix including the endocervix should be excluded.

Table 20.2: Causes of postmenopausal uterine bleeding

Cause of bleeding	*Percentage*
Endometrial atrophy	60-80
Estrogen replacement therapy	15-20
Endometrial polyp	2-12
Endometrial hyperplasia	5-10
Endometrial cancer	10

In a symptomatic patient, a strategy starting with transvaginal ultrasound (TVU) should be adopted.

If a thin endometrium measuring double thickness of 4-5 mm is seen, the patient can be reassured.

Saline infusion sonography will help to differentiate focal from diffuse lesions. Since focal lesions are highly likely to be malignant, hysteroscopy is the investigation of choice.

Generalized lesions can be sampled by endometrial aspiration biopsy or curettage. In a symptomatic patient whose curettage is negative or the endometrium is not properly visualized by TVS, hysteroscopy is the investigation of choice.

When TVS strongly suggests endometrial cancer hysteroscopy or saline infusion sonography is not required and preferably not done owing to risk of tumor spill. Endometrial sampling is sufficient for diagnosis

20.6.2 Signs

Usually these patients will be obese and hypertensive. Enlarged lymph nodes in the groin or supraclavicular fossa may be elicited on examination. Metastatic focus is to be looked for in the suburethral region. The entire vagina and cervix must be carefully inspected and palpated to exclude causes other than endometrial cancer. Bimanual examination should be performed to evaluate the uterus for size and mobility. The adnexa should be evaluated for masses. Pelvic examination is often unremarkable because most of these patients present at early stages of the disease. A rectovaginal examination should also be done to look for parametrial involvement and cul-de-sac deposits. Rarely patients present with metastatic disease.

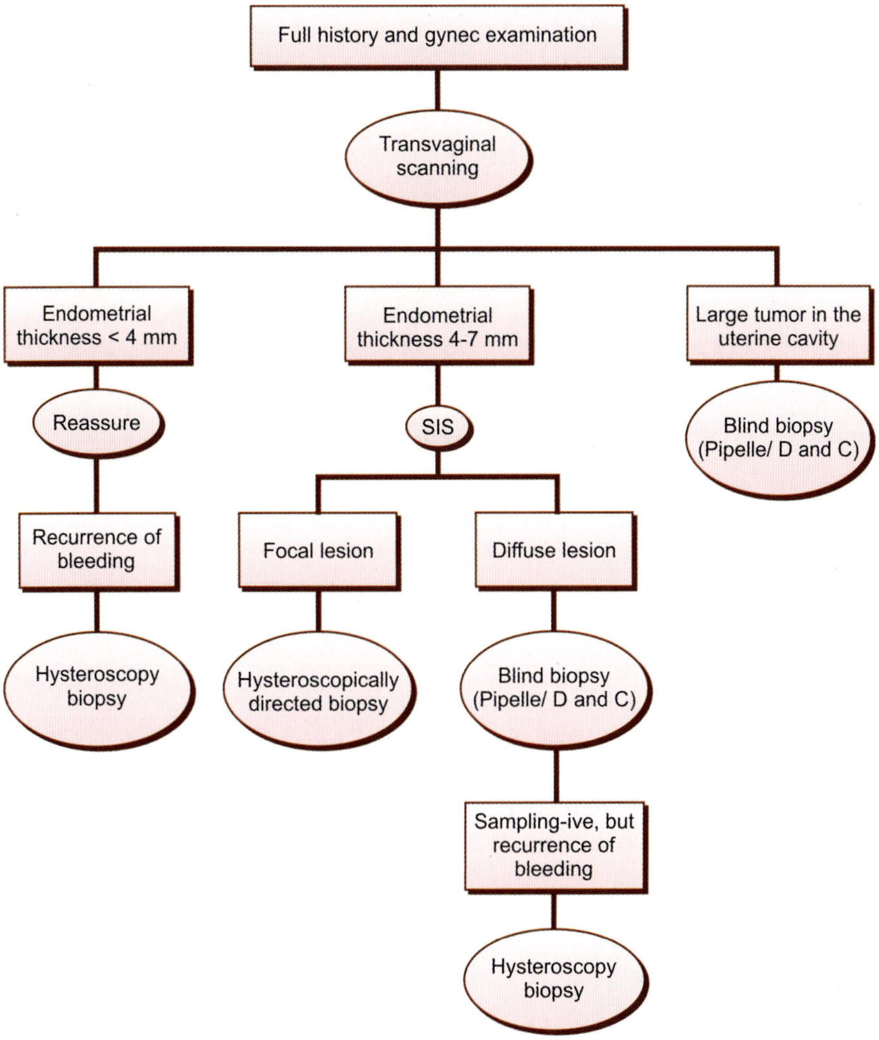

Fig. 20.2: Protocol for evaluation of postmenopausal/perimenopausal bleeding

20.6.3 Outpatient Endometrial Sampling (Fig. 20.2)

Traditionally, women with postmenopausal bleeding were being evaluated with dilatation and curettage. Since the last two decades, with the evolution of transvaginal ultrasound and hysteroscopy, approach to patients with postmenopausal bleeding has drastically changed.

Transvaginal ultrasonography should be done prior to endometrial sampling.

Depending upon TVS finding, the patient should be taken up for additional investigations. If a growth is seen filling the uterine cavity, she can be taken up for endometrial aspiration cytology. Hysteroscopy is dangerous in this situation because of chances of perforation as well as tumor dissemination. Moreover, hysteroscopy is not at all necessary in such a situation.'If TVS shows an endometrial thickness of 4-7 mm saline infusion sonography should be done to differentiate focal lesion from diffuse lesion. In the presence of focal lesion, hysteroscopically directed biopsy is the choice of investigation and endometrial sampling with Pipelle or dilatation and curettage should be the choice in the presence of diffuse lesion. A negative aspiration cytology needs evaluation by hysteroscopy (Figs 20.3A and B).

Outpatient endometrial biopsy is generally accepted as the first-step office procedure for the histopathological diagnosis of endometrial cancer and should be coupled with endocervical curettage. The procedure is definitive, if results are positive for malignancy.

Outpatient endometrial sampling can be done using a pipelle. It can be easily inserted and the endometrium sampled using a suction pipette. Most studies have shown that this instrument detects endometrial carcinoma and atypia with acceptable reliability (Stovall et al 1991).

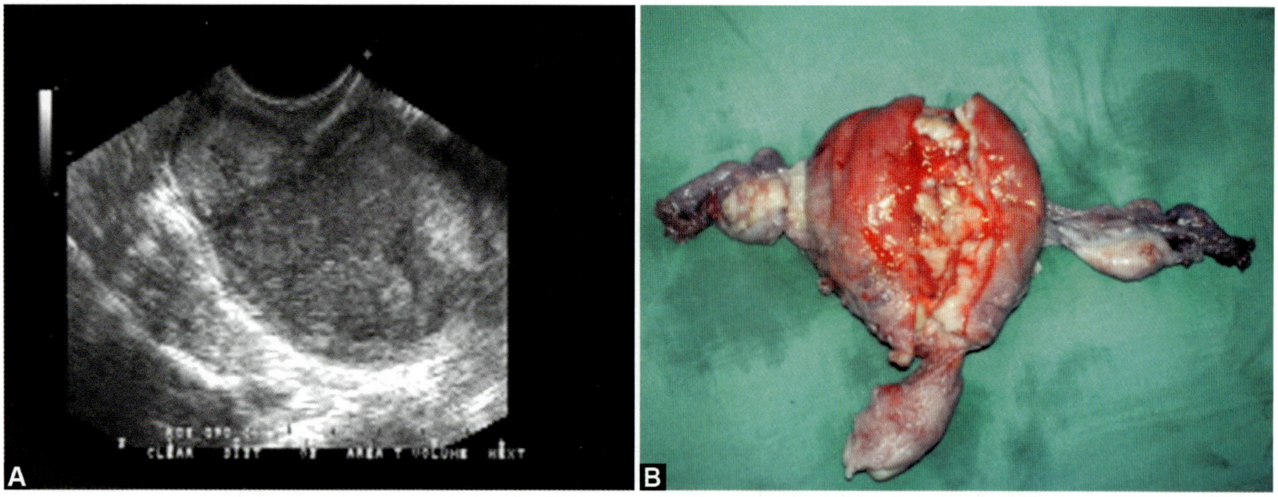

Figs 20.3A and B: TVS showing large volume tumor filling the uterine cavity (A). Hysterectomy specimen of the same patient (B)

When endometrial sampling does not yield a conclusive histologic diagnosis and adequate evaluation is precluded by cervical stenosis or limited patient tolerance, traditional fractional curettage may be necessary as it provides the largest amount of endometrial tissue. This procedure is preferably performed under anesthesia in the operating room. The procedure includes initial circumferential scraping of the endocervical canal and subsequent systematic curettage of the entire endometrial surface. Cervical and endometrial specimens are evaluated separately to determine if endometrial cancer has invaded the cervix and to allow detection of occult endocervical cancer. Availability of hysteroscopy directed biopsy has largely replaced fractional curettage (Figs 20.4 and 20.5).

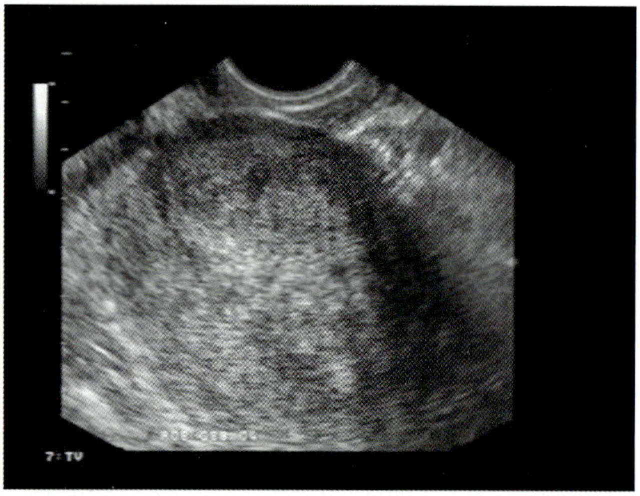

Fig. 20.4: TVS showing 3 × 2.5 cm tumor in the uterine cavity

20.6.4 Role of Hysteroscopy

With the advent of modern instruments it is possible to perform hysteroscopy as an outpatient procedure. Hysteroscopy is particularly useful in diagnosing small endometrial cancerous growths when a patient reports with bleeding after a negative curettage or endometrial aspiration (Fig. 20.6). It is useful in evaluation of the endocervix also. If the endocervix is seen to be involved, fractional sampling should be done for confirmation.

The biopsy specimen should be examined for histologic type, histologic grade, DNA ploidy, proliferative index and steroid receptor status.

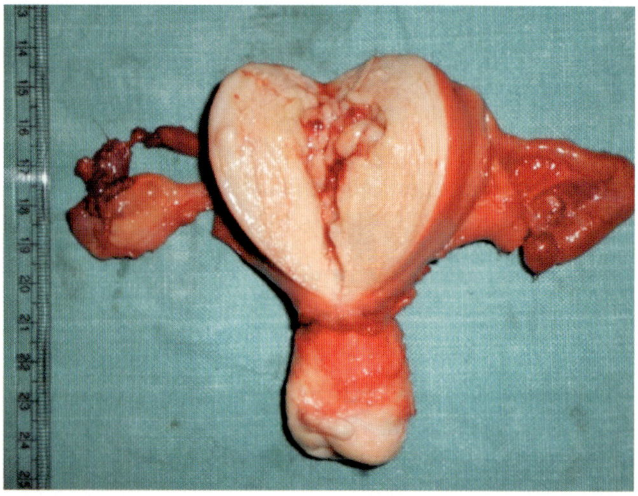

Fig. 20.5: Surgical specimen of uterus (cut open) of the patient shown above

20.7 PRETREATMENT EVALUATION

Pretreatment evaluation helps determine the best and safest approach to the management of the disease.

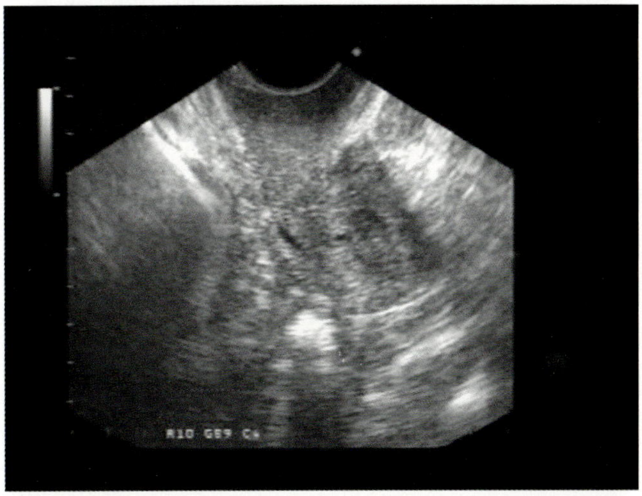

Fig. 20.6: TVS of a 65-year-old lady who presented with postmenopausal bleeding showing endometrial thickness of 6 mm. Endometrial curettage was negative. Hysteroscopy revealed a growth which on biopsy showed well differentiated adenocarcinoma

20.7.1 Physical Examination

A thorough general and pelvic examination should be done to discern the extent of the disease.

The patient whose disease is clinically not suspected to involve the cervix can be singled out for surgical staging. If clinically gross cervical involvement or parametrial spread is detected, the treatment approach is different. This emphasizes the need for thorough pelvic examination. *Clinical examination is complimentary to ultrasound examination.*

Routine preoperative evaluation should include ECG, X-ray chest, complete blood count, renal and liver function tests, blood type and urinalysis.

20.7.2 Assessment of Deep Myometrial Invasion

Assessment of deep myometrial invasion can be done with both USS and MRI with fairly high degree of accuracy.[4]

Knowledge about the degree of myometrial invasion is important in planning the extent of surgical procedure. The patient who has deep myometrial invasion needs para-aortic node sampling.

Histopathologic features of the tumor and clinical findings at presentation influence the choice of further imaging modality for preoperative staging of endometrial cancer. Kinkel et al provided clinical practice guidelines for staging based on a meta-analysis of the usefulness of MRI, CT, and US in imaging patients with endometrial cancer.

- Patients with grade 1 tumor, a clinically normal-sized uterus, and no clinical evidence of coexisting pelvic disease generally require no preoperative imaging except ultrasound because, the risk for myometrial, cervical, or lymph node disease is low. If the clinical evaluation is inconclusive or coexisting pelvic disease is suspected, then CT or MRI may be used for the initial imaging evaluation.
- In patients at risk for disease dissemination and lymph node involvement at presentation (because of tumor grade, histologic cell type, or clinical findings) CT or MRI of the abdomen and pelvis should be performed to determine the extent of tumor spread.
- Patients in whom cervical invasion is suggested clinically or in whom endocervical curettage was inconclusive, MRI should be done as MRI can depict cervical and parametrial invasion most accurately. MRI is superior to CT in detecting enlarged lymph nodes, but CT is considerably superior to MRI in detecting and distinguishing intraperitoneal, omental, and mesenteric metastases from bowel.

Routine preoperative evaluation should include an effort to diagnose the extent of spread to myometrium, cervix, parametrium, pelvis and upper abdomen. Knowledge of the histologic type and grade determined in a biopsy specimen and of the extent of spread is important in planning treatment—lymphadenectomy.

CT is clinically advocated in the evaluation of patients with poorly differentiated or high grade tumor, serous papillary carcinoma, or clear cell carcinoma due to the high risk for advanced disease and metastatic lymphadenopathy at the time of presentation. CT is also advised for patients who have abnormal liver function test results, elevated serum CA 125 levels, clinical suggestion of advanced disease, or inconclusive clinical evaluation.

Other investigations like cystoscopy, colonoscopy, IVP and barium enema are not advocated routinely but may be performed if indicated. MRI has a distinct advantage in patients who are not taken up for surgical staging (either because of tumor spread or because of contraindications for surgery) in evaluating the extent of disease.

20.7.3 Role of Tumor Markers

Serum CA-125 is elevated in most patients with advanced or metastatic endometrial cancer.[5] CA-125 is elevated in patients with extrauterine disease as well as lymph node involvement. Therefore, preoperative measurement of CA-125 may help to determine the extent of surgical staging. If elevated, it can also be used as a tumor marker in assessing the response to treatment.

20.7.4 Clinical Staging (Tables 20.3 and 20.4)

In the initial examination and evaluation, if the patient is found to have gross disease in the cervix, parametrial spread, invasion of the bladder or rectum, distant metastases or if she is unfit for surgery due to poor medical conditions, the disease is staged clinically.

20.8 SURGICAL STAGING

Due to the gross inaccuracy of clinical staging, FIGO advocated surgical staging in 1988. Surgical staging should be offered to all patients, who on clinical examination have no macroscopic cervical involvement or parametrial involvement and are fit for surgery.

The advantage of surgical staging is that it helps to make out the extent of the disease, so that postoperative treatment (radiation) can be tailored to the extent necessary. Most patients with endometrial cancer present when the disease is clinically confined to the uterus. A subgroup of these patients will have deep myometrial invasion, para-aortic node involvement, involvement of general peritoneal cavity or extension to the cervix and pelvic lymph nodes. This disease extension cannot be determined clinically. By surgical staging, patients who need postoperative treatment can be sorted out from those who do not. The extent of radiation treatment required can also be more precisely determined. Thus, unnecessary radiation treatment can be avoided. Evidence dictates that 70% of patients can thus be spared of radiation.

Before proceeding to surgical treatment, the patients who will need para-aortic node dissection can be predicted to an extent by the findings of deep myometrial invasion, poor grade tumor, large tumor volume or histological types – clear cell and papillary serous. This correlation between clinical staging and surgicopathological staging might not hold true always. Tumor histology and grade have been found altered after surgical evaluation. In a GOG series, 22% of the 621 patients with clinical Stage I endometrial cancer had evidence of extrauterine spread including lymph node metastasis, adnexal spread, peritoneal implants and positive peritoneal cytology. Surgical staging was found to be the most important factor affecting prognosis.

Surgical staging includes laparotomy, sampling of peritoneal fluid, exploration of the abdomen and pelvis, biopsy or excision of extra-uterine lesions suggestive of metastasis, extrafascial hysterectomy and bilateral salpingo-oophorectomy. The uterine specimen should be cut open and the size of the tumor, depth of myometrial invasion and isthmus—cervix extension must be assessed.

Table 20.3: FIGO clinical staging of endometrial carcinoma 1971

Stage	*Characteristic*
Stage I	Confined to the corpus
Ia G123	Uterine cavity < 8 cm
Ib G123	Uterine cavity > 8 cm
Stage II	Involves the corpus and cervix, but has not extended outside the uterus
Stage III	Extends outside the uterus, but not outside the true pelvis
Stage IV	Extends outside the true pelvis or obviously involves the mucosa of the bladder or rectum
IVa	Spread to adjacent organs
IVb	Spread to distant organs

Table 20.4: Revised FIGO staging for carcinoma of the endometrium (International Journal of Gynecology and Obstetrics 2009;105:103-104)

Stage	*Characteristic*
Stage I*	Tumor confined to the corpus uteri
IA*	No or less than half myometrial invasion
IB*	Invasion equal to or more than half of the myometrium
Stage II*	Tumor invades cervical stroma, but does not extend beyond the uterus**
Stage III*	Local and/or regional spread of the tumor
IIIA*	Tumor invades the serosa of the corpus uteri and/or adnexae#
IIIB*	Vaginal and/or parametrial involvement#
IIIC*	Metastases to pelvic and/or para-aortic lymph nodes#
IIIC1*	Positive pelvic nodes
IIIC2*	Positive para-aortic lymph nodes with or without positive pelvic lymph nodes
Stage IV*	Tumor invades bladder and/or bowel mucosa, and/or distant metastases
IVA*	Tumor invasion of bladder and/or bowel mucosa
IVB*	Distant metastases, including intra-abdominal metastases and/or inguinal lymph nodes

* Either G1, G2, or G3.

** Endocervical glandular involvement only should be considered as Stage I and no longer as Stage II.

Positive cytology has to be reported separately without changing the stage.

FIGO recommends pelvic and para-aortic lymphadenectomy for all patients as a part of surgical staging. As patients with lymphatic involvement may not always have enlarged nodes, palpation is not an alternative to lymph node sampling. Patients at high risk for pelvic and para-aortic lymph node involvement are the following:

- Adnexal or cervical involvement.
- Tumor >2 cm
- Deep myometrial invasion
- Moderately/poorly differentiated tumor
- Clear cell/papillary serous
- Extrauterine disease

Since papillary serous and mixed mullerian tumors have a propensity for intra-abdominal spread and upper abdominal recurrence, partial omentectomy should be done for those patients whose tumor histology is either of these.

20.8.1 FIGO Surgical Staging of Endometrial Carcinoma (Table 20.5)

Table 20.5: FIGO surgical staging of endometrial carcinoma

Stage		*Characteristics*
Ia	**G 123**	Tumor limited to endometrium
Ib	**G 123**	Invasion <half of myometrium
Ic	**G 123**	Invasion >half of myometrium
IIa	**G 123**	Endocervical glandular involvement only
IIb	**G 123**	Cervical stromal invasion
IIIa	**G 123**	Tumor invades the serosa and/or adnexae and/or positive peritoneal cytology
IIIb	**G 123**	Vaginal metastasis
IIIc	**G 123**	Metastasis to pelvic and/or para-aortic lymph nodes
IVa		Tumor invades bladder and/or bowel mucosa
IVb		Distant metastases intra-abdominal and/or inguinal lymph nodes

FIGO Definition for Grading of Endometrial Carcinoma

Grade	*Characteristics*
G1	< 5% nonsquamous or nonmorular growth pattern
G2	6%-50% nonsquamous or nonmorular growth pattern
G3	>50% nonsquamous or nonmorular growth pattern

Notes on pathologic grading: Notable nuclear atypia, inappropriate for the architectural grade, raises a grade I (GI) or grade 2 (G2) tumor by one grade. In serous adenocarcinoma, clear cell adenocarcinoma, and squamous cell carcinoma, nuclear grading takes precedence. Adenocarcinomas with squamous differentiation are graded according to the nuclear grade of the glandular component. *FIGO, International Federation of Gynecology and Obstetrics*

20.9 PROGNOSTIC VARIABLES

The stage of the disease is the most important prognostic factor. A number of other individual prognostic factors for disease recurrence or survival have been identified (Table 20.6).

Table 20.6: Prognostic variables in endometrial carcinoma

- Age
- Histological types
- Histological grade
- Myometrial invasion
- Lymph vascular space invasion
- Isthmus cervix extension
- Adnexal involvement
- Lymph node metastasis
- Intraperitoneal tumor
- Tumor size
- Peritoneal cytology
- Hormone receptor status
- DNA ploidy/proliferative index
- Genetic/molecular tumor markers

20.9.1 Age

Age is an independent prognostic variable. Endometrial cancer occurring in women less than 50 years of age has better prognosis than that occurring after 70 years. The lesser survival in the older age group is because of the increased incidence of extrauterine invasion and deep myometrial invasion at the time of diagnosis which is due to higher incidence of grade 3 tumors and unfavorable histological types (papillary serous and clear cell).

20.9.2 Histologic Type

Clear cell and papillary serous types of endometrial cancer are associated with increased risk for development of invasive disease and metastasis than endometroid type.[6] The overall survival for patients with these aggressive subtypes is only 33% as against 92% for patients with endometrioid type tumors.[7]

20.9.3 Histologic Grade

Patients with grade 3 tumors were more than 5 times likely to develop recurrence than those with grade 1 and 2.

It has been reported that the 5 year survival for patients with grade 1 and 2 disease was 92% when that of grade 3 disease was 64%. As the tumor grade increases chances for deep myometrial invasion, cervical extension, lymph node metastasis, local recurrence and distant metastasis increase.

20.9.4 Myometrial Invasion

As tumor invades the outer myometrium, the access to the lymphatic system increases. This explains the increased incidence of lymph node involvement and extrauterine disease in the presence of deep myometrial invasion. Of patients with no myometrial invasion the incidence of pelvic node involvement is found to be only 1% whereas when there is deep myometrial invasion, the pelvic node involvement is found to be 25% and para-aortic node involvement is found to be 17%. It is the distance between the tumor and the serosal surface that is the most sensitive indicator of the extent of myometrial invasion. Patients with noninvasive or superficially invasive tumors have an 80-90% survival compared to 60% survival in patients with deep myometrial invasion.

20.9.5 Lymph Vascular Space Invasion

Lymph vascular space invasion is another independent risk factor for recurrence. Overall incidence of lymph vascular space invasion in early endometrial cancer is 15%. One study reported 83% 5-year survival in patients without LVSI compared to 64.5% in whom LVSI was present.[8]

20.9.6 Isthmus and Cervix Extension

Extension of the tumor to the uterine isthmus, cervix or both is associated with increased incidence of extrauterine disease, lymph node metastasis as well as recurrence. It was found that if the fundus of the uterus alone is involved the recurrence risk is 7% whereas if the isthmus or cervix is involved, with occult tumor, the risk is 43%.[9]

20.9.7 Adnexal Involvement

If adnexal spread is the only high risk factor, the survival rate is reported to be 85%. But most patients with adnexal spread have other poor prognostic factors because of which they have high recurrence rate.

20.9.8 Peritoneal Cytology

Positive peritoneal cytology as a risk factor for tumor recurrence is a controversial issue. There are studies reporting significant relations between malignant peritoneal cytology and increased tumor recurrence. In contrast to these reports, there are equal number of studies that have found no significant relationship between positive peritoneal cytology and increased incidence of recurrence. Positive peritoneal cytology seems to have an adverse effect on survival if the endometrial cancer has spread to the adnexa, peritoneum or lymph nodes. Positive peritoneal cytology will not increase the risk of recurrence if the tumor is otherwise confined to the uterus.

Positive peritoneal cytology in the absence of other evidence of extrauterine disease or other poor prognostic factors does not seem to have significant effect on recurrence.

20.9.9 Lymph Node Involvement

Lymph node involvement is the most important prognostic factor. When the lymph node is involved, the recurrence rate is 6 fold. Among patients with clinical stage I disease, about 10% will have pelvic and 6% para-aortic node metastasis. The 5-year disease free survival rate for patients with lymph node metastasis was 54% when compared with 90% for patients without lymph node metastasis. GOG found the presence or absence of para-aortic lymph node metastasis as the most important factor determining prognosis. Histological type of tumor and the depth of myometrial invasion are the two most important factors determining the risk of lymph node metastases. The incidence of lymph node metastasis in clinical stage I is- 3% in Grade 1, 9% in Grade 2 and 18% in Grade 3. Lymph node involvement in patients without myometrial involvement or superficial (< 50%) myometrial invasion is 5%. When there is deep myometrial invasion (> 50%) ; the lymph node involvement will be above 20%. Cervical involvement is associated with a 15% risk of pelvic or para-aortic node involvement. When the tumor size is <2 cm, the lymph node metastasis is only 4%. When the tumor size is >2 cm, it is 15% and when the tumor fills the entire cavity, it is 35%. Presence of adnexal metastases also increase the risk of pelvic and para-aortic nodal metastases to 32% and 20% respectively. If the peritoneal cytology is positive for malignant cells the risk of pelvic node metastasis is 25% and para-aortic node metastasis is 19%.

20.9.10 Intraperitoneal Tumor

Intraperitoneal metastasis occurs in 4-6% of clinical stage I patients. The presence of gross peritoneal spread correlates with lymph node metastasis. The 5-year disease free survival rate with non-lymphatic extrauterine disease was 50% compared with 88% in other patients.[10]

20.9.11 Tumor Size

As the tumor size increases, the chance of lymph node metastasis also increases. The 5-year survival rate was 98% with tumor size 2 cm or smaller, 84% for tumors larger than 2 cm and 64% for patients with tumors involving the whole uterine cavity.[11]

20.9.12 Hormone Receptor Status

Patients whose tumors are positive for estrogen and/or progesterone receptors have longer survival than patients whose tumors lack the receptors. Progesterone receptor levels appear to be stronger predictors of survival than estrogen receptors.

20.9.13 DNA Ploidy and Proliferative Index

The proportion of aneuploid tumors increases with the stage, lack of tumor differentiation and depth of myometrial invasion. Similarly, higher the proliferative index worse is the prognosis.

20.9.14 Genetic and Molecular Markers

A large number of genetic and molecular markers have been identified, the presence of which predicts outcome (poor/better). The presence of Kras oncogene mutation appears to be an unfavorable prognostic factor. Reduced expression of E cadherin is related to advanced stage disease. Over-expression of HER 2-neu oncogene is frequently associated with metastatic disease. Mutations of p53 gene have been found to be associated with papillary serous cell type, advanced stage and poor prognosis. Expression of MIB 1 (ki 67) has been associated with extrauterine spread and decreased survival. Mutations and deletions of PTEN gene is seen in well differentiated tumors and is a marker of good prognosis. Microsatellite instability is found to be associated with other molecular features that predict a favorable outcome including PTEN mutation and absence of p53 alteration.

20.10 MANAGEMENT OF CLINICAL STAGE I ENDOMETRIAL CANCER (FIG. 20.7)

20.10.1 Abdominal Hysterectomy

Exploratory laparotomy, extrafascial total abdominal hysterectomy and bilateral salpingo-oophorectomy is the primary operative procedure. Removal of adnexa is mandatory because of two reasons:

1. There may be microscopic metastases
2. There may be simultaneous ovarian cancer

Removal of vaginal cuff is not advised as vaginal metastasis is not prevented by removal of the vaginal cuff but by postoperative radiation.

20.10.2 Surgical Technique

Abdomen is opened by either a vertical incision or a lower transverse muscle dividing incision (Maylard's) or a muscle detaching incision (Cherney's). After opening the abdomen the operability is assessed and peritoneal washings are taken from paracolic gutter, subdiaphragmatic area and pelvis with 200 ml saline and sent for cytology. The abdominal contents are carefully examined with special attention to the omentum, liver, under-surface of diaphragm, pouch of Douglas and adnexa. Extrafascial hysterectomy with bilateral salpingo-oophorectomy and biopsy of suspicious lesions should be done. Adnexal removal is recommended because of the possibility of micrometastases. Removal of the vaginal cuff or parametria are not recommended because it will not prevent vaginal vault recurrence. The uterus is opened up in the theater and myometrial invasion is assessed.

20.10.3 Lymphadenectomy

FIGO recommends lymphadenectomy for all patients as a part of surgical staging. The therapeutic benefit of lymphadenectomy is controversial. Some case control studies have shown therapeutic benefit in women with positive nodes.[12, 13]

The MRC ASTEC trial, which randomized women undergoing surgery for clinical stage I endometrial cancer to pelvic lymphadenectomy or no lymphadenectomy did not show a therapeutic benefit.

Lymphadenectomy can be deferred in patients who are at very low risk for nodal metastasis-small volume (<2 cm) tumor, well differentiated with no myometrial invasion or only superficial myometrial invasion and no evidence of extrauterine spread. Most patients with endometrial cancer are obese and elderly. They may also be diabetic and hypertensive. Hence, it is prudent to defer lymphadenectomy in such patients who carry high risk with extensive surgery.

Para-aortic sampling should be done in the following situations:

- Suspicious aortic or common iliac nodes
- Grossly positive adnexae
- Patients who have grade 3 disease

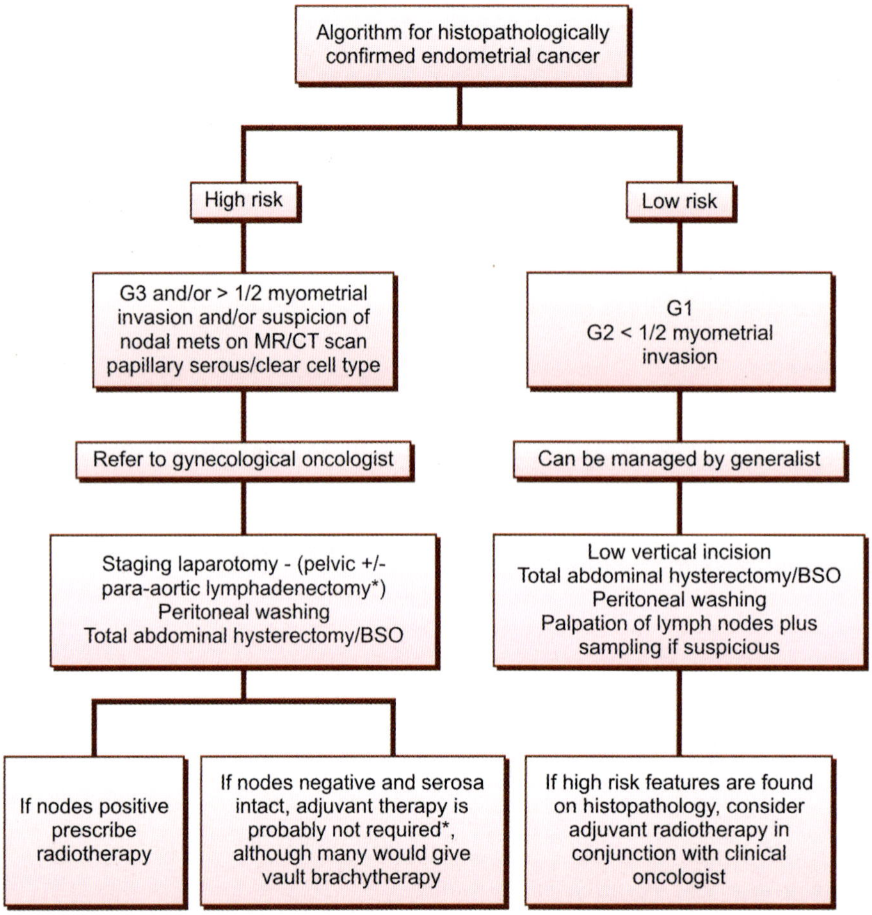

Fig. 20.7: Management algorithm for histopathologically confirmed endometrial cancer (FIGO)
*Randomised trials are needed to provide conclusive evidence regarding the clinical effectiveness of lymphadenectomy and adjuvant radiotherapy in the presence of high risk factors.

- Patients who have clear cell or papillary serous carcinoma diagnosed by histopathology
- Large volume tumor
- Deep myometrial invasion diagnosed by preoperative imaging.

20.10.4 Vaginal Hysterectomy

Patients who have small well differentiated tumors having low metastatic potential and who are obese may be taken up for vaginal hysterectomy. The disadvantages are the difficulty in removing the adnexa, the inability to explore the abdomen and perform lymphadenectomy.[14]

20.10.5 Laparoscopic Hysterectomy

Previously, laparoscopic management was not advised because of inadequate lymph node dissection and observation of port site recurrence in laparoscopically managed patients. Recently there are several reports documenting the feasibility of laparoscopically assisted vaginal hysterectomy[15] with laparoscopic retroperitoneal lymph node sampling for staging and treatment of endometrial cancer. One randomized controlled trial comparing LAVH with abdominal hysterectomy in patients with endometrial cancer showed blood loss and transfusion rates to be lower in the laparoscopically managed patients. The overall recurrence-free survival did not differ in the two groups. Currently, GOG is conducting a large trial comparing laparoscopic assisted hysterectomy with abdominal hysterectomy as a treatment modality for endometrial cancer.

20.10.6 Radical Hysterectomy

For patients with stage I disease, radical hysterectomy does not improve survival compared with extrafascial hysterectomy and bilateral oophorectomy. Since intraoperative and post-operative morbidity for radical hysterectomy is more, it is not advised for clinical stage I endometrial cancer.

20.10.7 Postoperative Adjuvant Therapy

Postoperative adjuvant therapy is determined by factors which are assessed preoperatively, supplemented with the findings at surgery and the histopathology report of the operated specimen. Based on these assessments patients can be classified into three treatment groups:

1. **Low risk:** Patients having grade I or II disease without myometrial invasion and a small tumor are at low risk for recurrence and hence do not need any postoperative treatment.[16]
2. **Intermediate risk:** Patients who have grade II disease with superficial myometrial invasion and grade III disease with no myometrial invasion should be given vaginal radiation. These patients if given brachytherapy, are found to have excellent progression-free survival with minimal morbidity.
3. **High risk:** Patients with cervical extension or deep myometrial invasion should be considered high risk and need loco-regional radiation treatment.

20.10.8 Radiation Therapy

Three important trials evaluated the role of pelvic radiotherapy in stage I endometrial cancer:

1. Norwegian trial
2. PORTEC trial
3. GOG 99 trial

The GOG 99 trial provided the essential information that helped to finally end the major controversies over the indications for pelvic radiotherapy and the extent of surgery in the treatment of endometrial cancer. Contrary to the other two trials, in the GOG 99 trial, surgery consisted of TAH with BSO, peritoneal cytology and pelvic and para-aortic lymphadenectomy. In the 8-year period from 1987 to 1995, 440 patients were randomized. 202 individuals were randomized for no adjuvant therapy (NAT) which comprised the low risk group and 190 were randomized for pelvic radiation (RT). Surgically staged Ib, Ic and II occult were also included. The two year vaginal and pelvic recurrence rate was 12% in NAT group and 3% in RT group. The pelvic failure rate was 8.9% in the surgery alone group, compared with 1.6% in the postoperative pelvic irradiation group. Overall survival rates also were improved in patients receiving postoperative pelvic irradiation compared to those treated with surgery.

This study confirms the substantial reduction in locoregional recurrence by pelvic RT.

Following surgical staging, hysterectomy and bilateral salpingo-oophorectomy, individualized radiation therapy is planned, tailored to the extent necessary and thus unnecessary radiation is avoided, optimizing survival rates.

Patients with Stage Ia, grade I and II have excellent prognosis and do not require postoperative therapy.

Patients with disease other than stage Ia, grade I and II require postoperative management which includes:

- Vaginal vault radiation
- External pelvic irradiation
- Extended field (pelvic and para-aortic) irradiation
- Whole abdomen irradiation
- Progestins
- Systemic chemotherapy

20.10.9 Vaginal Vault Irradiation

Postoperative vaginal radiation is given as an outpatient treatment, using high dose rate iridium source by afterloading technique. Morbidity is less for vaginal vault irradiation. Patients who are most likely to benefit from vaginal irradiation are those who have surgical stage I, grade 1 and 2 with superficial (< 50%) invasion or grade 3 with no invasion and stage IIc (occult), grade 1 and 2 with superficial myometrial invasion.

Postoperative vaginal irradiation

- Stage I—GI and G2 with superficial invasion, G3 with no invasion
- Stage II (occult)—GI and G2 with superficial myometrial invasion

  Dose: High dose rate Iridium or low dose rate Cesium source via colpostat to deliver 6000–7000 cGy

20.10.10 External Pelvic Irradiation

Patients who have cervical stromal involvement, positive pelvic nodes, adnexal or parametrial disease and patients with stage I grade 3 with any degree of myometrial invasion and patients with grade 1 and 2 with any myometrial invasion and large tumor (>2 cm), grade 2 or 3 and superficial myometrial invasion or any grade tumor with lymph vascular space involvement are advised external pelvic irradiation. Irradiation usually involves delivery of 4500-5040 cGy in 180 cGy daily fractions over 5-6 weeks to cover the upper half of vagina and pelvis. The vaginal apex is boosted to 6000-7000 cGy.

Patients who are at high risk of recurrence due to factors like poor tumor grade, deep myometrial invasion, extension to the cervix, parametrial spread, pelvic node involvement etc are those who would benefit from whole pelvic irradiation.

External pelvic irradiation

- Stage I G3 with any degree of myometrial invasion
- Stage I GI and 2 with deep myometrial invasion
- Large volume tumor
- Any tumor with lymph vascular space invasion

  Dose: 4500-5040 cGy over 5-6 weeks

20.10.11 Extended Field Irradiation

Some patients who need whole pelvic irradiation may have para-aortic node involvement as well. If they are not found to have disease spread outside the pelvis other than para-aortic nodes, they are treated with extended field irradiation to the para-aortic area. The dose given is 4500- 5000 cGy. 5-year survival rates of 43- 47% have been reported. The 5-year survival rates were seen to be better for patients with microscopic nodal disease than those with gross nodal disease.

Extended field irradiation

Patients with positive para-aortic nodes as the only evidence of spread outside the pelvis

Dose: 4500-5000 cGy

20.10.12 Whole Abdomen Irradiation

Patients who have positive residual upper abdominal disease and those who have papillary serous and clear cell tumors, which have a propensity for upper abdominal recurrence, are treated with whole abdominal irradiation. The recommended dose is 3000 cGy in 20 daily fractions of 150 cGy. The kidneys are shielded to 1500-2000 cGy. Patients who have gross residual intraperitoneal disease cannot be treated with whole abdominal irradiation as 3000 cGy will not be sufficient to treat gross disease. They have to be treated with progestagens or chemotherapy.

The treatment of patients with positive peritoneal cytology as the only evidence of disease spread outside the uterus is controversial.

Whole abdominal radiation

- Papillary serous and clear cell tumors which have a propensity for upper abdominal secondaries
- Patients with adnexal and upper abdominal disease which has been surgically excised
- Should not be given for gross residual intraperitoneal disease

  Dose: 3000 cGy in 20 fractions

20.10.13 Progestagens

Progestagens were used to treat metastatic endometrial cancer. But a Cochrane review of several large randomized placebo controlled studies has failed to identify benefit for adjuvant progestin therapy.[17]

20.10.14 Chemotherapy

For patients with bulky upper abdominal residual disease as well as for patients with advanced disease who are at high risk for surgery (stage III and IV), chemotherapy is the choice. But for patients who have undergone maximal surgical resection to <2 cm, chemotherapy is found to have minimally improved 2 year progression-free survival compared with patients who had postoperative whole abdominal irradiation.[18]

20.11 MANAGEMENT OF CLINICAL STAGE II ENDOMETRIAL CANCER

It is important to distinguish between clinical stage II and surgical stage II disease. Clinical stage II is macroscopic involvement of the cervix. Surgical stage II is microscopic involvement of the cervix diagnosed by histopathology of the hysterectomy specimen. The treatment of surgical stage II has been discussed earlier. When endometrial carcinoma extends to the uterine cervix, it is difficult to distinguish clinically between stage I and stage II. If the cervix is involved (stage II) there is a 35% incidence of pelvic node metastasis. Hence management of stage II endometrial cancer involves treatment of pelvic nodes as well.

The literature pertaining to the management of clinical stage II endometrial carcinoma is limited. There are no fruitful randomized control trials and no definite treatment plan has been formulated for clinical stage II disease so far.

The incidence of para-aortic node involvement, adnexal involvement and upper abdominal spread are higher in stage II than stage I. Treatment of stage II should include surgical evaluation of the abdomen and treatment of extrapelvic disease (surgical removal or radiotherapy) to the extent possible.

Three treatment approaches have been proposed for the management of clinical stage II disease:

1. Radical hysterectomy, pelvic and para-aortic lymphadenectomy.
2. External pelvic irradiation and intracavitary radiation followed 6 weeks later by total abdominal hysterectomy with bilateral salpingo-oophorectomy and postoperative radiation, as required.
3. Initial exploratory laparotomy, extrafascial hysterectomy followed by appropriate postoperative radiation.

An initial surgical approach has the advantage of obtaining accurate surgico-pathologic information. But unfortunately, most of the patients with endometrial carcinoma will be obese, elderly or hypertensive making them unsuitable for a radical surgery. The reported results for radical surgery are not better than initial radiation followed by a less radical surgery.

The most common traditional approach to the management of clinical stage II endometrial carcinoma is external radiation and intracavitary radiation followed by extrafascial hysterectomy. Patients who are medically unfit for surgery are treated with radiation therapy alone.

Stage II disease can also be managed by initial surgery followed by irradiation. The rationale behind this is that when fractional curettage shows positive endocervical curettings, it need not necessarily imply that the patient has cervical involvement as it could be falsely positive. Radiation is equally effective when given postoperatively. Explorative laparotomy, extrafascial or modified radical hysterectomy, bilateral salpingo-oophorectomy, peritoneal washings, resection of grossly enlarged lymph nodes and selective common iliac and lower para-aortic lymphadenectomy are performed. Results reported are excellent for postoperative radiation following surgical staging.

20.12 MANAGEMENT OF CLINICAL STAGE III ENDOMETRIAL CANCER

It is important to differentiate between clinical stage III disease and surgical stage III disease. Surgico-pathological stage III disease is a clinically occult disease process which is detected at surgery. Stage III disease implies involvement of the parametria, uterine serosa, adnexa, para-aortic lymph nodes or the vagina. About 5–10% of patients with stage I and II will have subclinical stage III which are detected at surgery. 5-year survival is better in patients with surgical stage III than those with clinical stage III (40% – 80% and 15% respectively).

Postoperative Radiation or Chemotherapy?

After surgery for endometrial cancer stage III and IV, with the maximum size of residual disease limited to 2cm, 388 patients were r and omly assigned to cisplatin and doxorubicin chemotherapy for seven courses or whole-abdominal radiotherapy with 30 Gy in 20 fractions and a pelvic boost of 15 Gy. Although recurrences were frequent (55%) in the pelvis and abdomen in both groups, 2-year progression-free survival was better with chemotherapy as was the overall survival[19] (59% vs. 46%).

20.13 MANAGEMENT OF CLINICAL STAGE IV ENDOMETRIAL CANCER

Rarely, endometrial carcinoma may be detected in stage IV. Stage IV disease implies involvement of bladder, rectum or distant metastasis. Treatment involves a combination of surgery, radiation therapy and systemic hormonal therapy or chemotherapy. Surgery is done to relieve the symptoms of pain and bleeding. If the patient is fit for radical surgery and the disease spread is only to the bladder or rectum, exenteration may be considered.

20.14 FOLLOW-UP AFTER TREATMENT

After complete treatment patients should have follow-up every 3-4 months in the first two years and every 6 months thereafter. Recurrences are most effectively diagnosed from history and detailed examination. Chest X-ray should be evaluated every 12 months. Other radiological investigations are not routinely advised as a part of follow-up. Those who have initial high values of CA-125 can be followed-up with periodic assessment of CA-125 levels.

20.15 TREATMENT OF RECURRENT DISEASE

In spite of adjuvant therapy 10-15% of patients with early endometrial cancer will relapse. About 50% of patients will have an isolated pelvic relapse, 30% will relapse at distant sites. Patients with pelvic recurrence present with pelvic pain or vaginal bleeding and 20% will have recurrence at both pelvic and distant sites. For patients who have isolated central pelvic recurrence who are otherwise healthy an exenteration procedure is a choice.

The usual sites of distant metastases are lung, abdomen, lymph nodes (aortic, supraclavicular, inguinal) liver, brain and bone. Patients with lung metastasis can be treated with progestins. Others can be treated with a combination of chemotherapy and radiotherapy. A few patients with intraperitoneal recurrence may benefit from laparotomy to relieve intestinal obstruction. Laparotomy may also be done for tumor reduction so that they may respond better to radiation.

HRT after treatment

Several non randomized studies have addressed the safety of estrogen replacement after treatment for early stage endometrial carcinoma. Safety was confirmed in a large randomized GOG137A study.

20.16 SURVIVAL BY STAGE

Approximate 5-year uterine cancer survival by stage is as follows. More than 75% of surviving patients are either Stage I or II. These stages are determined after surgery, as described above.

- Stage IA - 91%
- Stage IB - 90%
- Stage IC - 81%
- Stage IIA - 79%
- Stage IIB - 71%
- Stage IIIA - 60%

- Stage IIIB - 30%
- Stage IIIC - 52%
- Stage IVA - 15%
- Stage IVB - 17%

Fertility Preservation in Endometrial Cancer

The problem of fertility preservation in endometrial cancer occurs when young women develop the disease, which is a possibility among those with chronic anovulation. Conservative management in the form of large doses of progestagens may be thought of in younger patients with well differentiated endometrial cancer, without evidence of myometrial or cervical involvement made out by MRI. In a study by *Seli E et al* Medroxyprogesterone at a dose of 200-800 mg was given continuously for 3 months and endometrial sampling repeated. Resolution was found to occur in 50-80% but recurrence was seen in 30-40%. Progestagens incorporated intrauterine system have also been studied in such situations in small studies. These serve only to delay definitive treatment till pregnancy is completed.[20-22]

20.17 AREAS OF CONTROVERSY AND RESEARCH

- Newer drugs like erlotinib that blocks a protein needed for a cancer cell to grow
- Trastuzumab (Herceptin) - a monoclonal antibody which is a drug designed to attach to and block a growth factor protein called Her 2.
- The role of three-dimensional ultrasonography in the diagnosis of endometrial cancer
- Cost-benefit analysis of tests done in women with abnormal uterine bleeding.
- Microarray analyses and proteomics to further disentangle molecular pathways
- Distillation of prognostic and predictive factors from molecular findings
- Conservative management with antioestrogens or local progestagens to conserve fertility
- Long-term safety in relation to local and port-site metastases of laparoscopically assisted vaginal hysterectomy
- Accuracy of sentinel procedure for lymph-node staging
- Pelvic versus local radiotherapy to decrease local relapses
- Survival benefit of correct surgical staging (lymphadenectomy) and mode of radiotherapy
- Role of pure antioestrogens (fulvestrant) and newer selective estrogen-receptor modulators
- Tibolone and endometrium
- Role of ultrasonography in the detection of recurrent disease.

20.18 UTERINE SARCOMA

Sarcomas are relatively rare tumors of the uterus which originate from the mesoderm and constitute about 2-6% of uterine malignancies. They are the most malignant tumors of the uterus. With regard to clinical presentation, the pattern of spread and management, they differ from endometrial cancer.

20.18.1 Classification

Uterine sarcomas can be broadly classified into three main groups

- Endometrial stromal tumors
- Leiomyosarcoma
- Carcinosarcoma (Malignant mixed mullerian tumors)

20.18.2 Endometrial Stromal Sarcoma

Endometrial stromal sarcoma usually occurs in perimenopausal or postmenopausal women. The incidence of these tumors is not related to parity, other associated diseases or radiation exposure. The usual presentation is with abnormal uterine bleeding. In the presence of uterine enlargement, the patient can present with pressure symptoms. Pelvic examination usually shows an enlarged uterus. Since these women undergo endometrial sampling in view of postmenopausal bleeding, preoperative diagnosis will be usually possible. However, from the endometrial sample, diagnosis between leiomyosarcoma and endometrial stromal sarcoma is usually not possible. Imaging usually shows a vascular growth in the uterine cavity. During surgery, uterus will be seen filled with hemorrhagic necrotic material (Fig. 20.8).

On the basis of mitotic activity, vascular invasion and prognosis, these tumors are classified into three types:

1. Endometrial stromal nodule
2. Endometrial stromal sarcoma
3. High grade/undifferentiated sarcoma

Management is surgical. Total abdominal hysterectomy and bilateral salpingo-oophorectomy should be performed as the adnexa is likely to be involved by tumor extension. Estrogen is supposed to have a stimulatory effect on the growth of these tumors. Postoperative pelvic radiation is advised for inadequately excised tumors. Adjuvant treatment with progestagens is found to be effective in patients with low grade tumors. For patients with high grade or undifferentiated sarcoma, postoperative treatment with

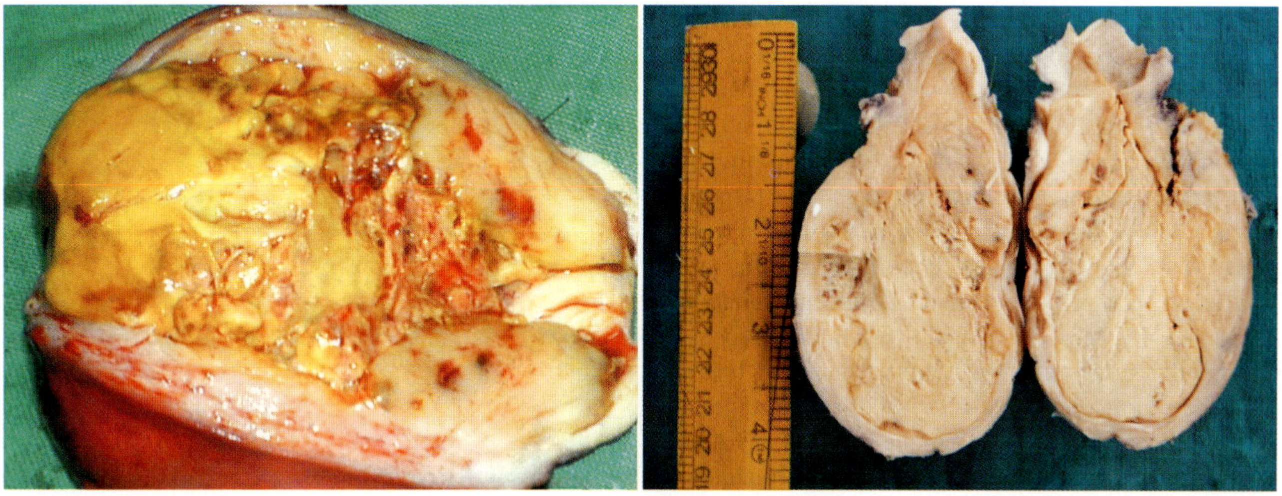

Fig. 20.8: Cut section of the uterus showing hemorrhagic necrotic tumor filling the uterus. The patient was a 65-year-old lady who presented with irregular vaginal bleeding. Histopathology revealed endometrial stromal sarcoma

chemotherapy as well as radiation is advised. The high grade type will not respond to progestin therapy.

20.18.3 Leiomyosarcoma (Fig. 20.9)

Leiomyosarcomas are also common in postmenopausal and perimenopausal women. There is no association with parity or other factors like endometrial adenocarcinoma. Increased incidence is noted among women who have had prior pelvic radiation. These tumors are not thought to occur as a consequence of malignant transformation of leiomyomas. The most common presenting symptom is abnormal bleeding. An abdominal mass or pressure symptoms may be complained of if the tumor is large enough. Clinical examination shows an enlarged uterus. Sarcoma should be thought of in the event of rapid enlargement of an uterine mass suspected to be a myoma and in presence of pelvic pain. Endometrial biopsy may be positive for malignant cells if the lesion is submucosal and the patient presents with vaginal bleeding. Spread occurs to the neighboring structures as well as to distant organs through blood vessels and lymphatics.

The number of mitoses/high power field is the most reliable indicator of malignant behavior. Tumors with >10 mitoses/10 high power field are frankly malignant and have poor prognosis. Tumors with 5-10 mitoses/10 high power fields are classified as smooth muscle tumors of unknown malignant potential (STUMP) and their clinical behavior is unpredictable. Severe cytological atypia and coagulative tumor cell necrosis are characteristic of sarcoma. DNA ploidy also has been found to be a prognostic factor with aneuploid tumors carrying poor prognosis. Tumors confined to the uterus have better survival whereas tumors with extension beyond the uterus are associated with poor prognosis.

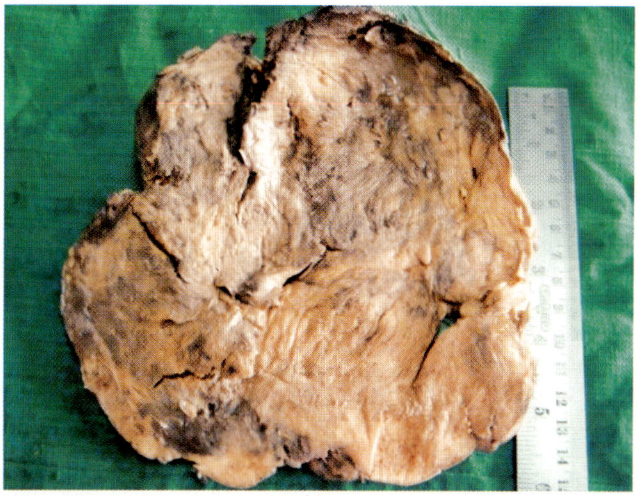

Fig. 20.9: Cut section of growth removed from the uterus showing areas of hemorrhage. Microscopy showed leiomyosarcoma

Management is surgical. After surgical staging total hysterectomy and bilateral salpingo-oophorectomy is performed. Postoperative adjuvant chemotherapy should be given. Gemcitabine-docetaxel combination is being evaluated as adjuvant therapy.

20.18.4 Carcinosarcoma (Malignant Mixed Mullerian Tumor)

These are a combination of carcinomatous and sarcomatous elements. They are grossly classified into homologous and heterologous (Fig. 20.10).

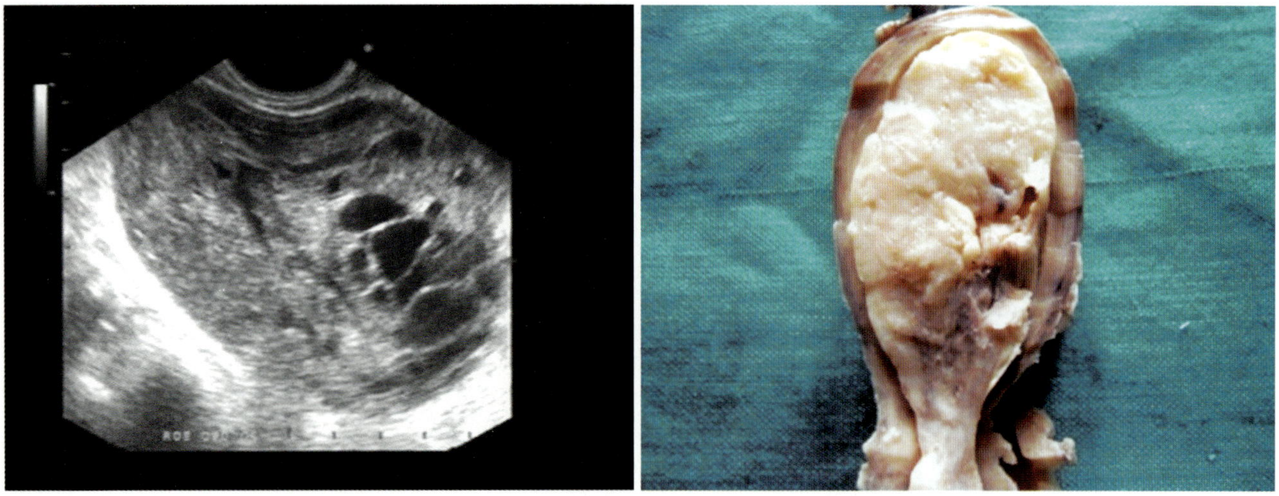

Fig. 20.10: TVS showing carcinosarcoma. Note the solid and cystic mass arising from the fundus and filing the uterine cavity extending to the cervical canal. Sagittal section of the specimen is seen on the right side

Homologous

Here the carcinomatous element is usually glandular and the sarcomatous element resembles normal endometrial stroma.

Heterologous

These tumors consist of carcinomatous elements from endometrial glands and sarcomatous elements which are not normally found in the uterus such as cartilage, bone or striated muscle and hence the name. The different types of mesodermal elements are likely to be derived from totipotential endometrial stromal cells. Spread usually occurs to the pelvic lymph nodes, peritoneal cavity and distant organs. These tumors behave more aggressively than endometrial adenocarcinoma. Upper abdominal spread is common at the time of diagnosis.

The presenting complaint is usually post-menopausal bleeding or vaginal discharge. As the tumor typically arises from the fundus of the uterus and project as polypoidal masses into the uterine cavity which sometimes extrude out through the cervix, they may be mistaken for polyps. Rarely the patient may complain of passing a fleshy mass. Diagnosis is usually made from biopsy of the polyp or endometrial curettage. Imaging shows large mass filing and distending the uterine cavity (Fig. 20.10). Surgico-pathological staging is advised as in endometrial adenocarcinoma. Age and depth of myometrial invasion are significant prognostic factors. Treatment is total hysterectomy, bilateral salpingo-oophorectomy and omentectomy followed by postoperative radiation in the presence of residual disease. The NCCN practice guideline recommends chemotherapy and radiation therapy as additional treatment options even for Stage I disease.

For stage III disease, aggressive surgical removal followed by adjuvant radiation and chemotherapy are advised. Prognosis depends upon the extent of tumor spread. Five year survival is reported as 75% in patients whose tumor is confined to the uterus. Tumor extension to the cervix and parametrium carries very poor prognosis.

20.19 CONCLUSION

Endometrial carcinoma is a relatively common female genital cancer. The role of estrogen in causing endometrial hyperplasia and carcinoma should be emphasized in young women who have chronic anovulation. These girls should be given progestagens for at least ten days in a month starting from adolescence so that they do not develop endometrial hyperplasia. Estrogen alone should not be given as HRT. Women with HNPCC gene mutation have a life time risk of 40-60% for the development of the disease. There is no effective screening strategy for detecting the disease in the premalignant or early malignant stage.TVS should be done for all perimenopausal as well as postmenopausal women who present with abnormal vaginal bleeding, as it can predict endometrial pathology to a very great extent. Histo-pathological confirmation either by endometrial aspiration or hysteroscopic biopsy is mandatory before treatment. Surgical staging is advised even for advanced disease as it will help to delineate the extent of spread, to perform optimal debulking and to plan postoperative radiation tailored to the particular extent necessary. Lymphadenectomy should be part of surgical staging unless the tumor is very small, well differentiated with no myometrial invasion or only superficial invasion. Patients who are detected to have extension to the cervix clinically can be better treated by preoperative radiation followed by surgery and adjuvant radiation. Cure rate of the disease is good for the endometrioid type of the tumor especially if well differentiated. Papillary serous and clear cell carcinomas which account for about 10% of the cases are highly malignant and carry high mortality rate. Prognosis depends on surgicopathologic staging, DNA ploidy and steroid receptor status.

20.20 CASE SCENARIOS

Case Scenario 1

M/s A 65-year-old lady presented with irregular bleeding per vaginum of 5 months duration. She also had pain abdomen since one week. She did not have loss of weight or loss of appetite. She is married for 40 years and has one 37 years old daughter. Her menarche was at 13 years of age and she attained menopause 23 years back. She had menorrhagia prior to menopause. She is diabetic for 20 years and hypertensive for 10 years. On examination she was found to be hypertensive. There was no generalized lymphadenopathy. Abdominal examination was unremarkable. Local examination revealed normal vulva, vagina and cervix. Bimanual examination showed a bulky uterus which was mobile and no mass in the fornices. Transvaginal ultrasound showed thickened endometrium (15 mm). The endometrial myometrial interface was irregular, pointing towards malignancy. Deep myometrial invasion could not be made out. Endometrial sampling was done with Pipelle. The histopathology report was endometrial adenocarcinoma well differentiated.

Is there any role for further imaging with MRI or CT?
If facilities are available MRI will help make out the extent of myometrial invasion. CT will be better in making out secondary deposits in the abdomen.

MRI pelvis (Fig. 20.11) was done which showed endometrial thickness of 14 mm. The endometrial myometrial interface was irregular. There was a tongue like extension of tumor tissue into the deeper area of myometrium up to the serosa. There was no extension to the cervix.

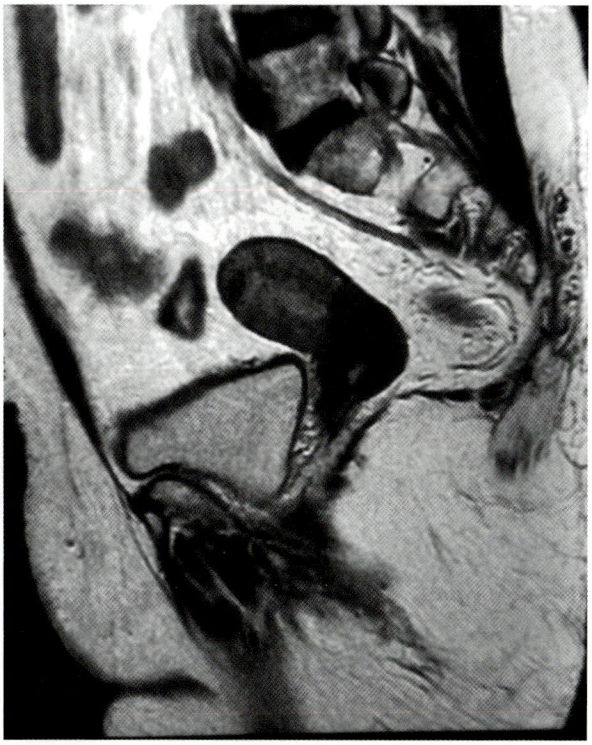

Fig. 20.11: MRI picture showing myometrial invasion in the fundo-anterior aspect

What should be the extent of surgical staging?
Along with extrafacial hysterectomy and pelvic lymphadenectomy, para-aortic node dissection should also be done as there is chance for para-aortic node involvement in view of deep myometrial invasion made out by MRI scan.

This lady had exploratory laparotomy, peritoneal fluid cytology, extrafascial hysterectomy and omentectomy. Pelvic and para-aortic lymphadenectomy were also done.

The histopathology report was as follows:

Uterus showing grade 1 endometrial adenocarcinoma infiltrating more than half of the myometrium. The cervix, lymph nodes and omentum were found to be negative for malignancy. Peritoneal cytology showed clusters of benign mesothelial cells and no malignant cells.

Is postoperative radiation indicated?
Even though the tumor according to the surgical stage is confined to the uterus, due to the presence of deep myometrial invasion, she needs to be treated with pelvic radiation.

Case Scenario 2

Mrs B, a 58-year-old postmenopausal lady with a history of adjuvant Tamoxifen therapy for 2 years following mastectomy for carcinoma breast, presented with vaginal spotting. General examination was unremarkable. Abdomino-pelvic examination revealed an irregularly enlarged uterus with an apparently normal cervix and vagina. Ultrasound examination showed multiple fibroids. The endometrial cavity appeared to harbor a mass which

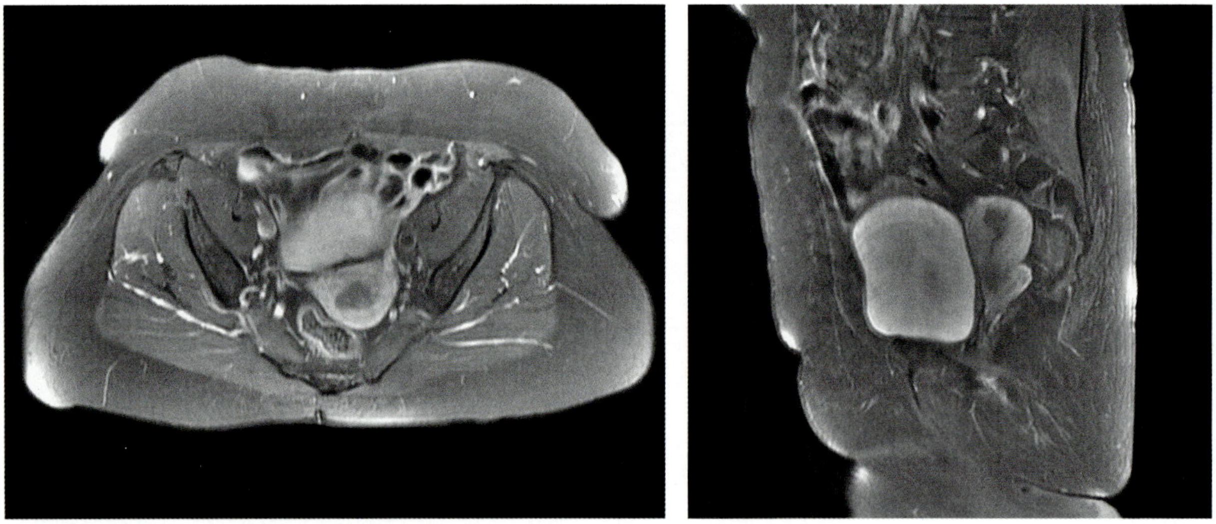

Fig. 20.12: MRI showing < 50% myometrial invasion which is better made out by dynamic contrast study

however could not be properly evaluated due to the presence of multiple fibroids. Endo-myometrial interface appeared irregular. Endometrial sampling revealed endometrioid adenocarcinoma Grade II.

What is the next imaging option which will give a definite idea about the size of the tumor and the extent of the disease?

MRI is the ideal imaging modality to make out the size of the tumor and its extent. This woman's MRI showed an enlarged uterus with multiple fibroids, an endometrial growth of 24 mm, disruption of the junctional zone s/o myometrial invasion (<50 % of its thickness) (Fig. 20.12) and no extension to the endocervix or pelvic lymph nodes.

What would be the clinical staging?

The clinical stage is I as the tumor is confined to the uterus.

What should be the treatment plan?

The treatment should comprise peritoneal fluid sampling, exploratory laparotomy and surgico-pathological staging.

Should lymphadenectomy be done?

Although mandated by the FIGO staging system, lymphadenectomy of the pelvic and para-aortic areas remain controversial. Para-aortic lymphadenectomy is reserved for patients with high risk features. Since this patient has no high risk features that warrant para-aortic lymphadenectomy, lymphadenectomy can be limited to the pelvic nodes.

If this patient had an enlarged lymph node which on frozen section showed malignant cells, should pelvic lymphadenectomy be proceeded with?

No, since the presence of an enlarged involved node necessitates pelvic irradiation, removal of further lymph nodes which are not enlarged is not warranted.

Her HPR came as endometrioid adenocarcinoma with < 50% myometrial invasion, no cervical extension and negative pelvic nodes. Does she require any adjuvant therapy?

Yes, in view of the myometrial invasion and the grade of the disease she needs vaginal vault radiation to prevent vault recurrence.

Case Scenario 3

Mrs P, 49-year-old postmenopausal lady presented with bleeding per vaginum for 3 months duration. General examination was unremarkable. Speculum examination revealed normal vagina and cervix. Uterus was found to be bulky on bimanual examination. Ultrasound showed uterine cavity to be filled with a tumor of about 4 cm size, but the extent of myometrial invasion could not be clearly made out. Doppler showed increased vascularity with low resistance flow. She underwent fractional curettage. There were no endocervical curettings. Endometrial curettings appeared cheesy and plenty. The histopathology report came as adenocarcinoma endometrium Grade II.

What is the clinical stage of the disease?

Clinically the disease is stage I.

What is the place of MR imaging in this lady?

The extent of myometrial invasion can be clearly made out. In the presence of deep myometrial invasion, para-aortic sampling should be planned.

MR imaging was done. The report- Polypoidal mass of 4.4 × 3 cm within endometrial cavity, Disruption of junctional zone, infiltrating < 50% of myometrium, Cervix normal, no enlarged pelvic nodes, post wall fibroid.

What is the management?

Since the disease is in clinical stage I, surgico-pathological staging should be advised.

She underwent surgical staging. The pathology report of the specimen is as follows.

HPR- Papillary growth extending to cervix, not infiltrating myometrium, multiple fibroids, Grade II adenocarcinoma- Stage II A

What is your comment?

Extension to the cervix was missed at fractional curettage as well as imaging.

What postoperative treatment should be advised?

In lieu of the extension to the cervix, she needs whole pelvic radiation.

REFERENCES

1. RJ Kurman, RJ Semin. Diagn Pathol 1988;5:154-71.
2. Goff BA, Kato B, Schmidt RA, et al. Gynaecol Onco 1994;54:264-68.
3. Dijkuizen FPHI.J, MolBWJ, Brolmann HAM, et al. Cancer 2000;89:1765-72.
4. Gordon AN, Fleiseher AC, Dudley BS, et al. Gynaecological Oncology 1989;34:175-79.
5. Niloff JM, Klug TO, Schaetzi E, et al. Am J Obstet Gynaecol 1984;148:1057-58.
6. Wilson TO, Podratz KC, Gaffey TA, et al. Evaluation of unfavourable histologic subtypes in endometrial adenocarcinoma. Am J Obstet Gynecol 1990;162:418-26.
7. Wilson TO, Podratz KC, Gaffey TA, et al. Evaluation of unfavourable histologic subtypes in endometrial adenocarcinoma. Am J Obstet Gynecol 1990;162:418-26.
8. Abeler VM, Kjorstad KE, Berle E Int J Gynecol Cancer 1992;2:9-32.
9. DiSaia PJ, Creasman WT, Boronow RC, Blessing JA. Risk factors and recurrence patterns in Stage I endometrial cancer Am J Obstet Gynecol 1985;151:1009-15.
10. Lurain JR, Rice BL, Rademaker AW, et al. Prognostic factors associated with recurrence in clinical stage I adenocarcinoma of the endometrium Obstet Gynecol 1991;78:63-69.
11. Schink JC, Rademaker AW, Miller DS, et al. Tumor size in endometrial cancer. Cancer1991;67:2791-94.
12. Kilgore LC, Partridge EE, Alvarez RD, Austin JM, Shingleton HM, Noojin F, 3rd, et al. Adenocarcinoma of the endometrium: survival comparisons of patients with and without pelvic node sampling. Gynecol Oncol 1995;56 (I):29-33.
13. Larson DM, Broste SK, Krawisz BR. Surgery without radiotherapy for primary treatment of endometrial cancer. Obstet Gynecol 1998;91(3):355-9. The MRC ASTEC
14. Chan JK, Lin YG, Monk BJ, et al. Vaginal hysterectomy as primary treatment for endometrial carcinoma in medically compromised women. Obstet Gynecol 2001;97:707-11.
15. Gemignani M, Curtin JP, Zelmanovich J, et al. Laparoscopically Assisted Vaginal Hysterectomy for endometrial Carcinoma clinical outcomes and hospital charges. Gynecol Oncol 1999;73:5-11.
16. Kong A, Johnson N, Cornes P, Simera I, Collingwood M, Williams C, Kitchener H. Adjuvant radiotherapy for stage I endometrial cancer. Cochrane Database of Systematic Reviews 2007, Issue 2. Art. No.: CD003916. DOI: 10.1002/14651858.CD003916.
17. Martin-Hirsch P L, Jarvis G, Kitchener H, Lilford R. Progestagens for endometrial cancer. Cochrane Database of Systematic Reviews 1999, Issue 4. Art. No.: CD001040. DOI: 10.1002/14651858.CD001040.
18. Randall ME, Brunetto G, Muss H, et al. Whole abdominal Radiotherapy vs combination doxorubicin cisplatin chemotherapy in advanced endometrial carcinoma, a randomized phase 3 trial of the Gynecologic Oncology Group Proc Am Soc Clin Oncol 2003;22.
19. Randall ME, Brunetto G, Muss HB, et al. Whole abdominal radiotherapy versus combination doxorubicin-cisplatin chemotherapy in advanced endometrial carcinoma: a randomized phase III trial of the Gynecologic Oncology Group. Proc Am Soc Clin Oncol 2003;22:2.
20. Seli E, Tangir J. Fertility preservation options for female patients with malignancies. Curr Opin Obstet Gynecol 2005;17(3):299-308.
21. Rackow BW, Arici A. Endometrial cancer and fertility. Curr Opin Obstet Gynecol 2006;18(3):245-52.
22. Fazio SB, Ship AN. Abnormal uterine bleeding. South Med J 2007;100(4):376-82.

21 Premalignant Diseases of the Cervix

B Presannakumari

21.1 INTRODUCTION

Cervical cancer, the second most common malignancy, in women has a long pre-invasive stage of 10-13 years. This long pre-invasive stage forms the basis of screening for cervical malignancy, by detecting the premalignant lesions of the cervix. In the 1940s and 50s, it was understood that pre-invasive lesions precede invasive cancer of the cervix.

George Papanicolaou, a Greek pathologist was indulged in studying exfoliated cells from the cervix and their transformations associated with menstruation. As one of his patients happened to be suffering from cervical cancer, he discovered that the abnormal cancer cells could be plainly detected on microscopic examination.

In 1941, Papanicolaou and H.F. Traut published their landmark discovery of diagnosing malignant and premalignant lesions by examination of exfoliated cells in the American Journal of Obstetrics and Gynaecology. This has led to the widespread application of the cervical smear testing popularly known as the Pap test (Papanicolaou smear test) which is the best cancer screening program available till now.

Papanicolaou classified exfoliated cells from the cervix into five classes.

Papanicolaou's Numeric Classification

Class I—Benign
Class II—Minor cellular abnormalities, considered benign

Class III—Cells suspicious - but not diagnostic of cancer
Class IV—Cells fairly conclusive of malignancy
Class V—Cells diagnostic of cancer

Since this classification lacked precision, new nomenclatures came into existence.

Dysplasia/CIN System of classification: Histopathologically, the premalignant lesions were originally named dysplasias. It was Richart who came forth with the terminology of cervical intraepithelial neoplasia (CIN) which signified that all types of dysplasias can progress to invasive cancer. Richart classified preinvasive changes of the cervix into - CIN-I, CIN-II and CIN-III.

This was based on the degree of:

a. Cellular immaturity
b. Cellular disorganization
c. Nuclear abnormalities
d. Number of mitotic activities

Squamous metaplasia should not be included under CIN as these changes are not precursors of cancer of the cervix.

Bethesda Classification System: The Bethesda system evolved from a National Cancer Institute workshop at Bethesda in 1989. This was modified in the year 1991 and later in 2001 as the Bethesda III system which is the presently followed system of reporting cervical smear. It was introduced in order to achieve better communication between the cytopathologist and the clinician. The Bethesda system is more precise than the previous two systems of reporting and allows better peer review and quality control. This would be dealt with in detail later.

21.2 PATHOLOGY OF PREMALIGNANT LESIONS OF CERVIX

Premalignant lesions of the cervix, otherwise called cervical intraepithelial neoplasia (CIN) are characterized by architectural and cytological changes. Architectural changes include abnormalities in differentiation, stratification and maturation (Fig. 21.1). Based on the proportion of the thickness of the epithelium showing differentiation seen in histopathology, CIN is classified into CIN I, CIN II and CIN III. In CIN I, the upper half of the epithelium usually shows differentiation and lower half shows abnormalities in stratification and maturation. In CIN II, more than half of the epithelium does not show differentiation. In CIN III, there is very little or no differentiation. Cytological

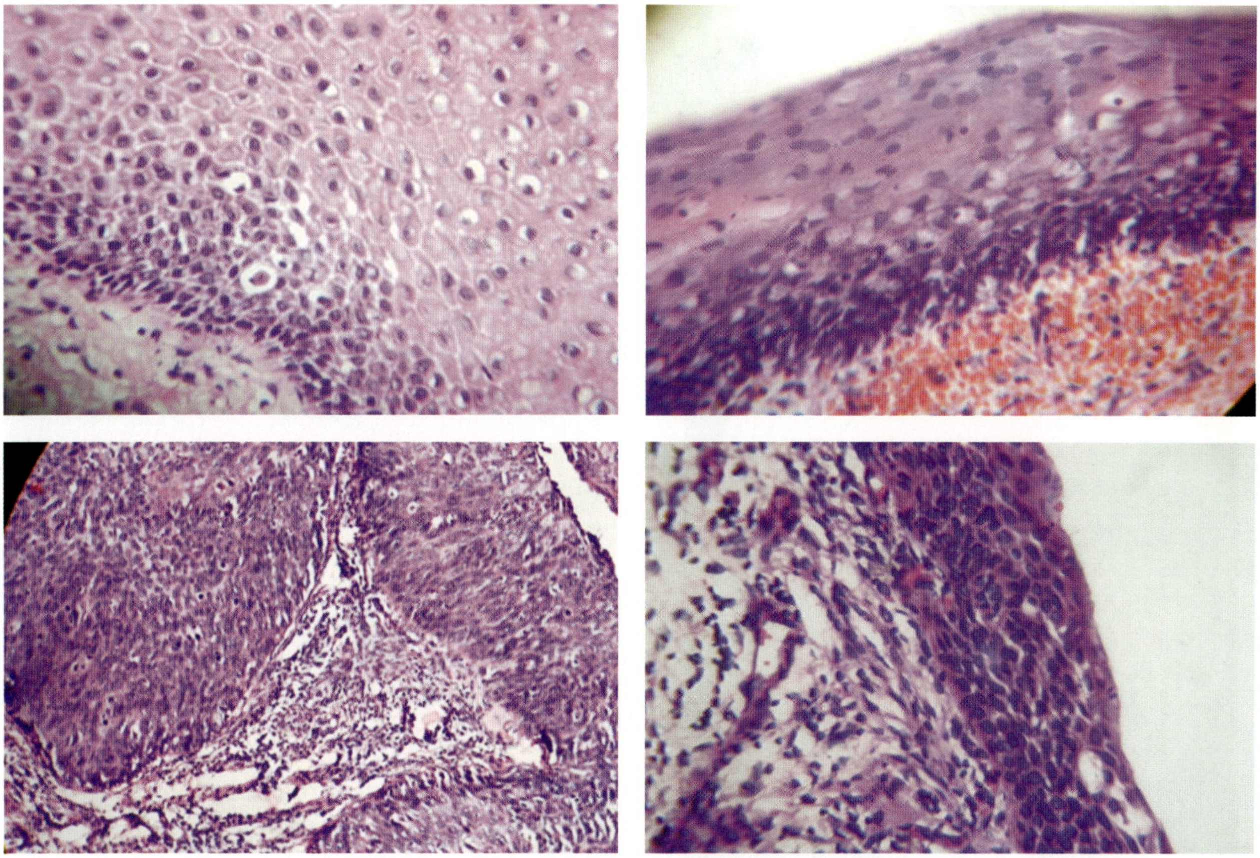

Fig. 21.1: (Clockwise from left) Normal histology of cervix, CIN-I, CIN-II and CIN-III

abnormalities are also important in assessing the severity of CIN. Nuclear cytoplasmic ratio, hyperchromasia, nuclear polymorphism and number of mitotic figures are also taken into consideration to classify CIN. CIN can affect the surface epithelium as well as the gland crypts. This is the basis of treating CIN by destroying up to 5 mm into the stroma. But most experts advise destroying up to 10 mm depth.

21.2.1 Transformation Zone

Cervical cancer almost always begins at the squamo-columnar junction (SCJ) and spreads externally to become exocervical cancer (80%) or spreads internally to become endocervical cancer (20%). Endocervical canal is normally lined by columnar epithelium and the exocervix by stratified squamous epithelium (Fig. 21.2). The point at which they meet is the SCJ.The SCJ is a dynamic area that changes in response to the hormonal influence at puberty, pregnancy and menopause. In the pre-pubertal period SCJ is located more externally. Estrogen production at menarche causes cells at the SCJ to undergo metaplasia. Metaplasia starts at the SCJ and proceed inwards towards the external os. This metaplastic area is called the TZ, which extends from the original SCJ to the physiologically active SCJ. The metaplastic epithelium matures into squamous epithelium taking the SCJ inwards. HPV infection is supposed to be the triggering factor for malignancy of the cervix. During the years of squamous metaplasia, the cells at the SCJ are susceptible to oncogenic stimuli because of the rapid turnover. HPV infection, occurring during menarche or after pregnancy when metaplasia is active is important in the pathogenesis of carcinoma cervix. During colposcopic evaluation of the cervix, the entire extent of TZ should be evaluated. If the upper extent of TZ cannot be visualized, it should be evaluated by endocervical curettage. After menopause because of the atrophy of cervix, the SCJ will be drawn into the endocervix making it difficult to evaluate the same.

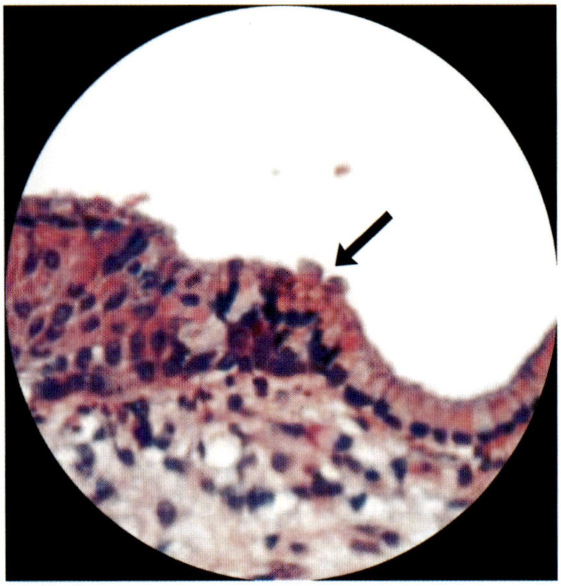

Fig. 21.2: Histology of transformation zone

21.2.2 Adenocarcinoma *in situ*

Adenocarcinoma in-situ (AIS) is the precursor of invasive adenocarcinoma. It is predominantly seen in younger women in the early 30s. AIS usually starts at the transformation zone and contiguous endocervical canal. When the endocervical curettage report indicates AIS, co-existing invasive disease can be present higher-up in the canal or as a skip lesion. Hence, patients reported as having AIS by endocervical curettage or colposcopically directed biopsy should have conization to exclude invasive disease elsewhere in the endocervical canal. There can be multifocal disease also. Loop excision in this situation is not the ideal procedure as it may miss lesions higher up in the endocervix. Hence a cold knife conization should be done. For a patient who wishes to conserve the childbearing function follow-up is enough, provided the margins are free of disease. If the margins are positive the chance of residual AIS or chance of co-existing invasive disease[1] is as high as 50%.

Even if the margins are negative, residual AIS might occur later at follow-up, which may represent multi-focal disease or another fresh lesion. Follow-up of AIS occurring in the endocervical canal is not as accurate as carcinoma-*in situ* of the exocervix. Hence, hysterectomy is advisable for women having AIS, who have completed family.

Adenocarcinoma *in situ*

AIS, on endocervical curettage can signify co-existing invasive disease higher up in the canal or a skip lesion. Hence, these patients should have cold knife conization to exclude invasive disease elsewhere in the endocervical canal.

For a patient whose cone biopsy shows AIS, it is advisable to offer hysterectomy if she has completed family, because follow-up of these women is not as effective as carcinoma-*in situ* of the exo-cervix.

21.3 CERVICAL CANCER SCREENING

21.3.1 The Pap Test

Papanicolaou and Traut's findings concluded that pre-malignant lesions and malignant lesions could be diagnosed by studying the morphology of the exfoliated cells. An ideal screening test should have reasonable sensitivity, specificity,

> **The Pap test**
> - The pap test is the most effective cancer screening test available till now.
> - The sensitivity ranges from 47%-62%.
> - The specificity ranges from 60%-95%.
> - The false negative rate of a single smear is as high as 50%.

> **Advantages of liquid based cytology**
> - Cell transfer from the spatula to the liquid medium is better than transfer from spatula to the slide.
> - Presence of obscuring material in the slide like blood, mucus, overlapping cells or inflammatory cells which reduce the ability to read the smear can be avoided.
> - Liquid based smear is easy to read which saves much time.

cost effectiveness, safety and also should have the ability to detect the disease in a treatable stage. The Papanicolaou smear test (Pap test) fulfills almost all of these criteria. In countries where regular Pap tests are being done, the incidence of invasive cancer of the cervix has been reduced by approximately 70%.

Dr. Papanicolaou's[2] initial method of collecting cervical cells was by using a glass pipette with a rubber-bulb at the end for suction effect. The cells were collected from the posterior fornix. Later in the year 1947, J. Ernest Ayre, a gynecologist from McGill University, Montreal, introduced wooden spatula for obtaining cells from the cervix. With this method, cells which were not already exfoliated could be collected, increasing the sensitivity.

After the introduction of the Pap test as a screening test for cervical cancer, both the mortality as well as morbidity due to cervical cancer has come down in developed countries where a regular screening program is available. However several publications have documented that the test lacks sensitivity as well as specificity. The sensitivity of a single Pap test in detecting CINII or greater lesions ranges between 47% and 62% and specificity ranges between 60% and 95%. The false negative rate of a single smear is reported to be as high as 50%. Hence, the sensitivity after 3 consecutive tests would be 86.8% only. The greatest reason for this high false negative rate is sampling error, another being the defective transfer of the sampled cells from the spatula to a slide in conventional smear. Presence of obscuring material in the slide like blood, mucus, overlapping cells or inflammatory cells also reduces the ability to fully evaluate the smear. This false negative rate is important in countries where there are poor resource settings and the patients cannot afford regular cervical smear, but can have minimal number of smears in their lifetime. Hence reducing the false negative rate of a single smear should be considered seriously.

21.3.2 Liquid based Cytology

The obscuring factors like blood, mucus or inflammatory cells in the conventional smear can be reduced by transferring the collected cells into a liquid media. Thus cell transfer to the medium can be improved. It is also easier to read the smear from a preparation of the cells in a liquid medium. In liquid based cytology the smear is collected with a plastic spatula and the spatula is vigorously agitated in a collection medium and the medium is then placed in a thin Prep 2000/3000 processor. In the processor the blood, mucus or debris is broken. The fluid containing the cells is drawn into a Thinprep filter resulting in a thin even layer of cellular material. The material from the filter is transferred to a glass slide and the slide is placed in a fixative bath. Thus a slide containing a circle of diagnostic material of 20 mm is prepared. This can be analyzed manually or by automated methods. These slides are much easier to screen, thereby reducing screening time. The remaining fluid in the vial can be tested for HPV DNA. Studies have shown that specimen adequacy of liquid based cytology is much superior to conventional smears. Available literature supports the fact that liquid based cytology can detect few more cases of HGSIL[3] (High Grade Squamous Intraepithelial Lesions) which might have been undetected.

21.3.3 Guidelines for Screening

The American College of Obstetricians and Gynecologists (ACOG), the American Cancer Society (ACS) and the American Society of Colposcopy and Cervical Pathology (ASCCP) recommend starting cervical cancer screening at age 21 or within 3 years of the onset of sexual activity. Screening before 18 years is no longer recommended. The reason being, most women become infected with HPV when they become sexually active. More than 70% of these infections clear by itself. If a smear is taken during active infection there is a high chance that low grade squamous intraepithelial lesions are detected leading to over-treatment. The ACS recommends subsequent cervical smear testing every year by conventional Pap or every 2 years by liquid based Pap. After the age of 30, testing every 2-3 year is enough, provided 3 consecutive smears are normal. Testing can be discontinued if 3 consecutive smear reports in 10 years are found to be normal. The recommendation of the

ACOG differs slightly. The test frequency is yearly irrespective of whether liquid based or conventional Pap is resorted to. There is no upper limit to discontinue screening.

If HPV DNA testing is combined with cervical cytology for women older than 30 years, the negative predictive value can be improved. If both HPV DNA and cervical cytology are negative, negative predictive value is >99%.

21.3.4 The Reporting System of Cervical Smear (Table 21.1)

Bethesda III System

As has been discussed earlier, the reporting system of cervical smear has changed from the original class system to the Bethesda system. The Bethesda system of reporting cervical smear was initially formulated in 1989 at the National Cancer Institute Workshop at Bethesda. In an effort to give clear significance to the various types of cytological abnormalities, it was revised in 1991 and later in 2001- The Bethesda III classification. Cervical smear is to be reported in the Bethesda system and histopathology of biopsy using the CIN terminology.

The Bethesda III report has the following sections:

a. Specimen type
b. Specimen adequacy
c. General categorization
d. Automated review
e. Ancillary testing - HPV DNA
f. Interpretation/Result
g. Educational notes and suggestions

Specimen type: The report should specify whether the smear was prepared in the conventional manner or by the liquid-based technology or collected from the vaginal cuff (post-hysterectomy).

Specimen adequacy: The report should specify whether the specimen is satisfactory or unsatisfactory for evaluation depending on the adequacy of the number of squamous cells and transformation zone (TZ) cells seen and also on the presence or absence of obscuring factors like blood. The number of squamous cells should be adequate for evaluation. Presence of RBCs will obscure the smear making it unsatisfactory for evaluation. Adequate specimens should have an estimated 8,000 to 12,000 well-preserved and well-visualized squamous cells. Liquid-based specimens should contain an estimated minimum of 5,000 well-visualized and well-preserved squamous cells.

General categorization (Figs 21.3 and 21.4): The term "within normal limits" is replaced by a more clear term - negative for intraepithelial lesion or malignancy. The Report should specify the grade of epithelial abnormality and also the type of abnormal epithelium found, whether squamous or glandular. The previously reported "benign cellular changes" is now referred to as "negative for intraepithelial lesion or malignancy. If there is any evidence of infection with Trichomonas vaginalis, Candida or bacterial vaginosis, it should be noted. Women with unsatisfactory slide should have a repeat Pap test done within 2-4 months. The report should make note of specimens taken from women 40 years or older. Endometrial cells after the age of 40, particularly in women who are perimenopausal or after menopause, may be associated with benign endometrium, hormonal alterations and, less commonly, endometrial abnormalities and may require further evaluation.

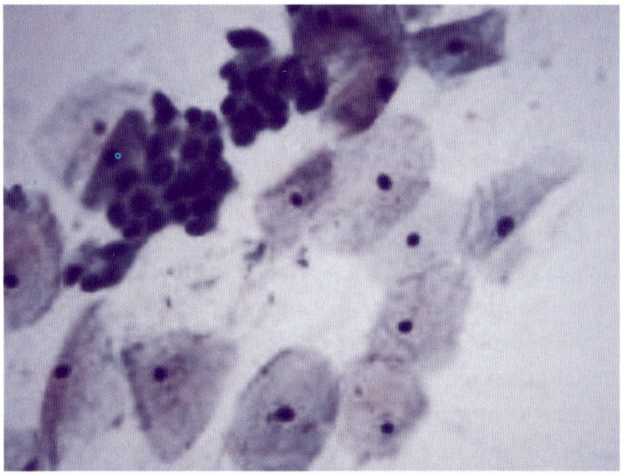

Fig. 21.3: Normal cervical smear

Table 21.1: Reporting systems of cervical smear and biopsy

Earlier terminology of reporting cervical smear	*Richart (1967) histopathology*	*Bethesda system cytology*
Mild dysplasia	CIN I and HPV changes	Low grade lesion
Moderate dysplasia	CIN II	High grade lesion
Severe dysplasia	CIN III	
Carcinoma-in-situ		

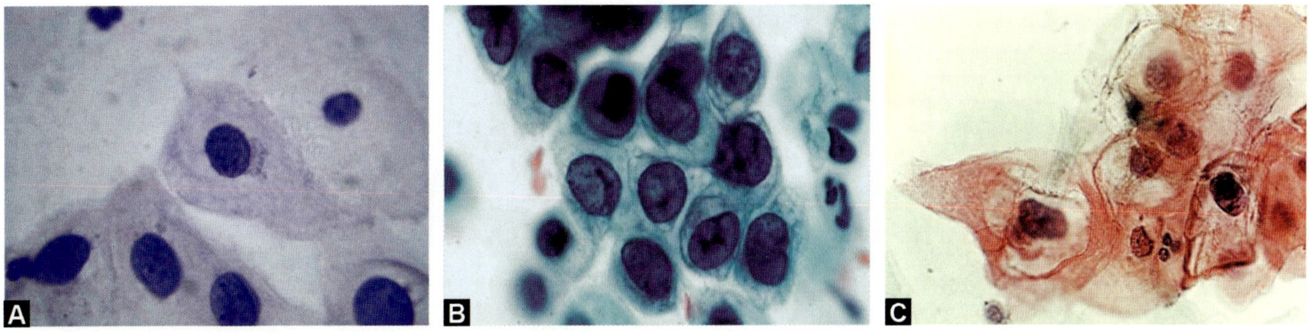

Figs 21.4A to C: Cervical smear showing LSIL (A), HSIL (B) koilocytic changes (C)

Under this system, potentially pre-malignant squamous lesions fall into 3 categories:

1. Atypical squamous cells-ASC
2. Low grade squamous intraepithelial lesions—LSIL (previously Mild dysplasia and HPV changes)
3. High grade squamous intraepithelial lesions—HSIL (previously moderate dysplasia, severe dysplasia and carcinoma *in situ*)

ASC is sub-divided into:

1. Those of unknown significance - ASC-US
2. Those in which high grade lesions should be excluded - ASC-H

Glandular Cell Abnormalities

The revision also included abnormal glandular epithelium, including atypical glandular cells. The abnormal glandular cells seen are classified under the following headings.

1. Atypical glandular cells
   a. Endocervical
   b. Endometrial
   c. Glandular cells not otherwise specified
2. Atypical glandular cells favor neoplasia
   a. Endocervical cells favor neoplasia
   b. Glandular cells favor neoplasia
3. Endocervical adenocarcinoma in-situ
4. Adenocarcinoma
   a. Endocervical
   b. Endometrial
   c. Extrauterine
   d. Not otherwise specified

Atypical Glandular Cell - AGC

The previously noted "Atypical glandular cells of undetermined significance" is replaced by the term "atypical glandular cells". If the glandular cells can be differentiated as endocervical or endometrial, it should be noted in the report. In a 5 year retrospective review of patients who had AGC on Pap smear, positive predictive value of high grade lesions were found to be higher than that of ASC. Hence it should be understood that although AGC are rare (1% of smears), if identified, approximately 48% patients have higher lesions like SIL, adenocarcinoma in situ and invasive carcinoma. In such instances, other than colposcopy, investigations like hysteroscopy or fractional curettage may be necessary.

When the smear shows adenocarcinoma cells, it should be reported as "adenocarcinoma not otherwise specified" if it is not clear whether it is endocervical or endometrial. The report should make a note of specimens taken from women 40 years or older. The presence of endometrial cells in cervical smear in such women needs further evaluation for endometrial abnormalities.

The most important revision is the ASC category. This facilitated triage of women for more intense screening when a true suspicion of a high grade lesion was present.

Automated Review

If the smear is examined by automated machine, the type of system and the results obtained should be specified.

Ancillary Testing

Ancillary molecular testing if done should be reported (e.g. HPV DNA). But it is ideal to report the ancillary molecular testing results concurrently with the cytology results which may not be always feasible.

Educational Notes and Suggestions

Educational notes, which comprise of the significance of the findings and the differential diagnoses, should be conveyed to the provider. The provider should be able to identify the patient who needs further management or repeat examinations. The term 'diagnosis' is to be replaced with 'results' which should be highlighted. The use of acronyms is discouraged for clarity purposes.

21.4 EVALUATION OF ABNORMAL CERVICAL CYTOLOGY

Patients who have abnormal cytological smear report should ideally undergo colposcopic evaluation of the cervix. Colposcopy is visualization of the cervix under magnification. It was Hinselmann who first described examining the cervix under magnification to locate biopsy site for detecting premalignant and malignant lesions in the year1925. With the help of the present day colposcope, a 3D image of external genitalia, exocervix and distal endocervical canal can be obtained under a magnification of 4× to 40×.

Premalignant lesions and malignancy cause changes in the cervix, due to the loss of cell to cell cohesion, neo vascularization and opacities due to keratinization. The underlying blood vessels are not usually visualized through the normal squamous epithelium. In premalignant lesions and malignancy, the new blood vessels formed are visible through the epithelium due to loss of epithelial integrity. These new blood vessels formed will make patterns in the cervical epithelium, which are visualized with the help of colposcope. The pattern is different in low grade lesions, high grade lesions and malignancy. By observing the pattern of blood vessels, one will be able to make out which areas are harboring low grade lesions, high grade lesions and malignancies to a great extent.

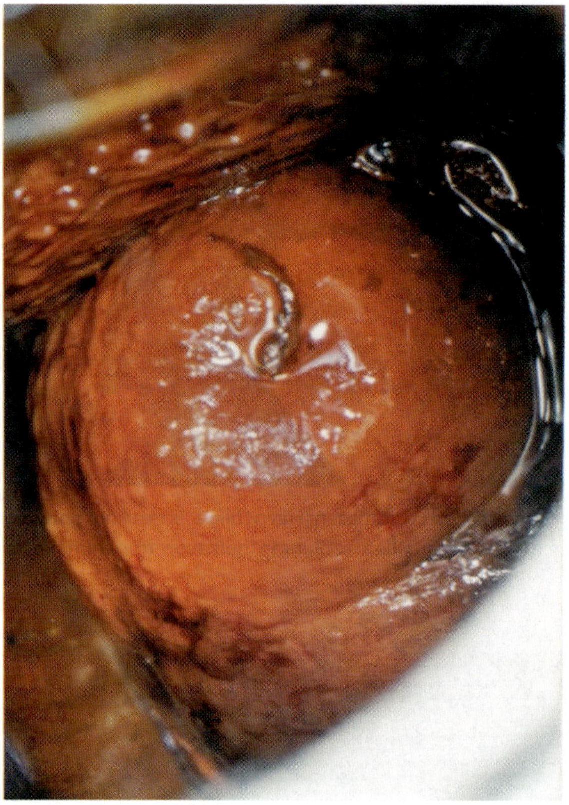

Fig. 21.5: Gross appearance of cervix showing evidence of HPV infection

21.4.1 Colposcopic Evaluation of the Cervix

The cervix should be exposed with the help of a Cusco's speculum. The cervical mucus is wiped off with a saline swab. The exocervix, the entire transfomation zone (TZ), the distal endocervix and the vaginal cuff are examined for abnormalities (Fig. 21.5). Since cervical malignancy almost always starts at the TZ and spreads externally or internally into the cervical canal, visualization of the TZ is very important. The cervix should be examined for areas of leukoplakia (Fig. 21.6). The importance of this is that there can be abnormal epithelium behind the areas of leucoplakia, which has to be biopsied. In post menopausal women, the TZ is drawn into the endocervical canal and sometimes cannot be visualized completely. Endocervical curettage should be done for such patients. Yet another situation which mandates endocervical curettage is when the cervical smear shows abnormal cells and no obvious lesion is noted in the exocervix, TZ or distal endocervical canal.

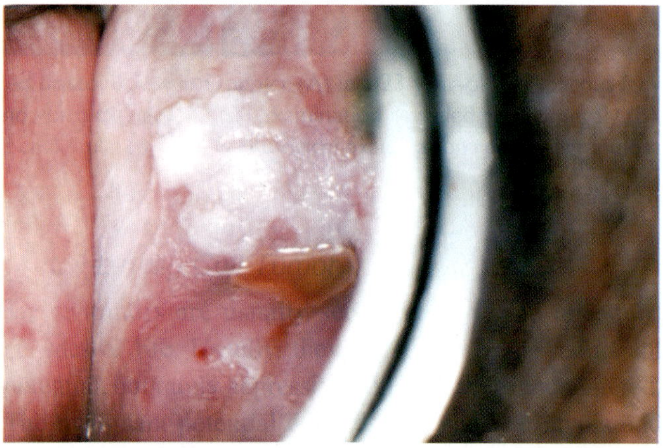

Fig. 21.6: CIN III masked by leukoplakia

The cervix is painted with 3-5% acetic acid and examined for acetowhite areas one minute after application of acetic acid. Acetic acid coagulates the proteins of the cells and makes the area white. The normal squamous cells which contain glycogen do not allow acetic acid to permeate inside.

Also, the normal squamous cells do not contain much protein, instead they contain glycogen. Hence after painting with acetic acid, normal squamous cells will be pink, whereas the abnormal areas which are deficient in glycogen and rich in protein will appear whitish due to the coagulation of protein.

Acetowhite areas can be a low grade lesion, high grade lesion, malignant lesion or immature metaplastic lesion. An experienced colposcopist will be able to differentiate these areas by studying the border, site and shape of the lesions.

Vascular Patterns

The new blood vessels formed, which shine through the abnormal epithelium produces different patterns in the cervix. The end-on view of blood vessels will emulate a pattern of punctation. The abnormally branched vessels will produce a mosaic pattern. In the low grade lesions, the mosaic and punctate lesions are fine and regular, whereas in high grade lesions, they are coarse and irregular. The blood vessels in invasive lesions are bigger and will sprout through the epithelium giving the appearance of comma or cork-screw (Fig. 22.4 provided in chapter on carcinoma cervix).

Cervix should also be examined after painting with Lugol's iodine. The normal areas will be stained brown due to the presence of glycogen. The endocervical epithelium, immature metaplasia, severe atrophy (postmenopausal), dysplastic areas and carcinomatous areas will not take up the stain and will be Iodine negative. These areas must be biopsied.

If squamocolumnar junction cannot be entirely visualized, colposcopic examination is classified as 'unsatisfactory'. In such situations, endocervical curettage should be combined with colposcopy.

21.4.2 Colposcopically Directed Biopsy

All abnormal areas singled out with colposcopy should be confirmed by biopsy and histopathological examination. The biopsy can be a punch biopsy or an excisional procedure like loop electrosurgical excision procedure (LEEP). In LEEP, an electrosurgical loop is used to remove a sample of tissue. Although LEEP is used interchangeably with large loop excision of transformation zone (LLETZ), LLETZ refers to the removal of entire Tz using electrosurgical loop in a single piece. Even though in theory, LEEP is removal of abnormal area of the cervix for diagnosis, in practice the entire transformation zone will be removed when it is performed.

In a 'see and treat' policy, cervix is examined under colposcope and LLETZ procedure is carried out at the same time as a part of treatment.

Indications for Cold Knife Conization

1. After the LLETZ procedure, if margins are not clear of abnormal areas
2. If endocervical curetting shows cells suggestive of high grade lesions
3 If a punch biopsy or LEEP shows microinvasion, a conventional cone should be done to exclude frank invasion elsewhere in the cervix.

Procedure of Cold Knife Conization

The cervix is painted with Lugol's iodine and the abnormal areas are delineated. 1% Lignocaine is injected along with vasoconstrictor norepinephrine or epinephrine for producing anesthesia and reducing hemorrhage. A cone shaped portion of the cervix with the apex of the cone at the level of the internal os is cut with knife and removed entirely. The specimen is marked at the 12 o' clock position for orientation.

Accuracy of Colposcopy

The clinical correlation between colposcopy and histopathology[4] has been reported variably in various studies. Overall accuracy of colposcopy is reported as 83.5%. If colposcopy is satisfactory, the accuracy is as high as 96.4%. Colposcopic accuracy increases as the grade of lesion and the area of lesion increases.

21.4.3 Cervicography

Cervicography is developed in an effort to evaluate large number of patients by a single trained person. A snapshot of the cervical appearance by colposcopy is taken by a non medical staff. The collected snapshots are analyzed by a trained person. Cervicography was found to be more sensitive than cervical cytology in detecting dysplasia. The sensitivity of cervicography was found to be 83% and that of cervical cytology to be 42% in one study. The specificity of the two methods was almost similar, 95% and 98% respectively.[5]

21.4.4 Telecolposcopy

The colposcopic findings are video recorded and the videos can be electronically transmitted to an expert colposcopist, who can interpret the findings. Thus patients living in rural areas can be evaluated by a colposcopist practicing at a distant place. The reported accuracy ranges from 43-93%.

21.4.5 Visual Inspection with Acetic Acid (VIA)

In countries with low resource settings, where routine colposcopy cannot be practiced, low cost methods have to be evolved for localizing abnormal area in patients with abnormal cytology. One such method is visual inspection after painting with acetic acid. Patients with abnormal findings should have biopsy done. Sensitivity of VIA is found to be comparable to conventional Pap screening. Specificity of VIA in detecting lesions is comparable to colposcopy.[6]

21.5 HPV TESTING IN CERVICAL SMEAR

The understanding that HPV is the primary cause of cervical cancer led to the identification of the high risk HPV types in the cervical cells. Presence of HPV is associated with 250 fold increased risk of HSIL. HPV infection is extremely common in sexually active women but most infections are transient and majority of women will clear the infection within a few months. Only 9% will have persistent HPV infection. Hence HPV testing is advised only for women 30 years or older.[7] Those who are found to be HPV positive need follow-up than those who are HPV negative.

Is HPV Testing Better than Pap-smear in Screening for Cancer Cervix?

This was studied in a large Canadian trial. More than 10000 non pregnant women participated in the trial. Participants underwent screening with both cytology and HPV DNA testing. Those with abnormal cytology or HPV DNA positive were referred for colposcopy. Random samples of participants with negative screening were also taken for colposcopy. The sensitivity of HPV testing in detecting high grade neoplasia was significantly higher than that of Pap test (94.6% vs. 55.4%). The specificity of Pap test was slightly higher than that of HPV testing (96.8% vs. 94.1%) Both tests combined gave a sensitivity of 100%.[14] Molecular testing for high risk HPV types is commercially available. But, the role of routine HPV testing is controversial.

In developing countries, there is a lack of effective screening programs for cervical cancer. In these countries, no clinically significant reduction in the incidence of cervical cancer has occurred during the past three decades compared to developed countries where 70% reduction was achieved. A single round of HPV testing compared with single Pap test and VI A in a cluster-randomized, controlled trial to evaluate the effectiveness in reducing the incidence of cervical cancer, was conducted in the Osmanabad district in the state of Maharashtra, India. After 8 years follow-up, it was observed that there was a significant reduction in the incidence of advanced cancers and deaths in the HPV tested group which probably reflects the higher sensitivity of HPV testing in detecting lesions with a high potential for malignant transformation than that of cytologic testing or VIA.[15]

21.6 MANAGEMENT OF SQUAMOUS INTRAEPITHELIAL LESION (FIG. 21.7)

The very idea of diagnosing pre-malignant lesions of the cervix by the Pap test is to manage and follow-up these lesions identified by cytology. The Bethesda system of reporting has clarified the terminology of reporting abnormal cervical cytology. In countries where regular cytology screening is practiced, these lesions can be identified well enough.

The American Society for Colposcopy and Cervical Pathology (ASCCP) in a consensus conference in September 2001, developed evidence based guidelines for the management of women with abnormal cervical cytology. Pap smear results are reported in the Bethesda system and histology results are often reported in the CIN terminology.

21.6.1 Management of ASC-US

There are three management options for ASC-US

1. Repeat cytology every 4-6 months till two consecutive negative smears. If ASCUS or more, patient should be referred for colposcopy.
2. Immediate colposcopy. If no CIN, follow-up smear yearly. If CIN treat.
3. DNA testing for high risk HPV types. If positive proceed for colposcopy. If liquid based cytology is used the same sample can be used for HPV testing. This is called 'Reflex' HPV testing.

Women who were reported to have ASC-US had a high incidence (10-20%) of later development of CIN II and III, diagnosed at cytological follow-up. This has led to clinical researches to find out the best method of sorting out women who are at risk of developing higher grade lesions. The ALTS trial addressed this issue. This was a follow-up study of women whose cytology report was ASCUS or LSIL. In the ALTS trial, women with cytology report of LSIL and ASCUS were triaged to 3 different management strategies—repeat cytology, colposcopy and HPV DNA testing. The trial made clear the natural history of such lesions as well as clarified the management options. It came to be understood that women who are positive for high risk HPV DNA are at high risk for the development of CIN II and III, compared with those who are negative for HPV DNA. The trial found that 26.9% of women who had ASCUS cytology

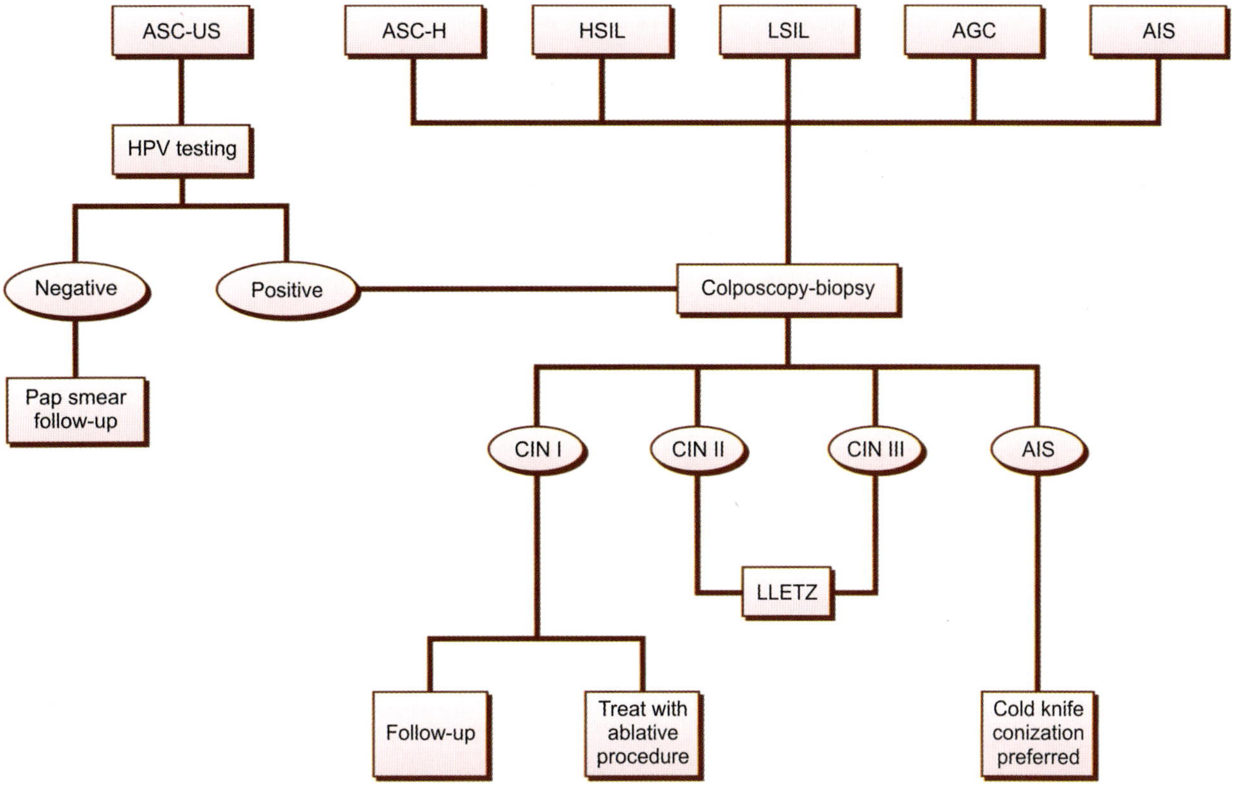

Fig. 21.7: Management algorithm for abnormal cervical cytology

report and positive for high risk HPV types developed CIN II or III in a follow-up period of 2 years. The ALTS triage study concluded that HPV testing is sensitive in detecting CIN II and III and can halve the need for colposcopy if HPV testing is done initially without directly going for colposcopy. Screening by cytology and HPV testing or reflex HPV testing is more effective in reducing the rate of cancer and will be less costly than annual conventional cytology.

However colposcopy should be done if HPV DNA is positive. After colposcopy if CIN II or III is diagnosed, the patient is to be treated accordingly. If CIN II or III is not present, either repeat HPV testing at 12 months or cytology at 6-12 months should be advised.

21.6.2 Management Protocol for ASC-H

As per ASCCP guidelines women with ASC-H should undergo colposcopy and directed biopsy as higher grade lesions are possible. If colposcopy is negative the specimen has to be reviewed and if still negative the patient only need regular follow-up. Patients with persistent ASC-H or any high grade lesion should have appropriate management.

21.6.3 Management Protocol for LGSIL

It is important to understand the natural history of women whose cervical cytology report is LGSIL as shown in Table 21.2.

Table 21.2: Natural history of LGSIL

Regress	57%
Persist	29%
Progress	11%
Invasive cancer	3%

Source: Ostor A. Natural history of cervical intraepithelial neoplasia: a critical review. Int J Gynecol Pathol 1993;12:186-192

FIGO Recommendation for LGSIL

Repeat cytology after 6-12 months, if LGSIL persists, perform colposcopy, or HPV testing and colposcopy if HPV high risk types are obtained.

As per ASCCP guideline, colposcopy is advised even when the cytology report is LGSIL because at biopsy 9-16% of women with cytology report of LGSIL was found to have a higher grade lesion (CIN-II or III). If at colposcopy no lesion is identified endocervical curettage should be done. If after satisfactory colposcopy and biopsy If only CIN I is identified, observation only is required, provided the patient is reliable for follow-up. 57% of CIN lesions regress spontaneously. During the observation period either repeat cytology at 6 to 12 months or HPV testing at 12 months should be done. If HPV DNA high risk types are identified or if the cytology report is atypical squamous cells or greater, colposcopy should be repeated. When the smear remains negative for 2 consecutive examinations or a single HPV testing is negative annual screening can be resumed.

In a prospective study of women whose cytology report was LGSIL it was found that about 23-55% of women who had LEEP when the cytology report was LGSIL, harbored a higher grade lesion.[8]

If the colposcopically directed biopsy shows CIN I, the patient should be on regular follow-up with regular cytology. Most lesions regress, but a few progresses to CIN II or III or invasive cancer. A comprehensive review showed that spontaneous regression occurred in 57%, progression to CIN II or III occurred in 11% and invasive cancer occurred in 3% (Table 21.2).[9]

Women who are not reliable or who are not willing for follow-up should have treatment of the lesion. Ablative therapy like cryotherapy, laser ablation, electrofulguration and excisional procedures like LEEP and cold knife conization are accepted therapies for LGSIL. Excisional procedure combined with endocervical sampling should be preferred when colposcopy is unsatisfactory.

Before deciding on ablative therapy, satisfactory colposcopic examination is a must.

Types of ablative therapy available are:

1. Cryotherapy
2. Laser ablation
3. Electrofulguration

There is a risk of missing a high grade lesion or an occult invasive lesion in the following situations

1. Colposcopy is unsatisfactory
2. When the endocervical curettage is positive
3. When high risk HPV infection or LGSIL is persisting for more than 2 years
4. Women older than 40 years

An excisional procedure like LLETZ is the preferred treatment in the above situations. In a follow-up of 77 women whose cytology report was LGSIL, and had one or more of the above risk factors, 22% had a higher lesion (CIN II/III) in the LEEP specimen. Post treatment HPV testing has 100% sensitivity and specificity in diagnosing persistent and recurrent high grade lesion.[10]

LLETZ Procedure

The procedure was first described in the year 1989 by Prendiville who published his results of treatment. The procedure involves cutting and removing the entire transformation zone with the help of a large thin wire loop using electrocautery. The advantages of the procedure are the reduced complication rate and the less time required for the procedure compared to conventional cone biopsy. An electrocautery system capable of performing cutting and coagulation functions, an insulated hand piece and various size wire loops are required. Ball cautery is also required for controlling hemorrhage. The procedure can be performed under local anesthesia. 1% lignocaine along with 2-4 ml of 1/20 vasopressin should be injected into the cervical tissue. The loop is to be placed on the cervix in such a way that 1-2 mm of free margin is included in the removed portion.

A cone shaped portion of the transformation zone is excised by spooning the cervix as the hand is moved swiftly in a unidirectional curve. Bleeding points are coagulated and the sample is sent for histopathology.

21.6.4 Management Protocol of HGSIL

As in LGSIL, histopathological correlation by colposcopically directed biopsy is the standard practice. Since these lesions have a higher rate of progression to malignancy the approach should be more aggressive than that of LGSIL. Patients should be directly taken for colposcopically directed biopsy. There are reports of progression of CIN II to CIS and invasive cancer to the extent of 22%.[11] CIN III lesions may regress in up to 32% and 14% may progress to invasive cancer if not treated (Table 21.3). Patients with reports of HSIL in Pap smear should have the entire transformational zone removed in an excisional procedure. The entire transformation zone should be visualized and there should not be suspicion of invasive disease. Large loop excision of the transformation zone (LLETZ) is the preferred method because of the advantage of lesser complication rate. An ablative therapy is not at all recommended for HGSIL as an occult invasive lesion may be missed, since the specimen cannot be examined after ablative therapy.

However, ablative therapy may be chosen if the following conditions are met

1. No discrepancy between cytology, colposcopy and histology

Table 21.3: Natural history of HSIL

Regress	32%
Progression to III , CIS or Invasive cancer	22%
Progression to invasive cancer	14%

Mitchel MF, Tortorelo-Luna G, Wright T et al. Cervical HPV infection and intraepithelial neoplasia: a review. J Natl Cancer Inst Monogr1996;21:17-25.

2. No colposcopy finding suggestive of invasive disease
3. No obvious evidence of glandular lesion
4. Satisfactory colposcopy

Excisional procedure should be preferred in the following circumstances
1. Colposcopic finding of micro invasion
2. Endocervical curettage is positive for CIN
3. AIS is suspected
4. Discrepancy between cytology and colposcopically directed biopsy

Cold Knife Cone Biopsy

Cold knife cone biopsy is indicated to exclude invasion in the following situations:
- If micro-invasion is suspected in the removed specimen
- If the upper extent of the lesion could not be located
- If the margins are positive for the lesion.
- There is a discrepancy between Pap test and colposcopic impression

Hysterectomy

Hysterectomy was widely resorted to as treatment for cervical pre-invasive lesion. But with the advent of LLETZ, it is not the first line management. Hysterectomy may still be indicated in the following situations.
1. HSIL in a patient who has completed family.
2. After LLETZ the margins are positive and the patient has completed family.
3. HSIL in a postmenopausal patient.
4. HSIL co-existing with benign uterine pathology (e.g. fibroids) or the woman has other co-existing problem like menorrhagia.
5. AIS diagnosed by cone biopsy in a woman who has completed family.

21.7 HPV VACCINE

The important understanding that the human papilloma virus is the causative agent of cervical cancer, has led to the development of HPV vaccine. Screening for cervical cancer and its precursors has led to the marked reduction in the incidence of cervical cancer in countries where regular screening programs are available. The institution of a regular screening program needs high cost. This led to the development of strategies for primary prevention. If successful vaccine is evolved against high risk types of HPV, cervical cancer can possibly be eradicated. Even if vaccination is developed, it would take decades to prove its benefits because of the long latent period.

The history of development of HPV vaccine dates back to 1991. Zhan et al showed that HPV 16 L1 capsid protein, when expressed in a recombinant system, formed virus like particles (VLPs). These particles are highly antigenic without pathogenic effects. These VLPs can be easily synthesized using recombinant vectors.

HPV vaccine is developed with the following two aims:
- To prevent HPV infection in those who are not yet infected (primary prevention).
- To avoid further progression of the disease in those who have an established infection so that invasive therapeutic treatment like excision can be avoided (therapeutic).

L1 VLP can be produced by recombinant DNA technology using vectors. Even if preventive vaccination is given, the establishment of effectiveness will take several decades because of long latent period between the establishment of infection and development of disease. If immunologic targets are developed against early viral proteins E2, E6 and E7, it can be used as a therapeutic vaccine for patients who are already infected with HPV.

HPV vaccines based on VLPs are primarily prophylactic. As HPV infection progresses, the replicative process of the host genes are changed by the viral proteins in an orderly manner. The early proteins E6 and E7 promote apoptosis of cells. These proteins are produced throughout the life cycle of the virus. Hence, vaccines can be made using these proteins. The late proteins L1 and L2 are not produced until the virus comes to the most superficial layers of the epithelium.

21.7.1 Prophylactic Vaccine

The prophylactic vaccine is made of virus like particles with repetitive pentamers of L1 to enhance the magnitude and prolong the resistance against L1. The vaccinated individuals develop antibodies against L1 particles of HPV. The vaccine is advised for girls of age 11-12 years, so that they develop immunity before being exposed to HPV infection. The schedule is to give a series of 3 injections over a 6 months period. The second dose is given 2 months after the first and the third 4 months after the second. The vaccine offers naïve women protection against types of virus used in producing the vaccine. Cytology screening should continue for women already infected.

21.7.2 Therapeutic Vaccine

Development of cellular immunity is the important factor necessary for the clearance of HPV infection. The therapeutic vaccine will help to prevent the development of malignant change after cervical epithelial cells are clearly infected with HPV. The early proteins E2, E6 and E7 are the most attractive immunologic targets for the development of HPV therapeutic vaccines. E7 is the best studied among these. It induces cell mediated immunity against cervical dysplasia.[12,13]

Three separate trials have been performed to test the efficacy of various HPV vaccines. Each of these trials demonstrated the efficacy of the corresponding vaccines in preventing persistent HPV infection.

1. A randomized trial of experimental HPV 16 VLP vaccine versus placebo was conducted in 1533 women. The vaccine was administered on day 0, month 2 and month 6 with a median follow-up of 17.4 months. A decrease was noted in persistent and transient HPV 16 infection and in cases of CIN in vaccinated versus placebo women.
2. Another trial for the prevention of HPV 16 and 18 was using the bivalent L1 VLP vaccine in 1113 women. These women were followed up for 27 years. The vaccine had 85% efficacy in persistent infection and 93% in those with cytological abnormalities.
3. A phase 2 trial of Quadrivalent vaccine against HPV 6, 11, 16, 18 was found to be highly effective in reducing the incidence of persistent HPV infection.[16] The vaccine was also found to be highly immunogenic to each of these HPV type. The quadrivalent vaccine is presently available in the market (Gardasil™).

21.8 CONCLUSION

- Cervical cancer has a long preinvasive period
- Human papillomavirus is the most probable etiological agent
- Most HPV infections subside by itself. Those with persistent infection are at risk of development of cervical dysplasias and cancer.
- Infection with the virus starts with the initiation of vaginal sex.
- Exfoliative cytology of the cervix described by Dr George Papanicolaou is the best cancer detection test ever developed.
- Terminology for reporting of cervical cytology is at present based on the Bethesda III system 2001.
- HPV DNA positivity is the best predictor of the risk of recurrence.
- Women with cervical cytology report of LGSIL should be taken for either direct colposcopy and biopsy or HPV DNA testing. Those with HPV DNA positive should have colposcopy and those who are negative should have annual cytological screening.
- Those who are reported to have ASCUS can be followed up according to ALTS Triage.
- Women whose cytology remains as LGSIL need to be followed up only. Those who are not willing for follow-up or cannot be relied upon for follow-up should have therapy done, which can be one of the ablative methods.
- Women with HGSIL should have colposcopy and directed biopsy. Those with CIN II and III should have excisional procedure as treatment.
- The preferred excisional treatment is LLETZ which has a lower complication rate. Future fertility is not much affected by LLETZ procedure.
- HPV vaccine is evolving as a means for preventing HPV infection which will go a long way in preventing cancer of the cervix.

REFERENCES

1. CH Shin, JO Schorge, KR Lee, et al. Conservative management of adenocarcinoma in situ of the cervix. Gynaecol Oncol 2000;79:6-10.
2. Shaw PA. The history of cervical screening I: the Pap test. J Soc Obstet Gynaecol Can 2000;22:110-14.
3. Bergeron C, Bishop J, Lemarie A, et al. Accuracy of thin layer cytology in patients undergoing cervical cone biopsy Acta Cytol 2001; 45:519-24.
4. Tovell HM, Banogan P, Nash AD. Cytology and colposcopy in the diagnosis and management of preclinical carcinoma of the cervix uteri: a learning experience. Am J Obstet Gynecol 1976;124:924-34.
5. Coibion M, Guenier C, Miloiu A, et al. The value of screening using cervicography in dysplasia and neoplasms of the uterine cervix. Rev Med Brux 1990;11:16-20.
6. Sankaranarayanan R, Wesley R, Thara S, et al. Test characteristics of visual inspection with 4% acetic acid (VIA) and Lugol's iodine(VILI) in cervical cancer screening in Kerala, India. Int J Cancer 2003;106:404-8.
7. Moscicki A, Shiboski S, Broering J, et al. The natural history of HPV as measured by repeat DNA testing in adolescent and young women. J Paediatri 1998;132:277-84.
8. Spitzer M, et al. Management of histological abnormalities of the cervix. Am Fam Physician 2006;73:105-12.
9. Ostor A. Natural history of cervical intraepithelial neoplasia: a critical review. Int J Gynecol Pathol 1993;12:186-92.
10. Immaculada Alonso, et al. High-risk cervical epithelial neoplasia grade 1 treated by loop electrosurgical excision: follow-up and value of HPV testing Am J Obstet Gynaecol October 2007.
11. Mitchel MF, Tortorelo-Luna G, Wright T, et al. Cervical HPV infection and intraepithelial neoplasia: a revew. J Natl Cancer Inst Monogr1996;21:17-25.
12. De Jong A, O'Neill T, Khan AY, et al. Enhancement of human papillomavirus (HPV) type 16 E6 and E7-specific T-cell

immunity in healthy volunteers through vaccination with TA-CIN, an HPV16 L2E7E6 fusion protein vaccine. Vaccine 2002;20:3456-64.
13. Borysiewicz LK, Fiander A, Nimako M, et al. A recombinant vaccine virus encoding human papillomavirus types 16 and 18 E6 and E7 proteins as immunotherapy for cervical cancer. Lancet 1996;347:1523-7.
14. Mayrand, et al. Human Papilloma virus DNA versus Papanicolaou screening tests for cervical cancer. N Engl J Med 2007;357:1579.
15. Rengaswamy Sankaranarayanan, Bhagwan M. Nene, Surendra S. Shastri, et al. HPV Screening for Cervical Cancer in Rural India. NEJM 2009;360(14):1385-94.
16. Joura EA, Leodolter S, Hernanded-Avila M. Efficacy if a quadrivalent prophylactic human papillomavirus(types 6,11,16, and 18)L1 virus-like-particle vaccine against high-grade vulval and vaginal lesions: a combined analysis of three randomized clinical trials. et al. Lancet 2007;369: 1693-702.

22 Carcinoma of the Cervix

B Presannakumari

22.1 INTRODUCTION

Worldwide, cervical cancer is the fifth most deadly cancer in women. It affects about 16 per 100,000 women per year and kills about 9 per 100,000 per year. Over 470000 new cases are diagnosed annually worldwide. In the US it is the second most common cancer and the most common cause of cancer death among women (American Cancer Society, 2005).

In developing countries like India it is the second most common malignancy among women and is the most common female genital tract malignancy. The incidence in India is estimated at 1,30,000 and 80,000 women die from the disease every year. It is fortunate that cervical malignancy is an easily detectable and preventable disease. Human Papilloma Virus (HPV) infection has been identified as the causative agent. The latent period between infection and occurrence of the disease is about 25 to 30 years. This provides an excellent window for detecting and treating the disease. Early diagnosis means excellent prognosis. The discovery of the Pap test is an important landmark on the way to prevention of cervical cancer. The recently introduced HPV DNA test from the cervix is a further step forward in cancer prevention. Today we even have a vaccine to prevent this deadly cancer, even though it may take a few decades to prove its effectiveness. Needless to say, clinicians should be well aware of the screening methods, prevention, diagnosis and management of cancer of the cervix.

Risk factors for cervical cancer

- Human Papilloma Virus infection—E6 & E7 proteins cause neoplastic transformation
- Smoking—tobacco byproducts damage DNA of the cell.
- Chlamydia infection—higher association with HPV infection.
- Hormonal contraception—risk is more when OCs are used for more than 5 years
- Low socioeconomic status—inadequate utilization of health facilities.
- Diet—low in fruits and vegetables
- Diethyl Stilbestrol exposure in utero—clear cell adenocarcinoma of the cervix.
- Family history of cervical cancer—inherited condition that makes women less able to fight off HPV infection than others.

22.2 EPIDEMIOLOGY AND RISK FACTORS

Cervical cancer usually occurs in the fifth or sixth decade of life and the mean age estimated is 54 years. Multiple sexual partners, high parity, race, low socioeconomic class and cigarette smoking influence the incidence of the disease. Based on data obtained in the year 2002, 83% of the cases occur in developing countries; whereas only 3.6% of new cases occur in the developed countries. In developing countries cancer cervix accounts for 15% of female cancers. The highest incidence occurs in Sub-Saharan Africa, South Central Asia and Latin America (Table 22.1). The isolation of Human Papilloma virus (HPV) from cervical cancer tissue is one of the important landmarks in the knowledge about cancer cervix. HPV has been isolated from 99.7% of cervical cancer[1,2] tissue.

Table 22.1: Incidence and mortality rates of cervical cancer by race

Race/ethnicity	*Incidence/ 100,000 women*	*Mortality/ 100,000 women*
Hispanic/Latino	16.2	3.6
African American	11.8	5.6
Asian/Pacific Islander	9.5	2.8
White	8.9	2.6
American Indian/Alaskan Native	6.0	2.8

Source: SEER Database

The most important risk factor for the development of the disease is early (adolescence and early adulthood) sexual intercourse. Before the introduction of screening techniques, the incidence was comparable in developing as well as developed countries. This stresses the impact of screening in preventing cancer of the cervix as well as detecting the disease in the early stages. The incidence of the disease correlates with human development index (HDI). HDI is a measure of education, life expectancy and gross domestic product. As HDI increases, the incidence of cancer cervix decreases.

22.2.1 Role of HPV in the Causation of Cervical Cancer

Infection with HPV is established as the initial causative event in the development of cancer cervix. The virus commonly infects the skin and the mucosa of the respiratory and anogenital tracts. Even though 30 different types of HPV have been found to cause infection in the lower genital tract, about 15 to 20 types are found to be oncogenic. These different types of HPV vary in their ability to cause malignancy. Low risk varieties 6 and 11 are associated with viral condylomata and mild dysplasia. High risk types 16 and 18 are associated with severe dysplasia, carcinoma *in situ* and invasive cancer. Types 16 and 18 are thought to cause 70% of cervical cancer. Other oncogenic types are 45, 31, 33, 52, 58 and 35.

HPV infects the cells by penetrating through the epithelium. The genome gets incorporated into the host DNA. This is considered to be an important step in malignant transformation. The viral proteins E6 and E 7 produced by high risk types of HPV binds to P53 and Rb proteins, which are the tumor suppressor proteins of the host cell and inactivate them. This inactivation leads to dysregulated entry of cells into S phase causing malignant transformation. In a minority of patients the p53gene is mutated leading to malignancy.[3]

Natural History of HPV Infection of the Cervix (Flow Chart 22.1)

HPV infection is common in sexually active women. More than 90% of the infections are spontaneously cleared by the host immune system within one year. Persistent infection after one year develops in about 10% of women. Cellular changes caused by HPV progress to LSIL and subsequently to HSIL and to invasive cancer. Some LSIL may directly progress to cervical cancer. Some initial HPV infection may progress directly to HSIL. About 1/3 to 2/3 of women with HSIL will progress to cervical cancer if left untreated. However, about 60% of low grade lesions regress without treatment. Another 30% will persist, 10% progress to CIN II and CIN III and roughly 1% progress to invasive cancer.

22.3 PREVENTION

The landmark discovery by Papinicolaou and Traut in the year 1941 that by studying the morphology of the exfoliated cells, pre-malignant lesions and malignancy can be diagnosed, led to cervical cytology screening. The cervix is easily accessible for cytological sampling. This led to the strategy of preventing cervical cancer by diagnosing the pre-invasive lesions as well as invasive disease in its early stages by cytological screening, popularly known as the Pap test.

The peak incidence of pre-invasive disease is observed between the ages of 25 to 40 and invasive disease between 40 to 55 years. This shows that cervical cancer has a long pre-invasive period, and detection of abnormal cytology by Pap test can make cervical cancer a largely preventable disease. The introduction of screening programs has led to reduced incidence and down staging of the disease in developed countries,[4,5] to the extent of 70%.

Cytological screening followed by colposcopy needs elaborate infrastructure and trained personnel, incurring high cost. Due to economic constraints, screening programs for cervical cancer cannot be instituted on a population basis in developing countries like India. Technologies with minimal resource requirements such as visual inspection of the cervix after painting with acetic acid (VIA) or with Lugol's Iodine (VILI), have to be developed as screening methods in developing countries with low resource settings. Evidence shows that a 25% reduction in life time risk of developing cervical cancer can be achieved by screening

Flow Chart 22.1: Natural history of cervical cancer (IARC: with permission)

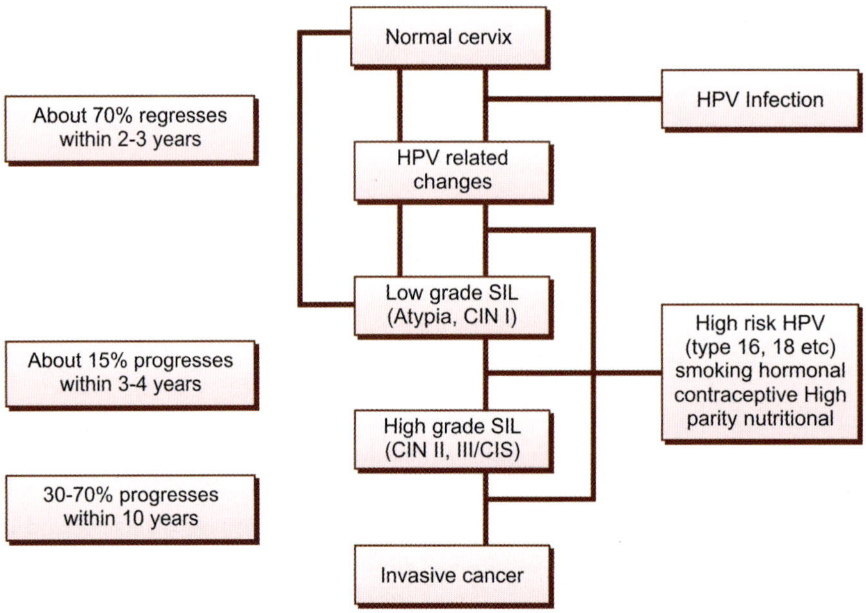

Table 22.2: Factors limiting pap test sensitivity

1.	Presence of inflammation and/or blood obscuring visualization of cell
2.	Inaccessible location of the lesion
3.	The lesion not being sampled
4.	The presence of only a few abnormal cells
5.	Small size of a lesion

with VIA.[6,7] Pap test is not absolutely perfect. Its sensitivity for the detection of high-grade cervical intraepithelial neoplasia (CIN) is in the range of 70 to 80 percent. The factors affecting sensitivity are given in Table 22.2.

22.3.1 Improvements in Cervical Cytology Screening

Liquid based cytology: After taking the smear, the cells are shaken off from the sample device in the vial of fluid. A thin layer of this preparation of cells is examined under the microscope. This reduces the number of inadequate smears.

22.3.2 HPV DNA Testing

Since the presence of HPV DNA in the cervical cells is closely associated with cervical cancer, testing for HPV improves the sensitivity of screening for cervical cancer. HPV testing is available in convenient kit-based systems which make screening possible on a population basis. In a low-resource setting, a single round of HPV testing was compared with cervical cytology and visual inspection with acetic acid. It was found that even a single round of HPV testing was associated with a significant reduction in the numbers of advanced cervical cancers and deaths from cervical cancer.[8] HPV testing can also be used to select patients with mild dyskaryosis in cervical smear for colposcopic directed biopsy. Those who are HPV negative need not undergo colposcopically directed biopsy.

22.3.3 The HPV Vaccine

The understanding that HPV infection of the cervix is the initial event in carcinogenesis of the cervix, led to researches for developing a vaccine against the high risk types of HPV. Even though 30 different types of HPV are known to be associated with cervical cancer, the vaccine which completed phase 3 trials and is available is the quadrivalent vaccine (Gardasil™) which is developed using L1 virus like particles (VLP) of HPV 6, 11, 16 and 18. Another bivalent vaccine containing VLP of 16 and18 will soon become available. (HPV vaccine is discussed in detail in the chapter on Premalignant lesions of the cervix) Since HPV is implicated in the causation of not only cervical cancer but vulval, vaginal as well as oral cancers, the vaccine gives protection from these cancers also.

The vaccine is advised for girls aged 11-12 years, so that they develop immunity before exposure to HPV infection. The schedule is to give a series of 3 injections, at 0, 2 and 6 months over a period of 6 months. The vaccine offers naïve women protection against infection by those types of viruses whose VLPs are used in producing the vaccine. Cytology screening should be continued for already infected women.

22.4 PATHOLOGY

The most common cancer of the cervix is squamous cell carcinoma, occurring in 75 to 80%, the rest being adenocarcinoma or adenosquamous carcinoma. Other malignancies of the cervix are sarcoma, malignant melanoma and neuroendocrine carcinoma. These are enlisted in Table 22.3.

Table 22.3: Pathological types of cervical malignancy

Squamous carcinoma
a. Large cell keratinizing
b. Large cell non-keratinzing
c. Small cell types
d. Rare types:
Verrucous
Papillary
Adenocarcinoma
a. Endocervical
b. Minimal deviation
c. Clear cell
d. Villoglandular
e. Adenocystic
f. Adenoid cystic
g. Adenosquamous
Sarcoma
a. Embryonal rhabdomyosarcoma (botryoid sarcoma)
b. Leiomyosarcoma
c. Mixed mesodermal tumors
d. Adenosarcoma
Malignant melanoma
Neuroendocrine carcinoma
a. Small cell
b. Large cell
c. Classical carcinoid
d. Atypical carcinoid

Types of Squamous Cell Carcinoma (SCC)

- Large cell keratinizing
- Large cell non-keratinzing
- Small cell types
- Rare types:
  Verrucous
  Papillary

Large cell keratinizing tumors are composed of cells with abundant eosinophilic cytoplasm. Their characteristic feature is the presence of keratin pearls in the cell nests.

In the large cell non-keratinizing type, individual cells show keratinization without the formation of keratin pearls. Generally, large cell types have better prognosis.

The small cell squamous carcinomas are poorly differentiated and anaplastic. The cells have scanty cytoplasm, small round nuclei and high mitotic activity. The small cell squamous carcinomas behave aggressively and will be associated with parametrial infiltration and pelvic lymph node metastasis, which affects prognosis adversely.

Verrucous carcinoma resembles condyloma accuminata. They are locally invasive but metastasis is rare.

The previously reported incidence of squamous carcinoma and adenocarcinoma was 95% and 5% respectively. It is seen that the incidence of adenocarcinoma is on the increase and the proportion reported is as high as 18.5 to 27%9.The recent Surveillance Epidemiology End Result (SEER) data for 1973 and 1988 shows that the age adjusted incidence of cervical squamous lesions decreased by 43% and 53% respectively, whereas adenocarcinoma and adenosquamous carcinoma increased by 32.3% and 32.9%. Several factors appear to be responsible for this difference. One is that the incidence of HPV infection is on the increase. Another is that the present screening programs are designed to detect lesions of the ectocervix, but the adenomatous type which is usually higher up in the endocervical canal fails to be detected.

Adenocarcinoma *in situ* (AIS) is the precursor of invasive adenocarcinoma. It is predominantly seen in younger women in the early thirties. AIS usually begin at the transformation zone and contiguous endocervical canal. When the endocervical curettage report shows AIS, co-existing invasive disease can be present higher-up in the canal or as a skip lesion. Hence patients reported as having AIS by endocervical curettage or colposcopically directed biopsy should have conization to exclude invasive disease elsewhere in the endocervical canal. There can be multifocal disease also. Loop excision in this situation is not the ideal procedure, as it may miss lesions higher up in the endocervix. Hence a cold knife conization should be done. For patients who wish to conserve the childbearing function, careful follow up is enough, provided the margins are free of disease. If the margins are positive, the chance of residual AIS or co-existing invasive disease is as high as 50%.[10] Even if the margins are negative, residual AIS might occur later at follow-up which may represent multi-focal disease or another fresh lesion. Follow-up of AIS occurring in the endocervical canal is not as accurate as ca-in-situ of the exo-cervix. Hence, hysterectomy should be advised for women with AIS, who have completed family.

22.5 PATTERN OF SPREAD

Cervical cancer almost always arises in the transformation zone between the squamous and columnar epithelium.

The common modes of spread of cervical cancer are the following:

- Lymphatic spread
- Direct invasion to neighboring structures
- Hematogenous spread
- Intraperitoneal implantation

22.5.1 Lymphatic Spread

Lymphatics from the cervix drain to the internal iliac, obturator, pre-sacral, external iliac and the common iliac groups of nodes. From the common iliac, lymphatics drain to the para-aortic group of nodes (Fig. 22.1). Lymphatic spread occurs early in the course of the disease by embolization and permeation through the lymphatics in the parametrium to the various nodes in the pelvis. Even in stage I, pelvic lymph nodes are involved in about 15% of patients. The spread is initially to the inter-iliac nodes, but can also occur to the internal iliac, obturator, presacral and common iliac lymph nodes. From these nodes, spread occurs to the para-aortic group. Spread to the supra-clavicular nodes signify advanced disease. Hence, presence of enlarged supraclavicular node warrants biopsy. Since the parametrial lymphatics and the pelvic lymph nodes are involved even in stage 1 disease, surgical treatment should include removal of the parametrial lymphatics and the pelvic lymph nodes or the same should be treated with radiation. Tumor factors such as stage of disease, depth of invasion, size and grade of the tumor and presence of lymph vascular space involvement influence the frequency of node involvement.

Sentinel node: Sentinel node is the first node to be involved during cancer spread. Identification of the sentinel node can be used as a marker of lymphatic spread. If the sentinel node is negative for malignant cells, extensive

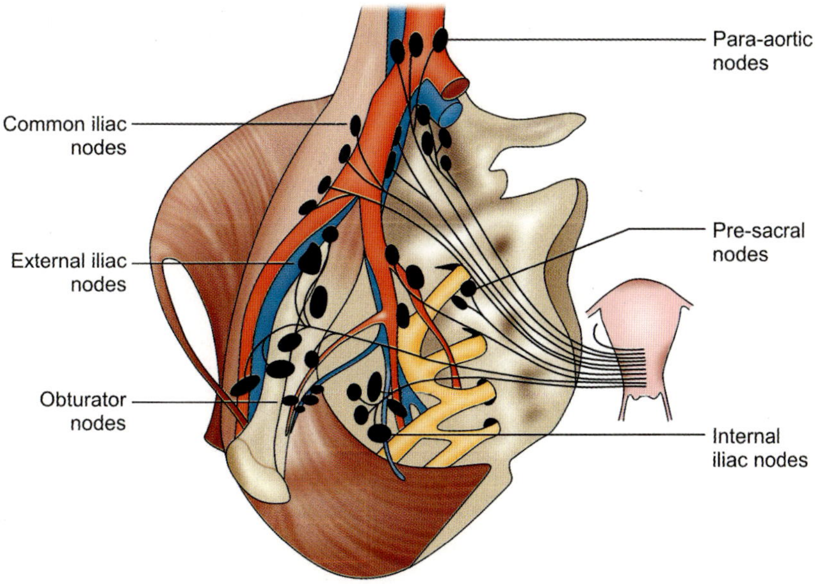

Fig. 22.1: Lymphatic drainage of the cervix

lymph node dissection which incurs morbidity can be avoided whereas if it is positive lymphadenectomy should be done.[11]

22.5.2 Direct Invasion to Neighboring Structures

From the cervix direct extension occurs in all directions. Lateral extension occurs through the parametrium to the pelvic sidewall. The ureter, which courses through the parametrium, can be affected resulting in hydroureter and hydronephrosis. Anterior spread can involve the bladder and can even result in a urinary fistula. Posterior extension through the posterior vaginal wall can involve the rectum, resulting in fecal fistula, which occurs only later, as the rectum is not in a close relation to the cervix as the bladder. Upward extension can occur to the endometrium which does not alter the stage. Spread to the ovary occurs in <1% of SCC whereas in adenocarcinoma the spread to ovaries is 7%. Spread can also occur downwards, to the vagina. Rarely, there can be multi-focal disease involving cervix and endometrium, cervix and vagina or cervix and vulva. Cervix can also be involved as a part of systemic spread from other malignancies like lymphoma, leukemia, and cancers of stomach, kidney or breast.

22.5.3 Hematogenous Spread

Blood-borne metastases occur only in advanced disease to the lungs, liver and bone. All patients should have a chest X-ray before planning treatment.

22.5.4 Intraperitoneal Implantation

Intraperitoneal spread is rare in cancer of the cervix, unlike cancer of the ovary.

22.6 SYMPTOMS

The most common symptom of cervical carcinoma is irregular vaginal bleeding. Postcoital bleeding is a sign of pre-malignant lesions and early cancer. Patients who have an obvious growth in the cervix will have blood stained and foul smelling discharge per vaginum. Very advanced disease may present with urinary or fecal fistula, cachexia, as well as pain due to involvement of pelvic nerve plexus. Rarely patients can present with a painful abdominal mass due to pyometra. The disease can be asymptomatic especially in the early stages. These patients are diagnosed during evaluation of an abnormal pap smear.

Symptoms
- Inter-menstrual bleeding
- Postcoital bleeding
- Foul smelling vaginal discharge
- Cachexia
- Pain

22.7 EVALUATION

Patients who present with post-coital bleeding or irregular vaginal bleeding should have a careful general examination.

The supraclavicular, axillary and the inguinofemoral lymph nodes should be examined. This should be followed by examination of the abdomen for masses, local examination of the vulva, and speculum examination (Fig. 22.2) of the vagina and cervix. A frankly invasive disease can be clearly identified by speculum examination. The four cardinal signs of cancer of the cervix are, friability, fixity, bleeding to touch and induration. Friability and bleeding to touch are elicited by a probe, if the patient does not have a telltale growth in the cervix. Fixity and induration are made out during bimanual examination.

At times a normal looking cervix may be harboring a neoplasm. A large endocervical growth produces a barrel shaped cervix (Fig. 22.3). Patients presenting with pyometra will have enlarged uterus which will be cystic and can be mistaken for an ovarian cyst especially in a postmenopausal patient. On evaluation of abnormal Pap smear, if no growth is seen, the exocervix is evaluated by colposcopy and the endocervix by endocervical curettage. If pathology is not identified in the cervix, the endometrium should also be evaluated because the cause of the abnormal bleeding could be an endometrial malignancy.

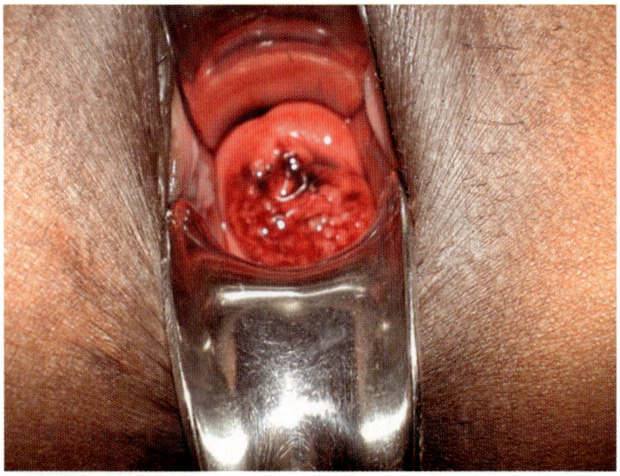

Fig. 22.2: Gross appearance of cervical cancer on speculum examination of a 45-year-old lady, who presented with irregular vaginal bleeding and watery discharge

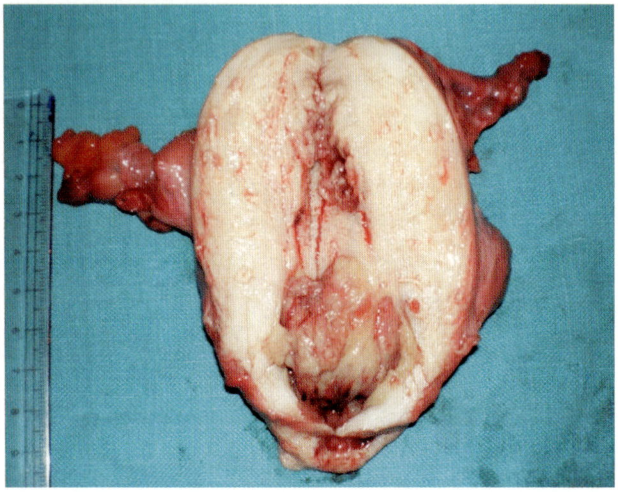

Fig. 22.3: Section of uterus showing growth in the endocervix resulting in barrel-shaped cervix. The malignancy was overlooked by the clinician preoperatively. Wertheim's hysterectomy should have been the surgical option

Bimanual examination can make out the hard nature of the cervix which is friable and the uterus will be fixed due to the involvement of the parametrium in advanced disease. A rectovaginal examination with the index finger in the vagina and the middle finger in the rectum can clearly make out the extent of parametrial involvement, which is important in staging.

22.7.1 Confirmation of the Diagnosis (Table 22.4)

When there is an obvious growth in the cervix, diagnosis can be confirmed by punch biopsy. The biopsy should be taken from the edge of the tumor, which should involve the normal cervix also. A cervical smear in this situation is not useful as it can be negative due to superficial inflammation. If the diagnosis is less obvious, a colposcopically directed biopsy is advised. Colposcopically directed biopsy helps to spot the sites of invasive disease so that cone biopsy to diagnose invasion can be avoided in a large number of situations. If the colposcopically directed biopsy shows microinvasion, cone biopsy should be done to exclude frank invasion elsewhere.

22.7.2 Colposcopic Findings of Invasion

When the cytology report suggests invasive cancer, but no frank growth is seen in the cervix, colposcopic examination of the cervix is mandatory. Cell proliferation and neovascularization which are features of malignancy can produce characteristic appearances in the cervix.

Atypical Blood Vessels

Malignant cells elaborate VEGF (vascular endothelial growth factor), PDGF (platelet derived growth factor),

Table 22.4: Confirmation of diagnosis

• Obvious lesion	Biopsy
• No obvious lesion	Colposcopically directed biopsy
• Biopsy shows microinvasion	Cone biopsy

EGF (Epidermal Growth Factor) and other cytokines which cause abnormal proliferation of vessels. The vessels push out from the surface epithelium and appear looped or cork screw shaped (Fig. 22.4). The normal vascular pattern of the cervix is like the tap root system with branching of the vessels at acute angles and progressively decreasing diameters. The abnormal vessels of invasive cancer branch out at obtuse or right angles and as they branch, the caliber of the vessels increases. There will not be any definite pattern, and hence it might appear like waste cotton threads. This abnormal vascular pattern produces a coarse mosaic or punctate appearance which are seen in high grade pre-invasive and early invasive lesions.

Irregular Surface Contour

The surface will be irregular due to lack of cohesiveness of cells, characteristic of malignancy. Even if irregular, if the consistency is soft and not bleeding to touch, it is unlikely to be a malignancy.

Chalky White Dense Areas

These areas are formed due to keratinization.

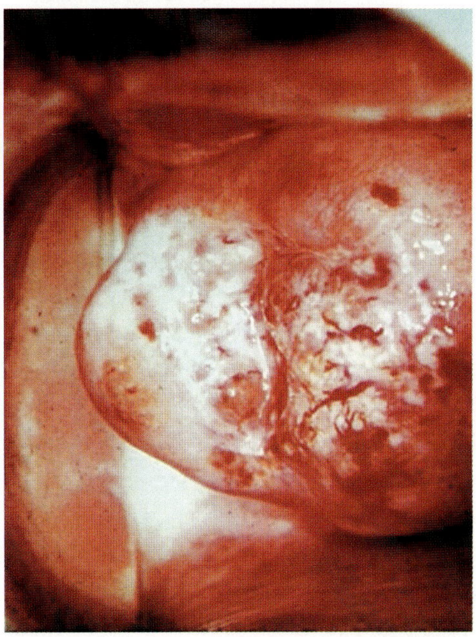

Fig. 22.4: Colposcopic appearance of the cervix showing atypical blood vessels

Colposcopic findings of invasion

- Comma-shaped vessels
- Irregular surface contour
- Coarse mosaic/punctation
- Chalky white dense areas

22.7.3 The FIGO Staging of Cervical Cancer (FIGO 1998) (Table 22.5 and Fig. 22.5)

Table 22.5: The FIGO staging of cervical cancer (with permission). FIGO 1998

Stage	*Description*
Stage 0	Preinvasive carcinoma (carcinoma in situ, CIN)
Stage I	Carcinoma confined to the uterus (corpus extension should be disregarded)
IA	Invasive carcinoma diagnosed only by microscopy. All macroscopically visible lesions even with superficial invasion are Stage IB/T1b
IA1	Stromal invasion no greater than 3.0 mm in depth and 7.0 mm or less in horizontal spread
IA2	Stromal invasion more than 3.0 mm and not more than 5.0 mm with a horizontal spread 7.0 mm or less*
IB	Clinically visible lesion confined to the cervix or microscopic lesion greater than IA2/T1a2
IB1	Clinically visible lesion 4.0 cm or less in greatest dimension
IB2	Clinically visible lesion more than 4 cm in greatest dimension
Stage II	Tumor invades beyond the uterus but not to pelvic wall or to lower third of the vagina
IIA	Without parametrial invasion
IIB	With parametrial invasion
Stage III	Tumor extends to pelvic wall and/or involves lower third of vagina and/or causes hydronephrosis or non-functioning kidney
IIIA	Tumor involves lower third of vagina no extension to pelvic wall
IIIB	Tumor extends to pelvic wall and/or causes hydronephrosis or non-functioning kidney
Stage IV	The carcinoma has extended beyond the true pelvis or has clinically involved the mucosa of the bladder or rectum. A bullous edema as such, does not permit a case to be allotted to stage IV#
IVA	Tumor invades mucosa of bladder or rectum and/or extends beyond true pelvis
IVB	Distant metastasis

* The depth of invasion should not be more than 5 mm taken from the base of the epithelium, either surface or glandular, from which it originates. The depth of invasion is defined as the measurement of the tumor from the epithelial-stromal junction of the adjacent most superficial epithelial papilla to the deepest point of invasion. Vascular space involvement, venous or lymphatic, does not affect classification.

\# The presence of bullous oedema is not sufficient to classify a tumor asT4.

Source: S. Pecorelli, U. Beller, P.A. Heintz, L.J. Benedet, W.T. Creasman and F. Peterson, The 25th FIGO Annual Report on the Results of Treatment in Gynecologic Cancer, Int J Gynaecol Obstet 83 (2003) (Suppl. 1), pp. 1-229.

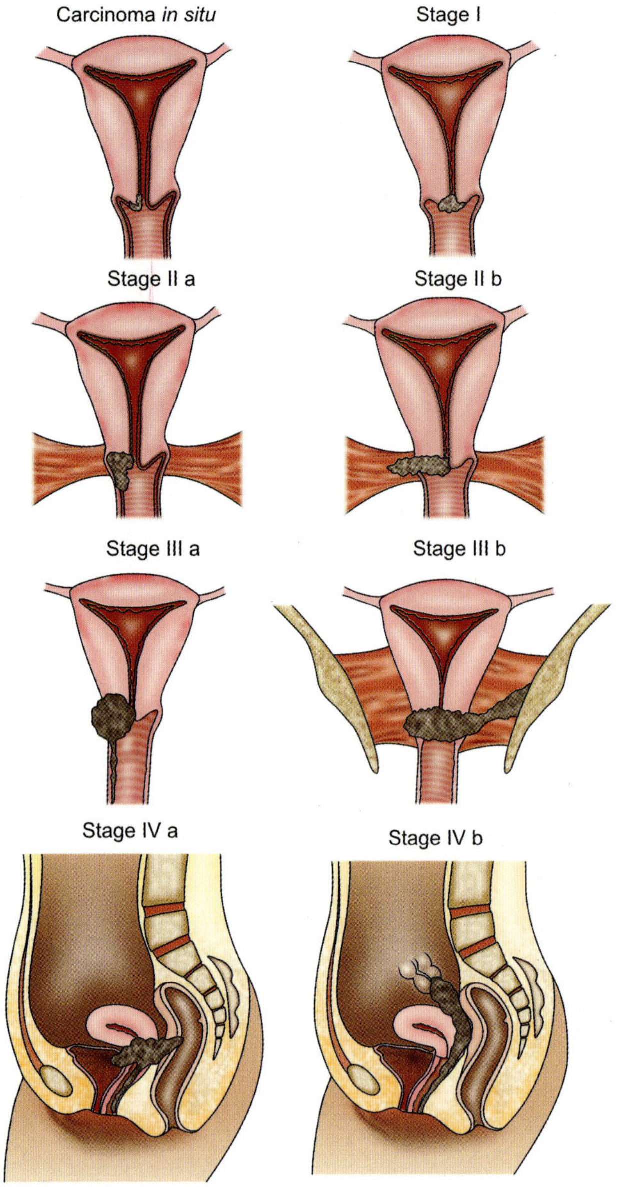

Fig. 22.5: Stages of cancer of the cervix

22.8 PRETREATMENT EVALUATION AND STAGING

After the diagnosis is established, the disease is staged clinically as recommended by FIGO (Table 22.6). Clinical examination is to make out the extent of invasion to the vagina, parametrium, rectosigmoid, urinary bladder and lymph nodes. Bimanual rectovaginal examination under anesthesia by two clinicians is recommended. Cystoscopy and proctosygmoidoscopy are recommended to make out bladder/rectosigmoid involvement. An intravenous pyelogram was previously recommended to exclude hydronephrosis and hydroureter. But it can be diagnosed by ultrasound. A chest radiograph should also be taken, even though distant spread is not common in early stage disease. Investigations like MRI, CT or PET scan is not advised by FIGO as these investigations cannot be routinely done in countries with poor resource settings. However, it can be done if available to know the extent of disease so as to plan treatment.

Table 22.6: Staging procedures

Physical examination[a]	Palpate lymph nodes
	Examine vagina
	Bimanual rectovaginal examination (under anesthesia recommended)
	Size of the growth
Radiologic studies[a]	Intravenous pyelogram
	Barium enema
	Chest X-ray
	Skeletal X-ray
Procedures[a]	Biopsy
	Conization
	Hysteroscopy
	Colposcopy (for microscopic lesions)
	Endocervical curettage (cervical smear shows malignant cells, but no growth seen in cervix)
	Cystoscopy
	Proctoscopy
Optional studies[b]	Computerized axial tomography
	Lymphangiography
	Ultrasonography
	Magnetic resonance imaging
	Positron emission tomography
	Radionucleotide scanning
	Laparoscopy

[a]Allowed by FIGO
[b]Information not allowed by FIGO to change the clinical stage

22.8.1 Staging Modalities

Since clinical staging cannot accurately make out node involvement as well as exact extent of parametrial spread, various investigators have resorted to other modalities to improve the accuracy of clinical staging.

Evaluation of lymph nodes by lymphangiography has high false negative rate of 50% as well as high false positive rate. Hence, lymphangiography12 is not practiced at present. Computed tomography has poor sensitivity but excellent specificity.

T2 weighted MR imaging is found to be 93% accurate in determining the size of the tumor to within 5 mm. The positive predictive value of identifying nodal disease is 66% and parametrial involvement is 67%. Hence, MRI is at present preferred to make out tumor size, lymph node status as well as local extension of the disease.[13]

Positron emission tomography (PET) might evolve as a means for better prediction of tumor size, extension and lymph node involvement because of better sensitivity and specificity.

These modalities are increasingly being used in developed countries, the results of which do not alter the clinical stage, but is useful in planning treatment.

For the staging of microcarcinoma (not clinically evident), colposcopically directed biopsy and cone biopsy may be required to make out the horizontal extension and extension below the basement membrane.

Adenocarcinomas are staged in the same manner as squamous carcinoma.

22.8.2 Surgical Staging

Even though FIGO recommends clinical staging of the disease, postoperative treatment is planned based on surgico-pathological findings. The most important prognostic marker is node involvement which is not taken into account in the FIGO system. The lymph glands can be assessed by laparotomy or laparoscopy. Assessment of node involvement prior to radical surgery can avoid multi modality therapy which incurs high patient morbidity. Patients with positive para-aortic nodes can be selected for primary chemoradiation rather than radical surgery followed by radiation. It is ideal to do pelvic lymphadenectomy before planning conservative surgical treatment like radical trachelectomy.[14]

Management of Stage I and Stage IIA

Management of cervical cancer depends upon:

a. Stage of disease
b. Patient factors concerning surgical risk
c. Fertility wishes
d. Age of the patient and need for preserving the vagina, for sexual function
e. Presence or absence of metastatic disease

The patient should be presented with suitable available options, as well as the advantages, disadvantages, complications and sequelae of each.

22.8.3 Management of Stage I Carcinoma of the Cervix

Stage I cancer is confined to the cervix. Extension to uterine body is disregarded in the present staging, but patients with

Table 22.7: Revised FIGO staging for carcinoma of the cervix (International Journal of Gynecology and Obstetrics 2009; 105: 103-104)

Stage I	The carcinoma is strictly confined to the cervix (extension to the corpus would be disregarded)
IA	Invasive carcinoma which can be diagnosed only by microscopy, with deepest invasion ≤ 5 mm and largest extension ≥ 7 mm
IA1	Measured stromal invasion of ≤ 3.0 mm in depth and extension of ≤ 7.0 mm
IA2	Measured stromal invasion of > 3.0 mm and not >5.0 mm with an extension of not > 7.0 mm
IB	Clinically visible lesions limited to the cervix uteri or pre-clinical cancers greater than stage IA*
IB1	Clinically visible lesion ≤ 4.0 cm in greatest dimension
IB2	Clinically visible lesion > 4.0 cm in greatest dimension
Stage II	Cervical carcinoma invades beyond the uterus, but not to the pelvic wall or to the lower third of the vagina
IIA	Without parametrial invasion
IIA1	Clinically visible lesion ≤ 4.0 cm in greatest dimension
IIA2	Clinically visible lesion > 4 cm in greatest dimension
IIB	With obvious parametrial invasion
Stage III	The tumor extends to the pelvic wall and/or involves lower third of the vagina and/or causes hydronephrosis or non-functioning kidney**
IIIA	Tumor involves lower third of the vagina, with no extension to the pelvicwall
IIIB	Extension to the pelvic wall and/or hydronephrosis or non-functioning kidney
Stage IV	The carcinoma has extended beyond the true pelvis or has involved (biopsy proven) the mucosa of the bladder or rectum. A bullous edema, as such, does not permit a case to be allotted to Stage IV
IVA	Spread of the growth to adjacent organs
IVB	Spread to distant organs

* All macroscopically visible lesions—even with superficial invasion—are allotted to stage IB carcinomas. Invasion is limited to a measured stromal invasion with a maximal depth of 5.00 mm and a horizontal extension of not > 7.00 mm. Depth of invasion should not be > 5.00 mm taken from the base of the epithelium of the original tissue—superficial or glandular. The depth of invasion should always be reported in mm, even in those cases with "early (minimal) stromal invasion" (~1 mm). The involvement of vascular/lymphatic spaces should not change the stage allotment.

** On rectal examination, there is no cancer-free space between the tumor and the pelvic wall. All cases with hydronephrosis or non-functioning kidney are included, unless they are known to be due to another cause.

extension to the uterine cavity will have increased chance of node involvement.

Stage IA

Stage IA cancer is a microscopic cancer diagnosed only by histopathological examination. Ever since Mestwerdt introduced the term microcarcinoma in 1947, there has been debate about the management of this condition. Cone biopsy should be done for all Stage IA disease diagnosed by punch biopsy whether colposcopically directed or not to exclude frank invasion elsewhere in the cervix. In the recent FIGO staging, stage IA is subdivided into A1 and A2. Stage IA1 has only negligible chance of lymphatic involvement and does not require radical treatment.

Management of stage IA1: Stage IA1 include, lesions with invasion ≤ 3 mm below the basement membrane. Chance of lymph node involvement is less than 1%.[15] If the patient wants to preserve the child bearing function, therapeutic conization would suffice as treatment, provided the surgical margins are free of disease. The patient should be on lifelong follow-up. For women who have completed family, hysterectomy is to be preferred.

If the cone biopsy specimen shows lymph vascular space invasion, there is risk of node metastases and central pelvic recurrence. The chance of lymph node involvement is 3.6% in such situations. Hence, they should be advised modified radical hysterectomy with pelvic lymphadenectomy[16-18] (Type II).

Stage IA1 Adenocarcinomas can also be treated by conization, but the upper extent should be free of tumor for about 2 mm. It should be borne in mind that follow-up after endocervical microcarcinoma is more difficult than exocervical lesions. The usual screening by Pap smear testing will fail to detect endocervical lesions.

Radical surgery following cone biopsy should be deferred till 4 to 6 weeks because immediate surgery after cone biopsy carries risk of severe hemorrhage.

Vaginal vault recurrence following treatment is usually due to failure in diagnosing the extent of lesion into the vagina before surgery. Therefore, the extent of lesion should be well delineated by colposcopy prior to definitive treatment.

Management of stage IA2: Stage IA2 is defined as tumor invasion >3 mm but <5 mm from the basement membrane and horizontal extension < 7 mm. The incidence of pelvic node metastasis is 3-8%.

For patients whose fertility should be preserved, radical trachelectomy and node dissection is the treatment of choice.[19] For patients who have completed their family, radical hysterectomy and pelvic lymphadenectomy is the treatment of choice. There is controversy about the extent of surgery. The standard recommendation is type III radical hysterectomy. Some authors recommend class II modified radical hysterectomy. Tumor volume is one factor that has been shown to correlate with the outcome. Tumor volume of <500 cu mm may be treated more conservatively. Brachytherapy, combined with pelvic radiotherapy is also an option (Point A dose 75-80 Gy).

Management of Stage IB

Stage IB cancer cervix is divided into stage IB1 and stageIB2. Stage IB1 is tumor size <4 cm and IB2 is tumor size > 4 cm.

Management of Stage IB1: If the tumor size is < 2 cm and the patient is desirous of preserving child bearing function, radical trachelectomy and pelvic lymph node dissection is an option.

Radical Trachelectomy (Fig. 22.6)

This is known as D'Argent procedure. This surgical option is a fertility sparing procedure for young women with cancer cervix stage IA1 with lymph vascular space involvement and stage IA2 and stage IB1 with tumor size < 2 cm. This can be done by the vaginal or abdominal route. The commonest one is the vaginal route. A 2 cm vaginal cuff is dissected out and the paravesical, vesicovaginal and rectovaginal spaces are opened after dividing the uterosacral, Mackenrodt's and vesicocervical ligaments at their mid points. The ureter is identified and dissected from the utero-vesical ligament. The vaginal branch of the uterine artery is ligated and cut. The cervix is transected at the isthmus. The removed specimen should contain at least 1 cm of the cervix, 1 cm of the vaginal mucosa and 1-2 cm of the parametrium. A prophylactic cervical circlage with No.1 prolene or nylon

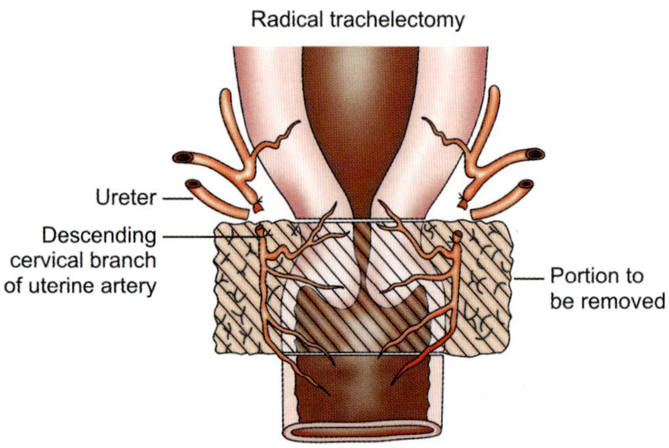

Fig. 22.6: Segment of cervix removed during radical trachelectomy

is placed around the cervical remnant. The vaginal epithelium is then sutured after leaving an opening in the center to communicate with the uterine cavity.

Later the woman may suffer from dysmenorrhea and if she conceives there may be problems in pregnancy, like abortion, preterm labor, etc. Radical trachelectomy can be done with laparoscopic assistance. Lymphadenectomy is done laparoscopically and the lymph nodes are subjected to frozen section. If the lymph nodes are negative for tumor cells, trachelectomy is completed vaginally.

For patients who have completed their family, whose tumor is < 4 cm (Stage IB1 and stage IIA disease), there are two options.

1. Type III radical hysterectomy with pelvic lymphadenectomy
2. Primary radiation. Presently radiation is given along with radio sensitizer cisplatin.

Patients with Stage IB2 disease have increased risk of lymph node involvement. Hence even if they are subjected to radical surgery, most of them need postoperative chemoradiation. This multimodal therapy carries high risk of intestinal and urinary tract morbidity. Hence, radical surgery and pelvic lymphadenectomy should be preferred in patients who are unlikely to have pelvic lymph node involvement and hence may not need postoperative radiation. The 5-year survival following radical surgery is nearly the same as that following radiotherapy.

22.8.4 Advantages of Surgery Over Radiotherapy

1. Surgery allows accurate surgical staging so that postoperative radiation can be better targeted and unnecessary radiation can be prevented.
2. In younger patients ovarian conservation is possible during radical surgery as shielding of ovary during radiotherapy is not very effective.
3. In younger patients vaginal stenosis can be avoided by surgery, in comparison to radiotherapy.

Advantages of surgical treatment

- Equal results as radiotherapy in expert hands
- Can retain ovarian as well as vaginal function
- Can accurately assess disease extent so as to plan adjuvant treatment and help decide prognosis
- Irreversible complications of radiotherapy can be avoided
- Better quality of life and psychological benefit

4. Urinary tract complications as a consequence of surgical treatment are more amenable to treatment than that following radiotherapy.
5. Patients will have psychological feeling of the disease being removed if surgery is done.

The final decision as to which mode of therapy is to be undertaken should be taken by the patient after having had full information about the advantages and disadvantages of each. The surgery preferred for Stage IB and IIA disease is type III radical hysterectomy.

22.8.5 Piver-Rutledge Classification of Hysterectomy for Cervical Cancer

Types of hysterectomy adopted for the treatment of different types of cervical malignancy described by Piver-Rutledge is shown in Table 22.8.

For stage IB and IIA, type III hysterectomy is the preferred surgical option.

Nerve sparing radical hysterectomy can be applied to both modified and radical hysterectomy. It involves careful identification and preservation of hypogastric plexus, leading to fewer bowel and bladder complications.

Main differences between original Wertheim's hysterectomy and type III radical hysterectomy are shown in Table 22.9.

22.8.6 Preoperative Preparation

The patient should be assessed medically after performing routine investigations. Risk of thrombosis should also be assessed. The stage of the disease should be confirmed if needed by examination under anesthesia. Chest radiograph should be taken as a part of metastatic work-up. Doubtful parametrial extension or node involvement should be investigated with MRI or PET whichever is feasible.

Bowel Preparation

Patient has to be on liquid diet 24 hours before surgery. If intestinal adhesions are suspected oral antibiotics should be started. Prophylactic antibiotic has to be given one hour before surgery.

Bladder should be catheterized and continuous bladder drainage maintained.

Incision

Abdomen can be opened with a midline incision or a low transverse Maylard or Cherney incision. The low transverse

Table 22.8: Piver-Rutledge classification of hysterectomy for cervical cancer

Type	*Description*
I	Extra-facial hysterectomy, removal of all peri-cervical tissue
II	Modified radical hysterectomy, removal of medial 50% of cardinal and uterosacral ligaments, uterine vessels are divided medial to ureter
III	Radical hysterectomy-Wertheim-Meigs operation, wide radical resection of the parametrium and paravaginal tissues, ureter dissected completely to bladder entry, uterosacral ligaments divided at origin, cardinals divided at pelvic side wall. Upper 1/3rd of vagina removed.
IV	Extended radical hysterectomy—Ureter divided from pubo-vesical ligaments, superior vesical artery ligated and upper two thirds of vagina excised.
V	Extended radical hysterectomy—More radical procedure with possible bowel, bladder or ureteric dissection

Table 22.9: Differences between Type II and Type III hysterectomy

Original Wertheim's Hysterectomy *Type II Hysterectomy*	*Wertheim-Meig's operation* *Type III Hysterectomy*
Medial half of cardinal and uterosacral ligaments only are removed. The cardinal ligament is divided near the ureteric dissection	Cardinal ligament is dissected near the pelvic side wall
Anterior vesicouterine ligament is divided	The anterior and posterior vesicouterine ligaments are divided and removed after dissecting out the ureters and rolling it laterally
Only enlarged lymph nodes are removed	Complete pelvic lymphadenectomy is done
A smaller margin of vagina is removed	Upper third of vagina is removed

incision gives good lateral exposure. After opening, the entire peritoneal cavity should be inspected and palpated. Tumor should be palpated to know its parametrial extensions, which can be best assessed by the thumb and index finger placed in the anterior and posterior aspect of the parametrium. Pelvic nodes should be evaluated in all patients and the para-aortic nodes for those with grossly enlarged pelvic nodes or bulky cervical tumors. If a suspicious para-aortic node is encountered it is to be removed by incising the peritoneum medial to the ureter above the bifurcation of the aorta and sent for frozen section. If para-aortic node is involved it is better to abandon the procedure and resort to primary chemoradiation.

The procedure begins with clamping and cutting the round ligaments at their midpoints. When the ovaries are not being removed the clamp is to be put medial to the ovary to include the ovarian ligament, fallopian tube and the round ligament. Peritoneal dissection is done starting from the cut round ligament. Anterior leaf of the broad ligament is opened and the pararectal and the paravesical spaces are opened by blunt dissection. The retained ovary is transposed to the abdomen and packed out of the surgical field along with the intestines. It is suggested that one of the ovaries can be transposed to a much higher site in the abdomen, as high as the lower rib and the other one left in the pelvis where it may function longer if the patient need not undergo post-operative radiation.

The peritoneal incision is carried anteriorly on to the uterovesical fold and the bladder is pushed down to ensure operability. After developing the pararectal and the para-vesical spaces the base of the broad ligament and the parametrium are again palpated to exclude parametrial extension. If enlarged lymph nodes adherent to the iliac vessels are encountered, it is better to abandon the procedure for primary chemoradiation. After excluding pelvic extension of the disease, surgery is proceeded with. If the ovaries are to be removed, the infundibulopelvic ligament is cut and the ovarian vessels isolated, clamped, cut and ligated. Lymphadenectomy can be done at this point or following hysterectomy, the latter being the usual preference. The posterior peritoneal incision is carried upwards lateral to the ureter and the ureter with the peritoneum is reflected medially.

Uterine Artery Ligation

The uterine artery is separated at its origin from the internal iliac artery and ligated. The branch to the ureter is sacrificed.

Ligation of the Uterosacral Ligament

The uterus is drawn forwards and the cul-de-sac peritoneum is opened .The rectovaginal space is opened and the rectum is pushed away from the vagina by blunt dissection. The uterosacral ligaments are identified and clamped close to the anterior wall of the rectum.

Dissection of the Lower Ureter

The lower ureter is separated from the peritoneal attachment from the level of the uterosacral ligament. The ureteric tunnel in the vesicouterine ligament is opened by sliding a curved clamp along the anteromedial aspect of the ureter with its curvature upwards. The anterior uterovesical ligament is clamped and cut. The ureter is dissected free from its attachment to the posterior aspect of the ligament and rolled laterally.

Transection of Cardinal Ligament

The cardinal ligament is clamped and ligated near the pelvic side wall after keeping the ureter laterally. The bladder is further dissected separate from the vagina downwards. The paracolpos is clamped and ligated. The vagina is clamped with right angled Wertheim's clamp and the specimen is removed without spillage of cancer cells into the pelvis. The vagina is closed.

Lymphadenectomy

Lymphadenectomy is the standard of care at present. Lymph node sampling alone is insufficient. As the number of nodes removed is increased, the number of involved lymph nodes detected will be more. Lymphadenectomy is started at the bifurcation of the common iliac artery. The common iliac group of lymph glands along with its connective tissue is removed from the bifurcation of the common iliac to the bifurcation of the aorta. When removing the glands at the bifurcation of the aorta, care should be taken not to damage the presacral vessels. Throughout the procedure the ureter should be retracted medially, preserving the attachment to the medial flap of the peritoneum. The external iliac group of lymphatics is removed by dissecting inferiorly to the inguinal ligament upto the point where the deep circumflex iliac vein crosses the external iliac artery. The external and common iliac veins are reflected carefully and posterior group of lymph nodes removed. The genitofemoral nerve is located lateral to the external iliac vessels and should not be injured. Sometimes an aberrant obturator artery which arises from the external iliac or inferior epigastric artery will be encountered.

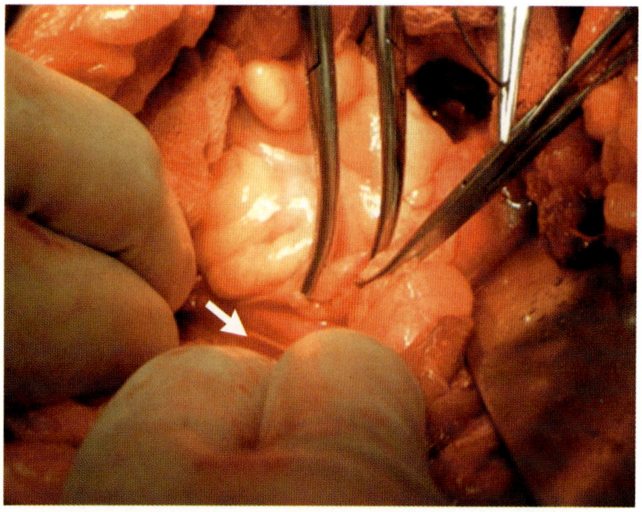

Fig. 22.7: The obturator nerve (arrow) is seen in the pelvic side wall after removal of the obturator group of nodes

The obturator group of nodes should be removed by reflecting the external iliac vessels medially. The obturator nerve and vessels can be seen entering the obturator foramen which should not be injured (Fig. 22.7). All the nodes in the obturator fossa and those along the internal iliac vessels are removed. If there is bleeding in the obturator fossa the obturator vessels can be clipped with hemaclips. If excessive bleeding is encountered from this space it can be controlled by hot mops. The procedure is repeated on the opposite side also.

Sentinel Lymph Node Evaluation

Detection of sentinel lymph node in cancer cervix is under evaluation. Sentinel lymph node is the first lymph node to be involved in malignant diseases. If sentinel lymph node is identified and found to be negative, further lymphadenectomy along with the associated morbidities can be avoided. Sentinel node can be identified intraoperatively by injecting blue dye into the tumor and by identifying the blue color in the lymph node. Another method is by injecting radio labeled Technetium 99 into the tumor and detecting the presence of radioactivity within the node by a hand held gamma probe. Sentinel lymph node can be detected by both laparotomy and laparoscopy in up to 80-100% of the cases.[20] The sensitivity is reported to be 65-87%. This method is still in the investigational stage. Presently, it cannot replace complete lymphadenectomy.

22.8.7 Laparoscopic Radical Hysterectomy and Pelvic Lymphadenectomy

The first report of laparoscopic radical hysterectomy and pelvic lymphadenectomy is by Nezhat. Recent reports reveal that laparoscopically assisted vaginal hysterectomy and pelvic lymphadenectomy has similar recurrence risk as abdominal radical hysterectomy.[21] The procedure is the same as the open technique. Argon beam coagulator is used for coagulation and the uterine artery is clipped. Inserting a drain does not seem to decrease infection or lymphocyst formation (Figs 22.8 and 22.9).

22.8.8 Complications of Radical Hysterectomy (Table 22.10)

Complication rates are much less in experienced hands with developments in surgical techniques. It is almost similar to that of hysterectomy done for benign disease.

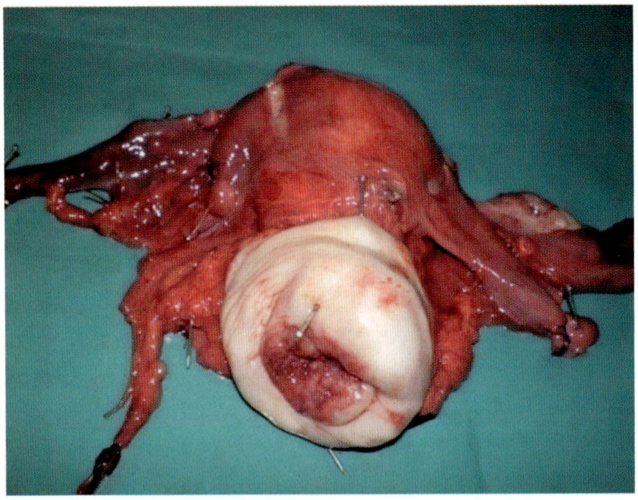

Fig. 22.8: Radical hysterectomy specimen with vaginal wall everted

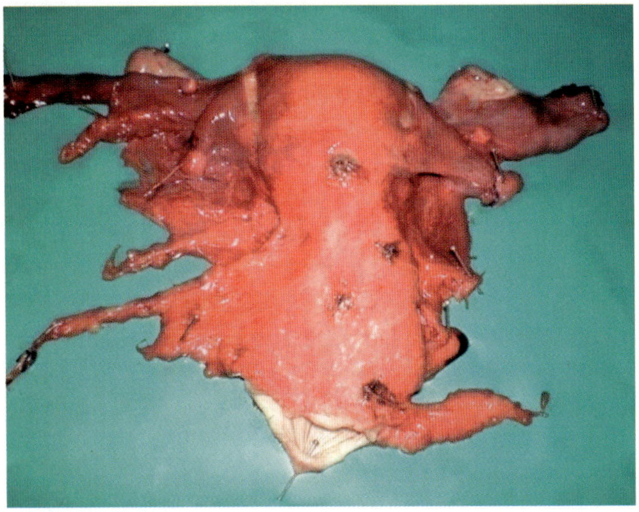

Fig. 22.9: Radical hysterectomy specimen (of the patient whose clinical photograph is given earlier)

Table 22.10: Acute complications of radical hysterectomy

Blood loss	0.8 liters (average)
Ureterovaginal fistula	1-2%
Vesicovaginal fistula	1%
Pulmonary embolism	1-2%
Small bowel obstruction	1%
Febrile morbidity	25-50%

Source: Boyce J, Fruchter R, Nicastri A. Prognostic factors in Stage I carcinoma of the cervix. Gynecol Oncol 1981;12:154-165.

Blood Loss

Meticulous dissection, keeping in mind the anatomy of the pelvis is important in preventing hemorrhage. But serious hemorrhage can occur from the pelvic side wall in the obturator fossa or from the presacral region. If the vessel cannot be identified pressure can be applied by placing a pack. This helps in reducing the blood loss and thereby identifying the vessel. The vessel can be clipped or ligated. It is safe to keep Bull Dog clamps ready so that, in case a vessel is torn these can be applied and the injury repaired.

Venous Thrombosis and Pulmonary Embolism

Extensive dissection during radical surgery releases thromboplastins into the circulation. Lymphadenectomy invariably causes damage to the venous walls. These factors supplemented with other patient factors can place the patient at high risk for venous thrombosis and thromboembolism. There is a place for prophylactic heparin therapy. Low Molecular Weight Heparin is as effective as conventional heparin in preventing thrombosis. Another method to reduce thrombosis is by pneumatic calf compression which can be started in the operating room and continued until discharge from the hospital. Deep breathing exercise as well as passive leg exercises should be taught preferably prior to surgery.

Ureteral Damage

Ureteral damage was previously reported as 12.5%. The recent reports of ureteral fistula and damage are less than 1%. The upper part of the pelvic ureter should not be separated from the medial flap of the peritoneum up to the uterosacral ligament to retain the vascularity. Injury to the muscular wall of the ureter should be avoided by meticulous dissection.

Subacute and Chronic Complications

Bladder dysfunction and lymphocyst formation

Bladder dysfunction can occur because of the inevitable denervation of the bladder. Nerve sparing radical hysterectomy is under investigation. Intraoperatively nerves can be identified by electrical stimulation and thus can be preserved.

The problem is that the same tissue which contains lymphatic channels may be harboring malignant cells which may also get retained instead of being removed. If a lymphocyst is formed, the patient will have discomfort and edema of the lower limbs. Large symptomatic lymphocysts should be drained by inserting a needle abdominally or vaginally. If lymphocyst formation occurs repeatedly, it can be sclerosed by injecting tetracycline into the cyst under CT guidance.

Ureteral stenosis is more common in patients who undergo postoperative radiation and in those who develop serious infection or lymphocyst formation. It should be diagnosed early as it can be treated, lest it can end up in nephrectomy. Ureteral stricture in the absence of radiation or lymphocyst should raise the suspicion of tumor recurrence. CT guided biopsy will help diagnose tumor recurrence.

Bladder hypotonia

The incidence of bladder hypotonia is reported to be as high as 50%. The patient experiences decreased bladder sensation and increased residual urine volume. Postoperatively the bladder should be continuously drained using suprapubic or transurethral catheter for 6-7 days. Later on the catheter can be clamped to check whether the patient appreciates bladder sensation. When the patient feels bladder sensation the catheter can be removed. Post void residual urine should be checked. Persistence of bladder hypotonia necessitates prolonged catheterization for 1-2 months by which time the bladder will regain its tone.

Fistula

Fistula is reported to occur in less than 1% of the patients. More than 1/3rd will heal spontaneously and the rest can be successfully repaired as against postradiation fistulas which are difficult to repair.

22.8.9 Adjuvant Therapy after Radical Surgery

Adjuvant chemoradiation is advised if any of these high risk features are found after surgery on histopathological examination.

1. Positive or close margins
2. Positive lymph nodes
3. Parametrial involvement

The most important prognostic factor is the status of the lymph nodes. Patients whose lymph nodes are negative, have a 5-year survival of 85-90% whereas if the lymph nodes are positive, the 5 year survival rate drops to 20-74%, depending on the group of lymph nodes involved (Table 22.11).

Table 22.11: Data on lymph node status and 5-year survival rates

Lymph node status	*5-year survival*
Tumor emboli in lymph node	82.5%
Unilateral pelvic node involvement	59-70%
More than 3 positive pelvic nodes	68%
Bilateral pelvic node involvement	22-40%
Common iliac nodes are positive	25%

Reference: Pillerom J, Durand J, Hamelin J. Prognostic value of node metastasis in cancer of the uterine cervix. Am J Obstet Gyanecol 1974;119:458-462

Piver M, Chung W. Prognostic significance of cervical lesion size and pelvic node metastasis in cervical carcinoma. Obstet Gynaecol 1972;114:964-62.

Patients with intermediate risk factors like greater than one-third stromal invasion, capillary lymphatic space invasion, and large clinical tumor diameter also will benefit from adjuvant chemoradiation. A GOG study evaluated postoperative radiation for patients who had radical hysterectomy, and in whom the nodes were negative, but had above mentioned risk factors. 277 patients were enrolled in the study. They were randomized to adjuvant radiation vs. no further treatment. The recurrence risk was 15% in the radiation therapy and 27% in the non-radiation therapy group.[22-24] Hence, adjuvant radiation should be considered for patients with 2 or more tumor related risk factors.

22.8.10 Follow-up after Radical Surgery for Cervical Cancer

Recurrent disease can occur in 5-20% of patients even after treatment of early stage disease. The reasons for recurrence are either incomplete removal of the tumor or incomplete lymphadenectomy. Recurrence usually occurs within 1 year of treatment and almost all occur within 3 years. The sites of recurrence are central, pelvic side wall; or it can be at distant sites or multiple sites. Hence, patients should be reviewed initially at least every 3 months for three years and every 6 months for the fourth and fifth years. They should be instructed about the warning symptoms of recurrence such as vaginal bleeding, discharge or pelvic discomfort. At the follow-up visits, she should be examined for lymphadenopathy, leg edema, abdominal masses and a rectovaginal examination should be performed to look for pelvic masses. Vault smear should be taken at each visit. If there is suspicion of involvement of rectum, bladder or pelvis, she should be subjected to the appropriate investigations like cystoscopy, proctoscopy, CT or MRI.

22.8.11 Radiotherapy (RT)

Radiotherapy is the other treatment option for stage 1B1 and IIA disease. For stage IB2, IIB, III and IV, radiation is the treatment of choice. The cervix can tolerate very high doses of radiation. This fact combined with the convenient position of the uterus in the center of the pelvis which allows intracavitary sources to be kept in the uterine cavity, makes radiation effective in the treatment of cancer of the cervix.

Advantages of Radiotherapy

Radiotherapy has the following advantages:

1. Treats the cervix along with the draining lymphatics and lymph nodes. Radiation to the whole pelvis takes care of all the pelvic nodes, which even the most radical surgery, cannot achieve without producing much morbidity.
2. Cure can be achieved with preservation of the organs
3. Primary mortality is almost nil.
4. Can be given when surgery is contraindicated due to other reasons.
5. Cure can be attempted even in advanced disease.

After the initiation of radiation therapy in the year 1903, radiation treatment has evolved enormously. The radiation source which was initially Radium has been changed to Caesium and Iridium. The dose of radiation is presently calculated in Gray (Gy). 1 Gray = 100 rads. 1 cGy = 1 rad. Radiation treatment is given as both intracavitary (ICRT) and External Beam Radiation Therapy (EBRT).

In the radiation treatment of cancer of the cervix, the tumor, parametrium and pelvic side walls (where the lymph nodes are situated) are irradiated by intracavitary source. The radiation to the pelvic side wall will not be enough from the intracavitary source. Hence, the pelvic side wall is irradiated with external beam mega voltage teletherapy using linear accelerator. Patients who have common iliac and para aortic node involvement need extended field radiation.

Either EBRT or ICRT can be administered first. However in the following situations, EBRT is preferred first.

a. Bulky tumors
b. Parametrial involvement (suboptimal dosimetry due to altered geometry if ICRT is administered initially)
c. Large necrotic tumors (Practical difficulty in carrying out ICRT)
d. Bleeding tumors (intracavitary administration can provoke bleeding).

External Beam RT (EBRT)

External beam RT is given using linear accelerator or a Cobalt 60 machine. The entire pelvis is treated by radiation. All tissues that are within the square marked by the green field on the X-ray are treated by EBRT (Figs 22.10A and B). The target tissues are the tumor, the parametrium, lymphatics and the lymph nodes in the pelvic side wall. However, toxicities to the bladder and the rectum which are also in the same field are the major concern. EBRT is given at a total dose of 40-45 Gray, usually in 20 fractions at a rate of 1.8-2 Gy/day, for 5 days a week. Treatment is given usually in a 4 field technique-1 anteroposterior, 1 posteroanterior and 2 lateral field. Treatment can also be given in 2 fields.

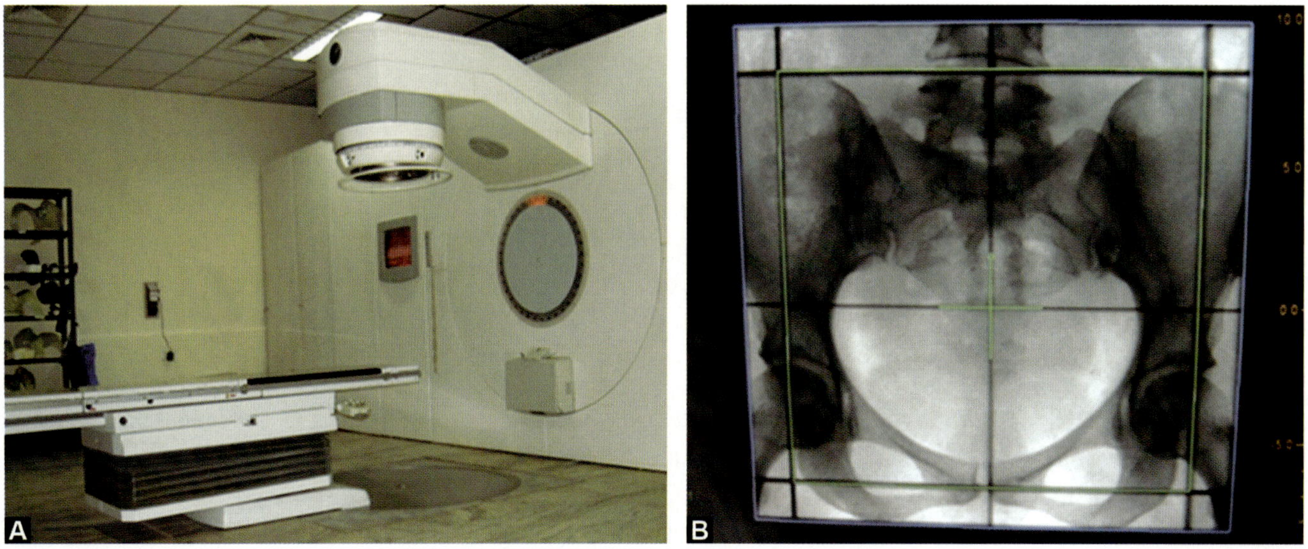

Figs 22.10A and B: Teletherapy machine for EBRT (A). X-ray picture showing field of whole pelvic radiation (B)
Courtesy: RCC Trivandrum

22.8.12 Intracavitary Radiation (ICRT/ Brachytherapy) (Figs 22.11A to C and 22.12)

The success of radiotherapy of cervical cancer lies in the extreme tolerance of the cervical tissue to high doses of radiation; as high as 200 Gy. Since the tumor in the cervix is approachable transvaginally, it can be irradiated by the intracavitary source. The dose of radiation given from the intracavitary source depends on the inverse square law. As the distance from the source increases the dose decreases. Hence, from the sources kept in uterine cavity and lateral vaginal fornix, the maximum radiation is delivered to the tumor and the parametrium. Part of the radiation would be delivered to the pelvic side walls where the lymph nodes are situated.

In the older method, the tubes which contain the radiation source are preloaded. The disadvantage of this method was the high radiation risk for medical and paramedical personnel.

To overcome this risk, the remote afterloading system was devised.

ICRT using afterloading Technique

ICRT is presently administered using high dose rate (HDR) isotopes, i.e. isotopes that produce radiation at high rates of more than 12Gy/hour. At these rates the biological effects produced by radiation is roughly 1.7 times that produced by the older isotopes. The radiation source used is Iridium 192.

In HDR ICRT, the sources are introduced into the patients' body through applicators. These applicators are hollow and are made of metal. They are usually available in a set of three. The one which is inserted into the uterine cavity is called the tandem. The other two are placed in the lateral fornices and are called the colpostats. The tubes are inserted, locked in place and further secured with gauze packing. These metal tubes are connected to flexible plastic tubes which in turn are connected at the other end to the device which houses the radiation source. The operator can load and unload the radiation source from the remote housing by providing signals. Thus, radiation to the operator is minimized.

Since the sources are kept in the uterine cavity and the lateral vaginal fornices, the primary tumor in the cervix and the parametrium are irradiated to the maximum. The anteriorly located bladder and posteriorly located rectum are comparatively spared of radiation. The pelvic side walls receive only minimal dose from ICRT. It will be taken care of by EBRT.

After securing the connections, a computer program calculates the radiation dose. The prescribed dose is calculated by the radiation given to point A. Point A is defined as a

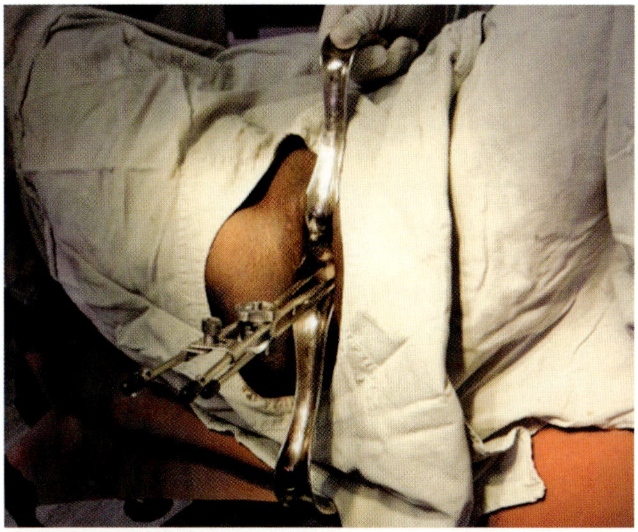

Fig. 22.12: Insertion of intracavitary applicators

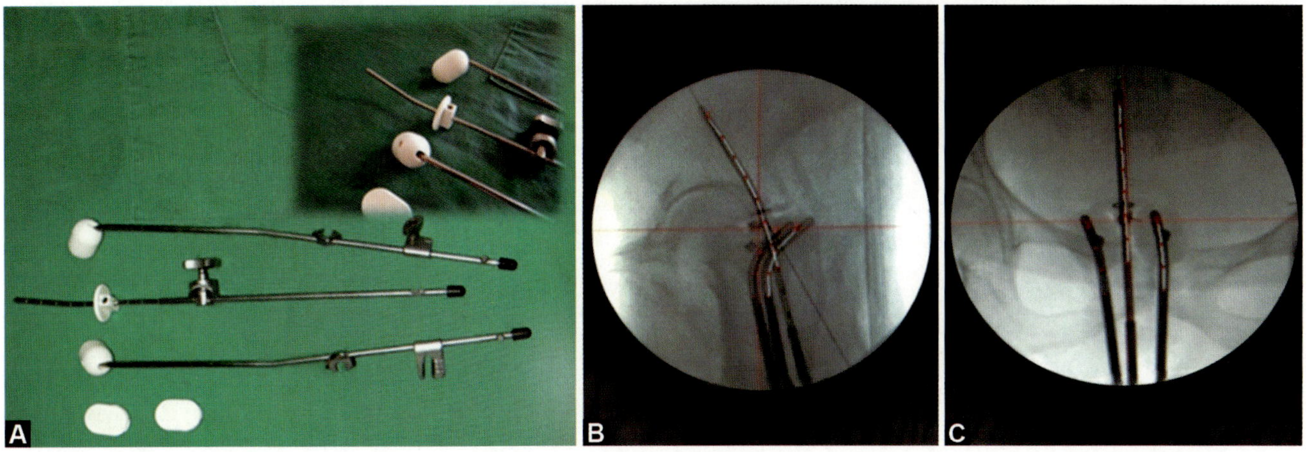

Figs 22.11A to C: Intrauterine and vaginal applicators (A). X-ray picture showing intracavitary applicators in place (lateral and anterior view) (B and C)

point 2 cm superior to the external os and 2 cm lateral to the middle of the cervical canal. Point A corresponds to the point where the uterine artery crosses the ureter. The usual dose prescribed is about 7Gy to point A weekly for 3 consecutive weeks. This amounts to a total ICRT dose of 35 to 40 Gy to the cervix. This, when combined with EBRT of 45Gy, amounts to a total of 80-100Gy. This total dose that the cervix receives is a critical dose above which the probability of viable tumor cells remaining is reduced to extremely low levels.

The dose received at point A correlates with the probability of local control because this is the site of the parametrium which is the most common site of invasion beyond the cervix. The dose received at point A helps predict the doses received at various other points within the pelvis. The tumor in the cervix receives approximately 3 times the dose calculated at point A. Point B is located 5 cm lateral to the midline and 2 cm superior to the external cervical os. Point B is described to calculate the dose received by the pelvic lymph nodes.

The computer program when activated directs radiation sources shaped like small balls, through the tubing systems into the metal tubes that are placed within the patient. These pellets are retained till the necessary dosage, prescribed by the radiation oncologist have been administered. Whenever the patient wants to communicate with the medical personal, she can give signals following which the sources can be retrieved. When the treatment is over, the computer redirects the radiation sources back into the secure housing. The tubes are disconnected. The metal tubes are removed and the patient discharged after a few hours observation.

Chemoradiation

In the radiation treatment of stage IB2 and IIA bulky tumors chemoradiation is preferred. This is confirmed by several studies by Gynecologic Oncology Group (GOG).[25] Here radiation is administered along with a chemotherapeutic agent usually cisplatin—concurrent chemoradiation. Cisplatin here acts primarily as a radiation sensitizer, i.e. it makes tumor tissue more sensitive to the destructive action of radiation. Another advantage of chemotherapy is that micrometastases outside the radiation field also will be taken care of. Cisplatin is given in a relatively low dose of 40 mg/ square meter weekly till the entire course of radiation is completed. Improved overall survival and reduced local and distant recurrence have been reported in a Cochrane review.[26-28]

22.9 MANAGEMENT ALGORITHM FOR STAGE IB1 (FLOW CHART 22.2)

Flow Chart 22.2: Management algorithm for stage IB1

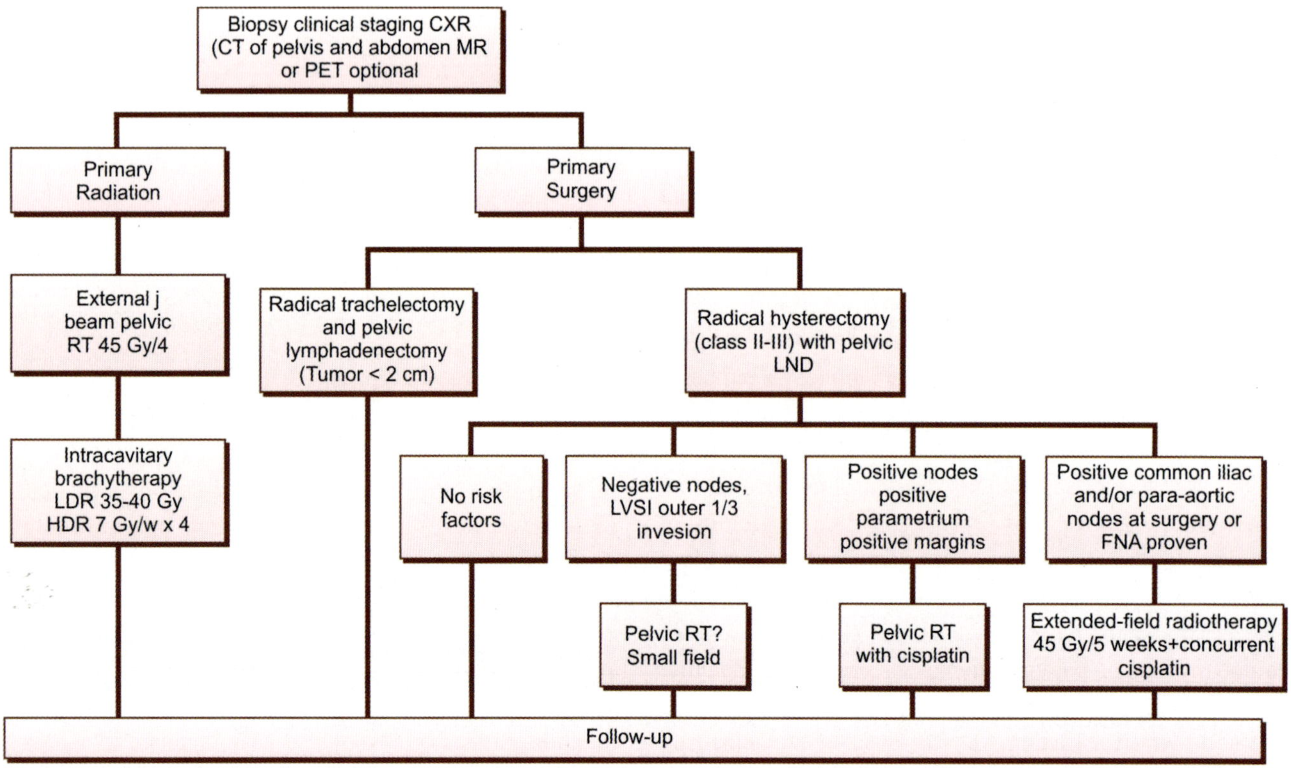

Flow Chart 22.3: Management algorithm of IB2 and Stage IIA

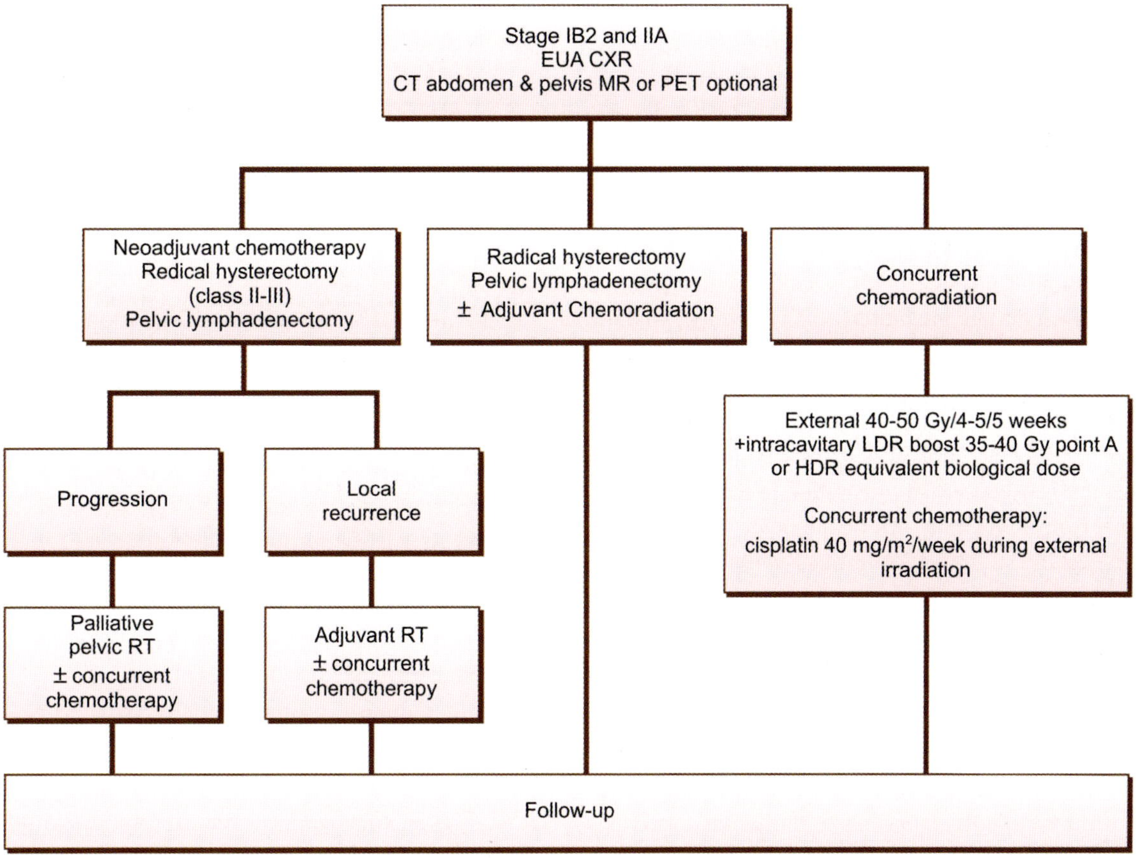

Management Algorithm for Stage IB2 and Stage IIA (Flow Chart 22.3)

22.10 MANAGEMENT OF STAGES IB2, IIB AND III

Radiation is the treatment of choice, for the treatment of bulky stage I B, IIB and III disease, as attempting surgery will result in leaving positive margins. Concurrent Chemoradiation with Cisplatin combined with EBRT and ICRT is the standard treatment.

Trials have been conducted with neoadjuvant chemotherapy followed by radical surgery for bulky stage Ib disease. A Cochrane review on this approach reveals that this has a potential to be beneficial in treating more women with surgery especially if they are young.[29] The benefit however has to be proved by proper RCTs.

22.11 MANAGEMENT OF STAGE IVA

Invasion of the bladder and rectum is an ominous finding. The curative dose of radiation in the presence of bladder or rectum involvement is well above the tolerance limit for the normal tissues. This dose will subject the patient at risk of developing vesicovaginal or rectovaginal fistulae. Surgery, if considered should be pelvic exenteration where urinary or fecal diversion is mandatory. If the patient presents with fistula, pelvic exenteration with urinary or fecal diversion is the choice. The decision to go for radiation or surgery depends upon the general condition of the patient and her choice. If the patient's general condition is good enough to withstand exenteration surgery, it should be preferred.

22.12 MANAGEMENT OF STAGE IVB

Metastatic disease is practically incurable. Radiation is primarily chosen to provide palliation, reduce pelvic pain and control bleeding. It also aids in relieving ureteric obstruction. In such situations, curative doses are not prescribed. Instead, lower total doses with high dose per fraction are prescribed which provides adequate palliation.

22.13 INTERSTITIAL BRACHYTHERAPY

While treating bulky cervical cancer, we may come across situations where, due to the bulk of the disease in the lateral aspect, there can be residual disease in the parametrium as a result of rapid fall off of dose from ICRT. Residual disease in the parametrium is usually treated by EBRT, as the radiation from the ICRT does not have enough range to reach deeper. Bulky disease need further dose of EBRT. Giving more EBRT is detrimental as this will lead to administration of doses far beyond the tolerance limit of the normal pelvic tissues (bladder and rectum). In such situations, interstitial brachytherapy is a safer alternative. In ICRT, radiation sources are applied into the natural body cavities (uterine cavity and the vagina). In interstitial brachytherapy, radiation sources are introduced directly into the parametrium through hollow needles inserted through the perineum. This requires a certain degree of surgical skill, but unfortunately facilities for this procedure are not widely available. Interstitial brachytherapy is used to treat infiltration to the vagina also, as the dose from ICRT may not be adequate to control the disease, especially in the lower third of vagina.

22.14 INTENSITY MODULATED RADIATION THERAPY

This is an advanced form of administering EBRT. Radiation from a linear accelerator is modified across a given field. The intensity of the dose across the field varies such that, the part of the field corresponding to the tumor receives a higher dose while normal tissues receive little or no radiation at the same time. Multiple fields are used providing a dose distribution that highly conforms to the tumor with adequate sparing of normal tissues. The entire process is computer controlled. The execution of such a complicated program needs exceptional quality control. It is predominantly used to boost parametrial residual disease, a large residual pelvic node or even residual vaginal involvement. Though IMRT is a highly conformed technique of administering radiation, it cannot replace ICRT; because it cannot attain the extreme degree of conformity that ICRT achieves.

Approximate 5-year survival depends upon stage (Table 22.12) (Cochrane data base).

Table 22.12: Five-year survival rate of cervical cancer

Stage	*5-year Survival rate (%)*
IA1/IA2	95
IB	90
IIA/B	65
IIIA/B	35
IVA	17
IVB	10

22.15 COMPLICATIONS OF RADIATION TREATMENT

Complications during Treatment (Table 22.13)

Uterine perforation can occur at the time of insertion of applicators. As a consequence of perforation, bleeding and infection can occur. In case perforation occurs, the applicators should be removed. The patient should be kept under observation and prophylactic antibiotic should be administered.

Table 22.13: Side effects of radiation treatment

Acute	*Chronic*
• Abdominal cramps	• Rectovaginal and vesicovaginal fistulas
• Diarrhea	
• Bleeding per rectum	• Proctosigmoiditis
• Increased frequency of micturition	• Small intestinal injury and adhesions leading to malnutrition
• Hematuria	• Ureteral stricture

Acute side effects during treatment

Effects of radiation on the epithelium of the bladder and bowel can cause diarrhea, abdominal cramps, bleeding per-rectum, increased frequency of micturition and hematuria. These can be managed conservatively. If symptoms are severe, treatment can be suspended for one or two weeks.

Chronic complications

As an effect of radiation, vasculitis and fibrosis can result, which compromise blood supply to tissues. Consequently, rectovaginal and vesicovaginal fistulae can occur. The reported incidence of rectovaginal fistula is 1.4% and vesicovaginal fistula is 5.3%. Proctosigmoiditis can persist after radiation therapy. Antidiarrheal medications and steroid enema will help to relieve the symptoms. Those who do not respond to conservative measures need temporary colostomy to provide rest to the bowel.

Rectovaginal fistula: Rectovaginal fistula following radiation treatment is not easily amenable to treatment. Tissue interposition can be tried with bulbospongiosus muscle flap or rectosigmoid. Repeated failures may need permanent colostomy.

Small bowel complications: Women who had previous laparotomies are prone for small bowel injury due to adhesion and fixity of the bowel. Persistent abdominal distention and pain will be the symptoms. This can result in malnutrition and anemia. After improving the general condition surgical correction can be done.

Vesicovaginal fistula: Vesicovaginal fistula occurs in 1-5% of patients. Compared to fistula following radical hysterectomy, radiation fistula is difficult to treat. Small fistula can be repaired by flap splitting method. Usually, fistulas are large and not amenable to repair. Urinary diversion is the only feasible management in such cases.

Ureteral stricture: Ureteral stricture following radiation treatment can be due to fibrosis or recurrence. CT guided FNAC will help in excluding recurrence. Laparotomy, ureterolysis and stenting may be needed to relieve ureteral obstruction due to fibrosis.

Follow-up

After treatment patients should be examined regularly every 3 months for 2 years and later every 6 months for the next 3 years. At each visit history suggestive of recurrence should be elicited. Enlargement of supraclavicular and inguinal lymph nodes has to be looked for. Careful pelvic examination should be done to make out the disappearance of the tumor, which is expected at the end of 3 months of completing treatment. Parametrium should be palpated by rectal examination. If there is any doubt about tumor recurrence, CT/MRI should be done. CT guided FNAC should be resorted to for confirmation.

22.16 RECURRENT CERVICAL CANCER

Management of recurrent cancer depends upon the performance status, type of initial treatment, site of recurrence (metastatic/local) and size of tumor. Management of those who have recurrence after initial radiotherapy is problematic. Selected patients who have small (≤ 2 cm) tumor size can be advised radical surgery as a curative measure. If it is a large volume tumor or metastatic disease, palliative chemotherapy is the only option.

Central recurrence following radical surgery is preferably treated by pelvic exenteration only if the patient is fit for the procedure. For recurrence involving the pelvic side wall, chemoradiation is the option.

Management of recurrent cervical cancer

- Palliation
- Pain relief- Analgesia ladder
- Hemostasis
  - Packing
  - Hemostatic radiation
  - Internal iliac artery embolization
- Colostomy for fistula

22.16.1 Management Algorithm of Recurrent Cervical Cancer (Flow Chart 22.4)

22.17 MANAGEMENT OF CERVICAL CANCER IN PREGNANCY

Rarely, cervical cancer is encountered during pregnancy. The reported incidence is 1.2 per 10,000 pregnancies.[30]

Speculum examination should be done for all women who presents with bleeding per vaginum during pregnancy. When an obvious lesion is encountered biopsy should be taken. As in the non-pregnant state biopsy report of

Flow Chart 22.4: Management algorithm of recurrent cervical cancer

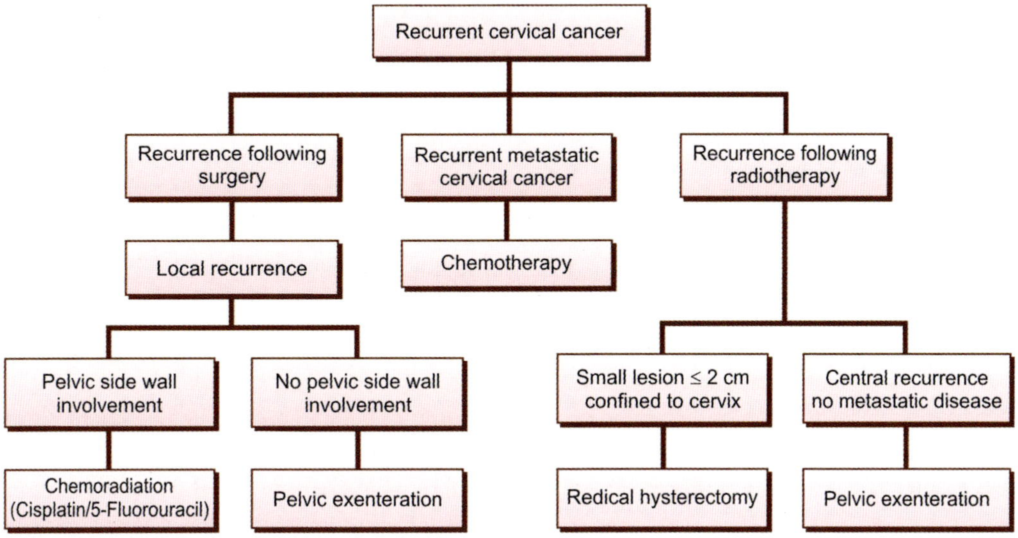

microinvasion should be confirmed by cone biopsy. Cone biopsy during pregnancy carries increased risk of hemorrhage, infection, abortion and preterm labor. To prevent pregnancy loss, cervical circlage can be combined with conisation. In the event of an abnormal cervical smear and no visible lesion in the cervix, colposcopic examination and endocervical curettage must be done. The only absolute indication for conization in pregnancy is to confirm or rule out microinvasive disease when such a diagnosis will alter the timing or mode of delivery.

Carcinoma in situ

Carcinoma in situ diagnosed in pregnancy can be managed conservatively till delivery. But patients should be followed up regularly.

Invasive cancer diagnosed in the first trimester

The possible treatment options are in situ radical hysterectomy and radiotherapy. For stage I or IIA disease in young healthy women, in situ radical hysterectomy with pelvic lymphadenectomy is the preferred procedure. Dissection is easier in pregnancy. For other stages external radiation will cause abortion after which treatment can be completed with ICRT.

Invasive cancer diagnosed in the second trimester

Termination of pregnancy before radiotherapy carries increased risk of recurrence. Radical hysterectomy with fetus in situ in the second trimester is technically difficult. Hence radiotherapy is preferred. EBRT is given initially, following which the patient will abort. Consequently, treatment can be completed by ICRT.

Invasive cancer diagnosed in the third trimester

Treatment can be delayed for 12 weeks if the stage of the disease is IB1 or less, so that the fetus will attain maturity, if the patient desires so. For stage IB2, the delay should not be more than 6 weeks.[31] A maximum delay of 6 weeks may not adversely affect maternal outcome. During this period the patient should be periodically examined. If the disease progresses definitive treatment should be resorted to immediately. This interval need not be strictly adhered to, but should be individualized.

After reaching viability classical cesarean is preferred to prevent hemorrhage as well as dissemination of cancer cells. For stage IB1 or IIA, along with classical cesarean, radical hysterectomy with pelvic lymphadenectomy is preferred. For all other stages chemoradiation is preferred after classical cesarean. Since women with cancer cervix who were delivered vaginally had greater recurrence rate compared to those who had classical cesarean,[32] vaginal delivery is not preferred.

22.18 INCIDENTALLY DIAGNOSED CERVICAL CANCER AFTER HYSTERECTOMY

Occasionally women are diagnosed to have invasive cancer of the cervix after hysterectomy done for benign disease. If the patient is young and parametrial disease is excluded by imaging, it is better to go for radical parametrectomy and upper vaginectomy sparing the ovaries. Lymphadenectomy should also be done. If gross parametrial disease is diagnosed by imaging, chemo-radiation is the treatment of choice.

22.19 CARCINOMA OF THE CERVICAL STUMP

Stump carcinoma developing after supracervical hysterectomy pose problems for surgery as well as radiotherapy. ICRT cannot be successfully given because of the inability to deliver adequate dose due to the short cervical stump. After hysterectomy the bladder and rectum will be closer so that radiation injury to these structures will be high. Since uterine tandem cannot be placed, ICRT can be administered only with vaginal ovoids. Parametrial disease is treated with EBRT through lateral ports rather than anterior and posterior ports, so that the bowel and bladder injury can be minimized. For early stage disease, radical trachelectomy with upper vaginectomy and lymphadenectomy should be resorted to. Because of distorted anatomy due to previous surgery, further surgery may be technically difficult.

22.20 CONCLUSION

Cervical cancer is the most common gynecological neoplasm in the developing countries and is a major health hazard. Human papilloma virus infection is identified as the causative agent for cervical cancer. Since there is a long window period between the virus infection and development of malignancy, there is sufficient time for detecting premalignant changes and preventing malignancy. The Pap test, the best cancer screening test available has made diagnosis of the disease in the premalignant or early stage possible. In the developed countries, the 70% reduction achieved in the incidence of the disease can be attributed to the Pap smear screening programs. Screening by HPV DNA is the next step forward towards screening which is yet to become popular. The disease is staged clinically. Modern investigations like MRI and PET if available can be used for treatment planning even though it is not recommended by FIGO. Early stage disease means excellent prognosis.

Stage I and IIA can be managed by either radical surgery or radiation. Quality of life is better after surgical treatment when compared to radiotherapy. Radiation treatment is presently combined with radiosensitizer cisplatin. With improvements in radiotherapy, there is reduction in the side effects and long-term sequelae. To optimize the outcome of surgical treatment, it is better that surgery is performed in specialized centers by experienced onco-surgeons. The management of late stage disease is by chemoradiation. HPV vaccine is another leap forward towards prevention of this common neoplasm. Since cervical cancer is preventable, there is a pressing need to educate women especially in countries where routine screening programs are not available, about symptoms of the disease and the need for seeking prompt health check up. Clinicians should be familiar with the screening techniques, diagnostic procedures and management of the disease.

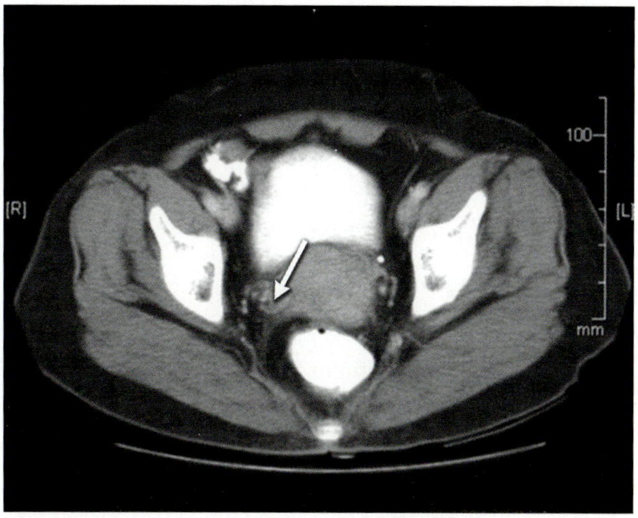

Fig. 22.14: CT picture of M/s B showing parametrial involvement. Note the loss of fat plane between the tumor and the parametrium on the right side (arrow)

22.21 CASE SCENARIOS

Case Scenario 1

M/s B aged 40 years presented with intermenstrual bleeding. On examination she was found to have a friable growth measuring about 3 cm arising from the anterior lip of the cervix (Fig. 22.13). Biopsy revealed large cell non-keratinizing squamous carcinoma. On clinical examination, there was doubtful parametrial involvement close to the cervix. There was no evidence of involvement of the bladder or rectum.

What is the stage of the disease?
If she has parametrial involvement, the stage is IIB.

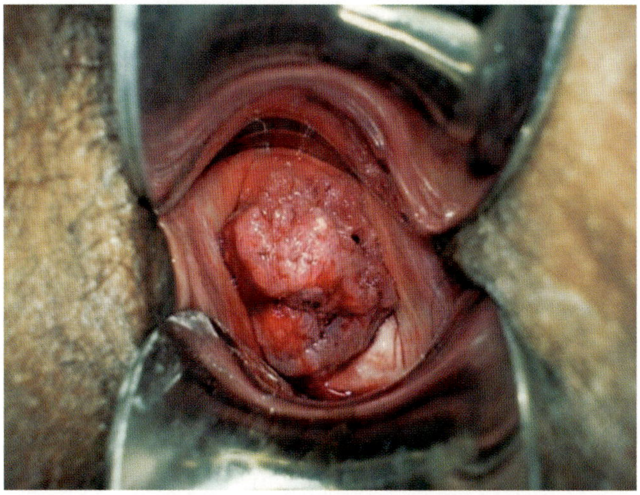

Fig. 22.13: Speculum examination showing the tumor arising from the anterior lip of the cervix

What is the mode of treatment?
The treatment options have to be decided based on the presence or absence of parametrial involvement. Even though FIGO does not recommend imaging by CT/MRI in the staging and treatment decisions of cancer cervix, since there is clinically doubtful parametrial involvement, MR imaging can be done for confirmation of parametrial involvement. Since the patient could not afford MR imaging, CT was done.

CT (Fig. 22.14) showed loss of fat plane between the tumor and the parametrium on the right side which signifies invasion into the parametrium.

Is CT the ideal imaging modality to delineate parametrial extension?
No, MRI is superior to CT in making out parametrial involvement.

If the patient prefers surgery, what would be your advice?
Surgery is likely to leave behind positive margins in the presence of parametrial involvement so that even after surgery, the patient will need radiation. Hence, radiation treatment is the choice.

Case Scenario 2

M/s A, a 42-year-old multiparous lady presented with intermenstrual bleeding of 2 months duration. On examination her general condition was found to be satisfactory. There was nothing positive on general examination. Examination of the abdomen also was unremarkable. On speculum examination, the cervix showed a growth at the level of the external os. The growth was friable and there was bleeding on touch. The growth measured 3 cm × 2.8 cm. The patient was examined under anesthesia for staging. Bimanual examination revealed induration of the cervix. Parametrium appeared normal on bi-digital examination. Biopsy of the growth revealed adenosquamous carcinoma.

What is the stage of the disease?
Stage IB1.

What are the management options which should be discussed with the patient?
She can be treated with either radiation or radical surgery. Advantages and disadvantages of each should be discussed. Since the cervix appears bulky the tumor can be bigger than what is assessed by speculum examination. There can be a big tumor in the endocervix which cannot be correctly measured by clinical examination. Since surgery is preferred if the tumor size is 4 cm or less and radiation is preferred if it is more than 4cms, it is better that the size be assessed by imaging. Imaging by MRI showed that the lesion to be measuring 3.2 cm. Since the stage was I b1, and the patient preferred surgical treatment, she was taken for Wertheim's hysterectomy. Her ovaries were transfixed to the upper abdomen during surgery.

Should she be given postoperative radiation?
The pathology report revealed no evidence of lymph node involvement. The margins were negative for malignancy and there was no deep stromal involvement. Hence, she need not be given radiation.

Case Scenario 3

M/s M, a 36-year-old multiparous lady, presented with post-coital bleeding. General examination and abdominal examination were unremarkable. Speculum examination showed a friable growth in the cervix involving both the anterior and posterior lips in the region near the external os. The lesion measured about 2.8 cm. Bimanual examination showed induration and an enlarged cervix. However, the uterus was mobile. There was no parametrial extension. Biopsy showed adenosquamous carcinoma.

What is the stage of the disease?
Since the tumor is confined to the cervix and <4cms, it is stage Ib1. However, since clinically the cervix appears enlarged, there can be a larger tumor in the endocervix.

How can it be assessed?
Since the patient is young, if the tumor measures <4 cm, she can be advised surgical treatment (Wertheim's).

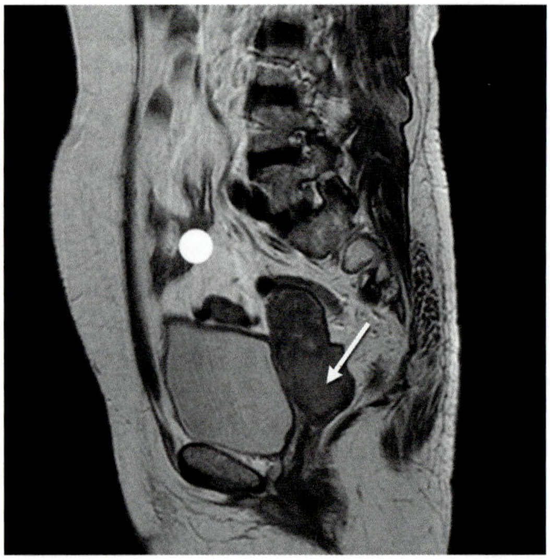

Fig. 22.15: T2 MRI image of the sagittal section of the pelvis and abdomen showing mass in the endocervical canal and both lips (arrow)

MRI/CT or PET scan can be resorted to for delineating the endocervical extent of the tumor and to plan treatment. She had MRI of pelvis which showed a large mass in the endocervix (Fig. 22.15).

Even though the patient was young and preferred surgical treatment, she was advised chemoradiation because of the large size of the tumor. She may need postoperative radiation if taken for surgery. Multi-modal treatment carries higher morbidity. She underwent external radiation followed by intracavitary radiation.

Why external radiation was given initially?
External radiation effect the shrinkage of the tumor causing more efficient brachytherapy with intracavitary source.

Case Scenario 4

M/s R, a 32-year-old Para 1 who came for a well woman check-up had a pap smear result reported as positive for squamous carcinoma cells. Her cervix was looking unremarkable on speculum examination. Bimanual examination was also unremarkable. She was temporarily separated from her husband as he was abroad.

1. **What further step should be taken after seeing this cervical smear report?**
   Malignancies of the cervix must be diagnosed based on histopathology as exfoliative cytology reports can be occasionally fallacious. Hence, the patient should be called back and counseled for biopsy.
2. **From where will you take the biopsy?**
   Since there is no obvious lesion, the biopsy should be taken ideally after colposcopic visualization. An

endocervical curettage must also be done as the cells exfoliated could be from a lesion in the endocervix.

Colposcopy was done which showed abnormal vascular pattern, cotton wool shaped blood vessels in an area on the posterior lip of cervix. Colposcopically directed biopsy was taken from this area. Endocervical curettage result came as negative.

The biopsy report came as carcinoma *in situ* with suspected invasion below the basement membrane.

3. **What should be the further evaluation?**

   Before deciding treatment, cone biopsy is indicated to differentiate between stage 1A1 and stage 1A2 and even stage 1B. If she has stage 1A1, cone biopsy will be sufficient treatment for her. But, if she has stage 1A2, she needs extensive surgery like radical trachelectomy or Wertheim's hysterectomy.

   Her biopsy report was: Microinvasive cancer of cervix with depth 5 mm below basement membrane and 6 mm horizontal extent. Hence, this is stage 1A2 carcinoma cervix.

4. **What would be the ideal treatment for this lady who is very keen to have one more child?**

   The lady should be counseled regarding surgical treatment. Radiotherapy is out of question as it will affect her fertility and may even cause menopause. Since she is keen to preserve her fertility, radical trachelectomy is the surgical treatment of choice for her. But, she must be counseled regarding the disadvantages of trachelectomy and the need for a preoperative pelvic lymph node assessment.

5. **If she asks whether she can delay treatment and complete her family within another 1 year, what should be your advice?**

   One year delay will definitely advance the stage of the disease and will adversely affect the cure rate.

   After proper counseling, the lady opted for radical trachelectomy. She had preoperative laparoscopic lymphadenectomy and it was found that lymph nodes were negative.

   Hence, radical trachelectomy was done for her.

REFERENCES

1. American Cancer Society, Cancer Facts and Figures 2002.
2. Bosch FX, Manos MM, Munoz N, et al. Prevalence of human papillomavirus in cervical cancer: A worldwide perspective. International biological study on cervical cancer (IBSCC) Study Group. J Natl Cancer Inst 1995;87:796-802.
3. Kurman RJ, Jenson AB,Lancaster WD. Papilloma virus infection of the cervix. Relationship to intraepithelial neoplasia based on the presence of specific viral structural proteins. Am J Surg Pathol 1983;7:39-52.
4. Devesa SS, Silverman DT, Young JL Jr, et al. Cancer incidence and mortalitytrends among whites in the United States, 1947-84. J Natl Cancer Inst 1987;79:701-70.
5. Koss LG. The Papanicolaou test for cervical cancer detection: a triumph and a tragedy. JAMA 1989;261:737-43.
6. S J Goblie, et al. Cost effectiveness of cervical cancer screening in five developing countries. N Engl J Med 2005;353(20):2158-68.
7. R Sankaranarayanan, et al. Visual inspection of the uterine cervix after application of acetic acid in the detection of cervical cancer and its precursors. Cancer 1998;83(10): 2150-56.
8. Sankaranarayanan R, Nene BM, Shastri SS, Jayant K, Muwonge R, Budukh AM, et al. HPV screening for cervical cancer in rural India. N Eng J Med Apr 2009;2;360(14):1385-94.
9. Kjorstad KE. Adenocarcinoma of the uterine cervix. Gynecol Oncol 1977;5:219-23.
10. CH Shin, JO Schorge, KR Lee, et al. Conservative management of adenocarcinoma in situ of the cervix. Gynaecol Oncol 2000;79.
11. Bidus MA, O'Boyle JD, Elkas JC. Sentinel lymph node detection in gynecologic malignancies. Postgrad Obstet Gynecol 2004;24(26);1-5.
12. Bipat S, Glas AS, Velden J, et al. Computed tomography and magnetic resonance imaging in staging of uterine cervical carcinoma: a systematic review. Gynecol Oncol 2003;91:59.
13. Donald G. Mitchell, Bradley Snyder, Fergus Coakley, Caroline Reinhold, Gillian Thomas, et al. Early Invasive Cervical Cancer: Tumor Delineation by Magnetic Resonance Imaging, Computed Tomography, and Clinical Examination, Verified by Pathologic Results, in the ACRIN 6651/GOG 183 Intergroup Study. Journal of Clinical Oncology 2006;24 (36):5687-94
14. Bipat S, Glas AS, Velden J, et al. Computed tomography and magnetic resonance imaging in staging of uterine cervical carcinoma: a systematic review. Gynecol Oncol 2003; 91:59.
15. Lagasse LD, Smith ML and Moore JG, et al. The effect of radiation therapy on pelvic lymph node involvement in stage I carcinoma of the cervix, Am J Obstet Gynecol 1974;119:328-43.
16. Schorge J. Stage IA1 cervical adenocarcinoma: definition and treatment. Obstet Gynecol 1999;93:219-22.
17. Östör A, et al. Microinvasive adenocarcinoma of the cervix: a clinicopathologic study of 77 women. Obstet Gynecol 1997;89:88-93.
18. Kasamatsu T, et al. Early invasive adenocarcinoma of the uterine cervix: criteria for nonradical surgical treatment. Gynecol Oncol 2002;85:327-32.

19. Covens A. preserving fertility in early cervical cancer with radical trachelectomy. Contemp Ob/Gyn 2003;48:46.
20. Angioli R, Palaia I, Cipriani C, et al. Role of sentinel lymph node biopsy procedure in cervical cancer: a critical point of view, Gynecol Oncol. 2005; 96:504-09.
21. Steed H, Rosen B, Murphy J, Laframboise S, De Petrillo D, Covens A. A comparison of laparoscopic-assisted radical vaginal hysterectomy and radical abdominal hysterectomy in the treatment of cervical cancer. Gynecol Oncol 2004;93:588-93.
22. Morely GW, Seski JC. Radial pelvic surgery versus radiation for stage 1 carcinoma of the cervix (exclusive of micro-invasion). Am J Obstet Gynecol 1976;126:785-98.
23. Martinbeau P, Kjorstad K, Iversen T. Stage 1b carcinoma of the cervix: the Norwegian Radium hospital. II. Results when pelvic nodes are involved. Obstet Gynecol 1982;60:215-18.
24. Hsu CT, Cheng YS, Su SC. Prognosis on the uterine cervical cancer with extensive lymph node metastasis. Am J Obstet Gynecol 1972;114:954-62.
25. Keys HM, Bundy BM, Stehman, et al. Cisplatin, radiation, and adjuvant hysterectomy compared with radiation and adjuvant hysterectomy for bulky stage IB cervical carcinoma. N Engl J Med 1999;340:1154-61.
26. Green J, Kirwan J, Tierney J, Vale C, Symonds P, Fresco L, Williams C, Collingwood M. Concomitant chemotherapy and radiation therapy for cancer of the uterine cervix. Cochrane Database of Systematic Reviews 2005(3)Art. No.: CD002225. DOI: 10.1002/14651858. CD002225.pub2.
27. PG Rose, BN Bundy, EB Watkins, et al. Concurrent cisplatin-based radiotherapy and chemotherapy for locally advanced cervical cancer, N Engl J Med 1999;340:1144-53.
28. Tambaro R, Scambia G, Di Maio M, et al. The role of chemotherapy in locally advanced, metastatic and recurrent cervical cancer, Crit Rev Oncol Hematol 2004;52:33-44
29. Neoadjuvant chemotherapy for locally advanced cervix cancer. Cochrane Database of Systematic Reviews 2004, Issue 1. Art. No.: CD001774. DOI: 10.1002/14651858. CD001774.pub2. ssue 1. Art. No.: CD001774. DOI: 10.1002/14651858.CD001774.pub2.
30. Duggan B , Muderspach L I, Roman LD, et al. Cervical cancer in pregnancy reporting on planned delay in therapy. Obstet gynecol 1993;82:598.
31. Nguyen C, Montz FJ, Bristow RE. Management of stage I cervical cancer in pregnancy.Obstet Gynecol Surv 2000;55:633-43.
32. Sood AK, Sorosky JI, Mayr N, et al. Cervical cancer diagnosed shortly after pregnancy: prognostic variables and delivery routes. Obstet Gynecol 2000;95:832-38.

23 Malignancies of the Vulva

B Presannakumari

23.1 INTRODUCTION

Carcinoma vulva is the fourth most common female genital tract malignancy. There has been an increase in the incidence in the past few decades. This can be attributed to the increased life-expectancy of the female population and the increased incidence of human papilloma virus (HPV) infection. DNA of HPV has been identified from pre-invasive as well as invasive lesions of the vulva. Chronic immunosuppression, systemic hypertension, diabetes mellitus and obesity are seen associated with vulvar cancer but no definite etiological link has been proved yet. It is reported that 13% of cases are associated with cancer in other sites like cervix, vagina and anal canal. This may be due to the common etiological factor, HPV infection. With better understanding of the lymphatic drainage of vulva, the surgical approach to vulvar cancer has drastically changed. The present surgical approach is more conservative. The advances in radiotherapy and chemotherapy have also contributed to the less radical surgical approach.

Squamous cell carcinoma (SCC) is the commonest form of vulvar carcinoma, amounting to 87%. The second most common being malignant melanoma (6%). The less common types of vulvar malignancies are Bartholin's gland adenocarcinoma, sarcoma, basal cell carcinoma and invasive Paget's disease.

23.2 SYMPTOMS

The usual symptom of vulvar carcinoma is pruritus; other symptoms being discharge, dysuria, pain and bleeding. 50% of the patients with early lesions are asymptomatic. Most women would be hesitant to seek medical advice. Vulvar carcinoma is usually diagnosed at an advanced stage possibly due to delay in reporting. This emphasizes the need for educating women to seek medical advice when they have any of the above symptoms.

23.3 SPREAD

There are three modes of spread:

- Lymphatic embolization
- Direct extension
- Hematogenous

23.3.1 Lymphatic Embolization

Tumor spread by embolization to the regional nodes is the commonest and the earliest way carcinoma vulva spreads. *When lymphatic embolization occurs, even when the regional glands are positive for malignant cells, the intervening part of the vulva between the lymph gland and the lesion will be free of the disease.* Understanding of this led to the treatment of vulvar SCC by separate incisions for tumor excision and lymphadenectomy.

Route of Lymphatic Spread (Fig. 23.1)

Lymphatic spread occurs initially to the superficial inguinal lymph nodes and from there to the deep femoral group of lymph nodes. But femoral nodes may be involved without the involvement of the inguinal nodes. The most cephalad of the femoral group of nodes is named as the Cloquet's or Rosenmuller's node. *Lymphatics of the vulva will not cross the labiocrural folds.* Intraoperative sentinel node mapping revealed that in 5% of the cases the sentinel node is the femoral group.[1] Hence superficial lymphadenectomy alone may not prevent the lymphatic spread of the disease. From the inguino-femoral group of lymph nodes further spread occurs to the external iliac group of nodes. From the midline lesions, lymph node involvement is bilateral but from lateral vulvar tumors, contralateral lymph node involvement is very rare. *From lesions of the clitoris, anterior labia minora and perineum, bilateral lymph node involvement should be anticipated.* From the clitoris and the Bartholin's gland, direct lymphatic channels to pelvic nodes are present, but direct spread to pelvic nodes without inguinal node involvement is very rare (0.6 %). This is an important point in planning surgical treatment. When the inguinal lymph nodes are involved, the incidence of pelvic lymph node involvement is 33%.

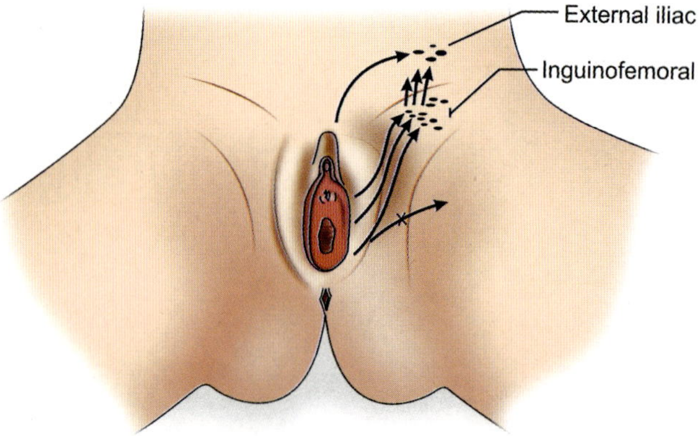

Fig. 23.1: Lymphatic drainage of vulva. The primary lymphatic drainage is to the inguinofemoral group of nodes from where it drains to the external iliac. From the region of the clitoris, direct spread to the external iliac nodes can occur. Lymphatics of the vulva do not cross the labiocrural fold

23.3.2 Direct Extension

Direct extension can occur to the neighboring urethra, vagina and anal canal.

23.3.3 Hematogenous

Hematogenous spread usually occurs late in the course of the disease. In the absence of pelvic node involvement, hematogenous spread is rare.

23.4 PATHOLOGY

Squamous cell carcinoma is the most common type worldwide. It is reported to be the type in 90% of the cases. Based on risk factors, there are three different forms of squamous carcinoma.

23.4.1 Bowenoid Type

The most common type is the bowenoid type which shows the same risk factors as cervical carcinoma like increased number of sexual partners, early age of first intercourse, abnormal Pap smear, presence of genital wart and tobacco use. HPV infection may also be an etiological factor. The bowenoid type of lesion may appear in different varieties. It can present as a whitish or pigmented region of thickened skin or as a verruciform (Fig. 23.3) or polypoidal lesion. The surface can be condylomatous or smooth.

23.4.2 Keratinizing Type

The keratinizing lesion will appear as hard crust like regions of thickened skin. These lesions are often surrounded by areas of squamous hyperplasia or lichen sclerosus. It is etiologically related to HPV.

23.4.3 Verrucous Type

The third common type of vulvar squamous cell carcinoma is verrucous carcinoma which occurs in older age group. No definite etiological factors are identified for this type. But the disease is seen associated with squamous hyperplasia and lichen sclerosus. It is found to be locally invasive but rarely metastatic. Lesions are usually large cauliflower like (Fig. 23.2). As depth of invasion is not uniform in this lesion, multiple biopsies are advised.

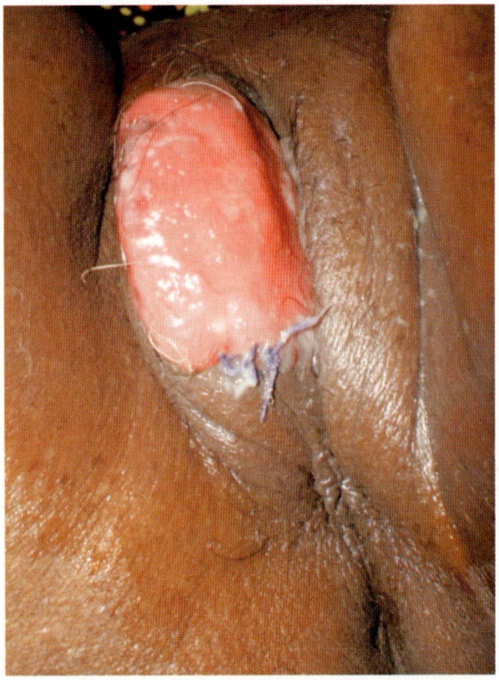

Fig. 23.2: Cauliflower like growth of the vulva in the right labium majus—Squamous cell carcinoma verrucous type in a 70-year-old lady who presented with discharge and bleeding PV

23.5 DIAGNOSIS OF VULVAR CARCINOMA

Women reporting with symptoms like pruritus, discharge or abnormal vaginal bleeding should have proper local examination of vulva, vagina and cervix. There will be recognized lesions in the vulva in most of the patients. Patients who complain of pruritus without any lesions of vulva should have colposcopic examination. The lesion is usually unifocal, but rarely multifocal. Suspicious areas should be biopsied. If there is a lesion, the *biopsy should be taken from the center of the lesion as well as from its periphery because in the periphery, the lesion may be preinvasive whereas in the center it may be an invasive one.*

23.6 DIFFERENTIAL DIAGNOSIS

The differential diagnoses of vulvar carcinoma are unilocular cyst, Bartholin's cyst, hemangioma, seborrhea, keratoma, hydradenoma and wart. Lichen sclerosus is one of the common conditions which presents with pruritus vulva. Since, there can be associated keratinizing squamous cell carcinoma, the vulva should be examined preferably with colposcopy and multiple biopsies should be taken. If there is a lesion the biopsy should be taken from the center of the lesion as well as from the periphery. Patients who have tumor with no distinct boundary, the biopsy can be directed after painting with acetic acid or toluidine blue. The abnormal area will be acetowhite when painted with acetic acid and bluish when painted with toluidine blue. In the case of Bartholin's gland adenocarcinoma FNAC may be preferred. PET scan is evolving as an imaging technique which provides information about depth of invasion which is important in staging.

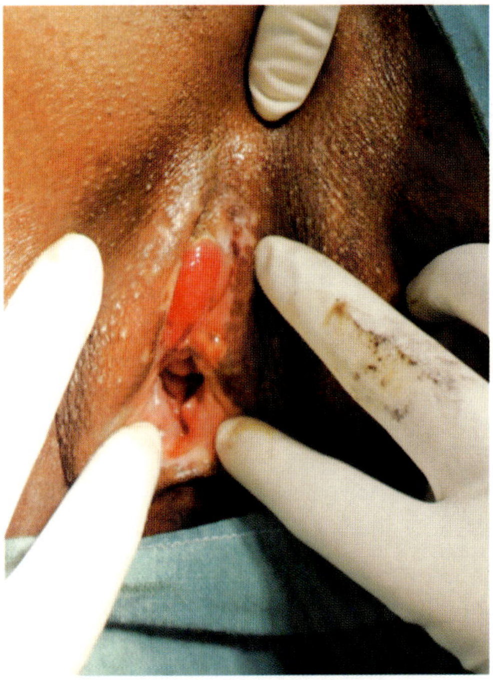

Fig. 23.3: Squamous carcinoma of the right labia minora with extension to the clitoris. Urethral opening is spared

23.7 STAGING

Since 1988, the staging of vulvar cancer is surgical. The final staging is based on the histopathological examination of the operated specimen. The staging was revised by FIGO in 1994 and 2009 (Tables 23.1 and 23.2).

23.8 PROGNOSTIC FACTORS

The most important prognostic indicator is lymph node involvement. Patients with negative lymph node involvement have 90% 5-year survival rate as compared to 50% 5-year survival rate for those with positive lymph node involvement.[6] Patients with microscopically positive lymph node status have disease progression rates similar to negative lymph node status.

Histological grade, tumor thickness, depth of stromal invasion and lymph vascular space involvement correlates with the degree of lymph node involvement. Hence these are not independent risk factors. As in other malignancies DNA ploidy is another prognostic factor, with aneuploid tumors having poor prognosis. Other poor prognostic factors identified are age, obesity, hypertension and smoking. Presence of other associated epithelial changes adjacent to the lesion mandates wider excision which should involve all abnormal areas. The alternative is to treat the abnormal areas with other treatment modalities.

23.9 MANAGEMENT

Surgery is the primary mode of treatment. The aim of surgery is to completely remove the tumor while conserving the vulva maximally and also identify the extent of the disease so as to plan additional treatment.

There has been a drastic change in the management of vulvar carcinoma. Previously, all patients with carcinoma vulva irrespective of the size or site of tumor were managed by radical vulvectomy which was pioneered by Taussig and Whey. Radical vulvectomy causes very high morbidity. Because of early detection of the tumors and the recent knowledge that small tumors with less depth of invasion are less likely to have bilateral lymph node involvement, they can be managed by radical local excision and ipsilateral lymph node dissection. *Radical vulvectomy is not resorted to uniformly in all patients especially in early stage disease.* The knowledge that lymphatic embolization is the early mode of spread led to the surgical management with separate vulval and groin incisions.

The recent modifications can be listed as follows:

1. More conservative vulvar dissection aiming at complete tumor removal with tumor free margin of 1-2 cm, at the same time conserving vulva as far as possible.

Table 23.1: Carcinoma of the vulva – FIGO staging

Stages		*Characteristics*	*TNM Categories*
		Primary tumor cannot be assessed	TX
		No evidence of primary tumor	TO
0		Carcinoma *in situ* (preinvasive carcinoma)	Tis
I		Tumor confined to vulva or vulva and perineum, 2 cm or less in greatest dimensions	T1
	IA	Tumor confined to vulva or vulva and perineum, 2 cm or less in greatest dimensions and with stromal invasion no greater than 1.0 mm*	T1a
	IB	Tumor confined to vulva or vulva and perineum, 2 cm or less in greatest dimension and with stromal invasion greater than 1.0 mm*	T1b
II		Tumor confined to the vulva or vulva and perineum, more than 2 cm in greatest dimension	T2
III		Tumour invades any of the following: lower urethra, vagina, anus and/or unilateral regional node metastasis	T3
IV	IVA	Tumor invades any of the following : bladder mucosa, rectal mucosa, upper urethral mucosa; or is fixed to bone and/or bilateral regional node metastases	T4
	IVB	Any distant metastasis including pelvic lymph nodes	

Regional lymph nodes (N)	
NX	Regional lymph nodes cannot be assessed
NO	No regional lymph node metastasis
N1	Unilateral regional lymph node metastasis
N2	Bilateral regional lymph node metastases

Distant metastasis (M)	
MX	Distant metastasis cannot be assessed
M0	No distant metastasis
M1	Distant metastasis

* *The depth of invasion is defined as the measurement of the tumor from the epithelial-stromal junction of the adjacent, most superficial dermal papilla, to the deepest point of invasion.*

Table 23.2: Revised FIGO staging of carcinoma of the vulva (International Journal of Gynecology and Obstetrics 2009;105:103-104)

Stage I	Tumor confined to the vulva
IA	Lesions ≤2 cm in size, confined to the vulva or perineum and with stromal invasion ≤1.0 mm*, no nodal metastasis
IB	Lesions >2 cm in size or with stromal invasion >1.0 mm*, confined to the vulva or perineum, with negative nodes
Stage II	Tumor of any size with extension to adjacent perineal structures (1/3 lower urethra, 1/3 lower vagina, anus) with negative nodes
Stage III	Tumor of any size with or without extension to adjacent perineal structures (1/3 lower urethra, 1/3 lower vagina, anus) with positive inguinofemoral lymph nodes
IIIA	(i) With 1 lymph node metastasis (≥5 mm), or (ii) 1-2 lymph node metastasis(es) (<5 mm)
IIIB	(i) With 2 or more lymph node metastases (≥ 5 mm), or (ii) 3 or more lymph node metastases (<5 mm)
IIIC	With positive nodes with extracapsular spread
Stage IV	Tumor invades other regional (2/3 upper urethra, 2/3 upper vagina), or distant structures
IVA	Tumor invades any of the following: (i) Upper urethral and/or vaginal mucosa, bladder mucosa, rectal mucosa, or fixed to pelvic bone, or (ii) Fixed or ulcerated inguinofemoral lymph nodes
IVB	Any distant metastasis including pelvic lymph nodes

* The depth of invasion is defined as the measurement of the tumor from the epithelial stromal junction of the adjacent most superficial dermal papilla to the deepest point of invasion.

2. Selective groin lymphadenectomy.
3. Lymphadenectomy and tumor resection through separate incisions in early lesions.
4. Whenever lymphadenectomy is indicated, both superficial and deep groin lymph nodes are removed.

23.9.1 Management of Early Vulvar Carcinoma (Flow Charts 23.1 to 23.4)

The management of vulvar carcinoma depends upon the site and size of the tumor, the depth of invasion and presence or absence of clinical node involvement.

As previously emphasized, radical vulvectomy (Whey's method) is no longer advised for early vulvar cancer. Recent studies have proved that radical local excision irrespective of depth of invasion gives a cure rate which is comparable to radical vulvectomy with much less psychosocial sequelae.[2]

Flow Chart 23.1: Management algorithm for early cancer vulva (FIGO)

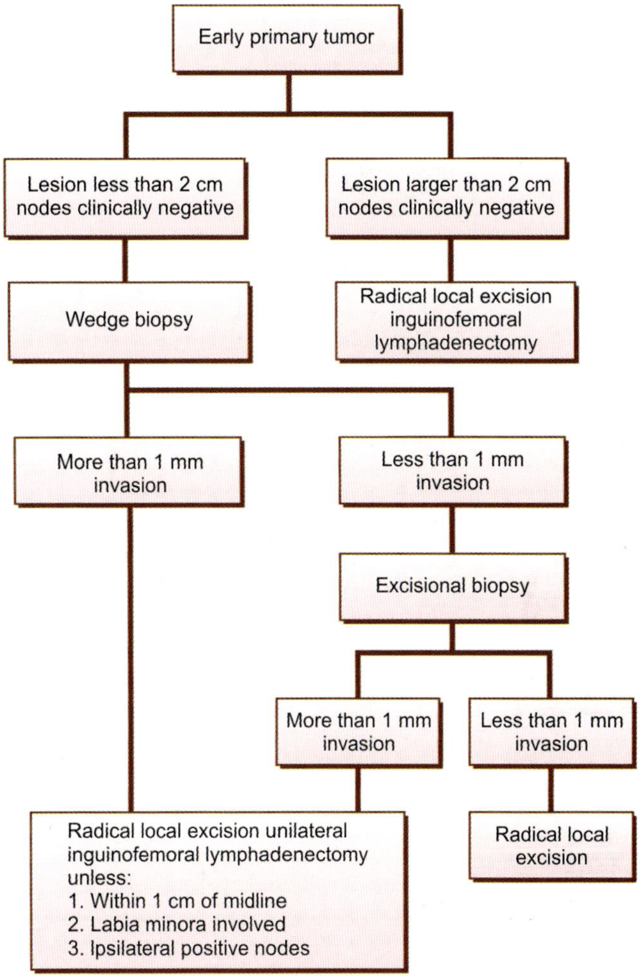

If there is associated VIN or lichen sclerosis, these areas may be superficially excised

Management of stage I lesion should be individualized. For patients with no clinically suspicious groin nodes, the preferred surgical management is conservative.

Management of Stage I A

If the tumor is <2 cm in size and the depth of invasion is <1 mm, wide radical excision should be preferred. Inguinofemoral lymphadenectomy is not advised for such a patient as the incidence of node involvement is negligible.

Management of Stage I B

A lateral lesion which is defined as a lesion 1 cm lateral to the midline is less likely to metastasize to contralateral

Flow Chart 23.2: Management algorithm for clinically suspicious groin nodes (FIGO with permission)

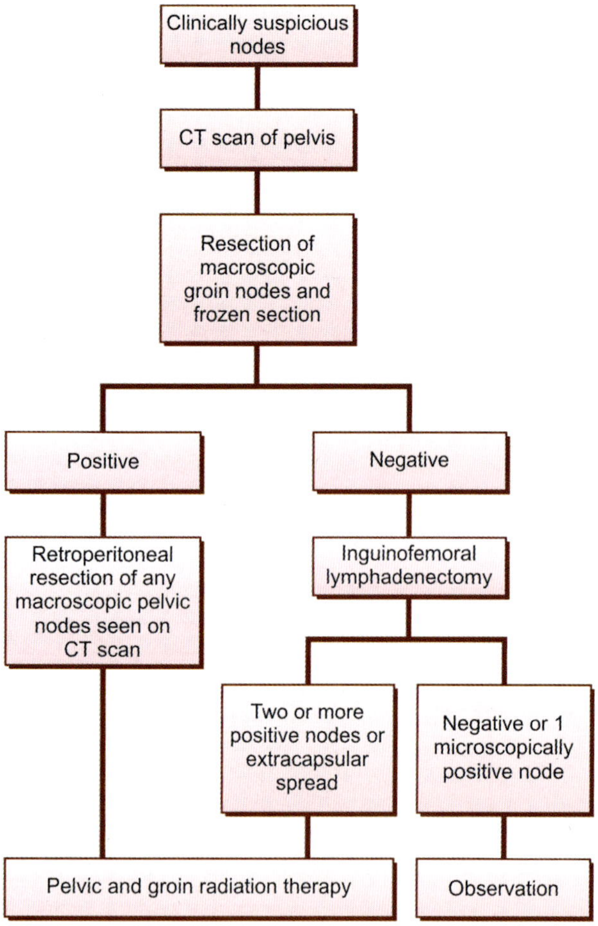

Flow Chart 23.3: Management algorithm for clinically obvious groin nodes (FIGO)

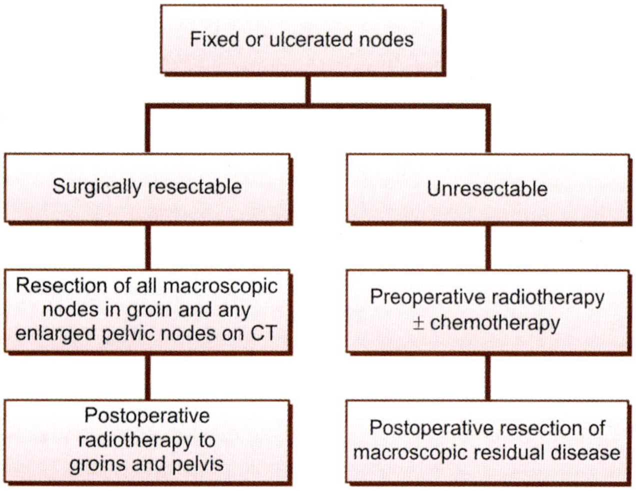

Flow Chart 23.4: Management algorithm for advanced primary tumor (FIGO)

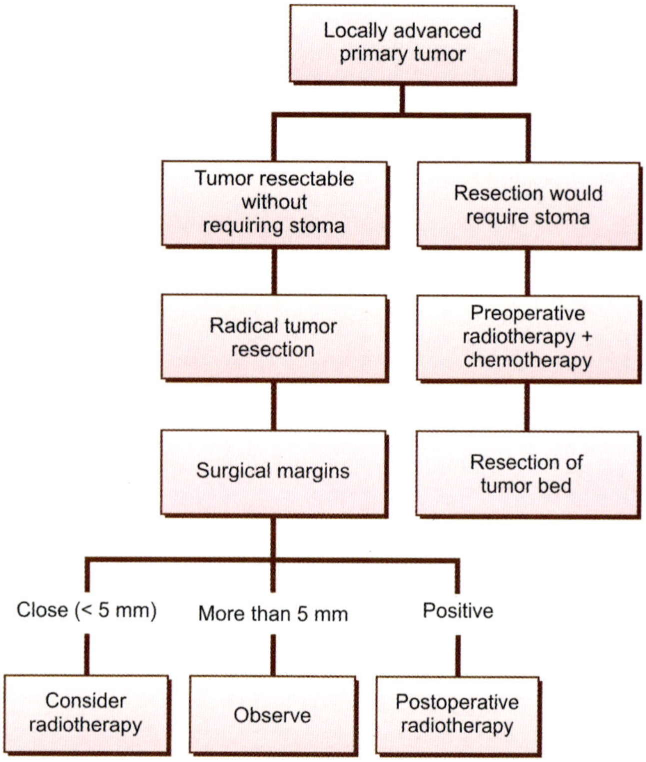

inguinofemoral lymph nodes (< 1%). If the lesion is < 2 cm in size and the depth of invasion is > 1 mm, lateral lesions are treated with radical local excision and unilateral inguinofemoral lymphadenectomy done through a separate groin incision.[3] This is based on the fact that metastasis rarely occurs in the skin bridge in patients without clinically involved groin nodes. Both superficial and deep nodes should be removed. If only superficial groin dissection is done, there is a high incidence of groin recurrence. This was proved in a randomized controlled study among 143 patients by Frederick Stehman[4] et al.

When radical local excision (Figs 23.4 to 23.6) is done for lateral lesions of the vulva, at least a 1 cm grossly negative margin should be obtained. The depth of excision should be up to the level of the inferior fascia of the urogenital diaphragm. For lesions involving the lateral or posterior aspects of vulva, radical local excision is ideal. For anterior lesions, clitoris-saving surgeries with tumor free margin of minimum 8 mm should be preferred. In a younger patient, if the lesion involves the clitoris, chemoradiation is an alternative.

If ipsilateral lymph glands are positive for malignant cells, chances of contralateral glandular involvement are 15%. Hence if ipsilateral lymph nodes are found to be

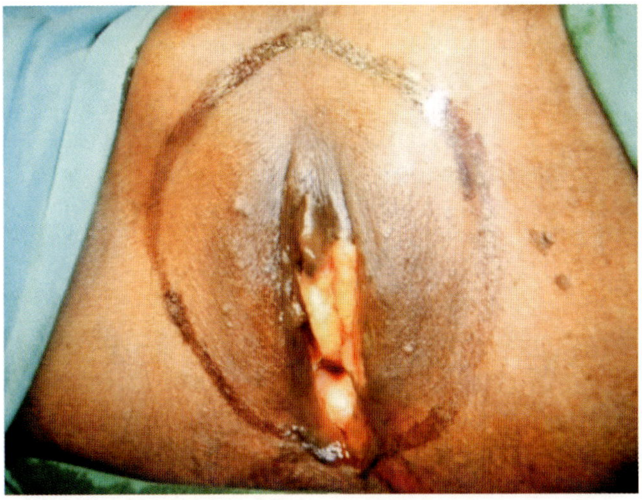

Fig. 23.4: Vulvectomy incision (growth on left labia minora)

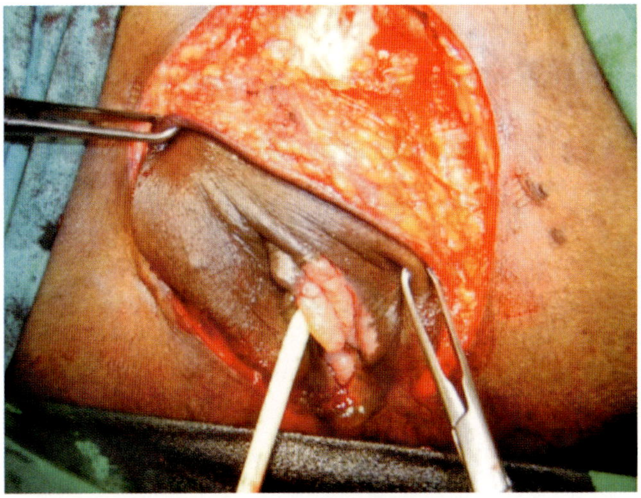

Fig. 23.5: Radical vulvectomy dissection up to inferior fascia of urogenital diaphragm

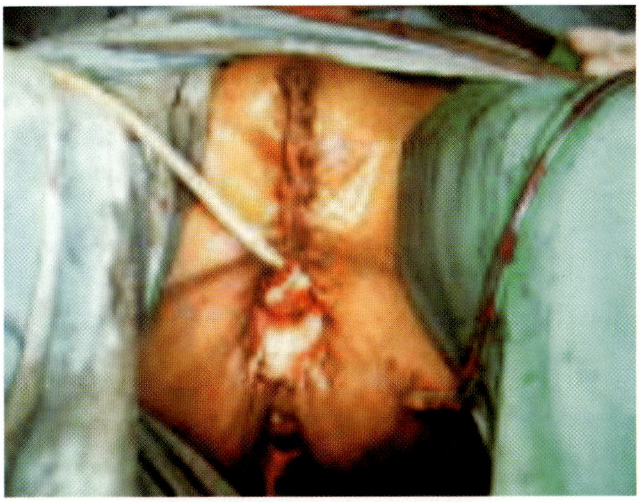

Fig. 23.6: Skin closure after vulvectomy

positive for malignant cells, bilateral lymphadenectomy should be done. Midline lesions are likely to metastasize to bilateral inguinofemoral lymph nodes and hence need bilateral lymphadenectomy.

If groin recurrence occurs, mortality is reported to be 90%. Patients who have 3 or more microscopically involved groin lymph nodes should undergo pelvic lymphadenectomy. An alternative is to give external radiation to pelvis and inguinofemoral lymph nodes. A randomized control trial by GOG group with surgery and radiotherapy for the inguinofemoral lymph nodes showed that, patients receiving radiotherapy had decreased groin recurrence.[5] Hence it is better to give adjuvant radiation if the unilateral groin nodes are found to be positive.

Patients who have associated nonneoplastic lesion like lichen sclerosus should be treated based on their age. In younger women, a conservative approach with radical local excision of the malignant lesion and topical steroids can be advised for lichen sclerosus or squamous hyperplasia. But if they have vulvar intraepithelial neoplasia (VIN), it requires superficial local excision of the lesion.

23.9.2 Lymphatic Mapping and Vulvar Cancer

Identification of the sentinel lymph node is being evaluated in vulvar carcinoma. The sentinel lymph node is defined as the first node in the lymphatic chain that receives primary lymphatic flow from the area of the lesion. This node is used as a representative of the entire lymphatic chain. Since this being the first site of metastatic disease and if it is found to be negative for malignant cells, complete lymphadenectomy is not necessary. The sentinel lymph node can be identified by injecting isosulfan blue dye or technetium 99. Using this technique, Decesare et al identified the sentinel node. All those who had negative sentinel node were found to be free of disease in the other nodes.

23.9.3 Treatment of Stage II and Stage III

Conservative surgery is advised even for stage II and stage III tumors. According to recent study, local recurrence rate for patients with stage II disease treated conservatively is the same as for patients with T1 lesions, provided surgical margin of at least 1 cm is obtained. So for younger patients with even T2 or T3 lesions, conservative surgery may be advised especially for lesions involving the posterior half of the vulva. For stage II lesions (T2 N0) lymphadenectomy also should be done as discussed earlier for stage I lesions. For lesions involving distal urethra, vagina or anus, it is preferable to give chemoradiation to allow less radical surgery.

Patients with clinically suspicious or *3 or more pathologically involved groin nodes should have treatment of pelvic nodes.* Pelvic nodes can be treated by pelvic lymphadenectomy which can be through an extraperitoneal approach. If the pelvic nodes are not enlarged, external beam therapy can be given instead of surgical removal. But enlarged lymph nodes should be removed surgically before radiotherapy, as *external beam cannot sterilize bulky positive lymph nodes.*

After radical local excision, small defects can be dealt with by primary closure. If more extensive dissection is required, the wound can be left open to granulate. Alternatively it may be covered with skin flaps.

23.9.4 Treatment of Advanced T3 and T4 Tumors

Because of the involvement of bladder and rectal mucosa, patients with advanced T3 and T4 tumors need pelvic exenteration, radical vulvectomy and inguinofemoral lymphadenectomy. To avoid the physical and psychological morbidity of the procedure, these patients are presently treated with chemoradiation followed by resection of the tumor-bed and removal of only enlarged lymph nodes. Because of extensive lymph node involvement, these patients will need radiation even if inguinofemoral lymphadenectomy is done. Lymphadenectomy and radiation can cause severe lymphoedema. Hence only enlarged nodes are removed.

23.9.5 Treatment of Recurrent Vulvar Cancer

Proper surgical management of the primary lesion will reduce recurrence of the disease. *The number of positive groin nodes is the most important prognostic factor in vulvar carcinoma. Groin recurrence carries poor prognosis.*

Local Recurrence

Local recurrence can be prevented by maintaining a tumor-free margin of 1 cm in the removed specimen during primary surgery. In case, after surgery close surgical margin is identified or the margin is involved, the patient should be given postoperative radiation.

Signs of recurrence are skin breakdown, ulceration, mass in the area of previous scar or a new groin mass. When isolated local recurrence occurs after treatment of large lesions, it can be treated by surgery. Chemoradiation along with interstitial radiation with needles has been tried to treat recurrences but the morbidity is found to be high.

Regional and Distant Recurrence

Survival is very poor in patients who have regional recurrence. For groin recurrence, external beam radiation can be given after removal of the enlarged nodes. Chemotherapy for recurrent disease is not found to be very effective.

23.10 5-YEAR SURVIVAL RATE

5-year survival is excellent for stage I disease while involvement of regional nodes carry poor prognosis (Table 23.3).

23.11 OTHER TYPES OF VULVAR MALIGNANCIES

23.11.1 Melanoma

Melanoma is the second most common vulvar cancer. It usually presents as a raised pigmented lesion. The commonest site of the lesion is the labia minora and clitoris. FIGO staging applicable to squamous cell carcinoma is not applicable to melanoma. The lesion is staged based on the vertical thickness of the lesion measured from the tip of the granular layer to the deepest point of invasion. Melanoma is a very small lesion and the prognosis depends on the depth of invasion rather than the diameter. Incidence of lymph node metastasis correlates with the vertical thickness of the lesion.

Several microstaging systems have been described for vulvar melanoma (Table 23.4).

Management

Wide radical excision with a 2 cm margin is the preferred mode of treatment. Lymphadenectomy can be deferred for lesions <0.76 mm thick with no lymph vascular space invasion. For patients with lesions larger than this, groin

Table 23.3: 5-year survival rate of carcinoma vulva

Stage	*Survival rate*
Stage I	+100%
Stage II	86.2%
Stage III	59.4%
Stage IV A	29.8%
Stage IV B	20%

Source: Origoni M, Dindelli M, Ferronid, Frigeni L, Rossi M. Surgical staging of invasive squamous cell carcinoma of the vulva: Analysis of treatment and survival. Int Surgery 1996; 81:67-70.

Table 23.4 Microstaging systems of vulvar melanoma

	Clark-level	*Chung-depth of invasion*
I	Intraepithelial	Intraepithelial
II	Into papillary dermis	<1mm from granular layer
III	Filling dermal papillae	1.1-2.0 mm from granular layer
IV	Into reticular dermis	>2 mm from granular layer
V	Into subcutaneous fat	Into subcutaneous fat

Source:

1. Chung AF, Woodruff JM, Lewis JL Jr. Malignant melanoma of vulva: A report of 44 cases. Obstet Gynaecol 1975;45:638-46
2. Clark WH, From L, Bernardino EA, et al. The histogenesis and biologic behavior of primary human malignant melanomas of the skin. Cancer Res 1969;29:705-27.

dissection is recommended. Patients who have deeply invasive lesion with more than 4 mm tumor thickness have high risk of systemic metastasis. Hence, they may not benefit from regional lymphadenectomy. Palliative radiation can be given for brain and bone metastases. The prognosis is not as good as squamous cell carcinoma and the overall 5 year survival rate is only 25-50%. Patients who have lesions invading 1 mm or less will have good prognosis but for patients who have greater invasion, prognosis is worse. Additional prognostic factors are age, presence of multiple lesions, tumor ulceration, midline location of tumor, histological growth pattern, aneuploidy and lymph vascular space involvement.

23.11.2 Bartholin's Gland Carcinoma (Figs 23.7A and B)

It is a very rare form of vulvar cancer. Primary tumor is very rare occurring in 2-7% of vulvar malignancies. It usually occurs in postmenopausal women. The bartholin's gland are situated posterolateral to the labia minora. The duct opens into the introitus at junction between the anterior two-third and posterior one-third of the labia minora. The duct is lined by stratified squamous epithelium and it changes to transitional epithelium at the distal end. Malignant tumors can arise either from the gland or the duct. Because there are several types of cells in the duct and the gland, several types of malignancies can arise. This can be adenocarcinoma, squamous carcinoma, transitional cell carcinoma, adenosquamous carcinoma or adenoid cystic carcinoma.

Signs and Symptoms

The initial symptom is usually a mass in the vulva and pain. Malignancies can be mistaken for benign cysts or abscesses which are more common.

Treatment

As in squamous carcinoma of the vulva, the management can be conservative. Wide local excision is advised for the primary tumor as the gland is situated deep in the vulva which entails deep dissection. Since it is difficult to maintain tumor free margin during the dissection, postoperative radiotherapy is advised. Prognosis is similar to that of squamous cell carcinoma.

23.11.3 Paget's Disease

Paget's disease of the vulva is usually an intraepithelial lesion. Rarely, it is found to be invasive. Usually it presents as an erythematous well-defined lesion with irregular

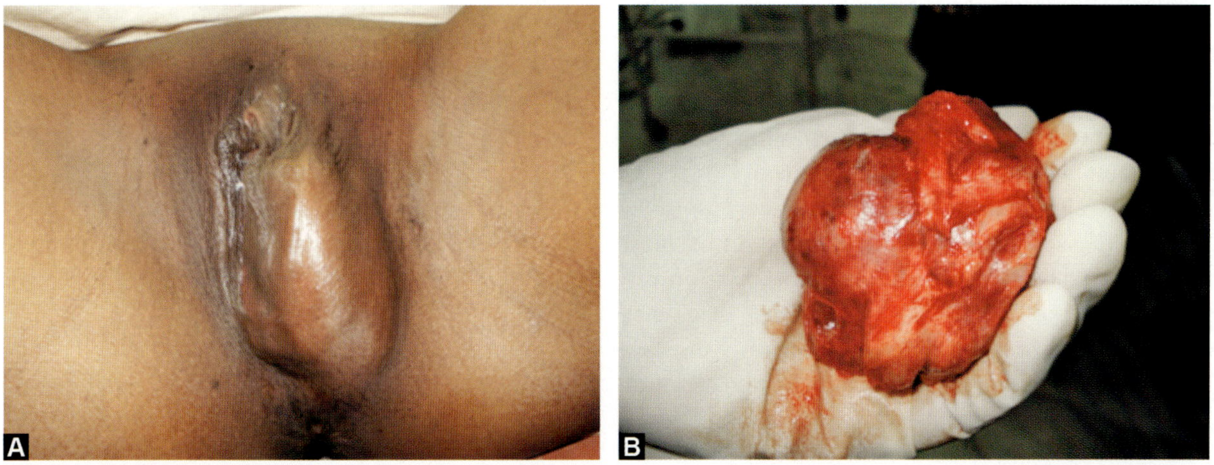

Figs 23.7A and B: Bartholin's gland carcinoma in a 36-year-old lady who presented with swelling in the vulval region (A). The swelling was excised without knowing that it is Bartholin's gland carcinoma. The diagnosis came as a surprise due to the younger age of the patient. The dissected specimen is shown on the right side (B). The patient was treated with postoperative radiation

borders. Microscopically, it is characterized by the presence of Paget's cells which are large eosinophilic cells. These cells are seen spread in the dermis or in the dermal appendages. Four clinical entities of Paget's disease are identified.

Noninvasive Paget's Disease

This is an adenocarcinoma *in situ*. It can be treated by wide local excision. The final diagnosis is by examination of the excised lesion.

Invasive Paget's Disease

In invasive Paget's disease, there will be invasion into the surrounding dermis and subcutaneous fat. Since there is invasion, groin nodes are involved in about 50% of cases. Hence groin lymphadenectomy is advised if the lesion is found to be invasive after excision.

Third Type

The third type of the lesion is found to be associated with underlying adenocarcinoma of sweat glands or Bartholin's gland.

Fourth Type

The fourth type is characterized by associated extragenital Paget's disease, usually of the breast or rectum.

Local recurrence is common after excision. This may be due to the associated malignancy of underlying sweat glands.

23.11.4 Basal Cell Carcinoma

These are rare tumors arising from skin or hair follicles of the vulva. They are invasive but rarely metastatic. Management is by wide local excision.

23.11.5 Sarcoma

Sarcoma of the vulva is a heterogeneous group of tumors, the commonest of which is leiomyosarcoma. This is usually seen in the labium majus as a large tender mass. Lymphatic involvement is rare. Treatment option is wide local excision.

Other rare sarcomas are epitheloid sarcoma and rhabdomyosarcoma. Epithelioid sarcoma may mimic Bartholin's cyst. They behave more aggressively than other sarcoma. Wide excision is the treatment for early disease. Rhabdomyosarcoma is usually found in children. Radical surgery was the standard approach previously but presently they are managed with wide local excision followed by chemoradiation. With this multi-model approach, 5-year survival rates have improved.

23.12 CONCLUSION

Squamous cell carcinoma is the commonest malignancy of the vulva. Early detection of vulvar carcinoma carries a good prognosis. Patients presenting with pruritus vulva should be evaluated carefully. It is advisable to examine the vulva with the help of a colposcope if no definite lesion is seen and the patient is symptomatic. If abnormal areas are found, it must be biopsied to diagnose malignancy as early as possible. The modern management of vulvar malignancy is more conservative. *Surgery can be individualized to minimize mutilation of the vulva.* Lymph node involvement is the most important prognostic factor. Patients who do not need groin node dissection should be identified so that unnecessary lymphadenectomy can be avoided. Those who have stage Ia disease need only radical local excision. Those whose tumor is Ib should have ipsilateral lymphadenectomy. The primary tumor in the vulva and groin nodes is dealt with through separate incisions. Lymphadenectomy should include removal of both superficial as well as deep femoral nodes. Those who have midline lesions need bilateral groin dissection. Groin recurrence which carries very poor prognosis can thus be minimized. If groin node is positive for malignant disease there is a very high risk of pelvic node involvement and hence pelvic nodes should be treated. Groin and pelvic lymphadenectomy carries the risk of lymphoedema. Hence such patients are better treated by chemoradiation. However, enlarged nodes should be removed prior to radiation. *Radiotherapy, with or without chemotherapy is used to manage unresectable disease, positive pelvic nodes or recurrence.* With individualized treatment of primary tumor as well as lymph nodes, vulvar conservation is achieved with minimum morbidity.

REFERENCES

1. Levenback C, Burke TW, Morris M, et al. Potential application of intraoperative lymphatic mapping in vulvar cancer. Gynaecol Oncol 1995;59:216-20.
2. Stehman FB, Bundy BN, Dvoretsky PM, et al. Early stage II carcinoma of the vulva treated with ipsilateral superficial inguinofemoral lymphadenectomy and modified radical hemivulvectomy: A prospective study of the GOG. Obstet Gynecol 1992;79:490-97.
3. Hacker NF, Leuchter RS, Berek JS, et al. Radical vulvectomy and bilateral inguinal lymphadenectomy through separate groin incisions. Obstet Gynecol 1981;58:574-9.
4. Frederick Stehman MD, Brein N Bundy Harrison Ball.Md Am J Obstet Gynaecol 1996;174;1128-33.
5. Homesley HD, Bundy BN, Sedlis A, et al. Radiation therapy versus pelvic node resection for carcinoma of the vulva with positive groin nodes. Obstet Gynecol 1986;68:733-7.
6. Hacker NF. Vulvar cancer in Berek JS, Hacker NF. Practical Gynaecolgic Oncology. 4th edition. Philadelphia. Lippincott Williams Wilkins 2005;40:543-83.

24 Gestational Trophoblastic Disease

NS Sreedevi, B Presannakumari

24.1 INTRODUCTION

Gestational trophoblastic disease (GTD) includes a spectrum of conditions ranging from various forms of hydatidiform mole through invasive mole and choriocarcinoma to placental site trophoblastic tumor (PSTT). The disease is unique due to the fact that it arises from chorionic tissue which is fetal in origin and hence foreign to the mother. The human placenta is hemochorial in type. The chorionic villi lie in the maternal pool of blood. This explains the presence of trophoblastic cells in the pulmonary circulation, and rarely, the systemic circulation also, in normal pregnancy. This embolization is exaggerated in the benign as well as malignant forms of trophoblastic disease.

Over the past few decades there has been great improvement in the prognosis of this disease. This can be attributed to several factors, which include the evolution of imaging techniques like ultrasound, CT and MRI, the sensitive radioimmunoassay techniques for estimating β-hCG, as well as the development of effective chemotherapeutic agents. In the present set up choriocarcinoma is one of the rare human malignancies that can be cured even in the presence of widespread dissemination.[1] Hertz and colleagues at the National Institute of Health Brewer in

Chicago and Bagshawe in London should be remembered for developing the chemotherapeutic approach to the management of malignant trophoblastic disease that would cure majority of patients with this fatal disease.

24.1.1 Definition and Terms

The term gestational trophoblastic disease (GTD) includes all aspects of this entity namely the benign forms of trophoblastic disease—vesicular mole (complete and partial) and the malignant counterparts—persistent trophoblastic disease, invasive mole, choriocarcinoma, and placental site trophoblastic tumor. The term gestational trophoblastic neoplasia (GTN) refers to the malignant forms only. According to FIGO, GTN replaces the terms like chorio-adenoma destruens (invasive mole), persistent trophoblastic disease, malignant GTD, and metastasizing mole. Chorioadenoma destruens and choriocarcinoma are pathological terms and PSTT is classified separately. Even though histopathological diagnosis is desirable, it is not essential for the clinical classification which is in use at present. World Health Organization has classified GTD (Flow chart 24.1) into premalignant and malignant disorders.

Gestational trophoblastic tumor most commonly follows a molar pregnancy, but they may occur after any gestational event including therapeutic or spontaneous abortion, ectopic pregnancy or term pregnancy. 9-20% of patients with complete hydatidiform mole (CHM) may develop GTN. This may be chemical only as evidenced by β-hCG titer or with associated evidence of invasive mole. If the disease is confined to the uterus, it is termed non-metastatic neoplasia. If metastases are detected in the lungs, vagina, brain, liver, kidney or elsewhere, it is termed as metastatic trophoblastic neoplasia. Non-gestational trophoblastic tumors include primary choriocarcinoma of the ovary.

24.2 EPIDEMIOLOGY

24.2.1 Geographical and Racial

The incidence of GTD varies dramatically in different regions of world. In Europe and North America it is very rare (0.6-1.1/1000 pregnancies). The disease occurs more frequently in South East Asia, Malaysia, Singapore, Hong Kong, Indonesia, Philippines, China and Japan. The incidence is highest at 1/200-1/300 live births in South East Asia.

24.2.2 Age

Maternal age more than 35 years has consistently been shown to be a risk factor for CHM. The risk of CHM is 2-fold among women older than 35 years and 7.5-fold among women older than 40 years.[2, 3]

24.2.3 Nutritional

The high prevalence of the disease in some populations is attributed to nutritional and socioeconomic factors. The disease occurs more commonly in "rice eaters". Low intake of carotene has been found to be associated with increased risk of CHM.[4] Deficiency of vitamin A is another contributory factor. The risk for partial hydatidiform mole (PHM) has been associated with the use of oral contraceptives and a history of irregular menstruation. There is no association between PHM and maternal age or dietary factors.[5]

24.3 RECURRENT MOLE

The incidence of recurrent mole is 1/76 after one previous molar pregnancy, 1/6.5 after two previous molar pregnancies and after three previous molar pregnancies it is almost 100%. A rare autosomal recessive condition of GTD is identified. Linkage analysis of candidate genes has

Flow Chart 24.1: WHO classification of GTD

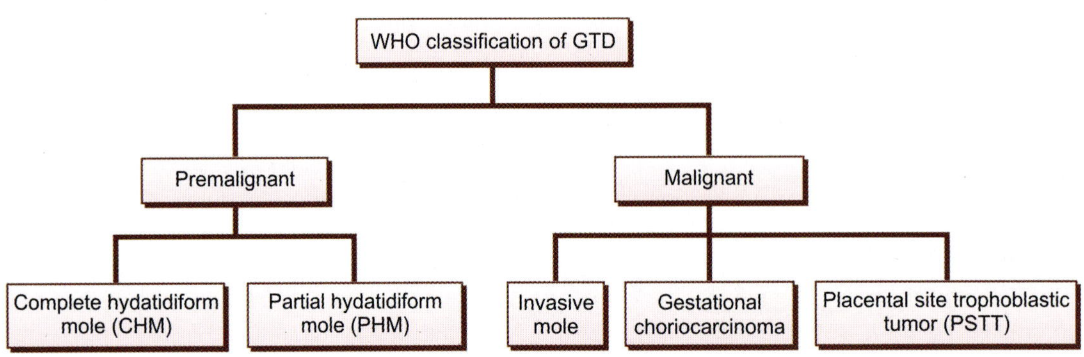

identified a gene, NLRP7 on chromosome 19q13.4 to be the causative gene in some families. An extremely rare familial syndrome of recurrent CHM has been recently identified; the defective gene is located on the long arm of chromosome.[19]

24.4 GENETICS OF HYDATIDIFORM MOLE

Vassilakos and Kajii, Szulman and Surti and Lawler[5] have clearly demonstrated that complete hydatidiform mole and partial hydatidiform mole are separate syndromes with different genetic background.[6-9] Several imprinted genes have been identified in man and some of these have been examined in molar tissue also. A maternally expressed gene CDKN1C (cycline dependent kinase inhibitor 1C) is highly expressed in normal human placenta whereas it is found to be clearly repressed in the cytotrophoblast and villous mesenchyme of CHM. Hence it can be used to discriminate CHM from non-molar miscarriages, when there is a doubtful clinical situation.

With advances in cytogenetics and molecular genetics, the etiology of hydatidiform mole is better understood. By genetic analysis and DNA fingerprinting the distinction between complete mole and partial mole has been validated (Table 24.1).

In complete hydatidiform mole (Fig. 24.1), the whole of the conceptus is converted into molar tissue. It is the result of fertilisation of "empty" ovum by one sperm, followed by endoreduplication resulting in a 46 XX androgenic conceptus. Fertilization may even be by two sperms resulting in XX or XY androgenic conceptus. The placenta develops hydatidiform changes and trophoblastic hyperplasia. Even though most CHM are androgenic, a rare subgroup of biparental diploid CHM (BiCHM) have been described. Recent studies have shown that this type of CHM is associated with familial recurrent molar pregnancies.

In partial hydatidiform mole (PHM) (Fig. 24.2), only part of the placenta shows molar changes. PHM generally has a triploid karyotype (69 chromosomes, i.e. 69XXX, 69XYY, 69XXY). Partial mole is recognized as a cause of early fetal loss. Many early first trimester abortions are recognized as due to triploid conceptus when examined cytogenetically and confirmed by flow cytometry. Clinically a fetus will be present and there will be hydatidiform changes in the placenta. The fetus will be morphologically abnormal showing features of triploidy, like syndactyly or hydrocephalus and will be growth retarded. Hence it is ideal to subject the products of conception to histopathological examination for all cases of missed abortion. If the pregnancy

Table 24.1: Features of complete and partial hydatidiform mole

Features	*Complete mole*	*Partial mole*
Fetal or embryonic tissue	Absent	Present
Hydatidiform swelling of chorionic villi	Diffuse	Focal
Trophoblastic hyperplasia	Diffuse	Focal
Scalloping of chorionic villi	Absent	Present
Trophoblastic stromal inclusions	Absent	Present
Karyotype	46, XX(90%)/ 46, XY	Triploid

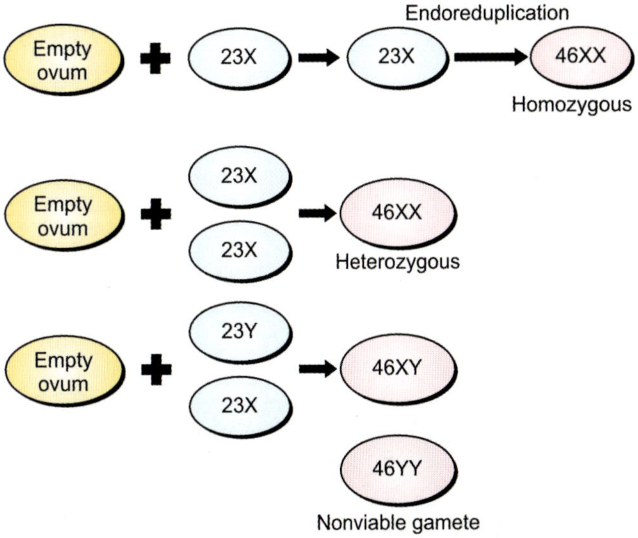

Fig. 24.1: Karyotype of complete hydatidiform mole

progresses pre-eclampsia occurs early. The incidence of neoplasia is reported as 4% after partial mole.

Hydatidiform degeneration without trophoblastic hyperplasia can occur in a poorly functioning early placenta associated with spontaneous abortion.

24.5 PATHOLOGY

Hydatidiform mole is a neoplasm of the trophoblast which involves both cytotrophoblast and syncytiotrophoblast in different proportions. The cells show proliferation and pleomorphism and nuclei are hyperchromatic and mitotic. The central core of vessels disappears and the villus swells to form a rounded cyst filled with watery fluid. In PHM, a fetus is formed but often dies *in utero* (Fig. 24.3). The fetuses which survive generally exhibit stigmata of triploidy.

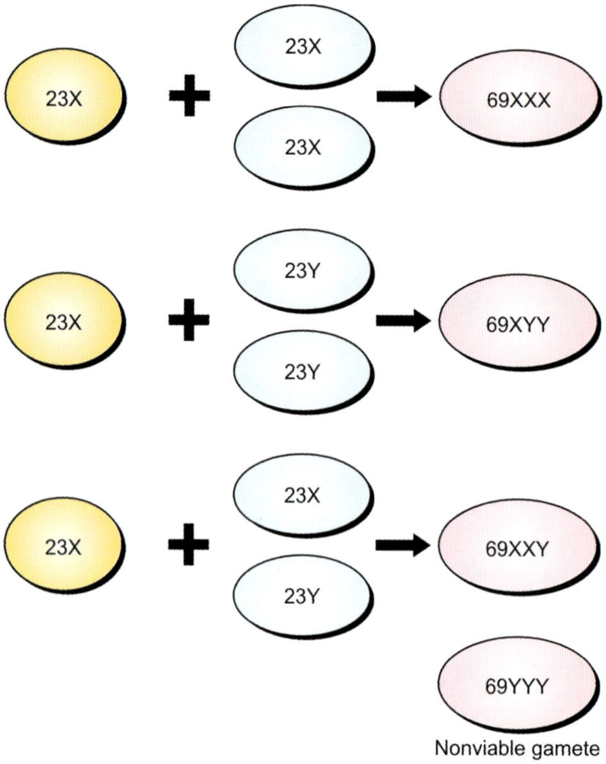

Fig. 24.2: Karyotype of partial hydatidiform mole. Note the contribution from both the parents—biparental genomic contribution

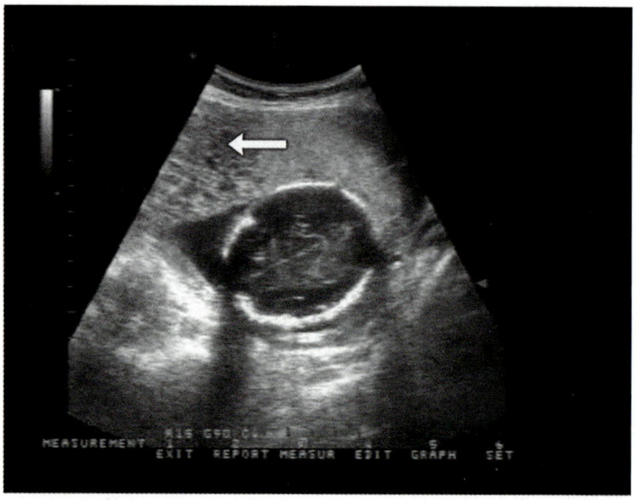

Fig. 24.3: Transabdominal scan showing partial mole. The fetal head and the placenta are seen. The placenta shows molar changes on the left side (arrow)

Even after fetal death, the mole continues to grow so that the uterus enlarges and may be bigger than that housing a normal pregnancy of similar gestational age. The excessive hCG acts on the ovaries to cause profound leutinization which may take the form of multiple theca lutein cysts. The theca lutein cysts are often bilateral and may attain large sizes in the presence of very high hCG levels.

24.5.1 Multiple Pregnancies with Mole and Coexisting Fetus

In a dizygotic twin gestation a normal fetus can coexist with a complete mole. The clinical presentation is that of hydatidiform mole with rapid enlargement of the uterus. Ultrasound examination will reveal a normal fetus, normal placenta and a separate molar tissue. In partial mole, the molar changes will be seen throughout the single placenta. The fetus in this pregnancy is normal compared to that of a partial mole where the fetus is abnormal. The identification of a separate normal placenta distinguishes it from partial mole. These patients are at high risk of developing pre-eclampsia. Their risk of developing GTN is higher than in other molar pregnancies. After proper counseling, if the woman chooses to continue the pregnancy, conservative management can be adopted unless pre-eclampsia or hemorrhage warrants termination of pregnancy.

24.6 CLINICAL FEATURES

With the extensive use of ultrasound, presently most of the cases of CHM are diagnosed earlier even before the classical symptoms and signs develop.

The usual presentation is vaginal bleeding following a period of amenorrhea. The bleeding can be heavy and prolonged or as a brownish discharge. If excessive uterine size is reached with very high level of hCG, pre-eclampsia, hyperemesis gravidarum and anemia can develop. Hyperthyroidism can also occur (in 7% of patients with CHM) because of the similarity between hCG with TSH.

Respiratory distress develops in 2% of patients with CHM, especially in those with excessive uterine size and markedly elevated hCG levels.

Uterine size more than the gestational age is one of the classic signs of CHM, which is however present only in 50% of patients. 50% of women with CHM have enlarged ovaries with theca lutein cysts $\geq$ 6 cm (Fig. 24.4). These theca lutein cysts usually regress spontaneously within 2-4 months. With early detection and evacuation of molar pregnancy, the classical presentation is seldom seen in the present scenario. The comparison between the clinical features in the past and the present is listed in Table 24.2.

The diagnosis is usually made by ultrasound.

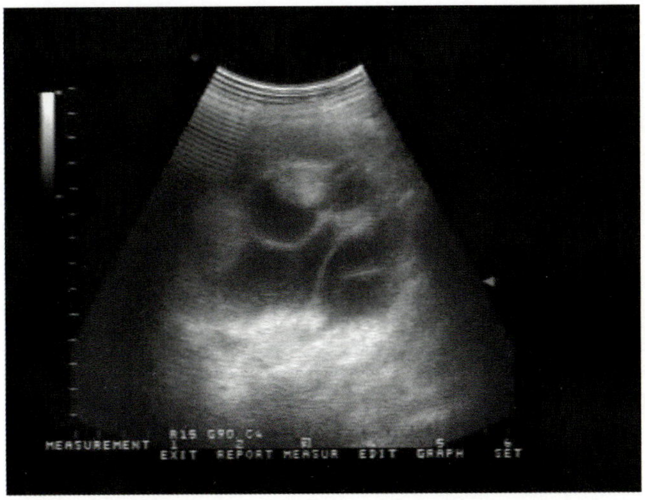

Fig. 24.4: TAS showing enlarged ovary with lutein cysts in a patient with molar pregnancy

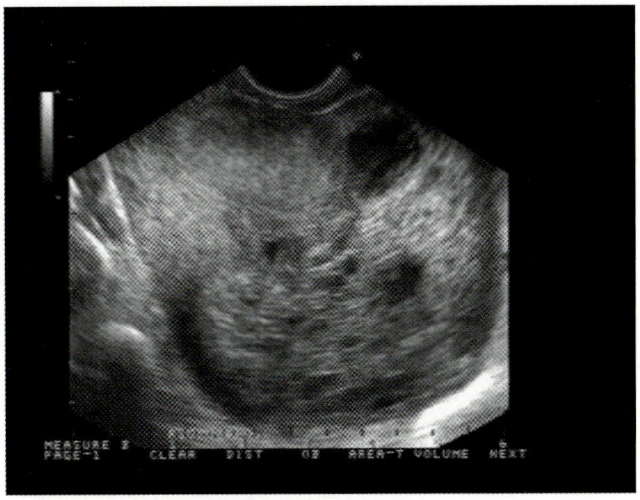

Fig. 24.5: Transvaginal scan showing complete molar pregnancy. Note the cystic spaces

Table 24.2: Clinical features of vesicular mole

Clinical features	*Previous incidence*	*Present incidence*
Vaginal bleeding	97%	84%
Excess uterine size	50%	28%
Pre-eclampsia	27%	1.3%
Anemia	50%	5%
Hyperemesis gravidarum	25%	8%
Hyperthyroidism	7%	0%
Trophoblastic embolization	2%	0%

Required investigations before evacuation

- Complete blood count
- Renal function tests
- Liver function tests
- Blood group and Rh type
- Serum β hCG
- Chest X-ray
- Coagulation studies (if indicated)
- Thyroid function test (If clinical hyperthyroidism is present)
- Digital oximetry, blood gases
- Lung scan (If pulmonary embolization is suspected)

24.7 PARTIAL HYDATIDIFORM MOLE

Partial hydatidiform mole usually presents as missed abortion in the first trimester. Rarely can they present in the second or early third trimester with a live fetus and partial molar changes.

24.8 DIAGNOSIS

Ultrasonography is the diagnostic method of choice due to its reliability, safety and sensitivity. In CHM, the typical 'snow-storm' appearance (Fig. 24.5) is seen even in the first trimester.

Estimation of hCG cannot be solely depended upon for absolute diagnosis of hydatidiform mole. Ultrasound and hCG are complementary to each other. Serum β-hCG level is especially important in the follow-up. Since partial moles can be misdiagnosed as missed abortion, it is ideal to perform histopathological analysis of product of conception after evacuation of missed abortions. Differentiation between complete and partial mole is difficult in some of the situations. The definite way to differentiate between the two requires identification of maternally expressed imprinted genes by DNA study. Maternally expressed imprinted genes are absent in complete mole whereas it will be present in partial mole. Ideally urinary hCG should be checked 10 weeks after evacuation of all miscarriages including termination of pregnancy, as GTN has been reported after such events.

24.9 MANAGEMENT (Flow Chart 24.2)

Evacuation of moles is the treatment of choice, once the diagnosis is made. The patient's condition should be stabilized by controlling pre-eclampsia, hyperthyroidism and anemia, if present.

Suction *evacuation preferably under anesthesia is the procedure of choice* for women who desire to preserve fertility. Tumor dissemination during evacuation is significantly less with the use of suction.

Very often the cervix is soft and permits the use of suction cannula without prior dilatation. Cervix maybe

Flow Chart 24.2: Guidelines for management of gestational trophoblastic disease (with permission from FIGO)

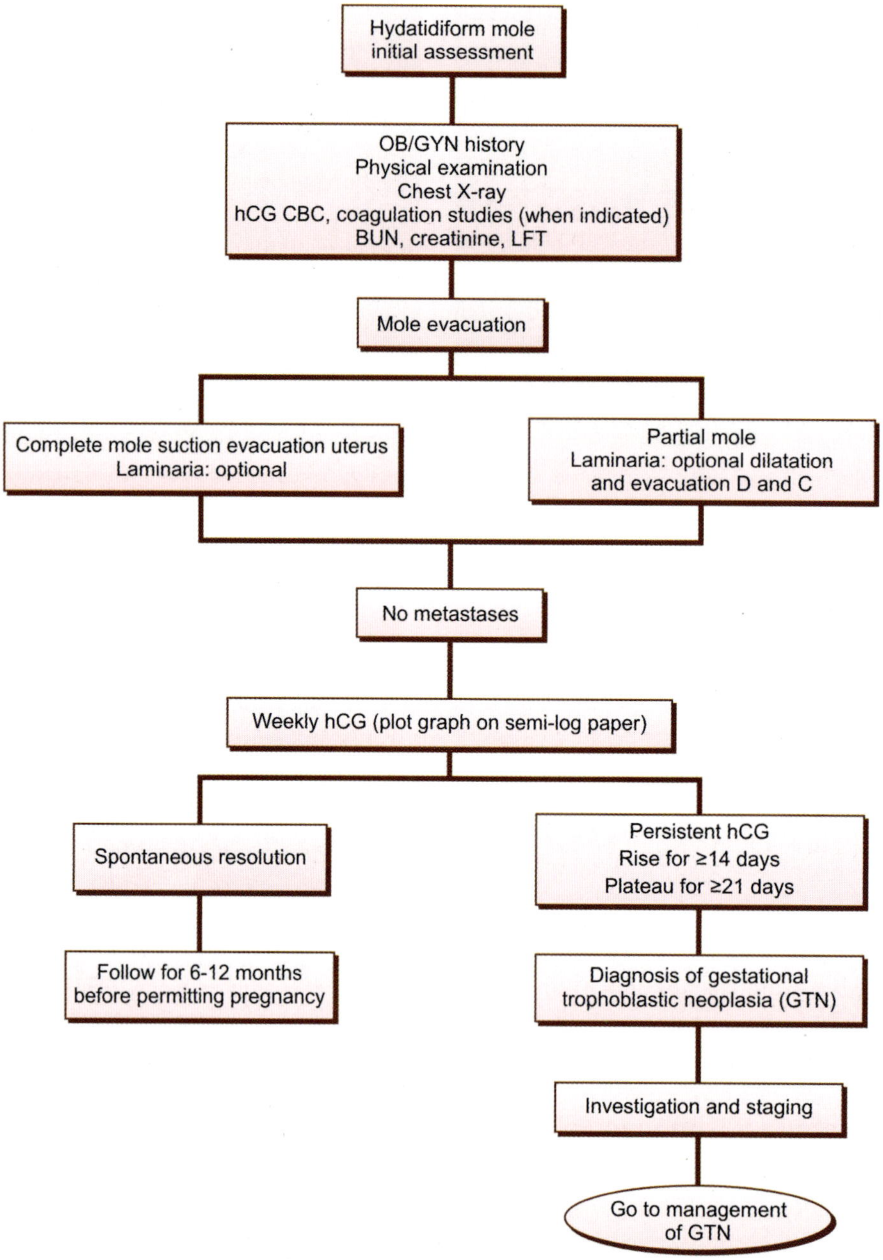

ripened with prostaglandins even though there is a theoretical risk of trophoblastic dissemination associated. This might particularly be needed in partial mole when the size of the fetal parts maybe expected to hinder evacuation.

Blood should be kept ready in the theater at the time of evacuation. Oxytocin infusion during evacuation helps to minimize bleeding without increasing the risk of persistent disease. The use of 12 mm cannula is advised to facilitate evacuation. When the size of uterus corresponds to >14 weeks, one hand should be placed over the abdomen and the uterus massaged to stimulate uterine contraction to reduce the risk of perforation.

At the end of suction evacuation, gentle sharp curettage is performed to remove any residual molar tissue. Patients who are Rh negative should receive Rh immunoglobulin at the time of evacuation.

Patient should be kept in the hospital for 48 hours after the evacuation. At the end of 24 hours β-hCG estimation should be repeated. Ultrasound should be done one week later to ascertain completeness of evacuation. Lutein cysts if present will regress spontaneously when the hCG level regresses. Complications like rupture, hemorrhage as well as torsion can occur, in which case surgical interference may be necessary.

24.9.1 Role of Hysterectomy

Hysterectomy with mole *in situ* is an option if the woman is above 40 or multiparous. Strict follow-up is essential even after hysterectomy.

24.9.2 Chemoprophylaxis

Routine prophylactic chemotherapy is not recommended as only 20% of patients need chemotherapy if selected by strict follow-up. In high risk CHM, when hCG measurements for follow-up are unavailable or the patient is unreliable for follow-up, chemoprophylaxis may be advised. The drug of choice for chemoprophylaxis is methotrexate which has to be administered till the β-hCG becomes normal.

24.9.3 Follow-up (Flow Chart 24.3)

About 20% patients will develop trophoblastic sequelae after molar pregnancy. Serum hCG is a faithful and sensitive tumor marker for the follow-up of patients after evacuation. Patients who have CHM and PHM should have follow-up as both are likely to develop trophoblastic sequelae.

Women who have the following features are at particularly high risk:

- hCG level > 100, 000 mIU/mL
- Excessive uterine enlargement
- Theca lutein cysts 6 cm in diameter
- Women who are older than 40 years

In a review of 858 patients who had any one of these signs were found to be at high risk for developing GTN. In this review it was found that local uterine invasion occurred in 31%, and metastases developed in 8.8% of the 352 high risk patients. For the 506 low risk patients, local invasion was found in only 3.4%, and metastases developed in 0.6%.[10,11]

A second curettage is not routinely advised. Approximately 80% of patients with high hCG values on follow-up, who undergo routine repeat evacuation will need chemotherapy. However, those who have vaginal bleeding may need repeat curettage. Those with mild elevation of hCG on follow-up will also get benefitted from repeat curettage as it could be due to the presence of recurrent trophoblastic tissue confined to the uterine cavity.

The hCG assay should be a reliable one which must measure all portions of the hCG molecule, particularly free β subunit, hyperglycosylated hCG, nicked hCG and hCG missing the terminal carboxyl segment. These subunits are more common in neoplasia than total hCG. If all these portions are not measured, it can result in false low values

Flow Chart 24.3: Follow-up algorithm of vesicular mole

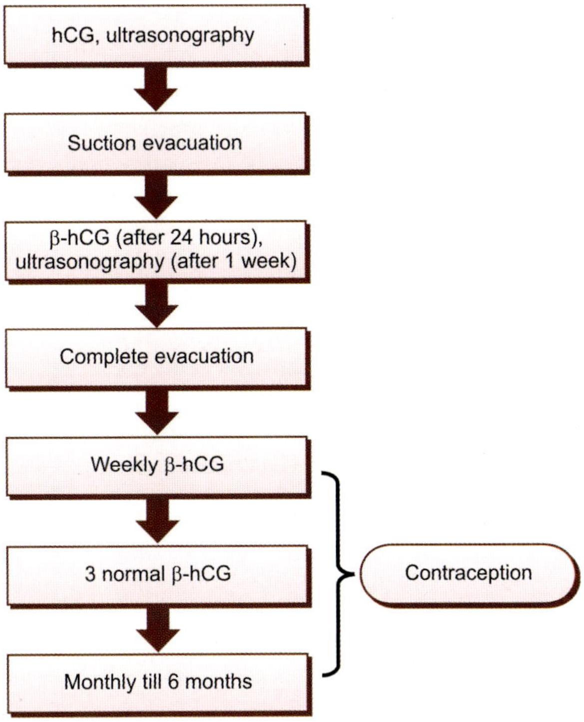

which can lead to inappropriate management. The assay should be sensitive to 2 mIU/ml or less. After evacuation all patients should be followed up by weekly hCG till normal levels are obtained. Meanwhile anemia or infection if present should be treated. Two further hCG tests are done at weekly intervals after hCG has become normal. Subsequent tests are done monthly for six months followed by two monthly tests for another six months to ensure that the hCG levels are maintained normal.

Reliable contraception should be advised following evacuation. Since, the incidence of post-molar persistent tumor has been reported to be increased among patients who used oral contraceptives before gonadotropin remission, after normalization of hCG hormonal contraceptive can be advised.[12,13]

Intrauterine contraceptive device may cause uterine bleeding which can raise the fear of choriocarcinoma. Insertion of IUCD before normalization of hCG carries the risk of perforation as well. After six months of follow-up, if the fall in hCG is logarithmic, the woman can be allowed to conceive. When the fall is very slow, a longer waiting period should be advised. If the woman reports with amenorrhea ultrasound should be done to confirm pregnancy and also to rule out repeat molar pregnancy. It should be kept in mind that the patient who develops persistent trophoblastic disease can also present as amenorrhea due to the high level of hCG.

24.9.4 Phantom hCG

Serum of some individuals may give false positive hCG results due to the presence of heterophilic antibody that reacts with antibody of certain assay kits. These women do not have trophoblastic disease or pregnancy associated events. This is called phantom hCG. Such patients do not require any therapy. They can be differentiated by performing hCG assay in dilution, which will give proportionate results in the presence of real hCG. Urinary hCG will not be elevated as these antibodies are not filtered by the glomeruli and hence not excreted in urine.

24.10 QUIESCENT GESTATIONAL TROPHOBLASTIC DISEASE

In some patients, following an episode of molar pregnancy the hCG level remains mildly elevated (50-100 mIU/ml). This is real hCG. Clinical findings and imaging may be negative and the low level persists in spite of chemotherapy or surgery. In a few patients (20%), after several weeks or years, hCG gets re-elevated and tumor become detectable. As soon as hCG rises, hyperglycosylated hCG, which is a variant of hCG with double-sized oligosaccharide side chains, will be elevated before clinical disease manifests. At this instance, treatment is indicated.

24.11 POSTMOLAR GTN

Following evacuation of vesicular mole, hCG level returns to normal by 8-10 weeks. The hCG level should be plotted on a semi-logarithmic paper. At each visit a detailed history suggestive of persistent or metastatic disease should be enquired. Even though metastatic disease is rarely encountered while on follow-up of molar pregnancy, it should always be kept in mind and chances excluded. Patient should be examined for the presence of suburethral nodule. The size of the lutein cysts should also be assessed. Regression of the cysts is a sign of decreasing hCG level.

In about 15% of patients after evacuation of a complete mole, locally invasive gestational trophoblastic tumor (GTT) develops. Infrequently it may arise after other gestations. The clinical features include:

- Irregular vaginal bleeding
- Persistence of theca lutein cysts
- Uterine subinvolution or asymmetric enlargement
- Persistently elevated hCG levels

Postmolar GTN is diagnosed on the basis of elevated hCG levels. In the presence of trophoblastic tumor either in the uterus or elsewhere in the body, hCG level could be elevated. *Histologic or radiologic evidence is not necessary for diagnosis.* Even in the absence of clinical evidence of metastasis or histological evidence of choriocarcinoma, persistently elevated hCG is an indication for chemotherapy.

24.11.1 Invasive Mole

GTD rarely presents as intra-abdominal bleeding caused by trophoblastic tissue penetrating the full-thickness of the myometrium. Pathologically this is same as post molar trophoblastic neoplasia. There is argument as to whether this should be classified as a separate entity or subclassified within GTN. The condition is stage I GTN. The degree of myometrial invasion can be specified as "o" for no myometrial invasion, "s" for superficial invasion, "I" for intermediate invasion, and "f" for full myometrial invasion. When the histology is molar, "M" may be added and "CH" if the histology is of choriocarcinoma.[19] The condition is usually diagnosed as persistent trophoblastic disease (Fig. 24.6). Most often a vascular lesion can be identified in the myometrium.

24.12 METASTATIC GTN

After evacuation of complete mole, metastatic GTN develops in about 4% of patients. It is more often seen when GTN develops after non-molar pregnancy. Common sites of metastases are given in Table 24.3.

Patients with pulmonary metastases may present with chest pain, cough, hemoptysis, dyspnoea or asymptomatic lesion visible by chest radiography. Chest radiography

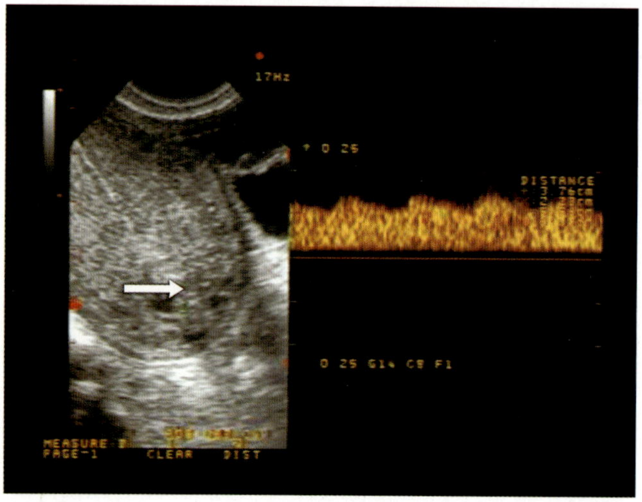

Fig. 24.6: Transvaginal scan showing persistent trophoblastic disease. Mixed echogenic lesion is seen in the myometrium (arrow). Note the low resistance flow in the spectral Doppler picture (right). The patient had hCG rise while on follow-up and needed 4 courses of methotrexate

Table 24.3: Common sites of metastases

Lung	80%
Vagina	30%
Pelvis	20%
Liver	10%
Brain	10%

reveals "cannon balls" or a "snow storm" appearance. It may be in the form of a pleural effusion or an embolic pattern. The condition may be mistaken for pneumonia, especially if it develops following non-molar pregnancy, a situation where choriocarcinoma is not anticipated. The presentation can be as pulmonary hypertension which develop secondary to pulmonary arterial occlusion by trophoblastic emboli.

Vaginal metastases usually appear in the suburethral region or at the fornices as bluish nodules which can attain a size of 3-4 cm (Fig. 24.7). Retrograde vascular spread explains this metastasis. This can lead to irregular vaginal bleeding or sometimes profuse bleeding from the disrupted surface of the nodule and can be difficult to control. A vaginal nodule may also be seen in patients presenting with vesicular mole.

Hepatic metastasis is usually encountered when there is a delay in diagnosis. Epigastric or right upper quadrant pain may develop if stretching of hepatic capsule ensues. Hepatic rupture can occur leading to exsanguinating intraperitoneal hemorrhage.

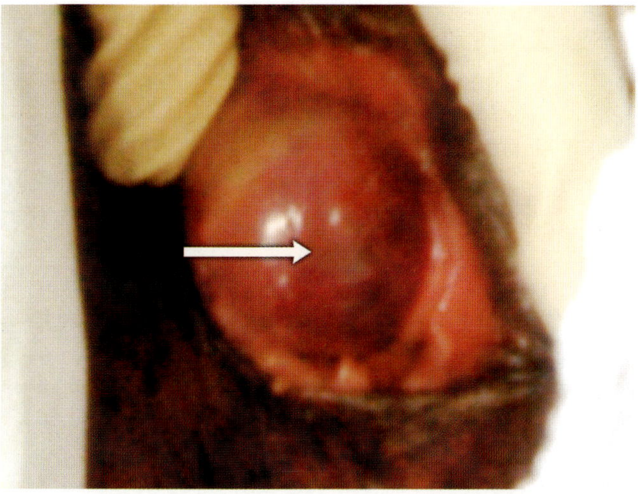

Fig. 24.7: Suburethral nodule in a 32-year-old lady who presented with irregular vaginal bleeding since 4 months. Her irregular bleeding followed an abortion evacuation. Her β hCG was 62,000 IU/L. She was given chemotherapy with methotrexate the same day. The nodule subsided without bleeding

Indications for chemotherapy after molar evacuation

- Rise in hCG (3 values over 2 weeks-1, 7, 14)
- Plateauing of hCG (4 values over 3 weeks 1, 7, 14, 21)
- hCG value >20, 000 IU/L after 4 weeks
- Persistence of hCG after 16 weeks
- Histological evidence of choriocarcinoma or clinical evidence of metastasis

All patients with brain metastasis have concurrent pulmonary or vaginal involvement or both. Patients may present with headache, convulsions or acute focal neurologic deficits.

24.13 MANAGEMENT OF GESTATIONAL TROPHOBLASTIC NEOPLASIA

In about 50% of cases, the condition is preceded by hydatidiform mole. In 25% cases, it follows an abortion or ectopic pregnancy, and in the remaining 25%, a delivery of normal fetus.

When a patient is found to have elevated hCG, irrespective of whether it follows molar pregnancy or non-molar pregnancy, it is mandatory to make out the extent of tumor dissemination so as to stage the disease and plan management.

Staging of GTN

For staging, the following studies are required to comprehend tumor dissemination.

- **Clinical examination** to look for vaginal metastasis.
- **Chest X-ray** or **preferably CT scan** to make out pulmonary metastasis: Chest CT scans may detect micrometastases which may not be visible on chest X-ray. Chest CT was found to demonstrate pulmonary micrometastases in about 40% of women who had normal chest radiograph.[14]
- If lung metastases are found, whole body CT is indicated to diagnose secondaries in the kidney, liver, bone and brain. *Secondaries in these sites are rare in the absence of lung secondaries.* All patients with lung metastasis should undergo lumbar puncture to estimate hCG level in CSF. CSF: serum hCG ratio of more than 1/60 signifies highly probable brain metastasis. Even in the absence of lung secondaries, if there is clinical suspicion of cerebral metastases, brain MRI/CT should be done.
- *Pelvic ultrasound:* TVS can reliably detect extent of uterine involvement and spot out patients who have resistant disease while on treatment and can be used to take decision for hysterectomy.

- *Biopsy from a suburethral nodule should not be tried* due to the grave danger of hemorrhage from the biopsy site.

After making out the extent of spread, the disease should be staged by the FIGO 2000 staging system, given in Table 24.4.

Hydatidiform mole should be registered, but not staged as stage 0. Staging applies only to trophoblastic neoplasia. Cases which do not fulfill the criteria for any of the given stages are listed as unstaged.

WHO scoring system (Table 24.5): WHO developed a scoring system for gestational trophoblastic neoplasia, based on prognostic factors. The score values are 0, 1, 2 and 4. Blood group is not included in the scoring system. Liver metastasis is given a score of 4. A score of *6 or less* is low risk disease treatable by single agent chemotherapy. A score of *7 or more* is considered as high risk disease that requires combination chemotherapy. There is no such category as medium risk.

In the year 2000, FIGO Committee on Gynecologic Oncology accepted the WHO scoring system based on prognostic factors which were originally formulated by Prof Kenneth Bagshawe. This was ratified in the FIGO announcement in 2002 and is the present FIGO staging and scoring system. The individual patient's stage and risk score is expressed by allotting Roman numerals for the stage and an Arabic numeral for the sum of all the risk factor scores, separated by a colon. Based on this, patients are divided into low risk and high risk (Table 24.6).

Table 24.4: FIGO 2000 staging system

Stage I	Gestational trophoblastic tumors strictly confined to the uterine corpus
Stage II	Gestational trophoblastic neoplasia extending to the adnexa or to the vagina, but limited to the genital structures
Stage III	Gestational trophoblastic neoplasia extending to the lungs, with or without genital tract involvement
Stage IV	All other metastatic sites

24.13.1 Management of Low Risk GTN (WHO Score ≤ 6; FIGO Stage I, II or III) (Flow Charts 24.4 and 24.5)

Hysterectomy Plus Chemotherapy

If the patient does not wish to preserve fertility, hysterectomy with adjuvant single agent chemotherapy may

Table 24.5: WHO risk factor scoring

FIGO (WHO) risk factor scoring	*0*	*1*	*2*	*4*
Age	<40	≥40	-	-
Antecedent pregnancy	Hydatidiform mole	Abortion	Term	-
Interval months from index pregnancy	<4	4-6	7-12	>12
Pretreatment hCG milli IU/ml	$<10^3$	10^3-10^4	10^4-10^5	$>10^5$
Largest tumor size including uterus	-	3-4 cm	≥5 cm	-
Site of metastases including uterus	lung	Spleen kidney	Gastrointestinal tract	Brain, liver
Number of metastases identified	-	1-4	5-8	>8
Previous failed chemotherapy	-	-	Single drug	Two or more drugs

Table 24.6: High risk and low risk GTN

Low risk GTN	*High risk GTN*
Non-metastatic gestational trophoblastic neoplasia Low risk metastatic neoplasia—Risk score ≤ 6 • FIGO stages I, II and III • Metastasis to lungs only • Duration less than 4 months from the index pregnancy • No prior chemotherapy • No antecedent term pregnancy • hCG <40, 000 mIU/L	FIGO stage I, II and III with risk score of 7 or more and FIGO stage IV • Duration >4 months since last pregnancy • Pretreatment hCG >40, 000 mIU/ml • Brain/liver metastasis • Antecedent term pregnancy • Prior chemotherapy failure

Flow Chart 24.4: Guidelines for the management of gestational trophoblastic neoplasia (with permission from FIGO)

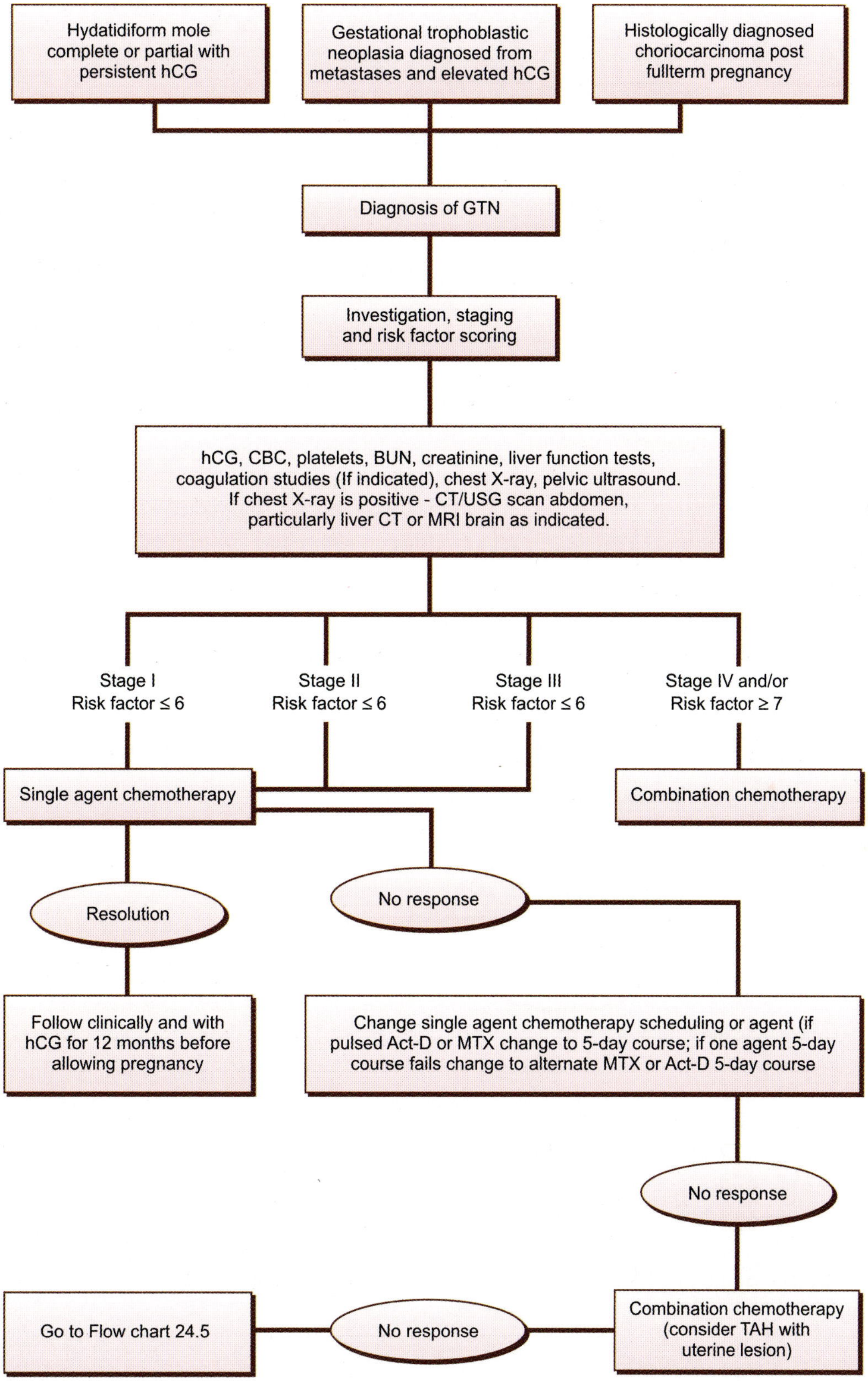

Flow Chart 24.5: Guidelines for the management of gestational trophoblastic neoplasia (with permission from FIGO)

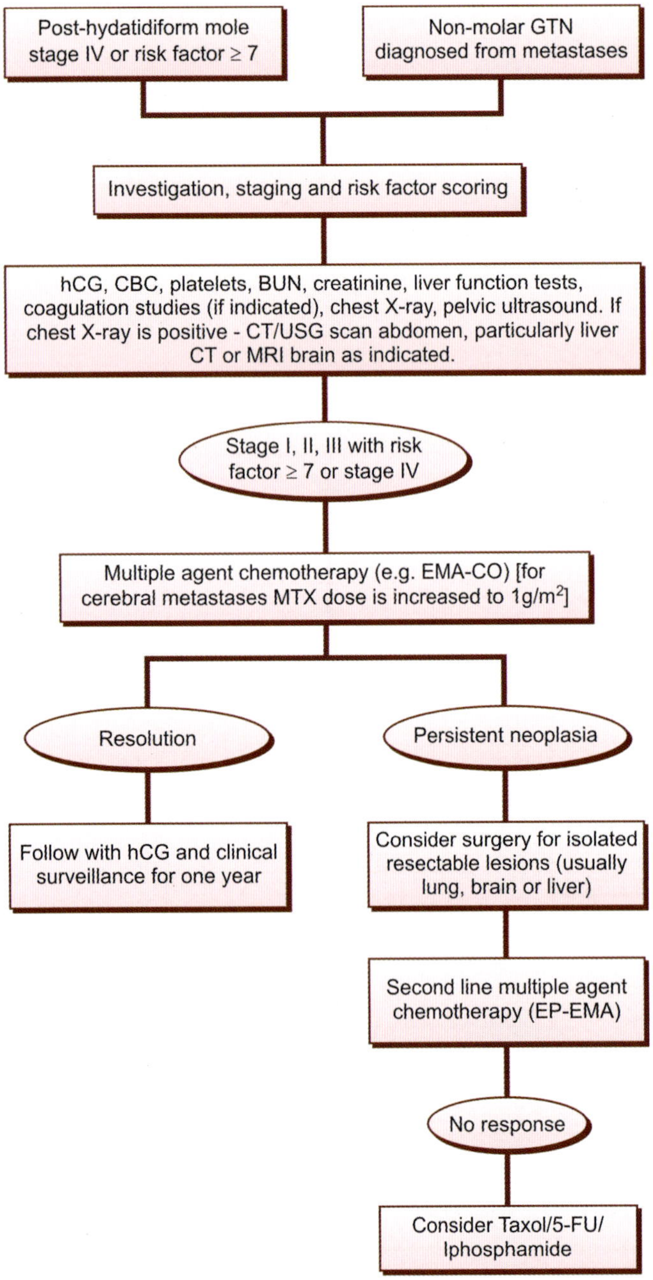

be performed as primary treatment. Adjuvant chemotherapy is administered for three reasons:

- To reduce the likelihood of disseminating viable tumor cells at surgery.
- To maintain a cytotoxic level of chemotherapy in the bloodstream and tissues in case viable tumor cells are disseminated at surgery.
- To treat any occult metastases that may already be present at the time of surgery. Chemotherapy can be administered safely at the time of hysterectomy without increasing the risk of bleeding or sepsis. In a series of 31 patients treated with primary hysterectomy and a single course of adjuvant chemotherapy, all achieved complete remission with no additional therapy.

Chemotherapy Alone

Single-agent chemotherapy is the preferred treatment in patients with stage I disease who desire to retain fertility. When primary single-agent chemotherapy was administered to 495 patients with stage I GTT, 452 patients (91.3%) attained complete remission. The remaining 43 resistant patients subsequently achieved remission after combination chemotherapy or surgical intervention. When patients are resistant to single-agent chemotherapy and desire to preserve fertility, combination chemotherapy is to be administered. If the patient is resistant to both single-agent and combination chemotherapy and wants to retain fertility, local uterine resection may be considered. When local resection is planned, a preoperative ultrasonography, MRI, or arteriography may help to define the site of the resistant tumor. Low risk GTN is treated with single agent chemotherapy. Methotrexate is the drug of choice. *Vaginal metastases may bleed profusely because they are highly vascular and friable.* When bleeding is substantial, it may be controlled by packing the vagina or by wide local excision. Infrequently, arteriographic embolization of the hypogastric arteries may be required to control hemorrhage from vaginal metastases.

Investigations before starting chemotherapy: Complete blood count and platelets, PT, APTT, fibrinogen, BUN, creatinine and liver function tests.

Drug schedules: single agent chemotherapy regimes

a. Methotrexate 0.4 mg/Kg IM for 5 days, repeated every two weeks. The primary failure rate is 10%.
b. Methotrexate with Leucovorin rescue: Methotrexate 1 mg/kg IM on alternate days for four doses with Leucovorin 0.1 mg/kg, 24 hours after each dose of methotrexate. The next course is given after an interval of 15-18 days. Primary failure rate is 20-25%. This is the most widely adopted regime.
c. Methotrexate 50 mg/m^2 IM weekly *(Pulse regimen)*. This is associated with 30% primary failure rate. If it fails methotrexate 0.4 mg/kg for 5 days can be given or the drug can be changed to Actinomycin-D 12 µg/kg for 5 days.
d. Actinomycin-D 1.25 mg/m^2 given every two weeks *(Pulse regimen)*. The failure rate is 20%.
e. Actinomycin-D 12 µg/kg IV daily for 5 days. Repeat every two weeks. This can be preferred in patients with

hepatic dysfunction. Primary failure rate is less – 8%.

f. Methotrexate 250 mg infusion over twelve hours *(Pulse regimen)*. It is associated with high failure rate of 30%.

The low dose methotrexate folinic acid regime is the most widely used regime with very high success rate. This regime is well tolerated. Side effects like alopecia or myelosuppression are very rare. Serum hCG value should be repeated weekly. After the first course of chemotherapy, the hCG value is expected to fall by one log or more. This could achieve remission in 87.6% of patients. A second course of chemotherapy is administered, if the hCG level does not decline by one log within 18 days of completion of the first course.

Before each course, complete blood count, platelet count, creatinine, BUN and SGOT should be done. After the first negative hCG level, 2-3 additional courses of chemotherapy should be administered.

The primary failure rate of the pulse regimens is greater than single agent 5 days course. The pulse regimens are intended to reduce the cost of therapy. If after a course of the pulse regime, the hCG level plateaus or rises, the 5 days regime should be adopted. The authors of a Cochrane review of RCTs, on this issue concluded that "pulsed" dactinomycin is superior to weekly parenteral methotrexate at the reported doses. However, the authors believe that well designed, multicentered, randomized double-blind trials are required to evaluate other chemotherapy regimens, most importantly "pulsed" dactinomycin with the widely used 8-day methotrexate-folinic acid.[15]

If the regression of β-hCG after 2 courses of MTX-FA regime is inadequate, actinomycin-D is substituted. If the decline of hCG is not adequate even after changing to actinomycin-D, the patient must be treated with combination chemotherapy.

Actinomycin should be given through a free-running IV infusion. Extravasation can cause severe sloughing. Failure of single agent regime is an indication to switch to combination chemotherapy. In single agent chemotherapy, remission is achieved with only one course in 81.5% of patients.[10] The overall success rate of therapy, which sometimes involves more than one line of treatment in low risk patients, is reported as nearly 100%.

24.13.2 Management of High Risk GTN

Single agent chemotherapy in high risk GTN has high failure rate. Hence the standard practice is to treat these patients with combination chemotherapy. EMA-CO is the widely accepted primary combination treatment regime with remission rates of 86%. The regime is listed in Table 24.7.

Table 24.7: EMA-CO regimen

Day	*Drug*	*Dose*
1	Etoposide	100 mg/m^2 IV over30 min
	Actinomycin D	0.5 mg IV push
	Methotrexate	100 mg/m^2 infusion in 1000ml 5% dextrose in 12 hours
2	Etoposide	100 mg/m^2 IV over 30 min
	Actinomycin D	0.5 mg IV push
	Folinic acid	15 mg IM every 12 hour for 4 doses beginning 24 h after start of Methotrexate
8	Cyclophosphamide	600mg/m^2 IV infusion
	Vincristine	1.0mg/m^2 push

Table 24.8: Long-term consequences of chemotherapy

1. Physical and psychological problems
2. Premature ovarian failure
3. Second malignancies especially in women treated with Etoposide
   - Hodgkins lymphoma
   - Myeloid leukemia
   - Carcinoma breast

Patients who have brain metastases need a very high dose of methotrexate. They should be treated with methotrexate 1gm/m^2. Granulocyte colony stimulating factor should be given to sustain white cells.

Patients who require more than 6 courses of EMA-CO are at risk of developing leukemia. Those who are resistant to EMA-CO may be treated by EMA–EP protocol. In this regime etoposide and platinum are substituted for cyclophosphamide and vincristine on day 8. Those with brain metastases should be given higher doses of methotrexate supplemented with fortnightly intrathecal methotrexate for the entire duration of therapy. Chemotherapy is continued until the patient achieves three consecutive negative values. After negative hCG all high risk patients should be treated with three further courses of chemotherapy. The rationale is that, even when the hCG value is negative there can be about 10^7 viable malignant cells in the body. Overall survival for high risk disease patients are reported as 86%.

Role of Surgery and Radiation

Hysterectomy can be chosen as the initial management in low risk patients who do not need uterine conservation as it reduces the number of courses of chemotherapy and consequently the duration of therapy. Patients who have severe vaginal bleeding can be managed by hysterectomy

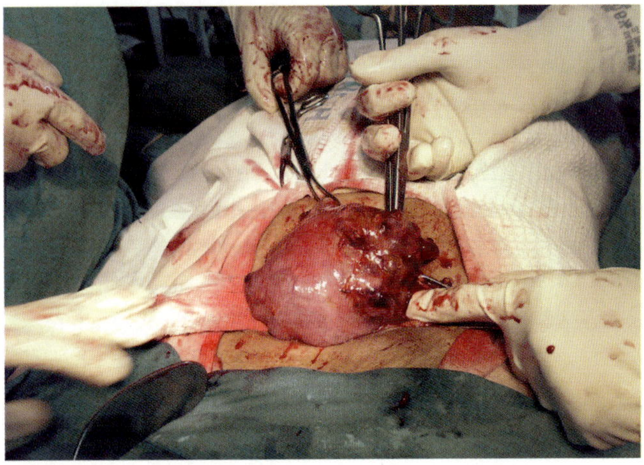

Fig. 24.8: Total hysterectomy and LSO specimen of a 32-year-old multiparous lady, showing choriocarcinoma perforating the uterine wall. Choriocarcinoma was diagnosed since her βhCG was 65,000 IU/L but this diagnosis was made only 2 years after her last delivery although she had several episodes of irregular vaginal bleeding. Hysterectomy was done for internal hemorrhage. Eventhough she was started on EMACO regime; she died due to the side effects of the chemotherapy

or uterine artery embolization. Hysterectomy may be required, also in patients who have sepsis or internal hemorrhage due to tumor perforating the uterus (Fig. 24.8). Furthermore, in patients with extensive uterine tumor, hysterectomy may substantially reduce tumor burden and thereby limit the number of courses of chemotherapy.

Metastatic sites in the liver, brain etc that do not regress with chemotherapy should be removed surgically. But it should be kept in mind that presence of radiological lesions when serological response is good need not be surgically interfered. Certain sites in the liver and brain which cannot be removed surgically can be treated with radiation. The aim of giving radiation is to prevent catastrophic hemorrhage rather than controlling the disease. Secondaries in the liver may be treated with 20 GY of radiation or hepatic arterial infusion of methotrexate. As already mentioned, sub-urethral nodule should not be excised due to the grave danger of hemorrhage. Even biopsy should not be tried as it is not necessary. The nodule will respond to chemotherapy.

24.13.3 Follow-up after Treatment of GTN

- Weekly hCG until normal for 3 consecutive weeks.
- Followed by monthly measurement until it is normal for 12 consecutive months.
- Effective contraception should be advised during the follow-up period.
- Women who have stage IV disease should have lifelong follow-up with β-hCG measurement in view of the chances of late recurrence.

While on follow-up, in the presence of persisting or rising hCG, if conventional imaging is negative, FDG-PET can be used to locate disease. Resistant disease should be excised if possible. Patients who do not respond even to second line treatment maybe offered high dose chemotherapy with stem cell rescue support. There are no randomized trials on this issue.

Vascular malformations like arteriovenous fistulae rarely follow treatment of the disease. This is detected at Doppler ultrasound following treatment. The condition can cause intraperitoneal or vaginal bleeding in which case either uterine artery embolization or hysterectomy may have to be resorted to.

Apart from the physical and psychological problems chemotherapy is reported to cause premature ovarian failure. Occurrence of second malignancies like Hodgkin's lymphoma, myeloid leukemia and carcinoma of the breast are also reported among these patients (Table 24.8).

24.14 PREGNANCY AFTER PERSISTENT TROPHOBLASTIC TUMOR

Future fertility is not affected by either the disease or chemotherapy. Women can be advised conception after 1 year follow-up since most relapses occur within this period. The risk due to possible teratogenicity of chemotherapy also will be over by this period. Premature menopause is a likely after effect of combination chemotherapy.

The outcome of pregnancy following chemotherapy is not different from the normal population.

24.15 PLACENTAL SITE TROPHOBLASTIC TUMOR (PSTT)

This is a rare form of trophoblastic disease which originates from the intermediate trophoblast. It can also develop following normal pregnancy, abortion or molar pregnancy. The tumor invades the myometrium and the blood vessels. Since it originates mainly from intermediate trophoblast, hCG is not produced significantly as in other trophoblastic tumors. Even though hCG is not markedly elevated it is still the reliable tumor marker for PSTT. *Human placental lactogen (HPL) can be demonstrated by immunohistochemical staining of the tumor tissue.* Recently it was found that free β-hCG is significantly higher in women with PSTT than in combined GTD.[16]

The clinical presentation is usually with amenorrhea and rarely irregular vaginal bleeding. Most women present with disease confined to the uterus but delayed extensive metastasis may occur. The uterine disease can be identified as a lesion in the myometrium (Figs 24.9 to 24.12 and Flow chart 24.6). *In the presence of a combination of uterine tumor, mild elevation of β hCG and amenorrhea, PSTT should be suspected.* The tumor is relatively insensitive to chemotherapy; hence *hysterectomy is the mainstay of treatment.* Hysterotomy, resection of tumor and adjuvant chemotherapy may be considered in women who wish to conserve childbearing function. Since there is a high chance of metastases, these patients should be on close follow-up. Before deciding on tumor resection, the patient should be adequately counseled about the chance of reccurrence. Prognosis for patients with disease confined to the uterus is good. High mitotic count in the tumor at microscopy is a poor prognostic factor. Those who have disease extension outside the uterus will have poor prognosis even after surgery and chemotherapy.

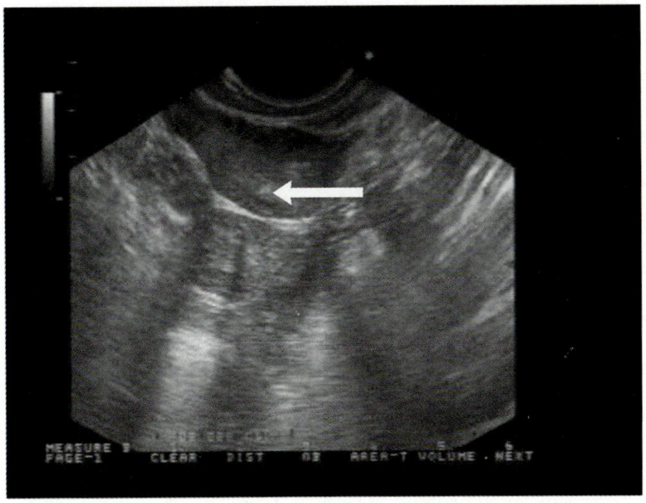

Fig. 24.9: Transvaginal scan showing echogenic lesion in the myometrium which later proved to be PSTT

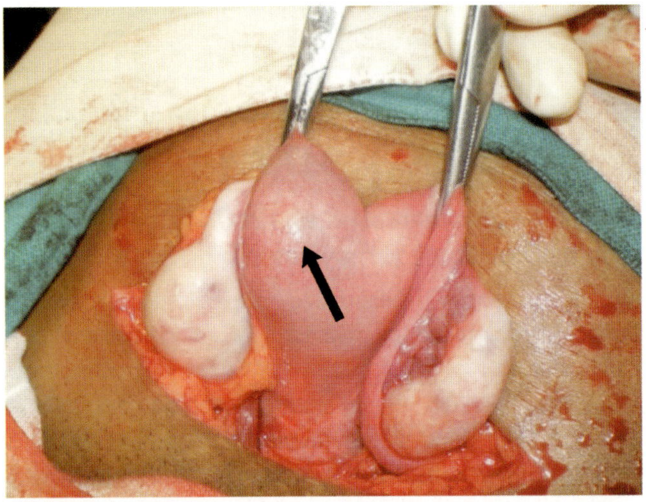

Fig. 24.10: External appearance of the uterus at hysterectomy of a 28-year-old lady who was diagnosed with PSTT in the curettage specimen. Note the asymmetric enlargement of the uterus due to the tumor (arrow). She presented with amenorrhea of 2 years following delivery

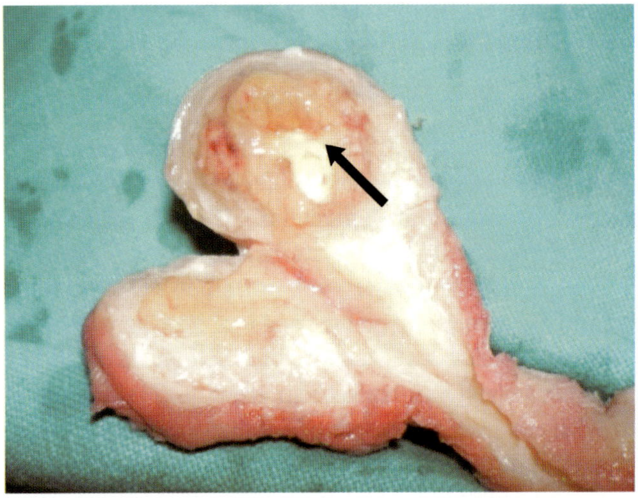

Fig. 24.11: Sagittal section of the uterus showing tumor (arrow) in the myometrium (PSTT)

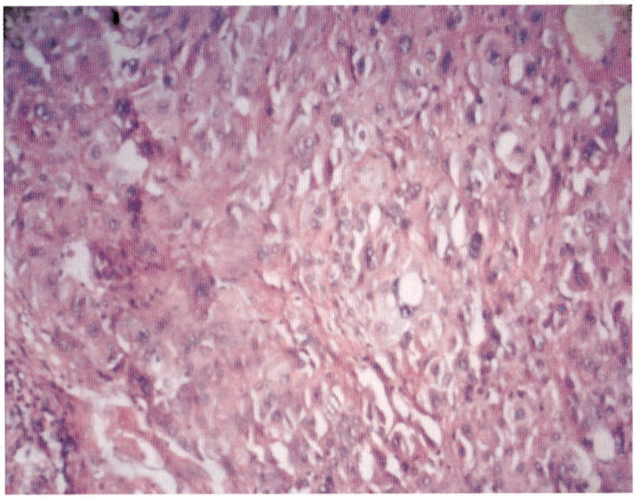

Fig. 24.12: Microscopic picture of the above specimen. Note the trophoblast cells invading the myometrium

Flow Chart 24.6: Guidelines for the management of Placental site Trophoblastic Tumor (with permission from FIGO)

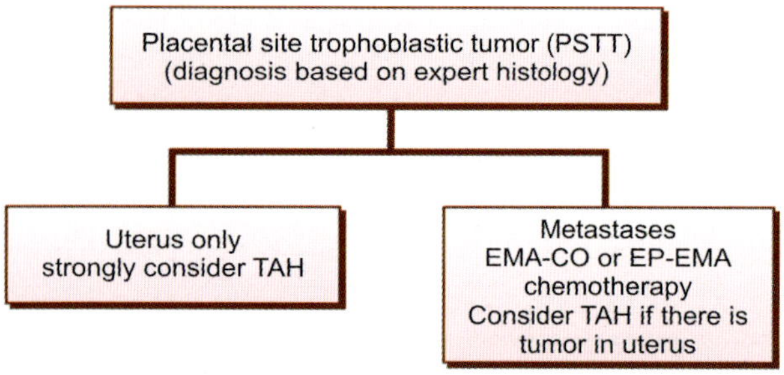

24.16 EPITHELIOID TROPHOBLASTIC TUMOR (ETT)

Epithelioid trophoblastic tumor is a recent addition to the types of trophoblastic tumors. This is very rare with very few cases reported in the literature. In the reported cases, the lesions were seen in the isthmus and endocervix. Histopathology revealed adenosquamous elements with trophoblastic cells. Levels of hCG were found to be moderately elevated. Their prognosis is better, with a single case of metastasis and one death among the five reported.[17]

24.17 CONCLUSION

The term gestational trophoblastic disease (GTD) includes all aspects of this entity ranging from the benign to the malignant forms, whereas gestational trophoblastic neoplasia (GTN) refers exclusively to those forms that are malignant and require chemotherapy. Following vesicular mole, all patients need follow-up with hCG. Chemotherapy is preferred only for patients diagnosed to have persistent disease. Gestational trophoblastic neoplasia can follow vesicular mole, abortion or term pregnancy. All patients are staged based on FIGO staging system, 2000. Treatment decisions are made after classifying the disease into low risk and high risk based on the scoring system developed by WHO. Low risk patients are treated initially with single agent chemotherapy, and those who are resistant are given combination chemotherapy. High risk patients are treated initially with combination chemotherapy. Prognosis for the disease is excellent with chemotherapy. Cure rate for low risk patients is nearly 100%. For the high risk, it ranges from 65 to 85%.

24.18 CASE SCENARIOS

Case Scenario 1

M/s D, a 24-year-old lady was referred from regional hospital after evacuation of vesicular mole. She had evacuation on 23/08/07. Her pre-evacuation hCG level was 2,09,200. She was referred to the trophoblastic clinic on 13/09/07. On examination, her vitals were stable. General examination was unremarkable. Speculum examination revealed nothing remarkable. Bimanual examination showed bulky uterus and no adnexal mass. She was followed up with weekly hCG level as routine. Her hCG levels were as follows:

13/09/07-1175 IU/L
20/09/07-1461 IU/L
26/09/07-2469 IU/L

She has not regained menstruation after evacuation.

Do you think her hCG regression is normal?

Ideally the hCG should be plotted on a semi-logarithmic graph. However, the values are abnormal as there is a rising titer and 3 consecutive values in 2 weeks shows doubling.

How will you manage?

Pelvic ultrasound should be done to make out whether the patient has retained molar tissue in the uterine cavity or she has stage I disease in the myometrium.

Pelvic ultrasound on 01/10/07 showed residual disease in the uterine cavity, she had a repeat evacuation on the same day. Moderate curettings were obtained.

What is the place of curettage?

Even though curettage is not recommended for persistent trophoblastic disease, it is reported that the hCG level comes down following curettage in some patients thus avoiding chemotherapy. Probably this is because these individuals have trophoblastic proliferation in the uterine cavity. However, if the patient has developed GTN either in the myometrium or elsewhere she will not benefit from curettage. This patient's hCG on 05/10/07 was 1488 IU/L.

Should she be started on chemotherapy at this point?

No. Because the hCG has fallen from 2469 IU/L to 1488 IU/L and it is only about 6 weeks postevacuation. She needs to be followed up as routine.

Her hCG on 18/10/07 was 5196 IU/L. Should she be treated?

Yes. She should be administered chemotherapy as her hCG level increased several times.

What is the chemotherapy regime?

The regime should be decided based on her stage and score.

What is her stage and score?

Staging is done after metastatic work up. Pelvic imaging and chest CT are the initial investigations. Pelvic ultrasound revealed vascular lesion in the myometrium measuring 2.3 × 1.9 cm. Chest CT was normal. Hence, the stage is I and score is 1. Hence she can be started on single agent chemotherapy. She was advised methotrexate. But she went home and returned on 25/10/07 only. Her hCG on the same day showed a rise. It was 12562 IU/L.

She had one course of methotrexate starting from 25/10/07. hCG on follow-up was as follows:
03/11/07- 6566
10/11/07-2484
17/11/07- 3488
Since the hCG level is not falling but shows a rise after an initial fall she needs to be given second course of methotrexate.

She was administered a second course of methotrexate. Her hCG after the second course was as follows:
24/11/07- 3632 IU/L
01/12/07- 3438 IU/L
10/12/07- 3501 IU/L

What is your comment about the regression?
The regression is not adequate as there is no fall of even 1 log.

What is the next line of management?
She should be changed to actinomycin D.
She was given actinomycin D.
On actinomycin also the regression was not adequate. Hence she was treated with combination chemotherapy using EMA. She responded to EMA regime. Presently she is 20 weeks pregnant.

Case Scenario 2

M/s N, 28 years, married for 6 months, LMP: *1.3.2009* following which she had an abortion on *21.3.2009* at a local hospital, the details of which including the pathology report are not available. Since she had bleeding PV following abortion, and the uterus appeared bulky, a D and C was done on *21.5.2009* in the same hospital. Since bleeding continued irregularly, she attended the tertiary center on *27.7.2009*. β-hCG was done which came as 87952 IU/L.

What is the probable diagnosis?
In the absence of a non growing pregnancy, β-hCG level of 87952 is to be taken as gestational trophoblastic neoplasia.

What is the management?
Metastatic work-up to stage the disease.

What is the metastatic work-up that is to be done?
Imaging of the pelvis and chest CT. Imaging of the pelvis will help in making out the size of the tumor in the uterus as well as its extension to other pelvic structures. Ultrasound is also sensitive in diagnosing the disease in the uterus.

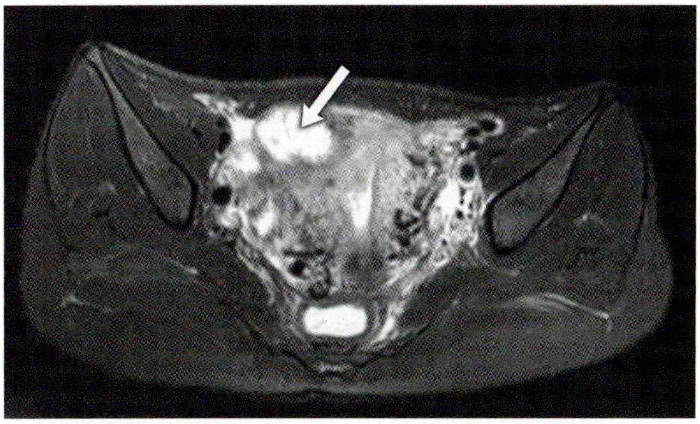

Fig. 24.13: MRI coronal section of pelvis showing lesion in the right side of the myometrium (arrow)

This patient had MRI of the pelvis which revealed ill-defined enhancing lesion in the myometrium towards the right lateral wall measuring 3.3 × 2.8 cm (Fig. 24.13).

What is the reason that chest CT is preferred rather than whole body CT?
If metastases are absent in chest CT, the patient is unlikely to have metastases in other sites. Hence in the absence of disease in chest CT, whole body CT need not be done. However, if symptom pertaining to any other site is present appropriate imaging should be done.

Her chest CT was unremarkable, what is the stage of the disease?
She has stage I GTN, as the disease is diagnosed to be confined to the uterus by metastatic work-up.

What should be the line of management?
Since the patient is young and wants to preserve the child bearing function and choriocarcinoma is a curable cancer, she can be treated with chemotherapy.

What should be the chemotherapy regime for this patient?
The choice of treatment between single agent and multiple agent chemotherapy depends upon her WHO score even though she has stage I disease. According to WHO scoring system her score is 4 (refer WHO scoring system). She need be treated with single agent chemotherapy-Methotrexate.

Case Scenario 3

27-year-old Ms B presented with vomiting, and amenorrhea of 2 months. She was a nullipara. Her periods were regular before, but recently became irregular. She gave a history of abortion about 6 months ago. In view of her amenorrhea, a pregnancy test was done which came as positive. Since her uterus was of normal size and ultrasound revealed no intrauterine pregnancy, she was referred to the tertiary center, suspecting unruptured ectopic pregnancy. On reaching the tertiary center, examination revealed no evidence of ectopic or intrauterine pregnancy. The patient was complaining of severe headache also.

How will you proceed?
hCG titer should be done.

Why?
Because this lady has amenorrhea, positive pregnancy test and empty uterine cavity, unruptured ectopic pregnancy is a possibility. Ectopic pregnancy can be missed on clinical as well as ultrasound examination. In the background of amenorrhea, recent history of abortion, absence of evidence of pregnancy, and severe headache a remote possibility of GTN with brain metastases should also be thought of. Her hCG titer came as 82,000 IU/L.

How will you proceed?
She has GTN. She needs metastatic workup. Since the patient has symptoms pertaining to brain metastasis, brain imaging, preferably MRI should be done initially.

Her brain imaging showed a hemorrhagic deposit measuring 3.5 cm.

What is the stage and score of the disease?
Stage IV; 9 (Refer WHO scoring system)

If brain metastases are absent on imaging, how can brain involvement be excluded?
hCG level in the CSF may be measured. If the ratio of plasma:CSF hCG is <60, it denotes presence of cerebral metastasis.

What is the role of pelvic ultrasonography in this patient?
The site and size of uterine tumor can be accurately determined noninvasively by ultrasound. The presence of extensive uterine tumor resistant to chemotherapy is an indication for hysterectomy.

How will you manage this patient?
She needs to be started on combination chemotherapy as the disease is in Stage IV with a score of 9 along with whole brain irradiation (3000 cGy in 10 fractions) as radiation is both hemostatic and tumoricidal. The latter helps prevent extension of cerebral hemorrhage and stroke, which this patient is prone for. The first line combination chemotherapeutic agent regime preferred is EMA-CO.

Is there a place for craniotomy?
Cerebral metastases which are resistant to chemotherapy can be treated with local resection. Usually cerebral metastases respond to combination chemotherapy without any residual neurological deficit.

Since she has only one secondary deposit in the left parietal cortex, is there a place for surgery?
Brain irradiation should be preferred over surgery as surgery in the left parietal region can endanger the Broca's area.

REFERENCES

1. Berkowitz RS, Goldstein DP. The management of molar pregnancy and gestational trophoblastic tumors. In: Knapp RC, Berkowitz RS, eds. Gynecologic oncology, 2nd edn, New York, NY: McGraw-Hill 1993;328-38.
2. Parazzini F, La Vecchia C, Pampallona S. Parental age and risk of complete and partial hydatidiform mole. Br J Obstet Gynaecol 1986;93.
3. Bagshave KD. Risks and prognostic factors in trophoblastic neoplasia. Cancer 1976;38:1373-85.
4. Berkowitz RS, Cramer DW, Bernstein MR, et al. Risk factors for complete molar pregnancy from a case control study. Am J Obstet Gynecol 1985;52:1016-20.
5. Jeffers MD, O'Dwyer P, Curran B, et al. Partial hydatidiform mole: a common but underdiagnosed condition. Int J Gynecol Pathol 1993;12:315-23.
6. Vassilakos P, Kajii T. Letter: Hydatidiform mole:two entities.Lancet 1976;1:259
7. Szulman AE, Surti U. The syndromes of hydatidiform mole, Cytogenetic and morphologic correlations. Am J Obstet Gynecol 1978; 131:665-71.
8. Szulman AE, Surti U. The syndromes of hydatidiform mole. Morphologic evolution of the complete and partial mole. Am J Obstet Gynecol 1978;132:20-7.
9. Lawler SD, Fisher RA, Dent J. A prospective genetic study of complete and partial hydatidiform moles. Am J Obstet and Gynecol 1991;164:1270-7.
10. Burkowitz RS, Goldstein DP, Bernstein MR. 10 years experience with methotrexate as primary therapy for gestational trophoblastic disease. Gynaecol Oncol 1986;23:111-8.
11. Hancock BW, Newlands ES, Berkowitz RS (Eds). Gestational trophoblastic disease. London, UK: Chapman and Hall, 1997:127-42.
12. Stone M, Dent J, Kardana A, et al. Relationship of oral contraception to development of trophoblastic tumour after evacuation of a hydatidiform mole. BJOG 1976;83:913-6.
13. Berkowitz RS, Goldstein DP, Marean AR, et al. Oral contraceptives and postmolar trophoblastic disease. Obstet Gynecol 1981;58:474-7.
14. Garner EIO, Garrett A, Goldstein DP, et al. Significance of chest computed tomography findings in the evaluation and treatment of persistent gestational trophoblastic neoplasia. J Reprod Med 2004;49:411-4.

15. Alazzam M, Tidy J, Hancock BW, Osborne R. First line chemotherapy in low risk gestational trophoblastic neoplasia. Cochrane Database of Systematic Reviews 2009, Issue 1. Art No: CD007102. DOI: 10.1002/14651858.CD007102.pub2.
16. Harvey RA, Pursqlove HD, Schmid P, et al. Human Chorionic Gonadotropin free b subunit measurement as a marker of placental site trophoblastic tumor. J Reprod Med 2008; 53(8): 643-8.
17. Shih IM, Kurman RJ. Epithelioid trophoblastic tumor: a neoplasm distinct from choriocarcinoma and placental site trophoblastic tumor simulating carcinoma. Am J Surg Pathol 1998;22:1393-1403.
18. BW Hancock, MJ Seckl, RS Berkowitz, LA Cole. Gestational trophoblastic disease, 3rd edition.

25 Ultrasound in Gynecology

B Presannakumari

25.1 INTRODUCTION

Ultrasound is a boon to the gynecologist. Transvaginal ultrasound (TVU) is a valuable adjunct to pelvic examination. The transvaginal probe can be advanced close to the pelvic structures to obtain valuable information regarding the uterus, adnexa and other pelvic organs. A wide range of gynecological disorders encompassing infections, benign and malignant lesions of the uterus, ovaries and other pelvic structures and pregnancy associated conditions can be diagnosed with high degree of sensitivity and specificity using TVS. The ability of TVS to diagnose ovulation by follicular tracking as well as by assessing the endometrium has been well understood and practiced. Previously the gynecological surgeon used to encounter surprises in the theater on opening the abdomen. What was thought to be a uterine mass may turn out to be an ovarian mass or a mass from some other structure. Quite often, malignancy may be encountered without prior clinical suspicion. Presently ultrasound is helping the surgeon in arriving at a highly accurate diagnostic prediction. A correct preoperative diagnosis will give the surgeon the opportunity to counsel patients and plan surgical management accordingly. Hence, it is imperative that gynecologists should have a thorough knowledge of ultrasound. The use of ultrasound in the diagnosis of the various gynecological conditions is discussed briefly.

25.2 SCANNING TECHNIQUES

Transabdominal ultrasound (TAU) should be performed prior to transvaginal ultrasound (TVU). TAS gives a global delineation of structures. For performing TAS, a low frequency probe of 3.5 MHz is used as it can delineate deeper structures. TAS can make out associated lesions in the upper abdomen in the presence of a pelvic mass, like hydroureter, secondary deposits in the upper abdomen, metastatic deposits in the liver, fluid in the hepatorenal pouch, etc. For transabdominal ultrasound the bladder must be full (so that an acoustic window is created which prevents scattering of the reflected sound waves) but not over distended, as an overdistended bladder will move the uterus away from the focal length of the transducer and hence cannot be well delineated. Partial voiding will make the uterus come comfortably nearer to the transducer. When a pelvic mass is identified either transvaginally or transabdominally, it is important to trace the mass to the uterine body and cervix to make sure that it is uterine in origin.

25.3 TRANSVAGINAL SCAN (TVS)

TVS is useful in evaluating masses confined to the pelvis. For TVS, high frequency probes can be used (7-9 MHz) as it can reach near the pelvis and can better delineate structures situated close to the probe. Because of beam scattering, structures situated away from the probe will not be well delineated. The high resolution of TVS helps in differentiating adnexal mass from uterine mass. TVS has a major role in detecting pelvic masses which escape detection on bimanual examination.

For performing TVS, the bladder should be empty. The patient is examined in the dorsal position. After proper counseling the probe covered with either a condom or a glove finger and coupling jelly is inserted into the vagina, directing backwards and downwards. Initially the uterus should be imaged. The uterus forms a prominent central landmark. Uterine body can be made out by the central cavity echo. Subsequently the bladder should be identified. The uterine wall near the bladder is the anterior wall and the wall opposite to it, the posterior wall. When the uterus is anteverted the fundus will be seen pointing towards the bladder. The fundus of a retroverted uterus will be seen pointing away from the bladder. The fundus, body, cervix and endometrium can be visualized in the midsagittal image. The transducer is moved in the parasagittal plane to image the rest of the uterus and the adnexa. The probe is angled laterally so that the internal iliac vein and artery are identified. The ovary is usually seen near the internal iliac vessels. Transverse scanning is then performed by rotating the transducer to 90° from the midsagittal plane. The ovaries can be imaged in this plane also on either side of the uterus. Sometimes the ovaries will be seen anterior (in the uterovesical pouch) or posterior to the uterus (in the Pouch of Douglas), instead of being lateral.

The size of the uterus varies based on parity, age and menopausal status (Table 25.1).

Table 25.1: Measurements of uterus and volume of ovary in different age groups

	Size of uterus	*Cervix: Uterine-body ratio*	*Mean ovarian volume (ml)*
Prepubertal	(1-3.3) × (0.5-1) cm	2:1	3
Nulliparous postpubertal	7 × 4 × 4 cm	1:3	9.8
Parous postpubertal	8.2 × 5.2 × 5.2 cm	1:3	9.8
Menopausal	(3.5-6.5) × (1.2-1.8) cm	Cervix shorter	5.8

The prepubertal uterus is small measuring 1-3.3 cm in length and 0.5-1 cm in width. The cervix to the uterine-body ratio will be 2:1. The endometrium is normally thin. The uterus of a nulliparous postpubertal woman measures 7 × 4 × 4 cm. The cervix to uterine body ratio wills be 1:3. In a multiparous woman, the uterus measures 1.2 cm greater in length, width and breadth compared to the nulliparous woman. In a postmenopausal woman, the uterus will be atrophic and the cervix will be shorter. The measurement ranges from 3.5 to 6.5 cm in length and 1.2 to 1.8 cm in thickness. The myometrial echotexture will be the same in the different age groups. However, in women several years after menopause, the myometrium usually show echogenic areas caused by calcified vessels.

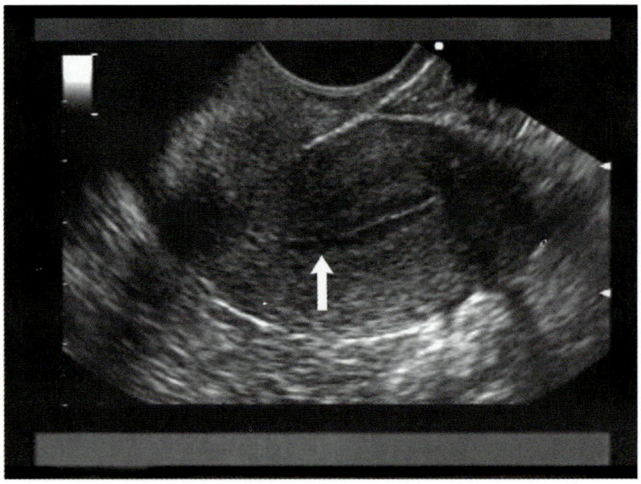

Fig. 25.1: TVS showing trilaminar proliferative endometrium (arrow)

25.4 EVALUATION OF ENDOMETRIUM

The thickness of the endometrium varies depending on the different phases of the menstrual cycle. The thickness of the broadest portion is measured in the midsagittal plane of the uterus. The anterior and posterior portions are measured together (Fig. 25.1).

Proliferative phase: Immediately after menses, the endometrium is constituted by the basal layer and will be thin, measuring < 4 mm in width (Fig. 25.2). As proliferative phase progresses, the endometrium increases in thickness. The fully grown proliferative endometrium measures 6-10 mm in thickness. The appearance is typically described as trilaminar. The central cavity line will be echogenic. On either side of the central cavity line the hypoechoic functional layer will be seen. The endometrial-myometrial interface will be hyperechoic. These three lines form the trilaminar pattern Figure 25.1.

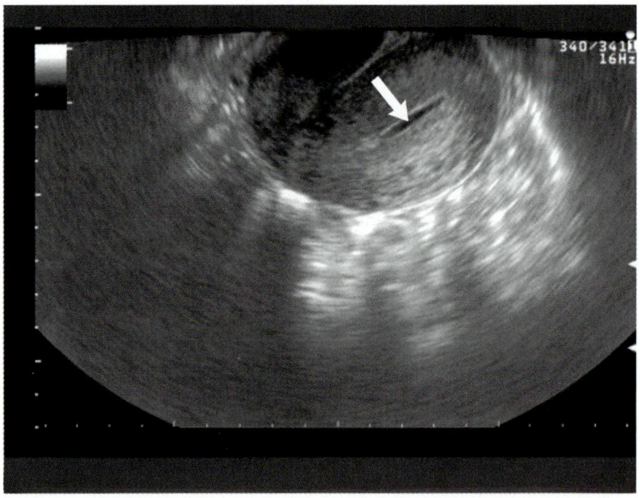

Fig. 25.2: Postmenstrual endometrium showing a small fluid collection in the uterine cavity (arrow)

Secretory phase: The endometrium thickens further in the secretory phase. The hypoechoic functional layer of the endometrium will become hyperechoic due to the presence of stromal edema. The change to hyperechoic appearance starts at the endometrial-myometrial interface and proceeds to the surface of the endometrium. In the mid secretory phase, the full thickness of the endometrium will be echogenic (Fig. 25.3). Thus, the trilaminar pattern will be lost in the secretory phase. The thickness of the normal secretory endometrium ranges from 7 to 14 mm. An endometrial thickness of more than 15 mm in the childbearing age group should be taken as abnormal and has to be sampled to exclude hyperplasia/malignancy.

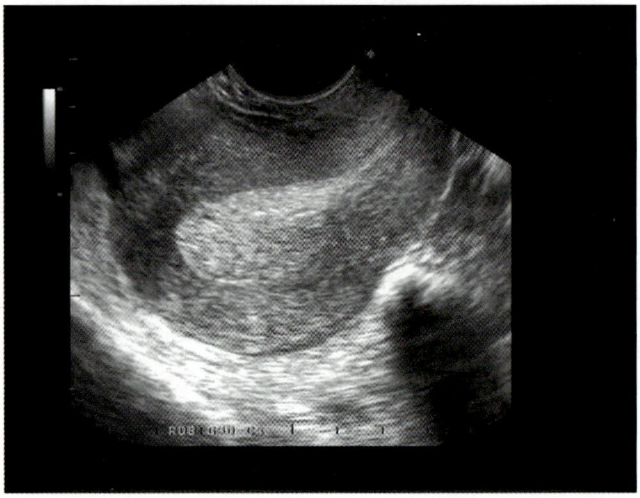

Fig. 25.3: TVS showing secretory endometrium. Note the homogeneous echogenicity

Postmenopausal phase: The mean endometrial thickness in asymptomatic postmenopausal women is 3.4 ± 2.5 mm (Carlson et al). A thickness > 4 mm is considered abnormal and is an indication to sample the endometrium. A meta-analysis of 35 studies found that an endometrial thickness < 5 mm will exclude endometrial pathology in the majority of women.[1] It is not unusual to find fluid in the endometrial cavity in postmenopausal women. Even though it does not always signify an abnormal endometrium, there is a high risk for pathology in such women. The presence of irregularity in the endometrial surface and the thickness of the endometrium excepting the fluid region will give a clue as to the presence of pathology. If the thickness including the fluid is 5 mm or less the presence of pathology is unlikely. Normally there will be a hypoechoic area between the endometrium and the myometrium—the subendometrial halo. This should not be included in the measurement of the endometrium (Fig. 25.4). This halo will be lost when there is malignancy invading the myometrium. In a postmenopausal woman the arcuate vessels will be calcified and multiple echogenic areas will be seen distributed in the myometrium. In the presence of extensive calcification it will be difficult to measure the endometrial thickness due to poor visualization.

Evaluation of the Cervix

The probe should be withdrawn 2-3 cm in order to visualize the cervix. The endocervical canal which is a continuation of the endometrial cavity will be seen as an echogenic line. Polyps and growths in the endocervix can be delineated (Fig. 25.5). In periovulatory periods mucus will be seen as a hypoechoic linear shadow. Nabothian cysts may appear as anechoic cystic areas in the cervix.

25.5 EVALUATION OF THE VAGINA

The upper part of the vagina can be seen in TAS. The vagina will appear as a hypoechoic structure, formed by the muscular walls with an echogenic line in the center, which is the cavity of the vagina.

25.6 EVALUATION OF THE OVARIES

The ovaries are usually seen in the ovarian fossae which can be identified by imaging the internal iliac vessels. Sometimes one or both of the ovaries will be seen in the pouch of Douglas. Very rarely it may be seen anterior to the uterus. The ovary is recognized by its oval shape and the presence of follicles. Follicles are usually absent in postmenopausal women making it difficult to identify the ovaries in them. When there is difficulty in imaging the ovaries in the parasagittal plane it can be imaged in the semiaxial plane by rotating the probe to 90°. The size of the ovary varies depending on the age, phase of the menstrual cycle and body status. In menstruating women the mean ovarian volume is 9.8 ml. In premenarchal girls, the volume is 3 ml and in the postmenopausal women it is 5.8 ml.

25.7 EVALUATION OF FALLOPIAN TUBES

The normal fallopian tubes cannot be visualized unless there is fluid in the pouch of Douglas. When the tube is enlarged due to hydrosalpinx, pyosalpinx or malignancy, it can be imaged.

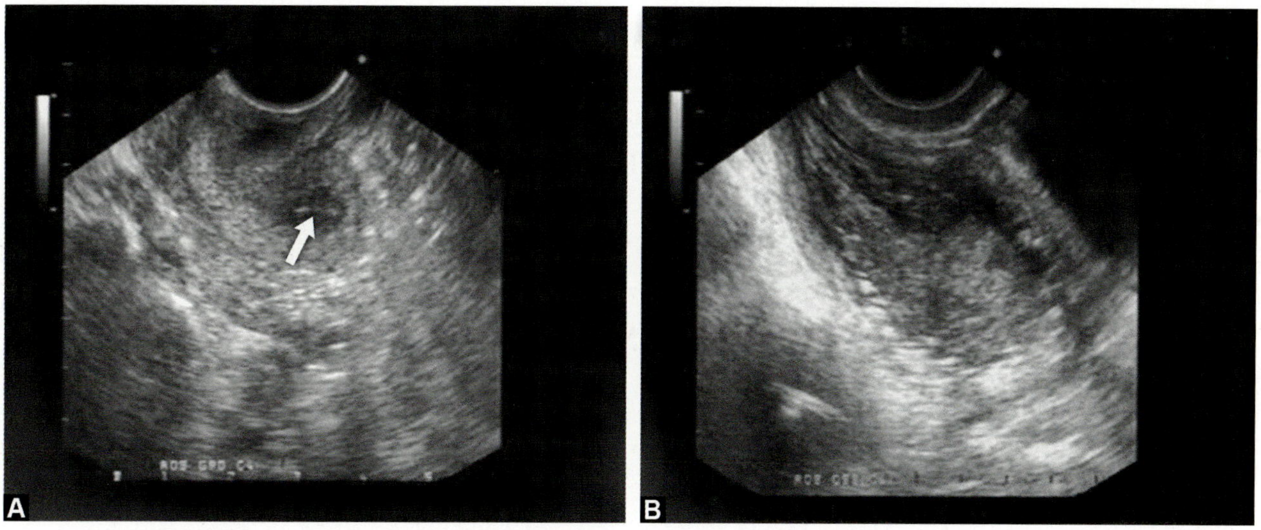

Figs 25.4A and B: Normal postmenopausal endometrium. Note the subendometrial halo (arrow) (A). Calcified vessels in a (postmenopausal) lady with pyometra (B)

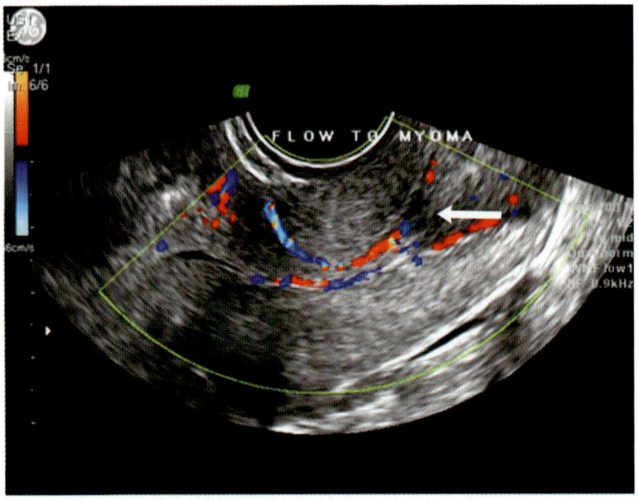

Fig. 25.5: TVS showing uterine cervix and polyp protruding from the cervix (arrow)

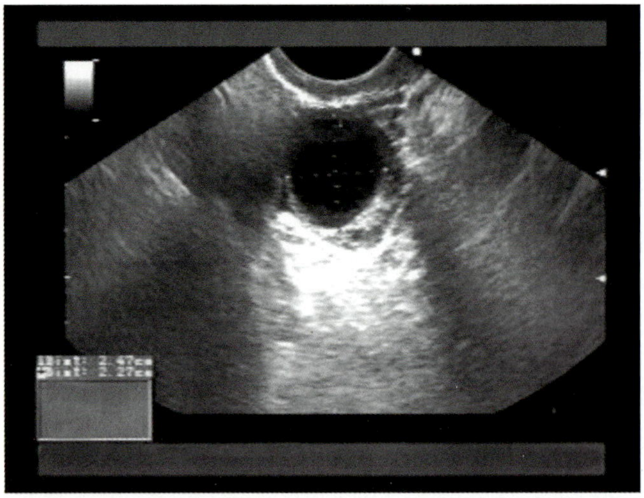

Fig. 25.6: Transvaginal scan showing mature follicle

25.8 FOLLICULAR STUDY

Ovulation can be documented by follicular study. An initial imaging should be done immediately after menses to make out the presence of functional cysts. A dominant follicle is recruited between day 8 to day 12 of the cycle. Hence, the follicular study should start by day 9. In the latter part of the follicular phase, the dominant follicle grows at the rate of 2-3 mm per day and reaches a mean diameter of 20 mm (16-28 mm) (Fig. 25.6). About 24 hours before ovulation the follicle will appear to have a double wall because of the separation of the granulosa layer from the theca. The cumulus oophorus may be visualized occasionally. After ovulation the follicle may either decrease in size and become echogenic or filled with fluid and appear as a cyst along with the presence of minimally increased fluid in the pouch of Douglas. A hemorrhagic corpus luteum will be larger and have a lacy appearance (Fig. 25.7).

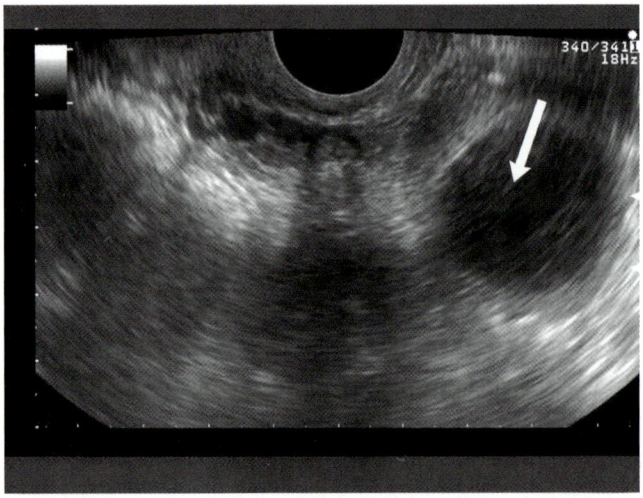

Fig. 25.7: TVS showing lacy appearance of corpus luteum (arrow)

25.9 INTRAUTERINE CONTRACEPTIVE DEVICE (IUCD)

When the thread of the IUCD is missing, the presence or absence of the device in the cavity can be made out with certainty by TVS (Fig. 25.8). If one or both transverse limbs or the vertical limb perforates the uterine wall, the exact position and extent of the device in the uterine wall can be made out. Devices completely extruded into the peritoneal cavity cannot be diagnosed by USS as it could be obscured by bowel loops. When TVS fails to detect the device in the uterine cavity or the myometrium, X-ray abdomen is indicated to exclude or diagnose the presence of the device in the abdomen.

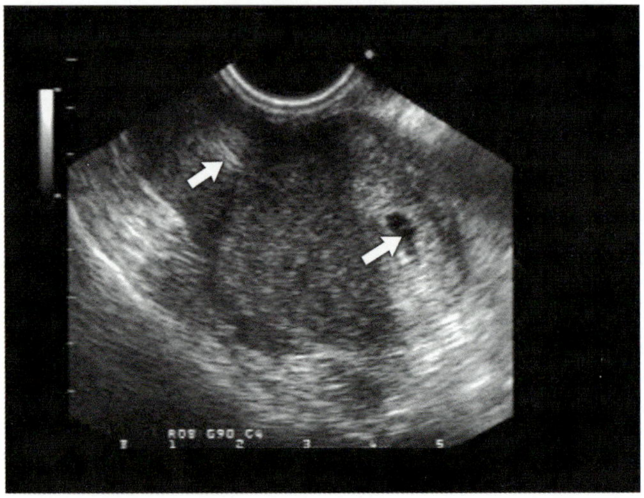

Fig. 25.8: TVS showing tiny intrauterine gestational sac (arrow-right) and part of Copper T (arrow-left) in the cervical canal

25.10 SONOGRAPHIC EVALUATION OF PELVIC MASS

For the evaluation of large masses which rise into the abdomen, the use of TV probe is limited. But details of a mass, like its nature and exact location in relation to other pelvic structures is better delineated by TVS. When evaluating a pelvic mass, ultrasound should be interpreted in the background of the history and clinical examination findings. Ultrasound helps to:

1. Confirm the presence or absence of a pelvic mass.
2. Make out the site of origin—uterine, ovarian, tubal or other pelvic structures.
3. Make out the presence or absence of features suggestive of malignancy.
4. Guide the site for aspiration biopsy.

By discerning the above features, the gynecological surgeon can make decisions appropriately regarding the following:

1. Whether to operate or not
2. The extent of surgery which depends upon whether the mass is malignant or benign
3. Whether multidisciplinary input is needed

Evaluation of these abnormal pelvic masses is discussed under separate headings.

25.11 ENDOMETRIAL CARCINOMA

The role of ultrasound in the evaluation of endometrial carcinoma is commendable. When women present with perimenopausal bleeding, if a growth is not identified in the vagina or exocervix, the endocervix and endometrium should be evaluated for abnormalities.TVS has an important place in evaluating the endometrium and endocervix in such situations. If the endometrial thickness is < 4 mm, endometrial evaluation by hysteroscopy can be deferred. However, if there is recurrence of bleeding, endometrial evaluation should be done, even if the thickness is < 4 mm. The presence of a large tumor filling the uterine cavity mandates endometrial sampling with pipelle. Resorting to hysteroscopy in the presence of a large tumor is unnecessary and dangerous as it will disseminate malignant cells. When the endometrium shows irregular thickening or a small lesion (Fig. 25.9), hysteroscopy is the investigation of choice. Blind curettage of the endometrium may miss a small malignant growth. Both hysteroscopy[2] and TVS are equally sensitive in detecting the presence of endometrial lesions. Ultrasound and Doppler cannot accurately distinguish malignancy of endometrium from nonmalignant lesions. Both may be associated with high vascularity. Whenever a lesion is seen

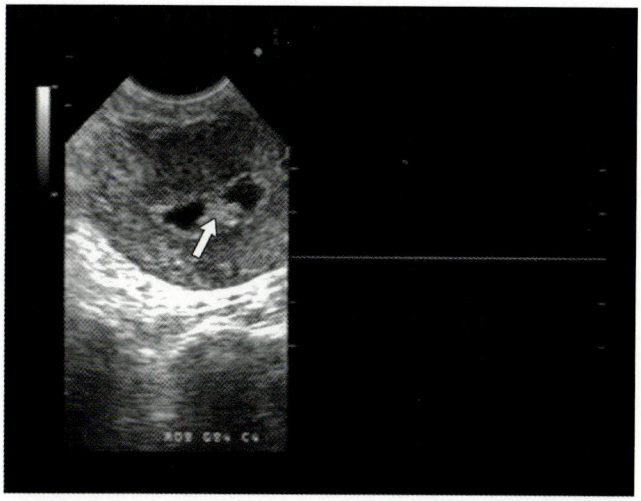

Fig. 25.9: TVS showing tiny endometrial lesion (arrow) in a postmenopausal lady who presented with irregular vaginal bleeding. This patient's endometrial malignancy was missed on fractional curettage but later diagnosed by a hysteroscopy directed biopsy

in the endometrium, histopathological confirmation by biopsy should be done by endometrial aspiration, fractional curettage or hysteroscopy directed biopsy.

The sensitivity of assessing deep myometrial invasion by TVS is 85% and specificity is about 65%. Associated adenomyosis, fibroids and calcification in the myometrial vessels can make assessment difficult (For ultrasound pictures refer Chapters 6 and 17).

25.12 DIAGNOSIS AND FOLLOW-UP OF GTD

25.12.1 Diagnosis of Vesicular Mole

The presence of a complete mole gives the classical picture of snow-storm appearance in USS with no evidence of fetal parts (For ultrasound pictures refer Chapter 21). In 50% of molar pregnancies, the ovaries may be enlarged and will give a soap bubble appearance caused by multiple theca lutein cysts. In the case of partial mole, a fetus can be identified and the placenta will show partial molar changes. Since triploidy of the fetus is associated with partial mole, the fetus should have targeted imaging for markers of chromosomal anomalies. Karyotyping of the fetus should be advised. Twin pregnancy with one normal fetus and the other being vesicular mole is also very rarely encountered.

25.12.2 Follow-up of Vesicular Mole

After molar pregnancy evacuation, completeness of the evacuation is assessed by ultrasound. Ultrasound also helps in diagnosing invasive disease. Multiple small cystic areas will be seen in the myometrium which show increased vascularity. Very rarely arteriovenous fistulas can be identified in the myometrium following treatment of trophoblastic disease.

25.12.3 Placental Site Trophoblastic Tumor (PSTT)

PSTT is a very rare form of trophoblastic disease which usually develops after term delivery. The tumor is composed of intermediate trophoblasts. The usual presentation is amenorrhea following term delivery. The tumor appears as a hypoechoic mass in the myometrium, which will show high vascularity. The combination of amenorrhea, a mass in the myometrium and mild elevation of hCG should raise the suspicion of PSTT.

25.13 FUNCTIONAL CYSTS

Functional cysts form a large percentage of adnexal masses in the childbearing age group. These cysts usually will not attain more than 6-8 cm in size. If there is nothing suggestive of malignancy, observation is all that is needed. A follow-up scan can be done after 6 weeks. Functional cysts will either disappear or reduce in size by this time.

Functional cysts can be follicular, corpus luteal or theca lutein cysts.

25.13.1 Follicular Cyst

Follicular cysts are thin and unilocular and occur in anovulatory cycles. Its size may reach up to 6-8 cm. These cysts are usually found to regress in 2-3 months and careful observation is all that is needed.

25.13.2 Corpus Luteum Cysts

Corpus luteum cysts can have different appearances. Usually the corpus luteum has a solid appearance after collapse of the follicle. Sometimes due to hemorrhage inside the corpus luteum, it will appear as a large mass (Fig. 25.10). As the clot begins to lyse, a reticular network can be seen inside the cyst giving it a lacelike pattern or honeycomb appearance.

25.13.3 Theca Lutein Cysts

These are multiloculated cysts that result from very high level of hCG. Hence, they are seen in trophoblastic disease. Rarely it occurs in pregnancy due to exaggerated response to hCG and is called *hyper-reactio luteinalis*.

Hyper-reactio Luteinalis

The ovaries are bilaterally enlarged and both will be of almost the same size or slightly asymmetrical. Multiple thin walled cysts without internal echoes will be seen. It is unwise to interfere surgically as trying cystectomy will result in mutilation of the ovary and unnecessary surgery in the first trimester. On careful observation, the size will be found to decrease. Rarely it persists throughout pregnancy and the size decreases and it gradually disappears only after delivery (Figs 25.11A and B). Unless this is kept in mind, it can be mistaken for neoplasm. Ascites is rare in these patients but in ovarian hyperstimulation syndrome (OHSS), fluid shift can cause ascites and pleural effusion.

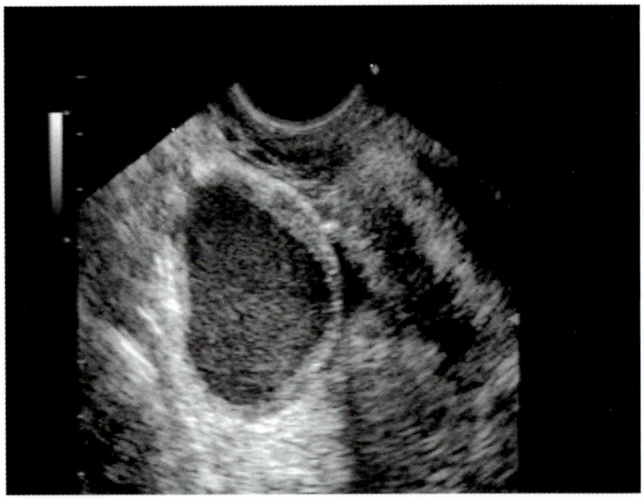

Fig. 25.10: Hemorrhagic corpus luteum resembling endometrioma. Repeat examination showed reduction in the size followed by disappearance

25.14 POLYCYSTIC OVARIES

It is pertinent to differentiate between polycystic ovaries (PCO) and polycystic ovarian syndrome (PCOS). PCOS is a spectrum of hyperandrogenism seen in lean normally menstruating women to obese women with hyperandrogenism and oligomenorrhea. PCO denotes polycystic ovaries and may be seen in 16-22% of normally menstruating women also. In PCOS, ovaries will be usually enlarged 2-5 times the normal size. Two types of ultrasound appearances are described based on the arrangement of follicles, either as multiple tiny cysts 2-8 mm in the periphery giving it a pearl necklace appearance or scattered in abundant stroma throughout the ovary (Fig. 25.12). According to Adam's criteria, the presence of 10 or more cysts measuring 2-8 mm in diameter in a single plane is evidence of PCO. This criterion was modified by Fox et al. According to them, the criteria are the presence of at least 15 cysts of 2-10 mm in diameter. In patients who have hypothalamic anovulation,

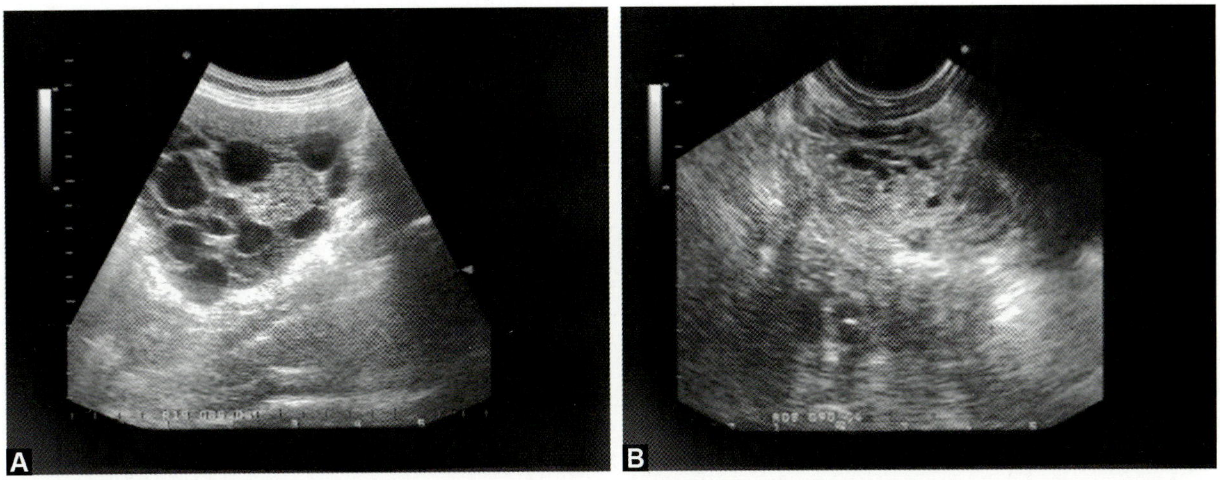

Figs 25.11A and B: Multiple lutein cysts in a primipara few days after delivery (A). The condition was diagnosed in the antenatal period. TVS showing ovary 6 weeks postpartum (B)

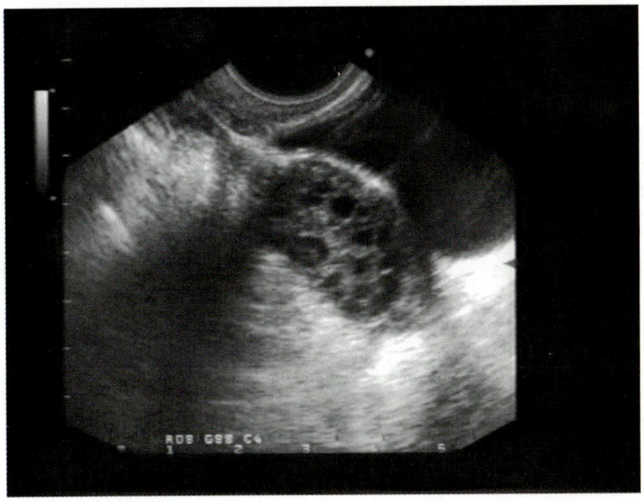

Fig. 25.12: TVS showing polycystic ovaries. The cysts are distributed throughout the abundant ovarian stroma

the ovaries will show multiple cysts but stroma will be normal as against abundant echogenic stroma in PCOS. Ovarian volume measurement is not given importance presently because approximately one-third of patients with a wide range of symptoms of PCOS were found to have normal ovarian volume.

25.15 OVARIAN TORSION

Torsion of normal ovary can occur in young women. Torsion can occur acutely or chronically. Due to obstruction as a result of torsion, the ovary will become edematous and will enlarge. Ultrasound scannig (USS) shows a solid mass which retains the shape of the ovary. Edema gives the characteristic uniform enlargement of the ovary.

25.16 CHARACTERIZATION OF OVARIAN TUMORS

Ultrasound is highly sensitive in differentiating benign from malignant ovarian tumor.[3] Adding color Doppler has been found to improve the sensitivity in diagnosing malignancy.[4] The different types of ovarian tumors can be differentiated to some extent by the ultrasound characteristics.

25.16.1 Epithelial Ovarian Tumor

Serous Tumors

Sixty percent of benign ovarian tumors and 80-90% of malignant ovarian tumors are epithelial in origin. Benign serous cystadenomas appear as thin walled well-defined anechoeic masses which are unilocular. Thin septations and papillary projections may be seen rarely (Fig. 25.13). Borderline tumors show multiple papillary projections. Cystadenocarcinoma shows multiple echogenic areas which are the solid components of the tumor. Doppler usually shows low resistance flow with RI < 0.4 and PI < 1.

Mucinous Tumors

Mucinous cystadenomas comprise 20-25% of all benign neoplasms. These are usually seen in the third or fourth decade of life. Mucinous tumors are usually multicystic with thicker walls than serous tumors. The contents show fine echoes due to the presence of mucinous material. The malignant counterparts show echogenic areas with increased vascularity and thicker septations (> 3 mm) (Fig. 25.14). Borderline tumors show mural nodules.

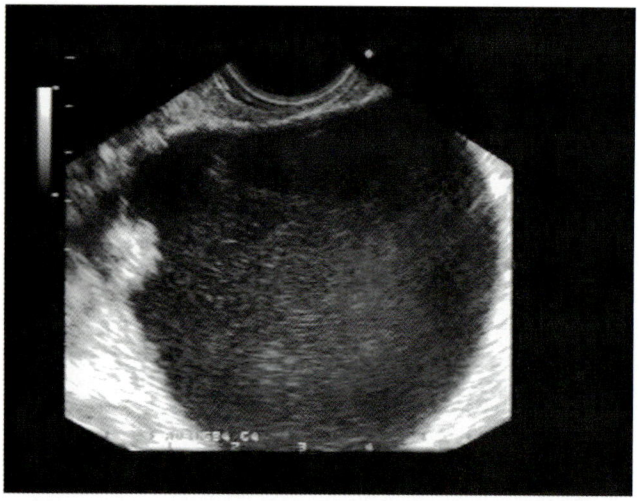

Fig. 25.13: TVS showing unilocular cyst with a small papillary excrescence in a papillary cystadenoma

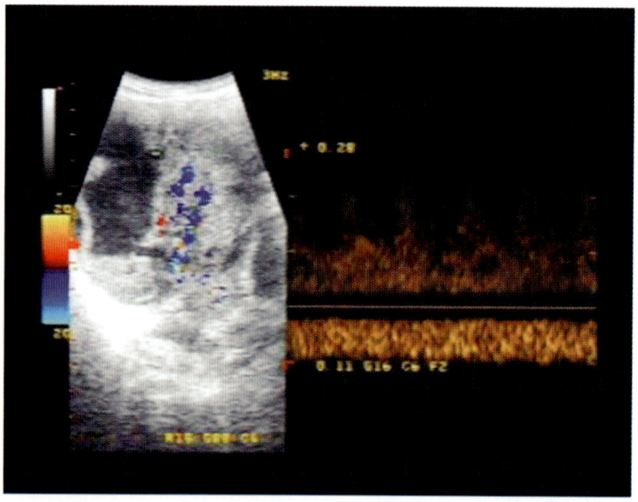

Fig. 25.14: Abdominal scan showing multiloculated cystic mass with fine internal echoes and thick septations with increased vascularity. The tumor was later found to be mucinous cystadenocarcinoma

Endometrioid Tumors

These are malignant solid tumors occurring in the 5th or 6th decade of life. Endometrioid tumors may be associated with endometrial malignancy. These tumors can arise from endometriotic areas in the ovary also. They are usually multicystic with solid areas. Rarely, it may be a predominantly solid tumor.

Clear Cell Tumors

They are the most aggressive ovarian tumors which usually occur in women in the 5th- 7th decade of life. They can also arise in endometriotic cysts. They do not have a characteristic ultrasound appearance. Usually the tumor will be predominantly cystic with solid areas.

Brenner Tumor

Brenner tumors are usually unilateral and benign. Ultrasound appearance is of a hypoechoic small solid tumor. Calcified areas may be seen. Cystadenomas might coexist rarely.

Germ Cell Tumors

Dermoid cyst: The most common benign tumor of the ovary is dermoid. It is usually seen in the childbearing age group and is mostly unilateral but may be bilateral in 15% cases. Dermoids normally grow to 5-10 cm in diameter but can rarely grow to very large sizes. It is predominantly unilocular. In one area of the cyst, an echogenic projection into the cyst may be seen (Rokitansky protuberance) (Fig. 25.15). Hair, bone, teeth, etc. of the dermoid cyst arises from this protuberance. The ultrasound picture is characterized by the presence of diffuse echogenicity in the cyst with posterior acoustic shadowing. Clumps of hair or fat can cause posterior acoustic enhancement. Fluid-fluid levels due to sebum and fluid is a common finding.

Immature Teratoma

Immature teratomas are predominantly solid and large echogenic tumors. It usually occurs in the first and second decade of life. There are no characteristic features that distinguish it from other solid ovarian tumors.

Dysgerminoma

Dysgerminomas comprise 3-5% of ovarian malignancies. It is commonly seen in the second and third decade of life and hence is the most common malignancy seen in pregnancy. The tumor shows multilobulated appearance on ultrasound. Lobules will be seen separated by fibrovascular

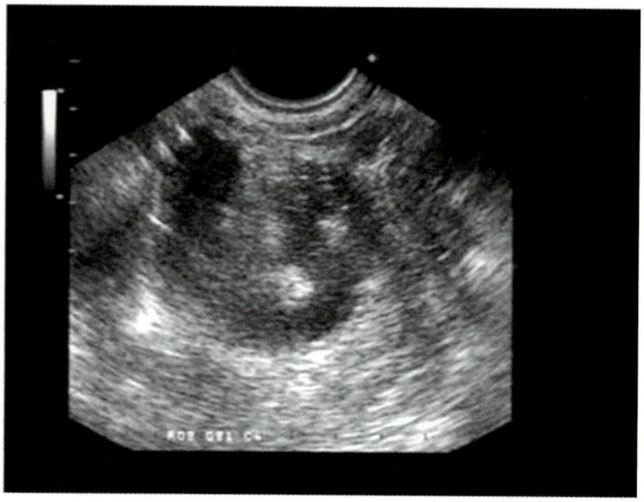

Fig. 25.15: TVS showing dermoid cyst

septa which are identified by the presence of vascularity in Doppler ultrasound.

Endodermal Sinus Tumor (EST)

EST usually appears as solid tumor. It lacks the fibrovascular septa characteristic of dysgerminoma.

25.16.2 Sex-cord Stromal Tumor

Fibroma

Fibromas comprise half of these tumors. The ultrasound appearance is that of fibroid. If it is very large, it is difficult to differentiate it from a subserous fibroid.

Thecomas

They are small solid tumors. No particular characteristic feature has been identified.

Granulosa Cell Tumor

These are solid tumors with mixed echogenic pattern (Ultrasound picture in Chapter 16).

Peritoneal Inclusion Cysts

These are accumulation of normal peritoneal fluid in cystic spaces formed by peritoneal adhesions. They usually result from infection, trauma or abdominal surgery. They can be small or large measuring up to 20 cm. They appear like uniloculated cysts. They can also be multicystic.

Hematometra

Hematometra usually occurs in adolescent girls who have fusion anomalies of the Mullerian duct. When the cervix is *non-canalized*, the uterus will be distended with blood and can be mistaken for ovarian cyst. In TAS, the mass can be traced to the *non-canalized* cervix and vagina. In imperforate vagina, collection of menstrual effluent in the vagina (hematocolpos) may also present as a cystic mass. Blood can get collected in the uterine cavity and the fallopian tubes also causing hematometra and hematosalpinx. Transverse vaginal septum can also cause hematocolpos, depending upon the level of septa. Hematometra can occur in a rudimentary noncommunicating uterine horn (Ultrasound pictures provided in Chapter 4).

25.17 ULTRASOUND IMAGING IN INFERTILITY

In the past, imaging in infertility consisted of hysterosalpingogram only. In recent years diagnosis of the various causes of infertility is made possible with the development of high resolution ultrasound. TVS is an adjunct to pelvic examination in every infertile woman. A clinician who understands and interprets the various ultrasound features would be able to manage the woman better.

25.17.1 Endometrial Evaluation

Different phases of the menstrual cycle like proliferative and secretory endometrium have distinctive sonographic appearances as described earlier. Luteal phase insufficiency can be diagnosed by the appearance of the endometrium in the secretory phase. Tuberculous endometrium can be suspected by the presence of multiple hyperechoic areas. Small submucous fibroids and endometrial polyps which may cause infertility may not be evident on pelvic examination but can be visualized on ultrasound. Intrauterine adhesions produce broken IUD appearance of the endometrium. Endometrial study by B Mode and Doppler has been used to determine luteal response in women who present with infertility and also before implantation in women undergoing IVF. However, the accuracy and reliability of clinical management of luteal phase defect based on US and Doppler have not been established.

25.17.2 Documentation of Ovulation (Figs 25.16A and B)

Ovulation detection by LH kit can be inconclusive. Documentation of ovulation by charting basal body temperature has several disadvantages. Ovulation can be documented as an office procedure by TVS. Follicular growth, number of follicles, endometrial changes and associated pelvic abnormalities can be detected by TVS.

25.17.3 Leiomyoma

Significance of leiomyoma in infertile women depends upon the size and location of the myoma. A submucous myoma even if very small, as well as myomatous polyps can cause infertility. Small submucous myomas (Fig. 25.17), polyps and adhesions will appear as small intracavitary lesions. The distinction and treatment can be done hysteroscopically.

25.17.4 Abnormalities of the Fallopian Tube

Tubal factors can cause infertility in 40% of women. Normal fallopian tubes are not visualized on routine TVS. The usual tubal factors are tubal obstruction or abnormal motility which are sequelae of pelvic inflammatory disease. Numerous tubal

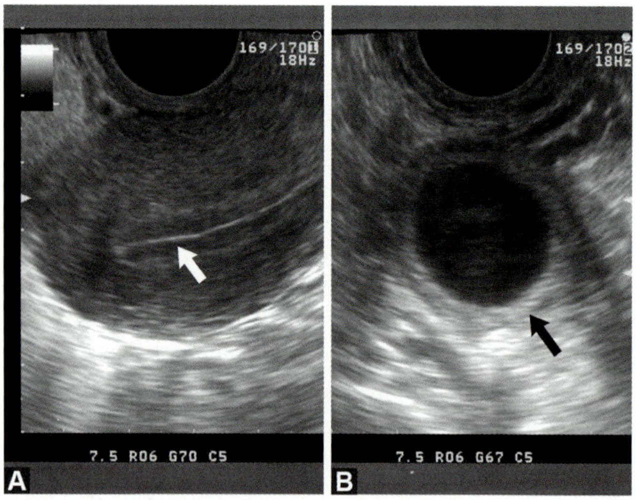

Figs 25.16A and B: TVS showing proliferative (three line; white arrow) endometrium (A) and mature follicle showing double walled (black arrow) appearance (B)

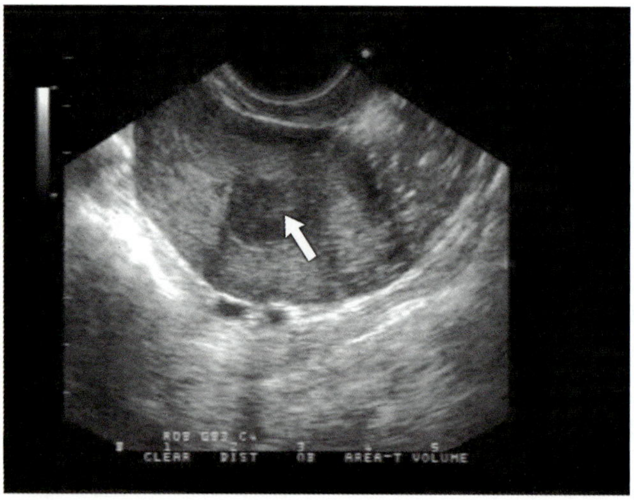

Fig. 25.17: TVS showing small submucous myoma (arrow)

conditions can be identified by USS. However, it should be kept in mind that a normal pelvic sonogram does not exclude tubal factor infertility. A tube blocked proximally by debris or adhesions will not be dilated, hence cannot be detected by USS. Distal tubal occlusion causes dilatation of the tube and hydrosalpinx. Hydrosalpinx will appear as a retort shaped cystic mass with incomplete septations giving a cog-wheel appearance. Saline sonohysterography is a method of tubal testing by USS. About 200 ml of saline is injected into the uterine cavity using No: 8 Foley catheter under ultrasound guidance and the fluid escaping through the fimbrial end into the peritoneal cavity is detected by USS. The optimal imaging technique for evaluating the internal structure and patency of fallopian tube is contrast hysterosalpingography which helps to estimate the correctability of tubal factor (Ultrasound pictures provided in Chapter 14).

25.17.5 Evaluation of Peritoneal Factor

USS imaging will not help diagnose flimsy peritubal adhesions or small endometriotic implants. However, extensive adhesion between the ovary and uterus can be suspected on TVS. By moving the probe the ovary can be seen to move along with the uterus if they are adherent whereas if there are no adhesions the ovary and uterus can be seen to be sliding between each other—*the sliding organ sign.*

25.17.6 Endometriosis

Endometriosis is a leading cause of infertility. Presence of chocolate cyst can be diagnosed with a high degree of accuracy by TVS. They are usually unilocular but can also be multilocular (Fig. 25.18). They have thick walls and fine internal echoes giving a ground glass appearance. The uterus will be fixed and the ovaries will be adherent to the uterus which can be made out by eliciting the sliding organ sign.[5,7]

25.17.7 Pelvic Inflammatory Disease (PID)

Sonographic findings are not much discernible in the acute phase of PID. Later when infection produces pathological changes like tubo-ovarian abscess, adhesions, hydrosalpinx, etc. it can be detected by TVS. Identification of hydrosalpinx is diagnostic of tubal factor infertility. These findings were described by Trimo Tritsch et al. The changes include:

1. Thickening of the tubal wall ≥ 5 mm
2. *Cog wheel sign:* The inflamed and dilated fallopian tube appears like cog wheel on cross-section due to the incomplete septal appearance produced by in folding of the tubal mucosa (Ultrasound picture provided in Chapter 14).

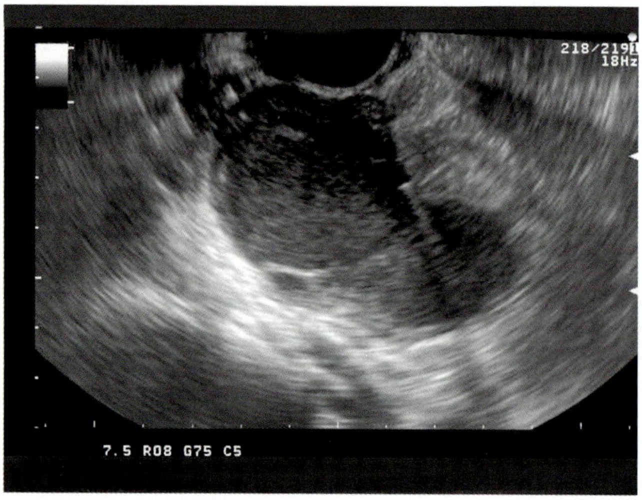

Fig. 25.18: TVS showing multiloculated endometrioma

25.17.8 Ovum Retrieval

In ART procedures ovum retrieval can be done by ultrasound-guided needle aspiration which has replaced the laparoscopic procedure.

Ultrasound thus has a very crucial role in the diagnosis and management of infertility.

25.18 DIAGNOSIS OF UTERINE ABNORMALITIES

25.18.1 Leiomyoma

Ultrasound is excellent in diagnosing leiomyoma. The typical lesion will be hypoechoic compared to the myometrium (Fig. 25.19). In a longstanding myoma, calcification can be visualized in the periphery. Cystic degeneration in fibroid will produce an irregular central echogenic area in a hypoechoic focus. The number of myomas and their location can be diagnosed by ultrasound prior to myomectomy. There are no particular characteristic features by which leiomyosarcoma can be differentiated from leiomyoma.

25.18.2 Adenomyosis

Adenomyosis usually causes pine-leaf appearance due to acoustic shadowing. Even though adenomyosis is a generalized disorder, it usually causes asymmetrical thickening of uterine wall (Fig. 25.20). Rarely, it can cause a localized lesion which is difficult to diagnose from leiomyoma. TVS has sensitivity and specificity of 86% in diagnosing adenomyosis. There can be tiny cystic spaces in the myometrium.[8]

25.18.3 Congenital Anomalies of the Uterus

With the evolution of TVU and 4D ultrasound, detection of congenital anomalies of the uterus is now possible by non-invasive methods. A subtle anomaly like arcuate uterus is more difficult to diagnose than bicornuate uterus. The scan should preferably be done in the secretory phase so that the endometrial echo and uterine cavity are better delineated. Fusion anomalies are better diagnosed in the *semiaxial* image. *It can be missed in mid sagittal image.* Septate uterus will have a broad uterine body. Two cavity echoes could be made out (Fig. 25.21). The myometrium and the contour of the uterus will not be divided. In semicoronal plane it gives a picture of *owl's eye appearance.* Two separate horns can be identified in bicornuate uterus in *semiaxial* plane (Fig. 25.22) and *semisagittal* plane. When the uterus is bicornuate bicollis and the vagina also is septate, the two cervices may not be evident in TVS. The probe will be in either half of the vagina and that particular cervix will be imaged. Since, the septum limits the movement of the probe the other cervix will not be imaged. Even though to some extent the two cervices can be imaged in TAS, a proper clinical examination will clarify the situation. A 'T' shaped uterus will have lesser volume compared to its normal counterpart and will be broader with a thinner fundus.

Uterine anomalies can cause recurrent abortion and infertility. For planning surgical treatment of Mullerian anomalies, accurate diagnosis is essential. With high resolution vaginal sonography accurate diagnosis is possible to a great extent. In situations where B Mode image is unsatisfactory 4D USS will sort-out the problem.

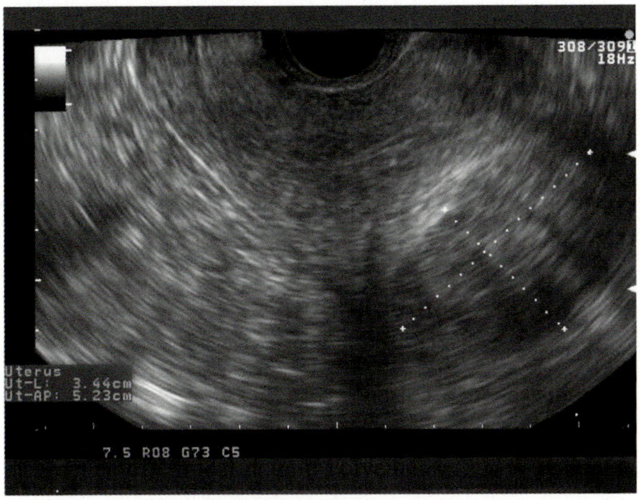

Fig. 25.19: TVS showing intramural myoma in the fundoposterior aspect

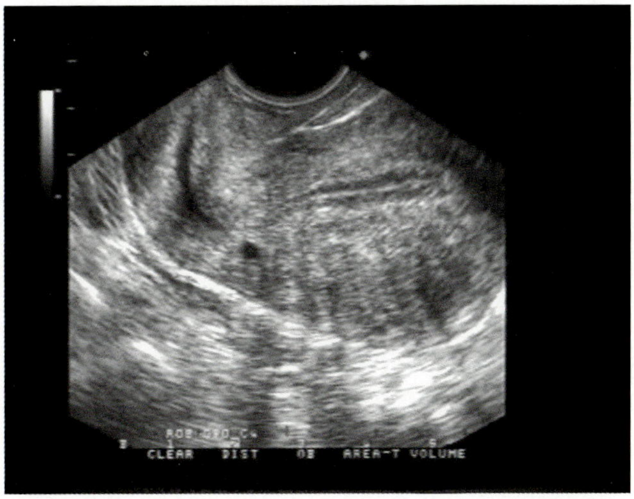

Fig. 25.20: TVS showing adenomyosis of the posterior wall of uterus. Note the asymmetrically thickened posterior wall with pine-leaf appearance

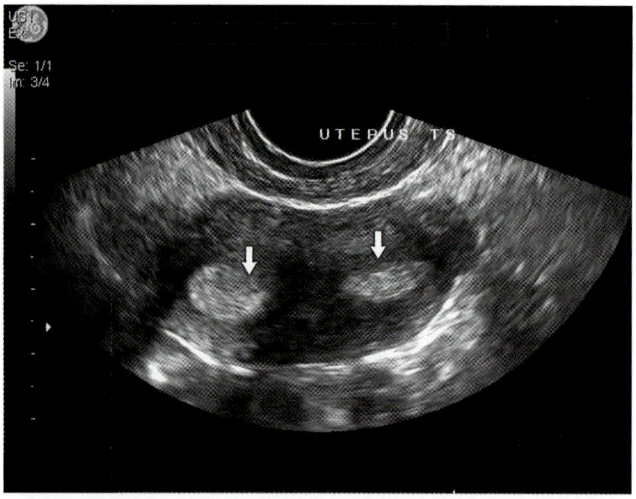

Fig. 25.21: TVS showing septate uterus. Note the two cavity echoes (arrows) simulating owl's eye

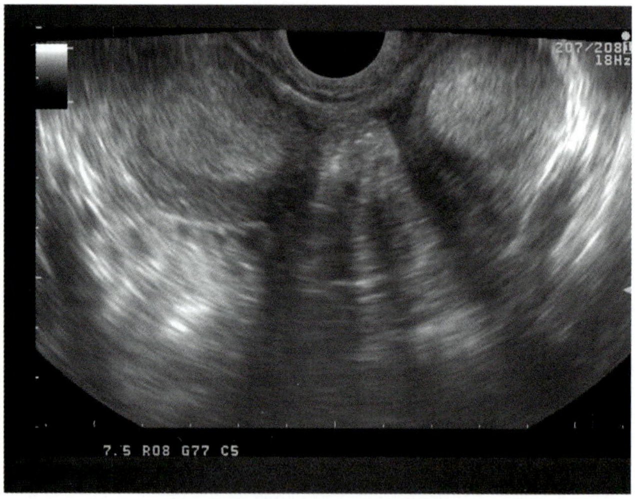

Fig. 25.22: TVS showing bicornuate uterus. Two separate uterine bodies can be identified

25.19 ECTOPIC PREGNANCY

With the evolution of highly sensitive hCG assay and high resolution USS, ectopic pregnancies are diagnosed at an earlier unruptured state so that an elective approach to management can be taken. Early diagnosis and management prevents tubal rupture, intraperitoneal hemorrhage, need for emergency surgery as well as mortality.

25.19.1 Sonographic Findings of Early Intrauterine Pregnancy and Ectopic Pregnancy

Approximately 26% of the patients with ectopic pregnancy will have a normal sonogram. When women present with symptoms like abdominal pain, pelvic tenderness or spotting per vaginum in early pregnancy, documentation of an intrauterine pregnancy excludes the likelihood of an ectopic pregnancy. However, heterotopic pregnancy which is a very rare occurrence (1/30000) should be kept in mind, especially in women undergoing ovulation induction where the incidence is quite high. Understanding early intrauterine pregnancy by TVS is important. The earliest sign of intrauterine pregnancy[6] is the appearance of gestational sac in the endometrium (intradecidual sign) which is eccentrically placed. Gestational sac of 2 mm or more can be visualized in TVS. In ectopic pregnancy, sometimes a small fluid collection can be seen in the endometrial cavity. This should not be mistaken for a gestational sac. A true gestational sac will be in the endometrium (intradecidual), eccentrically placed and will have an echogenic rim. The sac will have a double decidual sac sign. The double sac is formed by the inner echogenic rim of chorionic villi with decidua capsularis and outer decidua vera. This is highly reliable for the diagnosis of intrauterine gestation. Hence in situations where there is a high clinical probability of ectopic pregnancy, even if a small hypoechoic area is identified in the endometrium, a repeat scan should be done after a few days to look for double decidual sac sign for confirming intrauterine gestation. Presence of a yolk sac or embryo-yolk sac complex confirms the diagnosis of intrauterine pregnancy with confidence.

The distinction between an anembryonic pregnancy from pseudogestational sac is sometimes a difficult task. If the patient's history is suggestive of ectopic pregnancy, dilatation and curettage and histopathological examination of the curettings should be done. If chorionic villi can be identified a failing intrauterine pregnancy can be confirmed. Otherwise ectopic pregnancy should be kept in mind and the patient should be followed up.

The US findings in ectopic pregnancy depend upon the status of the ectopic pregnancy. An early ectopic gestation will appear as an anechoic cystic structure in the adnexa with an echogenic rim (Fig. 25.23). Corpus luteum also will be giving the appearance of a cystic mass with high vascularity and low resistance flow like ectopic gestational sac (Fig. 25.24). But the rim will not be as echogenic as gestational sac.

If a yolk sac or embryo can be identified inside the adnexal mass, the diagnosis of ectopic gestation can be confirmed. When the ectopic pregnancy is advanced the wall of the tube will be thick and can mimic an intrauterine pregnancy. By trying to trace the gestational sac to the cervix, intrauterine pregnancy and ectopic pregnancy can be differentiated. An intrauterine gestational sac will be

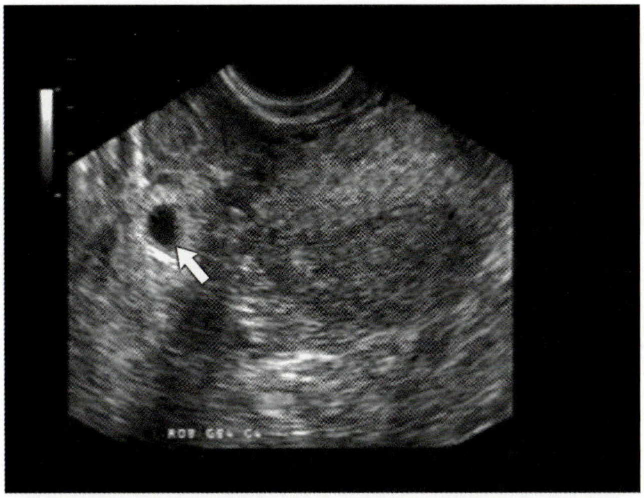

Fig. 25.23: TVS showing right adnexal ectopic gestational sac. Note the echogenic rim (arrow)

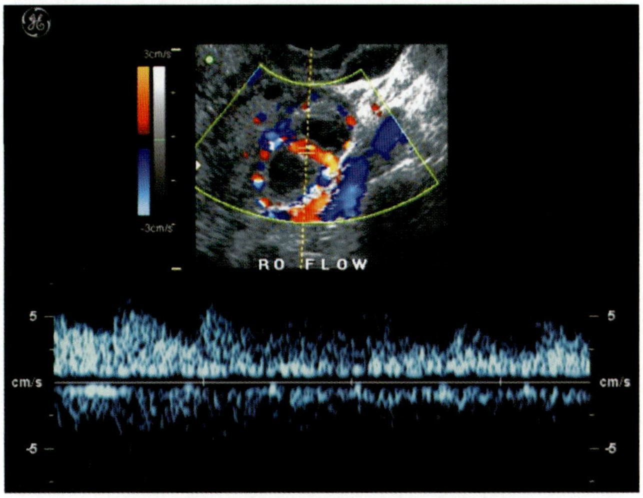

Fig. 25.24: TVS showing low-resistance flow in a corpus luteum

continuous with the cervix, whereas ectopic pregnancy sac will not be continuous. In a subacute ectopic, a tubal hematoma will form which will appear as a mixed echogenic mass in the adnexa.

25.19.2 Ruptured Ectopic Pregnancy

Ruptured ectopic pregnancy presenting with massive intraperitoneal hemorrhage is a clinical diagnosis. When there is a doubt about intraperitoneal hemorrhage, culdocentesis should be avoided as it would be extremely painful and may give false positive or false negative results.

Free blood in the peritoneal cavity can be clearly made out by ultrasound (Fig. 25.25) and a diagnosis of ruptured ectopic can be made by correlating with history, clinical examination and urine pregnancy test.

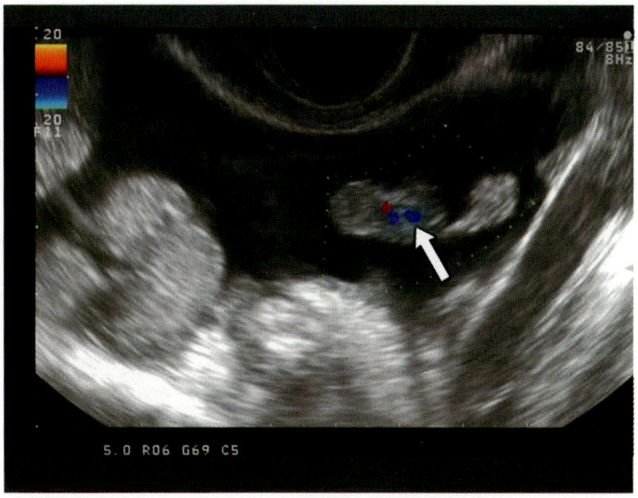

Fig. 25.25: TVS showing free fluid in the peritoneal cavity in a patient with ruptured ectopic pregnancy. The fallopian tube can be seen floating in the fluid (arrow)

25.19.3 Pregnancy of Unknown Location

When women present in early pregnancy with pain abdomen and bleeding per vaginum, ultrasound examination will usually be done. In the presence of a positive urine pregnancy test, if no intrauterine or extrauterine sac is seen, there are 3 possibilities:

1. A very early intrauterine gestation (too early to identify a gestational sac)
2. An unruptured ectopic gestation where the gestational sac is not visible
3. A complete abortion of early intrauterine pregnancy.

When no adnexal mass is seen an ectopic pregnancy cannot be excluded. History of passing a fleshy mass vaginally and pain subsiding subsequently will help diagnose complete abortion. TVS after complete abortion will give an irregular echogenic thin endometrium.

There is no characteristic finding of endometrium in ectopic pregnancy. It can be thin or thick. Decidual cysts, which are thin walled cystic areas in the endometrium, are common in ectopic pregnancy but are nonspecific. When in doubt the patient should be properly counseled and a follow-up scan should be arranged.

25.19.4 Role of Doppler USS

Low resistance flow can be demonstrated in the endometrium of intrauterine pregnancy. In ectopic pregnancy such flow will not be seen in the endometrium. When an adnexal ring is seen in a patient suspected to have ectopic pregnancy, low resistance flow can be demonstrated as ring of fire appearance. But a similar low resistance flow will be seen in the corpus luteum also. The echogenic rim

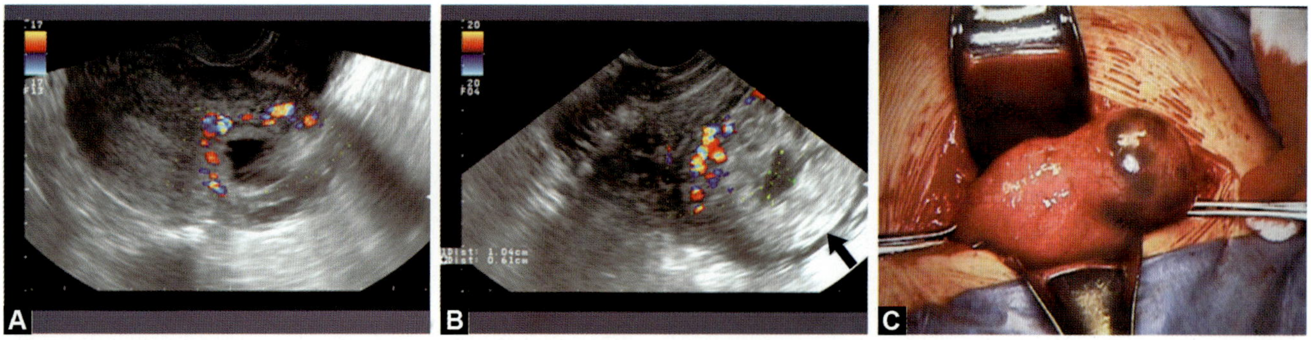

Figs 25.26A to C: TVS showing interstitial pregnancy. Note the gestational sac separate from the uterine cavity echo. The thin myometrial mantle is evident (arrow). The appearance at laparotomy is also shown

characteristic of ectopic pregnancy will help to differentiate it from a corpus luteum cyst.

25.19.5 Other Sites of Ectopic Pregnancy

Interstitial pregnancy (Figs 25.26A to C): 2-4% of ectopic pregnancy are interstitial. The morbidity and mortality of this condition is very high due to the late presentation and massive hemorrhage when rupture occurs. The diagnosis is made when a gestational sac is seen high in the fundal region and the myometrial mantle is less than 5 mm in thickness.

Cornual Pregnancy

True cornual pregnancies are located in the rudimentary horn of a bicornuate uterus. Here also rupture occurs late and hemorrhage can be profuse but the diagnosis can be easily made by TVS.

Cervical pregnancy: This is the rarest form of ectopic pregnancies accounting for 1% of ectopic pregnancies. When a gestational sac is seen with or without an embryo in the cervical canal, it could be cervical ectopic or inevitable abortion where the conceptus has reached the cervical canal. The presence of peritrophoblastic flow can be demonstrated in the cervical ectopic pregnancy whereas it will be absent in abortion. Moreover in spontaneous abortion, the sac size and shape will change on serial scanning (Rubin's criteria).

25.20 CONCLUSION

Ultrasound, especially the transvaginal scan has revolutionized gynecological diagnosis. Even though it is one of the cheapest investigations compared to other imaging modalities like MRI or CT, it gives very valuable information in the diagnosis of the various uterine as well as adnexal pathologies. The introduction of 4D ultrasound has further reduced the need for other imaging modalities. However, to make out deep infiltrating endometriosis, to diagnose the plane of separation of malignant ovarian disease, or to know the extent of tumor spread in cancer cervix, the gynecologist may have to resort to MRI or CT. It should never be forgotten that ultrasound should always be interpreted against the background of history and clinical examination findings. Ultrasound has become an essential diagnostic tool for the gynecologist so much so that it cannot be considered as an investigation, but should be viewed as a diagnostic aid like the pen torch of a physician. Hence, it is imperative that every gynecologist should know how to make best use of ultrasound for arriving at the correct diagnosis and planning the ideal management for their patients.

REFERENCES

1. Smith-Bindman R, Kerlikowske K, Feldstein VA, et al. Endovaginal ultrasound to exclude endometrial cancer and other endometrial abnormalities. JAMA 1988;280:1510-7.
2. Epstein E, Ramirez A, Skoog L, Valentine L. Transvaginal sonography: Saline contrast sonohysterography and hysteroscopy for the investigation of women with postmenopausal bleeding and endometrium >5 mm. Ultrasound Obstet Gynecol 2001;18:157-62.
3. Timmerman D, Schwarzler P, Collins WP, et al. Subjective assessment of adnexal masses with the use of ultrasonography: An analysis of interobserver variability and experience. Ultrasound Obstet Gynecol 1999;13:11-6.
4. Valentin L, Hagen B, Tingulstad S, Eik-Nes S. Comparison of pattern recognition and logistic regression models for discrimination between benign and malignant pelvic masses: A prospective cross validation. Ultrasound Obstet Gynecol 2001;18:357-65.
5. Mais B, et al. The efficacy of transvaginal ultrasonography in the diagnosis of endometrioma. Fertil Steril 199;60:776-80.
6. Yeh HC, et al. Intradecidual sign. Criterian of early intra-uterine pregnancy. Radiology 1986;161:463.
7. Eskenazi V, et al. Validation study of non-surgical diagnosis of endometrioma. Fertil steril 2001;76L:929-35.
8. Reinhold C, Atri M, Mehio A, et al. Diffuse uterine adenomyosis: Morphologic criteria and diagnostic accuracy of endovaginal sonography. Radiology 1995;197:609-14.

26 Laparoscopic Equipment and Techniques

Paul PG, B Presannakumari, Sejal Naik, Madhu KN

26.1 INTRODUCTION

Endoscopy is visualization of the interior of a viscus, space or organ with the help of a narrow telescope. In gynecology, endoscopes are used to visualize the peritoneal cavity (laparoscopy), or the uterine cavity (hysteroscopy). Even though laparoscopy has been in practice for almost than 100 years, the use of the procedure evolved as a means for surgery only during the past few decades. Presently laparoscopic surgery can be resorted to for performing most of the gynecological procedures. It is worth remembering the great people behind the evolution of this novel technology.

26.2 HISTORY

The presently practiced video-laparoscopy evolved from the hard work of several dedicated surgeons. Heinz Kalk (1929), a German gastroenterologist, is considered to be the founder of laparoscopy. Kalk developed a 135° lens system to visualize the peritoneal cavity. J Veress of Hungary (1938) developed the spring-loaded needle, deservingly known in his name, for creating pneumoperitoneum. Richard W Telinde (1939) was the first gynecologic surgeon to perform laparoscopy for visualizing the pelvic organs, approaching through the pouch of Douglas. However, this method was abandoned due to the disadvantage of encountering bowel enroute. In 1944, Raoul Palmer of France performed gynecological examinations using laparoscopy placing the patient in the Trendelenburg position and stressed the importance of continuously monitoring the intra-abdominal pressure. Kurst Semm (1960), a German gynecologist invented the automatic insufflator. Patrick Steptoe (1980), from England was the first to perform laparoscopic procedures. Video-laparoscopy was introduced in the year 1982, which made major surgery possible laparoscopically. The first video-laparoscopic surgery was a cholecystectomy performed by Phillipe Mouret (1987), in Lyons, France.

26.3 LAPAROSCOPY

Laparoscopy is currently not a diagnostic modality alone, but is being resorted to for performing major surgical procedures, most of which were previously performed through laparotomy. Laparoscopic surgery has several advantages compared to open surgery. It offers reduced pain, better cosmetic results, decreased adhesion formation, and above all, faster recovery. Since drying of tissues, direct peritoneal trauma and contamination are less; there is reduced chance for adhesion formation and infection. With experience in laparoscopic surgery, operating time can be made comparable to open surgery.

Even though laparoscopic surgery has the above mentioned benefits, it has several limitations and disadvantages. The learning curve is very steep. Long instruments have to be used through fixed ports only. Though hospital stay is less, the necessity of using expensive instruments and comparatively longer operating time makes the procedure expensive. There are innate risks of complications associated with the procedure. Complications like major vascular injury and those related to pneumoperitoneum occur almost exclusively during laparoscopic surgery. As a result of the greater use of thermal cautery, chances of injury to bowel or urinary tract are more common following laparoscopic surgery than open surgery. With the evolution of newer safer equipment which are of course expensive, complications are becoming less. Use of harmonic scalpel which avoids the risk of thermal injury is one such advancement. With adequate training, experience and practice of safe surgical techniques, complications of laparoscopic surgery can be minimized.

26.4 LAPAROSCOPIC EQUIPMENT AND TECHNIQUES

An organized and well equipped operating theater set-up can greatly add to patient safety and satisfaction. The set-up should be designed to optimize efficiency using a team concept. Good surgical training includes understanding of instruments and techniques involved. Hence, it is essential to have a thorough knowledge of the ideal theater set-up and equipment.

In operative laparoscopy, the peritoneal cavity is visualized by introducing a telescope inside the abdomen through a cannula. The peritoneal cavity is distended with carbon dioxide for facilitating visualization and surgery. Light is introduced into the peritoneal cavity, with the help of a fiber optic cable attached to the telescope. The image received by the telescope is transmitted to a monitor so that the surgeon and the assistants can coordinate the steps of the surgery. The quality of endoscopic surgery entirely depends on the quality of the image on the screen. The image quality depends on the laparoscope, light source, light cable, video camera and the monitor as well as the balance of interaction achieved between them. Tissues are severed using different types of energy sources. Knots can also be tied using special instruments. Irrigation of tissues can be achieved with the help of saline and the washed fluid can be removed from the peritoneal cavity using suction. Special instruments are needed for each of these procedures. Hence operative laparoscopy necessitates the use of several specially designed equipment.

The following description is intended to give an overview of the various equipment used in laparoscopy.

26.4.1 Veress Needle

A Veress needle is used for creating initial pneumoperitoneum to separate the internal organs and tissues from the abdominal wall so that the trocar can be inserted safely. Veress needle technique is the most widely practiced way of peritoneal access. The presently used needles are modifications of the hollow needle designed by Veress. It is available in reusable or disposable models containing a spring-loaded tip that retracts as it pierces the abdominal wall, allowing a blunt tip to engage on entry into the peritoneal cavity (Fig. 26.1). This is so designed to avoid damage to the bowel or other intra-abdominal organs. The needle is available in three sizes depending on the length; 80 mm, 100 mm and 120 mm.

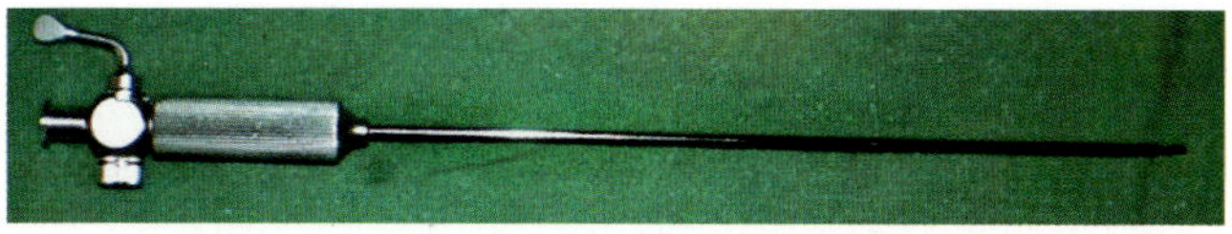

Fig. 26.1: Veress needle. The needle should be held like a dart at the time of insertion

Before using, the needle should be checked for its patency as well as spring action.

A small midline incision, just adequate for the introduction of the needle is made at the lower border of the umbilicus with a number 13 scalpel blade. The abdomen is maximally lifted either by grasping on either side lateral to the umbilicus or by lifting the middle of the abdomen below the umbilicus. In order to avoid injury to the major retroperitoneal vessels, the needle should be held by the shaft and directed towards the center of the pelvic cavity at an angle of 45° to the horizontal. Before connecting to the insufflator, the intra-abdominal position of the needle should be ascertained. This can be done by several methods which are listed below.

- As the needle enters the peritoneal cavity, there would be a hissing sound of air being sucked in.
- About 10 ml of saline can be instilled into the peritoneal cavity through the needle. If the needle is in the peritoneal cavity, the saline cannot be aspirated back as it falls into the dependant portion of the peritoneal cavity.
- In the hanging drop technique, a drop of saline instilled into the needle will be sucked in if the needle is in the peritoneal cavity, whereas it will remain there itself if it is extraperitoneal.

The needle is then connected to the insufflator through the tubing. Intraperitoneal placement can be ascertained by visualizing uniform distension of abdomen and obliteration of liver dullness. Even if the needle is in the peritoneal cavity, the liver dullness may not be obliterated in the presence of adhesions. If the needle is extraperitoneal, distention will be confined to the hypogastrium and the pressure recorded will be high.

Carbon dioxide is the choice of gas for insufflation. It has the advantage of being rapidly absorbed by blood, as it will be converted to carbonic acid which immediately dissociates to bicarbonate and hydrogen ions which prevent gas embolism. However, formation of carbonic acid in the peritoneal surfaces can cause pain in the postoperative period. The use of heated or hydrated gas has been advocated to prevent hypothermia during laparoscopy.

Gasless laparoscopy can be performed with the use of a mechanical lifting arm that attaches to a fanlike retractor along the peritoneal surface of the abdominal wall, obviating the need for distension using gas. Traditional instruments can be used in gasless laparoscopy. Some favor this approach in patients with cardiopulmonary risk factors.

26.4.2 Insufflators

High-flow CO_2 insufflators are a basic prerequisite for laparoscopy. Electronically controlled insufflators (Fig. 26.2) have become the preferred choice in this respect, as the intra-abdominal pressure can be maintained automatically during use of suction as well as change of instruments.

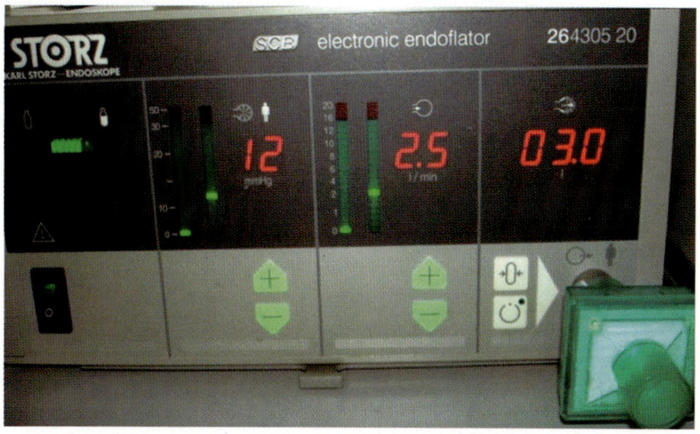

Fig. 26.2: Electronic carbon dioxide insufflators. The intra-abdominal pressure is kept at 12 mm of Hg (left). The flow rate is 2.5 L/min (middle). The total gas insufflated is 3 Liters (right)

A carbon dioxide gas insufflator should provide a continuous flow of gas to maintain an intra-abdominal pressure ranging from 10-15 mm of Hg. Most of the electronic insufflators provide a flow rate up to 10-20 liters/ minute continuously. Before the introduction of the primary trocar, a higher intra-abdominal pressure of 20 mm of Hg can be set to facilitate insertion of trocar as well as to increase the distance between the trocar and the retroperitoneal vessels. This higher pressure is avoided during the surgical procedure, as it can compromise diaphragmatic movement and decrease venous return by compressing the inferior vena cava. A higher intra-abdominal pressure can also increase the incidence of gas embolism. Hence after the insertion of the trocar, the pressure is reduced to 12-15 mm of Hg. Flow rate is ideally kept at 1 liter/minute during initial insufflation with Veress needle and increased to higher flow rates when connected to the trocar. Insufflation tubing with a 0.3-micron filter is recommended to prevent intraperitoneal contamination with bacteria, microparticles, and debris from the insufflator and gas tank. The insufflator display, which the surgeon should always be able to see, gives continuous information on the following data:

1. Patient's intra-abdominal pressure (actual value)
2. Flow rate
3. Total volume of CO_2 insufflated
4. Gas reserve

26.4.3 Trocars

The word 'trocar' is usually used to refer to the assembly of cannula and stylet, but the actual trocar is a stylet which is introduced through the cannula. Cannulae allow the insertion of laparoscopic instruments into the abdominal cavity. The most frequently used sizes of trocars are 5 and 10 mm (Fig. 26.3). The size of the operating instrument decides the size of trocar. Appropriate reducers must be used when smaller instruments are used through larger cannulae. Most trocar sheaths contain a Luer-lock port that attaches to the insufflation tubing. Trocars may have a pyramidal, conical, bladed, or blunt tip. Pyramidal tips are easier to insert. The sharp edges can sometimes damage smaller blood vessels and other organs. By using the blunt trocar tips, the blood vessels are pushed aside and protected to a large degree. However, greater pressure has to be exerted sometimes during insertion. To visualize the layers of the abdominal wall during placement, optical access trocars are available. Expandable trocar sheaths are also available that are initially placed with a Veress needle and then expanded to accept a 5 to 12 mm port (Step port, Inner Dyne). These offer the advantage of creating smaller abdominal wall defects and thereby reduce the risk of hernia later on as well as injury to the inferior epigastric vessels.

Trocars usually have 2 types of valves to prevent the escape of gas. Trumpet valves protect the telescope from contamination by tissue and blood particles during insertion. The valve has to be pressed during insertion. However, they grip the instruments and prevent its smooth movement. Hence flap valve trocars are generally preferred. A multifunctional valve combines the advantages of both.

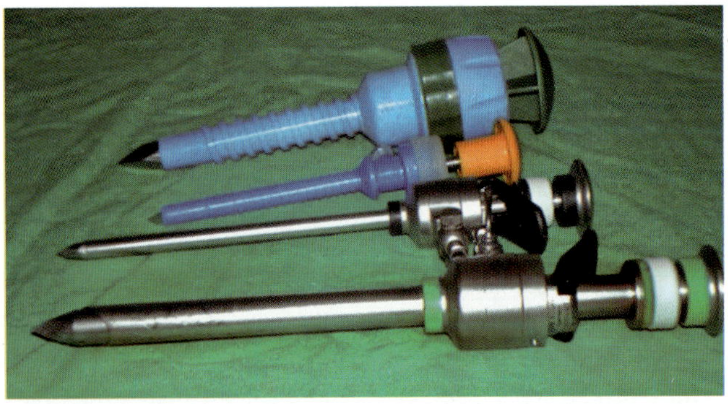

Fig. 26.3: 10 mm and 5 mm size plastic and metal trocars

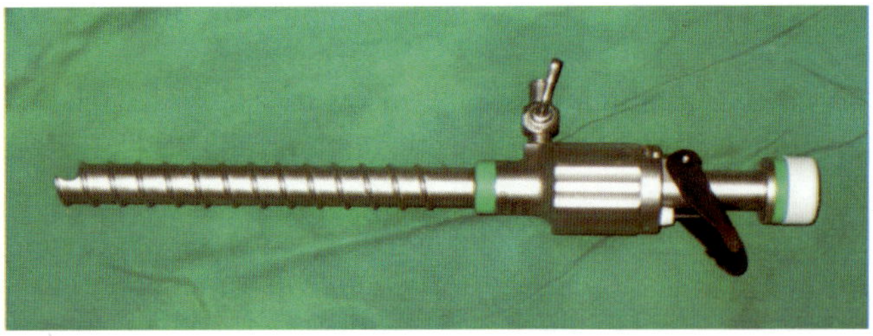

Fig. 26.4: Endotip

The Endotip (Fig. 26.4) is a sheath with screw threading. This is a new generation instrument for safe peritoneal entry under vision. In this method, the sheath which has a screw thread tip is inserted with the telescope inside so that, as the sheath is screwed in, the tissue layers can be visualized and inadvertent injury to the internal organs can be prevented. This is safe when adhesions are expected especially when the patient has had a previous laparotomy. The screwed endotip prevents it from slipping out of the intraperitoneal space.

26.4.4 Peritoneal Entry

The peritoneal cavity can be entered by an open or a closed technique. In the open, Hasson technique, the peritoneal cavity is entered through a mini-laparotomy incision which may be a transverse or vertical one in the subumbilical region. The cannula is directly introduced without prior insufflation of the peritoneal cavity. As the stylet is not used and blind entry is avoided, injury to major structures can be minimized. Gynecologists usually prefer the closed technique, where the peritoneal cavity is initially distended with carbon dioxide and the trocar is introduced blindly into the peritoneal cavity.

The primary cannula with stylet is usually inserted through the umbilical port and the telescope is introduced through the primary cannula. While introducing the primary cannula and trocar through the umbilical port, the patient should be in the supine horizontal position without the Trendelenburg tilt. This is necessary as tilting the patient head-end down will bring the aortic bifurcation more anteriorly and is likely to be injured.

Entry through Palmer's Point

The primary trocar can also be introduced through the Palmer's point, which is about 2 finger breadth below the left costal margin in the mid clavicular line. Prior insufflation of the abdomen with Veress needle is not necessary. After making a small incision about 1 cm wide in the Palmer's point the trocar is placed in the incision vertically. The abdomen is held by the left hand close to the trocar entry site and raised and the trocar and cannula can be pushed in directed towards the umbilicus. Once the feel of peritoneal entry is perceived, the trocar is removed and the cannula is pushed a little further. After introducing the telescope, intraperitoneal entry is confirmed and the gas tubing is connected. All the secondary cannulae used for introducing the instruments necessary for surgery are inserted under vision. While introducing the secondary cannulae, care should be taken to avoid injury to the major vessels of the abdominal wall. The superficial epigastric vessels can be transilluminated and the site could be identified and avoided. The deep epigastric artery lies between the peritoneum and the rectus muscle and hence cannot be transilluminated. It can be identified by locating the lateral umbilical ligament (obliterated umbilical artery) on the inner side of the anterior abdominal wall. The artery could be seen lateral to the lateral umbilical ligament (Fig. 26.5).

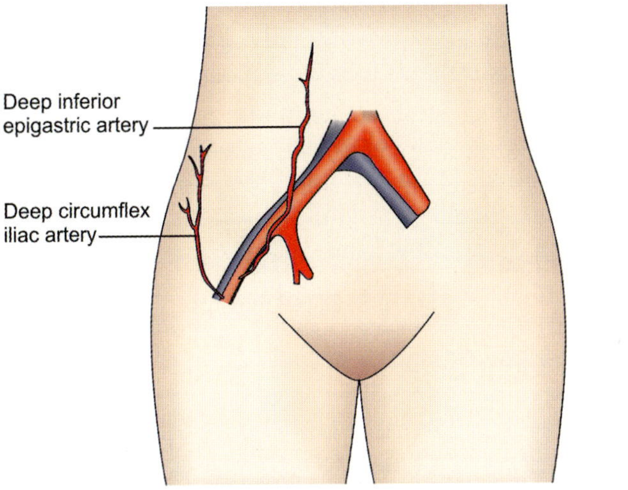

Fig. 26.5: Picture showing the anatomy of the vessels of the anterior abdominal wall

26.4.5 Laparoscopes

In laparoscopy, the peritoneal cavity is visualized through the telescope (laparoscope). Even though for diagnostic purpose direct visualization through the telescope is enough, for proper visualization and for performing surgical procedures video guidance is required. The image from the telescope is captured by the camera head connected to the telescope which in turn forwards it to the body of the camera which is placed away from the field of surgery, usually in the instrument shelf where the insufflator is also kept. The image will be processed by the camera and will be displayed in the monitor. The image quality achieved will depend on the amount of light transmitted through the endoscope, the output of light from the source, the quality of the camera, the light transmitting cable and the resolution of the monitor. The light sources currently available are 250-300 watts Xenon or Mercury halide bulbs. Narrow diameter telescopes (3-5 mm) transmit less light so that the image obtained will be of poor quality. The ideal illumination required for performing operative procedures is provided by a 10 mm telescope. However, the image quality can be improved by using more sensitive camera and more sensitive light source even when a smaller diameter (3-5 mm) telescope is used.

Depending on the viewing angle mainly 2 types of telescopes are used (Fig. 26.6):

1. *0° straight-forward telescope*: This telescope has the greatest application range, because it facilitates orientation and conveys an impression of the area inspected. The direction of view corresponds to the natural approach and the usual perspective. It is generally preferred in gynecological interventions.
2. *30° forward-oblique telescope*: This can be rotated to enlarge the field of vision. It can be advantageous during dissection in the Douglas' pouch and for visualizing partially obscured areas.

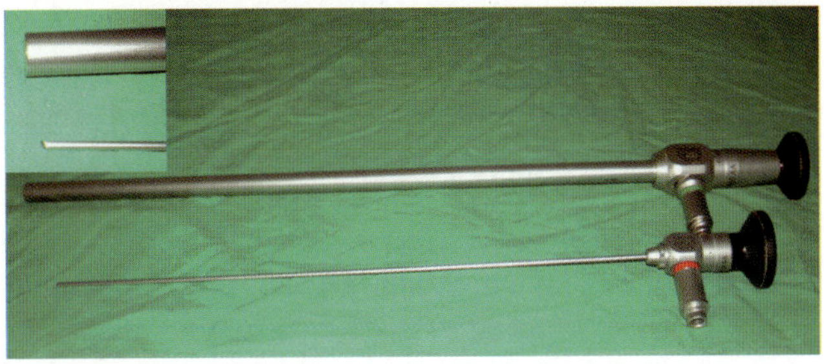

Fig. 26.6: 10 mm and 3 mm telescopes. 0° viewing angle of the 10 mm telescope and 30° of the 3 mm telescope are shown in the inset

Fogging is a common problem during endoscopic surgery. It most commonly occurs due to the presence of moisture between the telescope and the camera lens. Using a sterile camera cover instead of soaking in glutaraldehyde solution will partially solve this problem. Always wipe and dry the telescope head before connecting the camera. Washing the tip of the telescope with the irrigating fluid followed by rubbing on the bowel or uterus can clean and dry the lens when dirty ('car screen washing').

26.4.6 Video Camera

Most of the available endoscopic cameras are single chip CCD (charge couple device) cameras. Single chip means it contains a single solid state silicon computer chip, which consists of a large number of photoelectric cells. These cells produce a current when light strikes on them, which is converted to an image on the video screen. Each silicon element contributes one pixel unit to the image produced. The image resolution is dependent on the number of pixels on the chip. Most laparoscopic cameras have 250,000 to 380,000 pixels. Three-chip CCDs provide better image clarity but are more expensive, as they have a separate chip for each primary color, as opposed to the single chip CCD.

High-definition digital cameras are now available that are compatible with high-definition flat screen monitors having increased resolution capabilities. Image I HD is a new generation three chip digital camera (Fig. 26.7).

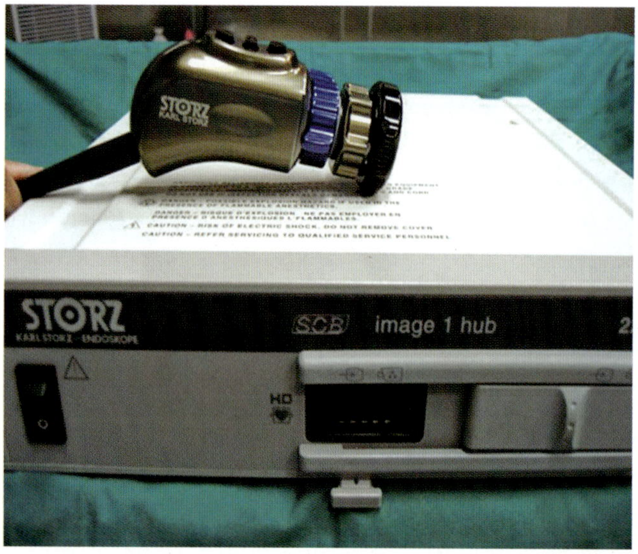

Fig. 26.7: Video Camera–Image I HD

All cameras have a white balance facility. Depending on the light source, color reproduction can vary. Hence before starting surgery, the camera has to be white balanced by showing a white object with light source on. The white light is composed of equal proportion of red, blue and green color and at the time of white balancing the camera sets its digital coding for these primary colors to equal proportion assuming that the target is white. Most cameras have white balance memory till there is a change in the light source. White balancing need not be done every time the camera is switched on.

Another important facility most of the cameras posses is automatic light intensity control to avoid glare. To test the efficiency of this mechanism, point the camera fitted to telescope with light on to a white object and move towards and away from it. There should either be no glare or glare that disappears very quickly.

26.4.7 Video Monitors

The quality of the image we see depends on the monitor also. It is better to use monitors with a higher resolution than the camera. High-resolution color monitors produce around 700 horizontal lines of resolution. Monitors are available in 14 and 20-inch sizes. Digital monitors are easier to handle (Fig. 26.8).

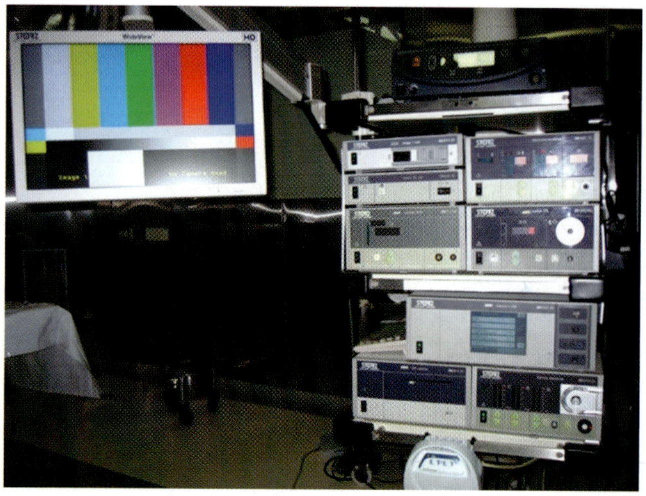

Fig. 26.8: Digital monitor

26.4.8 Light Generators

The quality of the light delivered to the endoscope depends on both the light source and the cable. High-intensity light sources should be used. The available light sources are:

1. Quartz halogen
2. Xenon
3. LED bulbs

The difference can be appreciated in the color obtained, the xenon having a slightly bluish tint. The light emitted by xenon lamp is more natural compared to halogen lamp. However, most of the cameras at present analyze and compensate these variations by means of automatic equalization of whites (2100 K to 10,000 K), which allows the same image to be obtained with both light sources. The commonly used light sources are 250 watts halogen or 175-300 watts xenon (Fig. 26.9).

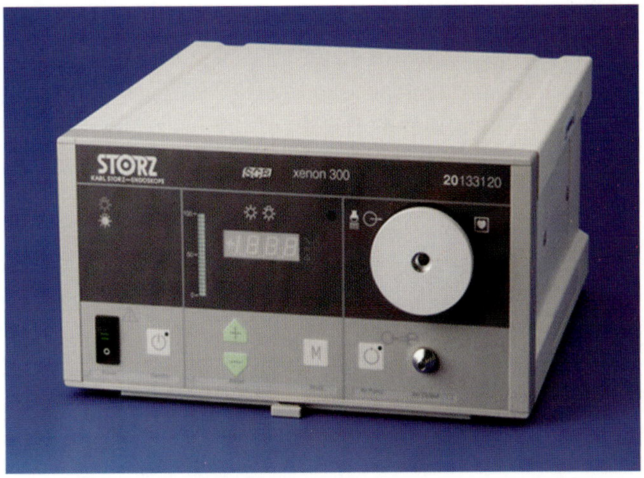

Fig. 26.9: Light source

26.4.9 Light Cables

Two types of light cables are available:

1. Cold light/fiber optic cable
2. Liquid crystal gel cable

Fiber Optic Cable

These cables are made up of a bundle of optical glass fibers of 3 μ in diameter, swaged at both ends (Fig. 26.10). The cable size used is usually between 10 and 25 mm in diameter. Light transmission occurs by total internal reflection. They have a very high quality of optical transmission, but are fragile. In fact, after repeated use, some optical fibers break. The loss of optical fibers may be seen when one end of the cable is viewed in daylight. The broken fibers are seen as black spots.

Distal end of fiber optic cable should never be placed on or under drapes, or near the patient when it is connected to an illuminated light source. The heat generated from the intensity of light may cause burns to the patient or ignite the drapes.

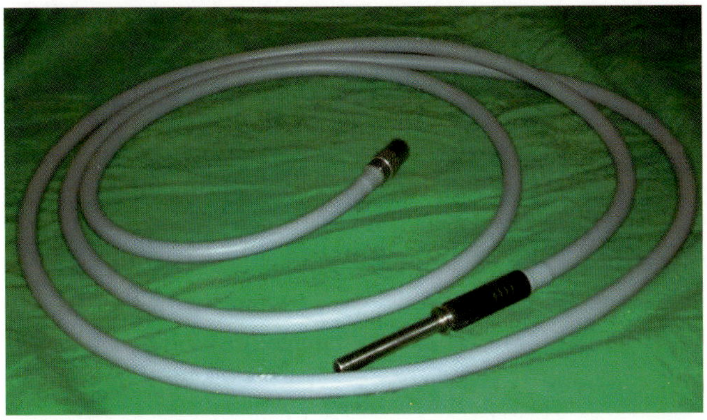

Fig. 26.10: Fiber optic light cable. The cable is made of a bundle of glass fibrils about 3 μ in diameter, clad with rubber. It should be handled carefully taking care not to bend so that the fibrils do not get damaged

Light carrying capacity of the cable depends on the number of fiber optic bundles. Video endoscopic surgery requires fiber optic cables of at least 4.5 mm diameter.

Gel Cables

These cables are made up of a sheath that is filled with a clear optical gel (Liquid crystal). Theoretically they are capable of transmitting 30% more light than optic fibers.

These cables are made more rigid by a metal sheath, which makes them difficult to maintain and store. They have the disadvantage of transmitting more heat than the optical fiber cables.

Cables filled with liquid alcohol transmit light somewhat more effectively than fiber optic cables. But these cables are heavily clad and hence are less flexible.

26.4.10 Suction-irrigation Cannula

An efficient suction cum irrigation cannula is one of the most important equipment for laparoscopic surgery, as it helps to make the operating field clear. Most of the surgeons use normal saline or Ringer lactate for irrigation. Heparinized saline can be used to dissolve blood clot to facilitate proper suction in the presence of excessive intra-abdominal bleeding, thus maintaining excellent vision. At the time of using suction and irrigation, the tip of the suction irrigation cannula should be dipped inside the fluid, otherwise the gas would be sucked out and visibility will be lost. Suction irrigation cannula with single hand control is the popular one (Fig. 26.11). Irrigation is usually achieved by gravity. Irrigation under pressure which is needed for hydrodissection can be achieved by using an infusion pump. There are different types of pumps to deliver the fluid for irrigation.

The stopcocks should have the same diameter as that of the tube itself to avoid clogging. 10 mm suction irrigation cannula is used for removing organized blood clots.

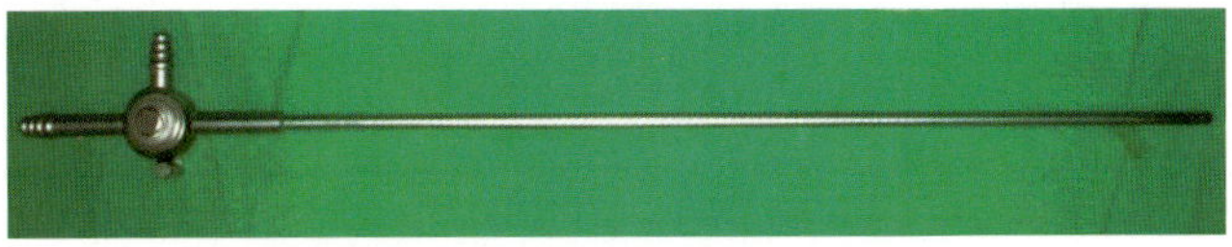

Fig. 26.11: Suction-irrigation cannula

26.4.11 Operating Instruments

Several factors should be considered at the time of choosing laparoscopic instruments including cost, availability and reliability. Reusable instruments are expensive initially but in the long run they are cost-effective.

Disposable instruments are comparatively less costly. The main advantage of disposable instrument is high performance due to its sharpness and reduced chance of disease transmission due to certified high-end factory sterilization. Even though disposable, biodegradability of these instruments will remain an environmental concern. Reuse of disposable instrument is not safe as cleaning and sterilization cannot be properly done.

Size: Laparoscopic hand instruments vary in diameter from 1.8-12 mm, but majority of the instruments are designed to pass through 5-10 mm cannula. They also vary in length from 18-45 cm (used in obese or very tall patients) but most have the same length of approximately 36 cm in adult and 28 cm in pediatric practice. For better ergonomics, half of the instrument should be inside the abdomen and half outside, so that it behaves like a class 1 lever, stabilizing the port and making surgery convenient.

Most of the laparoscopic procedures require a mixture of sharp and blunt dissection techniques, often using the same instrument in a number of different ways. Most re-usable instruments can be partially dismantled so that it can be cleaned and washed properly. Modular instruments in which the parts can be changed to suit the surgeon's favorite attachment like handle or working tip are also available.

Most of the hand instruments have three detachable parts.

1. **Handle:** Most laparoscopic instruments like graspers and scissors have basic opening and closing function. Many instruments have mechanism for rotating the tip which makes them capable of rotation up to 360° angle. Certain handles are designed to allow locking of the jaw which is useful when the tissue needs to be grasped firmly for a long period of time. They have ratchets allowing the jaws to be closed in different positions and at different degrees of pressure. Most of the laparoscopic instrument handles have attachments for unipolar electrosurgical lead and some have hand switches for cutting and coagulation.
2. **Insulated outer tube:** Instruments which have silicon or plastic outer tube prevents accidental electric burn to bowel or other viscera. Utmost care should be taken so that insulation should not be scratched by any sharp contact while cleaning. Even a pin hole breach in insulation may be dangerous at the time of electro surgery. Insulation of disposable instrument also can be torn easily which can lead to electrosurgical injuries.
3. **Insert which makes the tip of the instrument:** Insert of hand instrument varies only at the tip. It may be grasper, scissors, or forceps.

Grasping Forceps

There are two types of grasping forceps: traumatic and atraumatic. A variety of grasping forceps are required for different surgeries (Fig. 26.12). This grasper may have single action jaw or double action jaw. Single action jaw opens less than double action jaw but close with greater force thus, most of the needle holders are single action jaw. Graspers and dissecting forceps have wider opening jaws. Atraumatic dissecting and grasping forceps are particularly suitable for holding hollow organs. Atraumatic grasping forceps (multi-serrated) are designed for atraumatic and precise tissue grasping. Teethed grasping forceps are used to hold tissues to be removed like a cyst wall. The 10 mm claw forceps is useful for grasping and removing bigger specimens. A 10 mm spoon forceps is useful when fleshy tissues like ovarian cysts or ectopic pregnancy products are to be removed.

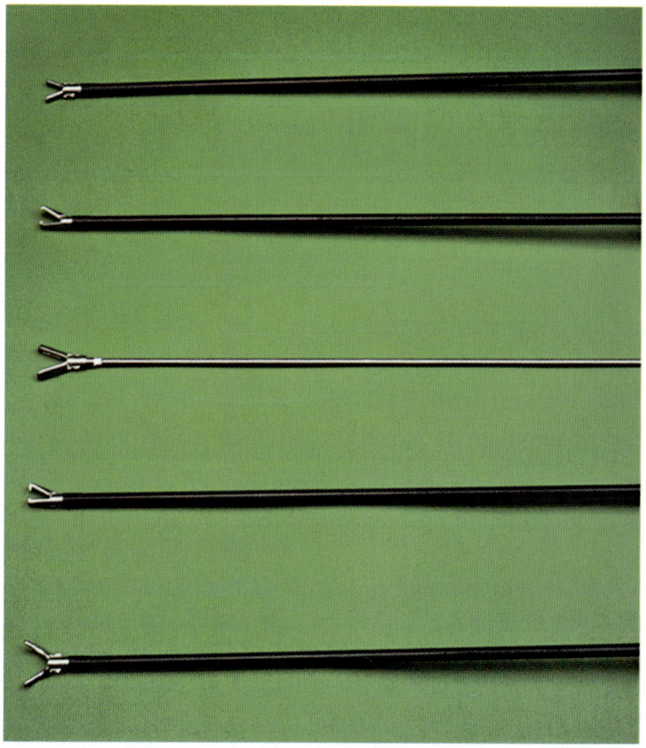

Fig. 26.12: Graspers with serrated and atraumatic blades

Scissors

Scissors are available in a multitude of forms—straight, curved or hooked (Fig. 26.13). Scissors become blunt rather soon. Straight scissors is widely used for mechanical and delicate dissection. They can give controlled depth of cutting as they have only one moving jaw. Hook scissors are particularly suitable for transecting ligature fibers and for cutting duct, artery, or nerve bundle in neurectomy.

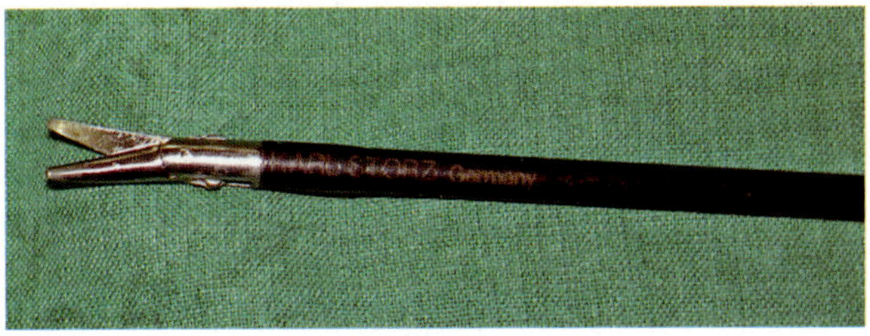

Fig. 26.13: Scissors

Curved scissors, in general, have the same features as straight ones. In some cases, they are easier for dissection, because the curvature changes the viewing angle. Serrated scissors prevent the tissue from slipping out of the blades. It is a useful instrument in cutting a slippery tissue or ligature.

Myoma Fixation Screw/spiral

This is used to fix a subserous or intramural myoma at the time of laparoscopic myomectomy. It is an important instrument used in performing total laparoscopic hysterectomy as it can be used to fix the uterus.

Needle Drivers

Laparoscopic suturing can be performed with specially designed needle drivers to drive needles through tissue, and knots may be tied outside the laparoscopic port (extracorporeal knot) or within the body (intracorporeal knot). Suturing devices of various designs are available. Needle holders are ergonomically designed for suturing (Fig. 26.14). Extracorporeal knots are usually performed as sliding square knots, pushed through the trocar sleeve to the tissue by multiple passes of a knot pusher, which serves as the surgeon's finger. These knot pushers are of either closed jaw or of open jaw type. Pre-tied loops are useful for free pedicles like appendicectomy.

Intracorporeal knots are tied within the abdomen by looping the suture material around the laparoscopic needle holders using the same technique as in open surgery.

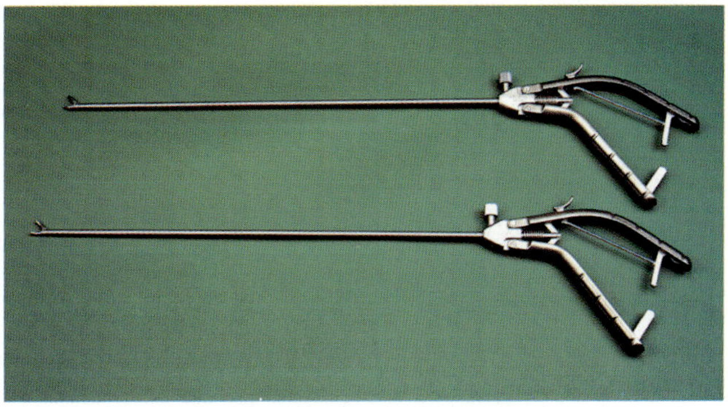

Fig. 26.14: Needle holder

Laparoscopic suturing requires considerable practice to load the needle into the needle driver and place sutures accurately. Staplers are presently available, the use of which needs less training.

Morcellators

One of the major difficulties in laparoscopic surgeries is to remove large volumes of tissues such as fibroids, ovarian tissue, or even the uterus from the peritoneal cavity.

Suprapubic minilaparotomy or transvaginal extraction through colpotomy are methods of tissue removal during laparoscopic surgery. Electromechanical morcellator is a novel instrument for removing large masses thus avoiding need for colpotomy or minilaparotomy. A variable speed motor drives the rotation of the sharp outer sleeve (Fig. 26.15). Cylindrical pieces of tissue can be removed very easily with this device. It is possible, with the aid of this morcellator, to extract even large amounts of tissue from the abdomen, using the size 15 trocar, in a short period of time. Because of the good quality cutting of the rotating morcellator, the tissue structure is minimally damaged enabling a reliable histological examination.

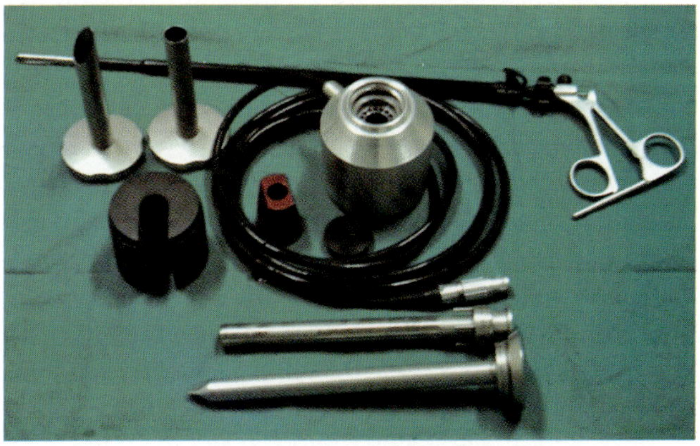

Fig. 26.15: Morcellator

Uterine Manipulators

A uterine manipulator (Fig. 26.16) may be used to improve access to the uterus, fallopian tubes, ovaries, and the posterior and anterior cul-de-sacs. These are available in reusable and disposable models. Some are inserted in a fixed position and allow limited uterine mobility, whereas others are hinged and allow the uterus to be moved anteriorly, posteriorly, and laterally. Many of these also offer the ability to perform chromotubation for evaluation of fallopian tube patency. A different type of manipulator is used for total laparoscopic hysterectomy. They not only manipulate the uterus, but also bulge the fornices for performing colpotomy. A vaginal blocker is also incorporated to avoid the leakage of pneumoperitoneum when colpotomy is made. Different designs are available like Clermont Ferrand model (Karl Storz).

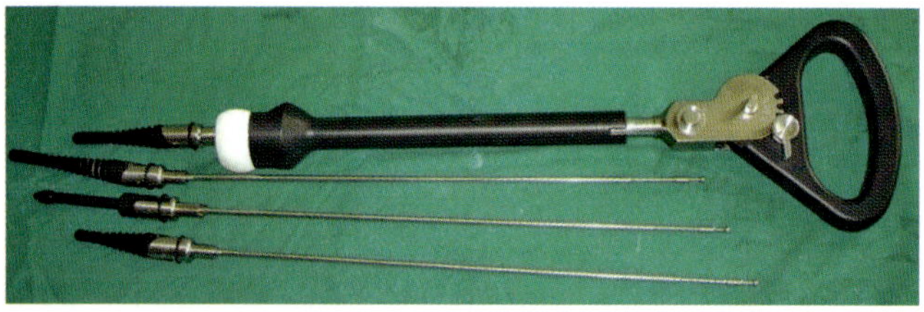

Fig. 26.16: Clermont Ferrand uterine manipulator

The list of instruments available for use in laparoscopy will never be complete. It is important for the surgeon to be aware of the basic instruments that are currently available and be familiar with their functioning and mechanism.

26.5 INSTRUMENTS AND ENERGY SOURCES FOR CUTTING AND HEMOSTASIS

Complex laparoscopic surgeries involving division of tissues and maintenance of hemostasis are possible by mechanical means or by the use of different energy sources.

The mechanical means are suturing, stapling, and the application of vascular clips.

The energy sources available for cutting tissues are:

1. Electrical energy
2. Laser
3. Ultrasonic energy

26.5.1 Electrosurgery

Monopolar and bipolar electrosurgical instruments are used to perform various types of surgeries and to obtain hemostasis (Fig. 26.17). The instruments include monopolar needles, hooks, and spatula forceps. Bipolar forceps of varying breadth and shapes are also available.

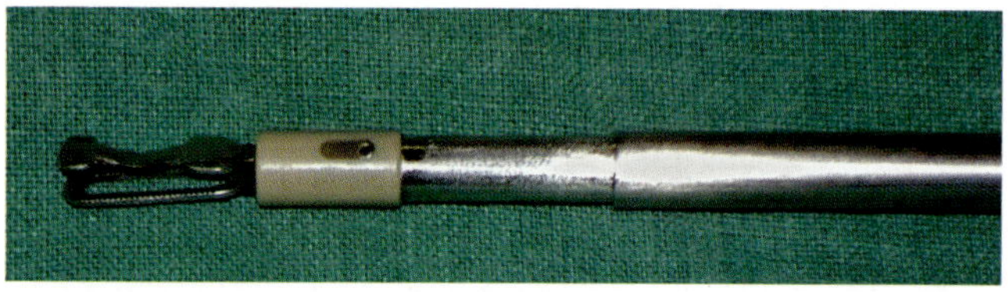

Fig. 26.17: The tip of the bipolar forceps. The tissue to be coagulated is caught with the jaws of the forceps

Diathermy is widely used in open surgery in standard settings. Use of diathermy in laparoscopic and hysteroscopic surgery necessitates knowledge about the settings as well as the hazards involved. Electrosurgery refers to both monopolar and bipolar diathermy. They are used for cutting as well as for hemostasis.

When household current is modified to a higher frequency of 200 Hz, ions are excited to produce a thermal effect. This is the basis of diathermy. The effect of diathermy depends on the following factors.

1. Density of the current
2. Type of wave form—cutting or coagulating
3. Type of tissue
4. Duration of application
5. Size and shape of the electrode used

Density of the Current

Tissue damage produced depends on the density of the current used. The current density will be concentrated at the tip of the needle electrode and hence will be very high at the tip. As the patient plate is very broad, the current density will be distributed and hence will not cause heating of tissue at the site of contact between the body and the patient plate. Hence, it is important to make sure that the patient plate should have a wider area of contact with the body. If the patient plate is not properly placed, it can result in burns. When tissue resistance is high, the current density automatically increases in most diathermy equipment. Hence when using diathermy on high resistance tissue, in the presence of insulation failure, capacitive coupling and direct coupling are likely to be more.

Current Waveform

Three types of electrical currents are used in electrosurgery:

1. Cutting
2. Coagulating
3. Blended

Electrosurgical instruments use household current that is transformed into radiofrequency current. The waveform of radiofrequency current can be altered.

In the cutting mode a continuous wave current (undamped) is used. The cutting current is a low voltage high frequency current. Here the temperature of the tissue is raised to the boiling point of water. The site of contact is vaporized and destroyed producing cutting effect, minimizing lateral thermal spread.

With waveform modification, current can be interrupted (damped) to varying degrees. The current waveform is modulated in coagulation mode in such a way that coagulation rather than vaporization occurs. Coagulation is caused by slower desiccation resulting in denaturation and charring (fulguration) to cause hemostasis with minimal cutting. The higher voltage produced by coagulation current carries higher risk of inadvertent discharge of energy.

If a mixture of these two types of waveforms is employed, then the advantages of both can be obtained. This is the blended current.

Type of Tissue

As the moisture content of the tissue increases the resistance as well as the current flow also increases. Tissues with lesser moisture content require only lower voltage.

Duration of Application

As the duration of application of current increases, the intensity of thermal injury increases.

Size and Shape of the Diathermy Electrode

When a pointed electrode is used, current intensity will be concentrated to a smaller surface. Hence, the sharp side of the scissors can be used for cutting and the blunt side can be used for coagulation. A spatula or ball electrode can be used for coagulation and a needle electrode can be used for cutting.

Monopolar Diathermy (Fig. 26.18)

Monopolar instruments use current that flows from an active electrode, through the tissue, achieving a cutting or coagulating effect. The circuit is completed through the patient's body. The current exits through a return electrode plate (usually placed under the patient's thigh or buttocks) to the electrosurgical unit. Monopolar current is usually used for cutting. However, if a spatula or a spherical electrode is used, it can be used for coagulation. Spatula and hook are the main electrodes used for monopolar cutting and coagulation.

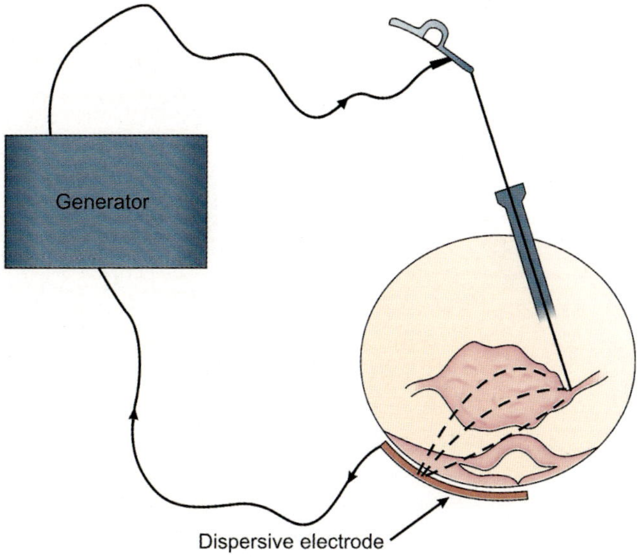

Fig. 26.18: Diagrammatic representation of the circuit in monopolar diathermy. Current flows from the generator through the cable to the laparoscopic electrode and reaches the tissue. The circuit is completed by the current flowing back to the generator through the dispersive electrode

Bipolar Diathermy (Fig. 26.19)

In bipolar diathermy, the current flows through the tissue between the two electrodes and the patient's body is not part of the circuit. It is safer compared to monopolar current because current travels only through the tissue held between the jaws. Both the jaws of bipolar instruments are insulated and the patient plate is not necessary. However, since both monopolar as well as bipolar instruments are used during laparoscopic surgery, it is necessary that the patient plate be kept in all surgeries.

Bipolar instruments, such as the Kleppinger forceps and the newer impedance-controlled bipolar systems, use current that flows from an active electrode, through tissue having a cutting or coagulating effect, and returning through a return electrode within the same instrument directly back to the electrosurgical unit. There is no need for a return electrode plate on the patient.

Bipolar instruments have undergone significant transformation in recent years. Simple bipolar systems, such as the ESU with a Kleppinger forceps, have evolved to devices that provide bipolar energy that senses tissue impedance to perform controlled energy delivery. These devices, such as Enseal (Surgrx), Plasma Kinetic dissection forceps (Gyrus Medical), and Ligasure (Valleylab), use pressure and pulsed current to seal vessels with minimal lateral thermal spread.

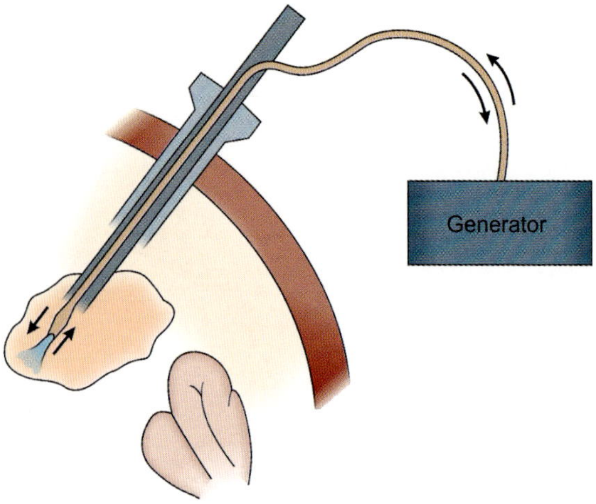

Fig. 26.19: Diagram showing circuit in bipolar diathermy. Current flows only between the prongs of the bipolar forceps

Diathermy Safety

Use of monopolar diathermy entails 3 major risks. Thermal injury can occur due to current diversion through an unintended path. This can occur due to insulation defect, direct coupling or capacitive coupling.

1. *Insulation failure:* Defects in the insulation of instruments are likely to cause a discharge of current especially when the power is increased. It can occur at any point between the unit and the active electrode. Damage of the insulation occurs due to friction between the instrument and the port. Hence, all diathermy instruments should be checked for damage to insulation before each use. Use of a metal port is safe in one way. It will cause the leaked current to be discharged in a wider area. When a plastic port is used the current may not get discharged instead it may flow to an adjacent bowel. The sigmoid colon is the most likely site of injury as it is close to the left adnexal region. Any part of the bowel may be affected. When using electrosurgical instruments especially monopolar, the shaft of the instrument should be away from viscera as well as other instruments.
2. *Direct coupling:* When an activated electrode touches a metal instrument like the laparoscope or metal cannula or a metal grasper, electrical energy can get conducted through the latter instrument and damage structures in contact with it. Hence care should be taken to see that an activated monopolar instrument is not touching the laparoscope, suction cannula or any other metal instrument when current is activated. The electrosurgical instrument should be viewed panoramically to ascertain this aspect of care.
3. *Capacitive coupling:* Capacitance is the ability of a conductor to establish an electrical current from an unconnected nearby circuit. An electrical field is established around the metal shaft of an electrosurgical instrument. This can make the shaft a capacitor. When the dispersive electrode is in proper contact with the patient and the current is of normal intensity, the electrical energy will be dispersed through a wider area in the abdominal wall and hence burning effect will not be produced. However, in the presence of a non conductive plastic retaining tube, current dispersal will not occur in a wider area and will result in dispersal to a nearby bowel or any other structure and can result in thermal injury. This type of injury can be avoided by not using hybrid cannula which is a mixture of metal and nonmetal cannula.

26.5.2 Laser Energy

Surgical lasers available for gynecologic use include CO_2, argon, potassium-titanyl-phosphate (KTP), and neodymium: Yttrium-aluminum-garnet (Nd-YAG). These have the ability to vaporize, cut, and, to varying degrees, coagulate tissue. Since, the equipment is expensive and its use needs special training laser is not widely used.

26.5.3 Ultrasonic Energy

The Harmonic Scalpel (Ethicon Endosurgery) uses vibration at the rate of 55,000 cycles per second as an energy source to break hydrogen bonds in tissue, resulting in cutting or coaptation of vessels. The Harmonic Scalpel is available as a 5 mm rounded scalpel with a blunt or hooked edge or as a 5 to 10 mm Harmonic Ace, which can be used to grasp tissue. Their use is advantageous as they result in minimal lateral thermal spread of energy, and there is no risk of electrical injury. Hence, it is fast replacing electrocautery in modern laparoscopic surgeries.

26.5.4 Staplers

The endo-GIA, originally designed for gastrointestinal anastomosis, is used in gynecologic laparoscopy as a stapling device for securing and dividing tissue. When the jaws of the instrument are closed over the tissue and the grip is fired, six staggered rows of staples, 3 cm in length and 1 cm in width, are placed. A knife blade simultaneously divides the tissue, leaving three rows of staples on each side of the incision.

26.5.5 Vascular Clips

Endoscopic vascular clips may be used to achieve hemostasis for bleeding vessels or pedicles. These offer the advantage of being used near vital structures to avoid lateral thermal injury by energy devices.

26.6 OPERATION THEATER SET-UP

The operating room should be sufficiently large to accommodate a variety of equipment, preferably 20 × 20 feet. Ceiling mounted instrument carts avoid gas tubing and electrical wires on the floor (Fig. 26.20). Suction irrigation device can be kept on a separate trolley for avoiding spillage of irrigation fluid on other equipment.

The equipment can be positioned according to the surgeons' preference.

One convenient positioning is to have a ceiling mounted high definition digital monitor placed at the leg end of the table on the right side of the patient. The theater nurse can occupy the space between the legs of the patient and can view the ceiling mounted digital monitor placed at the head end of the patient. Since, most of the gynecological surgical procedures necessitate use of instruments for vaginal manipulation, one trolley can be kept at the leg end of the patient for vaginal instruments. Laparoscopy instruments can be placed by the side of the surgeon (Fig. 26.21).

The ceiling mounted instrument cart should have a high definition digital camera (3 chip camera), carbon dioxide insufflator, Xenon light source, morcellator, endomat, harmonic generator, diathermy unit (Autocon II 400), pneumatic sequential compression device for DVT prevention and SCB computer for controlling the equipment remotely (Fig. 26.20).

26.6.1 Patient Positioning

Whenever vaginal manipulation is deemed necessary or is anticipated, the patient should be positioned in a semi-lithotomy position. The legs must be properly padded and supported. The legs should be positioned in such a way that the thigh makes a 160° angle with the abdomen. This will allow free movement of operating instruments. The modern stirrups like OR Direct allow easy positioning of legs by the surgeon (Fig. 26.22). The table should have capabilities for at least 45 degree Trendelenburg and reverse Trendelenburg positions, preferably motorized. The height of the table should be in the lowest position so that the patient's abdomen is below the waist of the surgeon. Short surgeons may still need stepping stools to achieve this.

26.7 COMPLICATIONS OF LAPAROSCOPY

Instrumentation in laparoscopy is often complicated and may lead to additional hazards. Good surgical training including

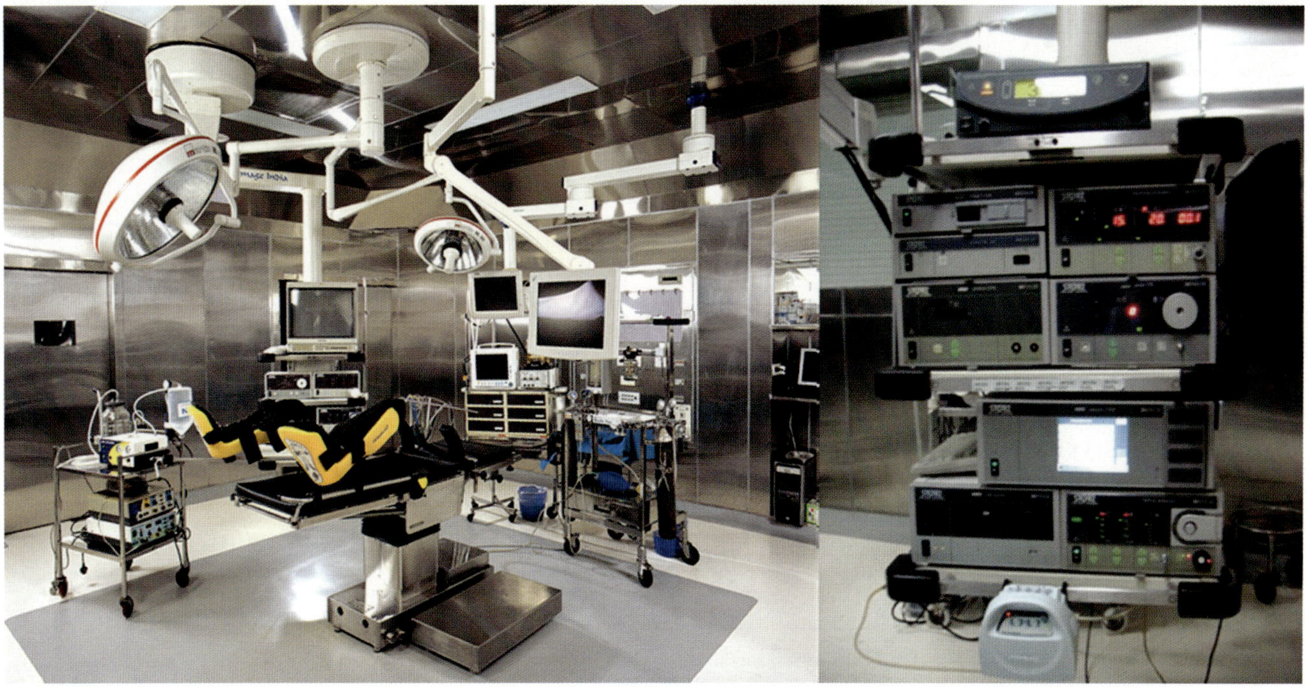

Fig. 26.20: Ceiling mounted instrument carts and monitor. Instrument cart is shown on the right side

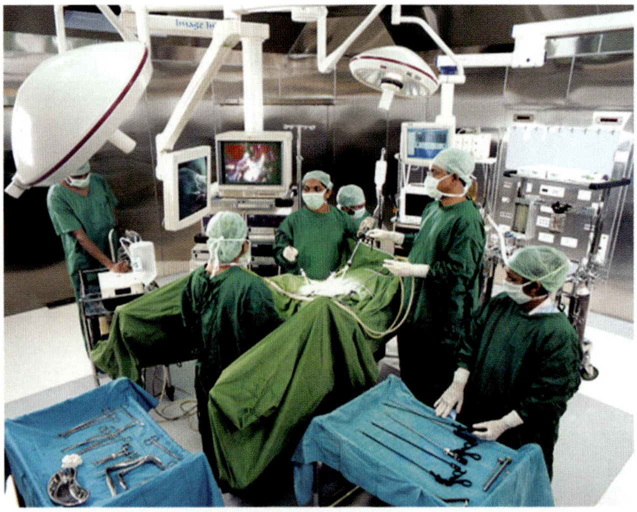

Fig. 26.21: Laparoscopy team

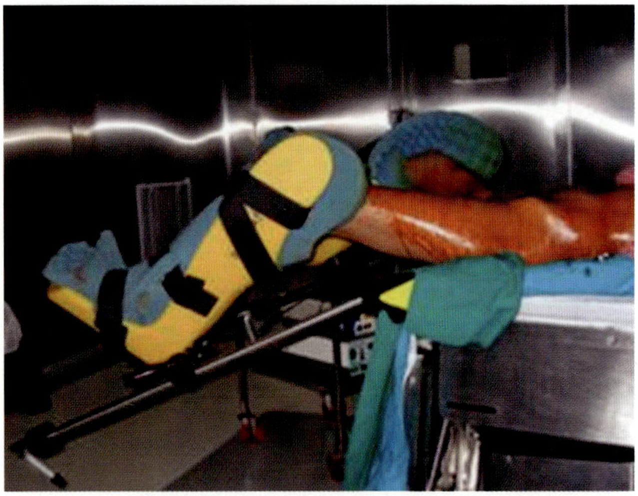

Fig. 26.22: Patient positioning

knowledge of instruments and techniques is very important before starting laparoscopic surgery. Overlooking these essential aspects is the reason for complications. Overall surgical risk is lower for laparoscopic procedures than laparotomy.

26.7.1 Risk Factors

1. **Obesity:** Thick abdominal wall makes insufflation as well as trocar entry difficult. Increased amount of extraperitoneal fat also add to the difficulty.
2. **Age:** As the age increases, concomitant problems like cardiovascular disease will also be present, which increase anesthetic risk.
3. **Previous abdominal surgery:** Adhesions involving bowel loops will be present in more than 20% of the patients who have had previous abdominal surgeries. Adherent bowel loops are at risk of injury by the Veress needle as well as trocars.

26.7.2 Pneumoperitoneum Related Complications

Gas Embolism

Gas embolism is one of the dangerous complications of laparoscopy. The incidence of gas embolism is much less when carbon dioxide is used for insufflation. Carbon dioxide is 200 times more soluble than air. Immediately after entering the circulation it will be converted to carbonic acid which dissociates to bicarbonate and hydrogen ions. However, carbonic acid formed in the peritoneal surface will cause shoulder pain postoperatively. Escape of large amounts of carbon dioxide can cause embolism. Various factors affect the incidence of gas embolism as well as other complications of pneumoperitoneum.

Insufflation volume and rate: The total volume of gas to be insufflated for introducing the needle is 2-2.5 liters. The rate of gas flow initially is set at 1 liter/minute and later may be increased to 2.5 -3 liters/minute. The intra-abdominal pressure at the time of Veress needle insertion is kept at 20 mm of Hg to help the insertion. After inserting the primary trocar and telescope, the pressure should be reduced to 12 mm of Hg. Maintaining intra-abdominal pressure more than 12 mm of Hg while performing surgical procedures can increase the risk of gas embolism as well as reduction of venous return and cardiovascular compromise. The capnograph will show increased end-tidal CO_2 level when there is hypercarbia due to prolonged absorption of CO_2 and restriction of diaphragmatic movement. Hence, it is mandatory that the anesthesiologist should monitor the end-tidal CO_2, heart rate, heart sounds as well as the color of the blood so that the early signs of CO_2 retention can be diagnosed. Sudden unexplained hypotension, cardiac arrhythmia, cyanosis and heart murmurs should raise the suspicion of gas embolism. There will be a sudden drop in CO_2 level when there is gas embolism or pulmonary embolism. If embolism is suspected or diagnosed, the surgeon should immediately evacuate the CO_2 from the peritoneal cavity and the patient should be kept in the left lateral position with the head end of the table below the level of the heart. A large bore central venous line can be inserted so that the gas can be aspirated from the heart.

Cardiac Arrhythmias

Hypercarbia and acidemia can cause cardiac arrhythmias. Maintaining a low intra-abdominal pressure < 12 mm of Hg greatly reduces the incidence of hypercarbia (CO_2 pressure > 65 mm of Hg).

Gastric Reflux and Aspiration

The stomach must be decompressed if distended. Always a cuffed endotracheal tube should be used. Obese patients and those with hiatus hernia are prone for aspiration. Use of preoperative *metoclopramide* along with H_2 blockers will reduce the risk of aspiration.

Extraperitoneal Insufflation

Extraperitoneal insufflation of gas usually occurs due to inadvertent placement of the insufflation needle in the pre-peritoneal space. Hence, checking proper placement of the insufflation needle as described earlier is important. Since, maintaining intra-abdominal pressure above 12 mm of Hg during the surgical procedure will push gas into the extraperitoneal space around cannula sites, it is mandatory that the pressure be kept at 12 mm of Hg or less. Mild subcutaneous emphysema does not need any aggressive management. If the edema extends to the neck, pneumomediastinum or pneumothorax might result. Pneumothorax can be treated by intercostal drainage.

26.7.3 Complications of Electrosurgery

Electrical injuries can occur due to direct or indirect electrical trauma. Direct thermal injury occurs due to direct extension of thermal effect when the zone of vaporization or coagulation extends to the neighboring structures like ureter, bowel, or urinary bladder. Bipolar instruments reduce the incidence of thermal injury, but will not completely avoid it. To avoid unintended activation of electrodes, the surgeon should be in control of the activation of the electrode. Electrosurgical instruments should not be retained inside the abdomen when not in use. While in use, the uninsulated part of the electrosurgical instrument should be completely under vision. Otherwise part of the electrode tip touching the viscera may not be seen and hence will not be noticed.

Thermal injury to the bladder, bowel or ureter should be managed immediately. Laceration injuries should be managed by suturing. If a zone of coagulative necrosis is identified at the time of laparoscopy, wide excision and repair should be done as the area of thermal damage might extend wider than the area of necrosis.

Thermal injury to the bowel can be unnoticed at the time of surgery. Necrosis of the site of injury and consequent leakage and peritonitis can occur from 2-10 days after the procedure. Hence, it is advisable to warn patients that they should report if they have pain, distention of abdomen or any other unusual symptom.

26.7.4 Vascular Injuries

Injury to the Abdominal Wall Vessels

Both superficial and deep inferior epigastric vessels can get injured while introducing secondary trocars. The superficial inferior epigastric vessel can be transilluminated and avoided. The deep inferior epigastric vessels lie between the rectus muscle and the peritoneum and cannot be transilluminated. It could be identified inside the abdomen lateral to the medial umbilical ligament which is formed by the obliterated umbilical artery (Refer Chapter 1, Fig. 1.16). Accessory trocars should be introduced under vision, avoiding the superficial as well as the deep inferior epigastric vessels. In the case of accidental injury to the vessel, it can be coagulated with bipolar forceps introduced through another accessory port. If this method fails, a Foley catheter can be introduced through the cannula which injured the vessel and tamponade can be effected by inflating the bulb and pulling on the catheter after removing the cannula. The Foley catheter can be removed after effectively controlling hemorrhage which may take a few hours.

Injury to Major Vessels

Major vessel injury is a catastrophic event in laparoscopy. Injury to the aorta, inferior vena cava, common iliac vessels, external iliac vessels and superior mesenteric vessels has been reported. Several factors have been identified as contributing to the injuries. Inexperience of the operator, dull trocar, inadequate pneumoperitoneum, failure to stabilize the abdominal wall, perpendicular or lateral direction of trocar, etc. have been suggested as causing these vessel injuries.

Resorting to proper technique is important in the prevention of these injuries. The Veress needle should be tested for its spring action as well as its patency before use. Patient should be in supine position while introducing the Veress needle as well as the primary trocar. Trendelenburg position will cause the aortic bifurcation to be rotated anteriorly and is more likely to be injured. Tilt should be given only after the insertion of the primary trocar and telescope. The needle should be held like a dart and thrust towards the center of the pelvis after raising the abdominal wall sufficiently outwards. The needle should not be directed perpendicular to the abdominal wall. The valve of the needle should be kept in open position. Aspiration of the needle should be done to exclude unintended placement inside vessel or bowel. When pre-peritoneal insufflation occurs, multiple attempts may be resorted to with increased risk of injuries. It is advisable to proceed to open laparoscopy (Hassan's technique) in such instances.

In the event of a suspicion of major vessel injury due to the presence of blood gushing through the Veress needle or cannula the abdomen should be immediately opened through a midline vertical incision. Bleeding should be controlled by digital pressure or with mops till the vascular surgeon comes for help.

26.7.5 Urinary Tract Injuries

Bladder Injury

The urinary bladder can be injured while introducing the accessory trocar if it is pulled up as in the case of previous cesarean section, myomectomy or endometriosis and when the bladder is full. The bladder can be lacerated while performing laparoscopic hysterectomy especially if the anatomy is distorted due to adhesions from a previous surgery. Suspected injury should be confirmed by methylene blue instillation. All injuries diagnosed during the procedure should be managed by suturing.

Thermal injuries may go unnoticed during surgery, but should be suspected if the patient shows any of the following symptoms:

- Hematuria
- Decreased urine output
- Mass in the abdominal wall
- Peritonitis

The bladder should be emptied before introducing the needle or trocar to prevent injury to a distended bladder. Before introducing the secondary trocar the upper limit of the bladder should be identified especially when the anatomy is distorted by previous surgery or tumors.

Trocar injuries which are very small, < 1 cm in width can be managed by postoperative continuous bladder drainage for about 7 days. Lacerations of the bladder wall should be repaired either through the laparoscope or by laparotomy. Injuries near the trigone should be sutured after inserting ureteric stents to prevent injury to the intramural portion of the ureter. The usual injuries occur in the region of the dome which does not need such precaution. Thermal injuries should be inspected through the cystoscope to make out the extent of thermal damage.

Ureteric Injury

Ureteric injuries can occur in patients with extensive endometriosis, pelvic inflammatory disease or broad ligament myomas. Even though ureteric injuries can occur anywhere in the course of the ureter, majority of them were seen in the vicinity of the uterosacral ligaments.

The common situations in which ureteric injuries occur are the following:

1. While an adherent ovary is being dissected from the pelvic side wall
2. When the uterosacral ligament is transected
3. While coagulating or transecting the uterine arteries
4. When trying to control bleeding in the pelvis
5. While enucleating a broad ligament myoma
6. Releasing endometriotic adhesion or coagulating endometriotic implants over the peritoneum in relation to the ureter.

To prevent ureteric injuries, the ureter should be identified before dissection. Aqua-dissection should be preferred over sharp dissection near the ureter. To prevent thermal injury due to lateral spread of heat, always use bipolar diathermy near the ureter and avoid monopolar diathermy. Even when using bipolar diathermy, try to include only small chunks of tissue. Trying to coagulate large amount of tissue with bipolar diathermy will cause more lateral spread of heat and if the ureter is nearby it can be damaged. Catheterization of the ureter with illuminated stents can be resorted to when ureteric damage is anticipated, as in open surgery.

Most ureteric injuries are diagnosed postoperatively when urine collects in the peritoneal cavity and distends the abdomen. Thermal injuries can cause ureteric stenosis which will lead to hydronephrosis and hydroureter several weeks after the surgery.

Injuries sustained during surgery can be diagnosed by injecting indigocarmine. These injuries should be repaired by suturing the lacerated ends over a stent passed retrograde through the bladder. Minimal damage might heal over a ureteric stent without suturing.

Postoperatively injuries can be diagnosed by IVP. Urologist should be consulted and injury should be repaired.

26.7.6 Gastrointestinal Injuries

Gastrointestinal injuries can occur during laparoscopic surgery. The stomach, colon or small bowel can be injured. Bowel injuries can occur due to the presence of bowel adhesions sustained during previous laparotomies. The stomach can be injured when it is unduly distended due to improper intubation. In the presence of inadvertent intubation into the stomach, it should be decompressed before proceeding to Veress insertion. The colon can get injured while placing the accessory trocars. If intestinal or gastric injuries are detected immediate suturing is required with either laparotomy or laparoscopy depending upon the expertise available. When bowel adhesions are anticipated, preoperative mechanical preparation should be done.

26.7.7 Neurological Injury

Neurological injuries usually occur due to improper positioning of the patient. The common peroneal nerve can get compressed against the stirrup. Excessive flexion or external rotation of the hip can overstretch the femoral or the sciatic nerve. Proper positioning is important in preventing these types of injuries. The arm can be kept in the adducted position by the side of the body or by proper padding to prevent brachial plexus injuries. The legs should not be unduly abducted or laterally rotated. Most injuries recover spontaneously. Full recovery usually occurs in 3-5 months time. Recovery can be hastened by physiotherapy.

26.8 OPERATIVE LAPAROSCOPIC PROCEDURES

The advances achieved by refinement of technical skills and technological improvements in endoscopic equipment have made possible most of the gynecological procedures to be done laparoscopically. A few of the procedures commonly resorted to are discussed below.

26.8.1 Ectopic Pregnancy

Conservative surgical treatment via operative laparoscopy is preferred over laparotomy except for cases in which the patient is hemodynamically unstable due to internal hemorrhage.

Salpingostomy

The contemporary surgical approach in a hemodynamically stable patient is operative laparoscopy. With adequate practice and surgical experience in operative endoscopy, most patients with ectopic pregnancies can be treated by laparoscopy, regardless of the gestation size, location, number of gestations or the presence of tubal rupture.[1]

Instruments

Apart from the usual laparoscopic diagnostic instrumentation the following instruments are required.

- Atraumatic grasper
- Unipolar needle
- 5 mm suction irrigation cannula
- Microbipolar forceps
- Scissors
- 10 mm suction

Technique

1. A 10 mm primary trocar at the umbilicus and three 5 mm suprapubic trocars are introduced.
2. Clean the blood clots and fluid blood from the pelvis with a 5 mm suction irrigation cannula. Blood in the peritoneal cavity is the greatest enemy of vision. A 10 mm suction irrigation cannula may be used when there are blood clots.
3. Identify the affected fallopian tube and the ectopic site (Fig. 26.23). The unaffected fallopian tube may also be distended with blood and should be differentiated from the one harboring the ectopic.

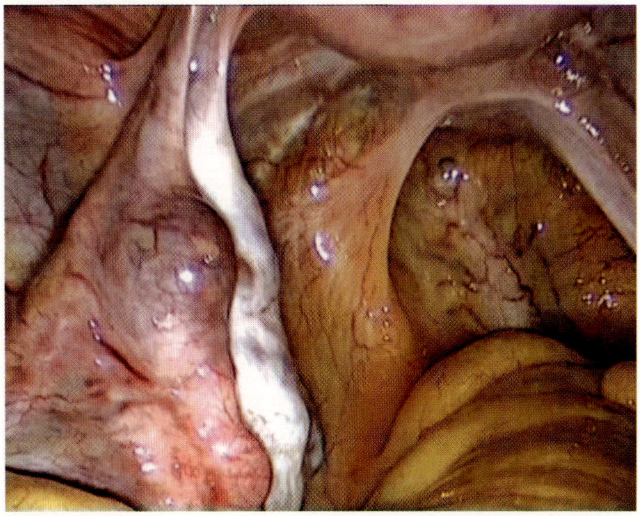

Fig. 26.23: Laparoscopy depicting an ampullary ectopic pregnancy

4. Introduce the atraumatic grasper through the ipsilateral port and hold the tube just proximal to the ectopic.
5. Introduce a unipolar needle through the contralateral secondary port and try to make an imaginary incision exactly on the anti-mesenteric border.
6. Activate the electrode after proper setting of diathermy in the cutting mode and make an incision of 1 to 1.5 cm starting from the bulging portion of the tube (Figs 26.24A to D). Always keep a small air gap between the tip of the electrode and the tube to produce a small spark.
7. Remove the unipolar needle and introduce the 5 mm suction irrigation cannula. Use aqua-dissection to dislodge the ectopic from the endosalpinx. The extruding product of conception is removed with a grasper taking care to avoid injury to the endosalpinx. Sometimes products of conception (POC) will be adherent to the implantation site with vascular connections. This is coagulated before removing the tissue. With suction irrigation all floating chorionic tissues are identified and removed.
8. Irrigate the base of the ectopic with saline and coagulate with a microbipolar forceps (Fig. 26.25), only if an active bleeder can be identified. Oozing from the tube is common but usually stops spontaneously.

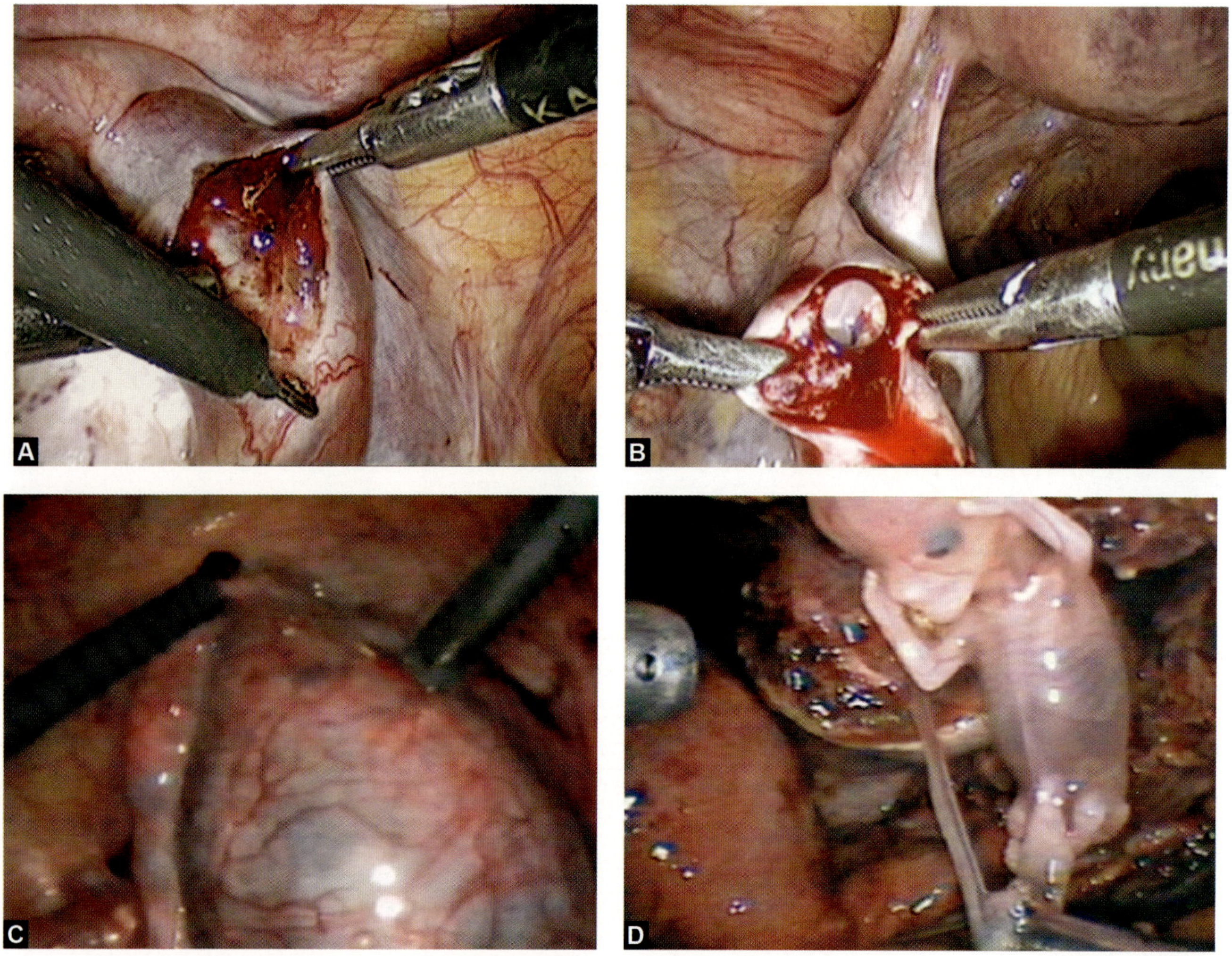

Figs 26.24A to D: Laparoscopic salpingostomy showing products of conception (A and B). Laparoscopic salpingostomy for ampullary ectopic, live fetus visible after salpingostomy (C and D)

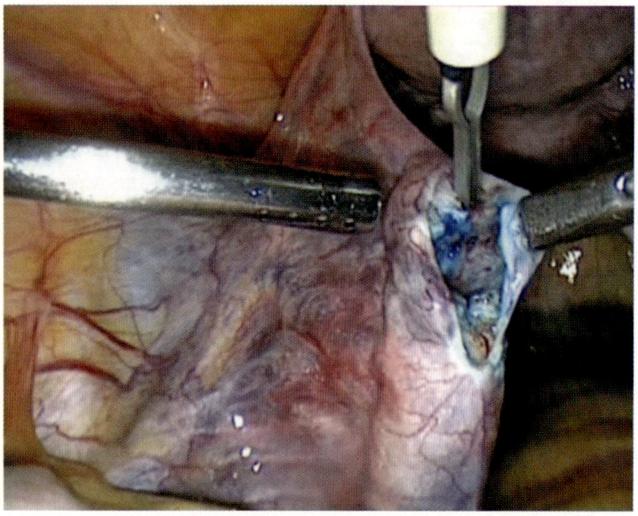

Fig. 26.25: Achieving hemostasis with microbipolar forceps

9. The edges of the tube can be held in approximation with an atraumatic grasper (Fig. 26.26) for a few minutes.
10. Remove the products of conception through either a 5 or 10 mm cannula. Clean the upper abdomen with the suction irrigation cannula in the reverse Trendelenburg position
11. Do chromopertubation to see the patency of the other tube. Remove atraumatic forceps and look for any active bleeding (Fig. 26.27).

Difficulties

Removal of blood clots: 10 mm suction cannula can be used when the clots cannot be sucked out with 5 mm suction irrigation cannula. Another technique to remove clots with 5 mm suction irrigation cannula is as follows. First push the trocar sleeve deep into the peritoneal cavity and then try to

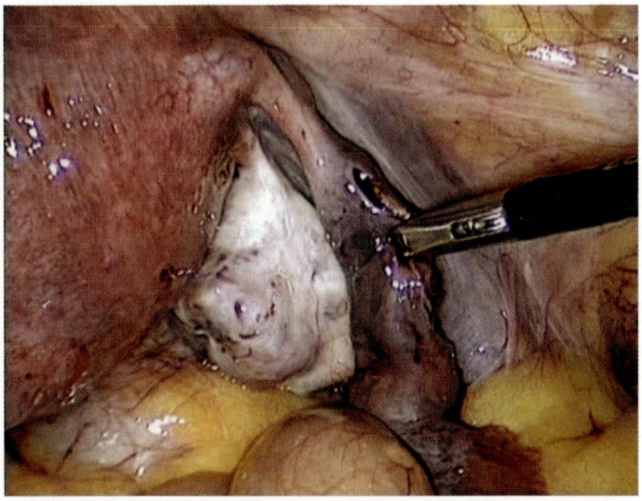

Fig. 26.26: Approximation of tubal edges with atraumatic grasper

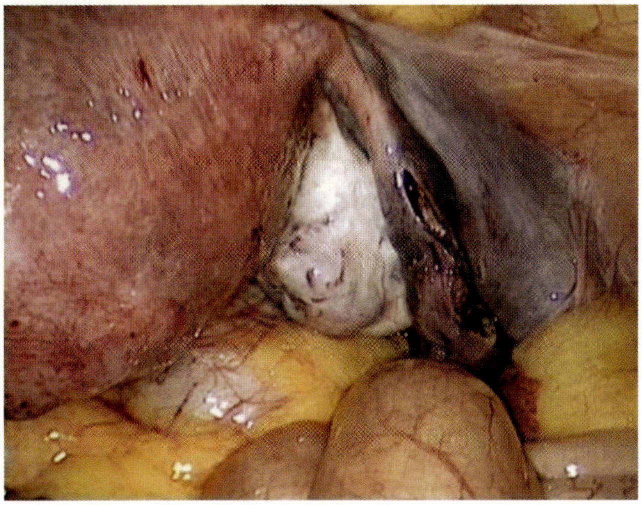

Fig. 26.27: Salpingostomy right side

suck the blood clot first in to the sleeve with the suction irrigation cannula and then suck the clot from the sleeve. This technique is repeated till all the clots are removed.

Active bleeding from the base: Do not debride the implantation site of ectopic aggressively with a grasper. Irrigate the base profusely and remove only the floating chorionic tissue. Coagulate any visible bleeding vessel while irrigation is on. Use 1.5% glycine in difficult situations for irrigation because one can coagulate the bleeder while irrigation is flowing. Coagulation of mesosalpingeal vessels feeding the ectopic site is the alternative.

Active bleeding from the tubal edges usually results from an oblique incision of the tube. Always make a perpendicular incision in the anti-mesenteric border. Sometimes the coagulated tissue sticks to the forceps and starts bleeding when the bipolar is taken out from the coagulated tissue. Hence, it is better to keep the diathermy pedal pressed while the forceps is taken out. Occasionally the bleeding site will not be visible because the implantation site is proximal to the salpingostomy site and hence always start the salpingostomy incision from the beginning of the ectopic bulge on the tube. Bleeding will be very difficult to control if the ectopic is live or has already eroded the serosa. Salpingectomy is required if bleeding cannot be controlled by the above measures. Few studies have proved that if the contralateral tube is healthy, the pregnancy rate is not affected whether salpingostomy or salpingectomy is done on the affected side.

Follow-up

Around 5-10% of patients who had undergone salpingostomy will have persistent ectopic.[2] This is because some amount of live chorionic tissue remains active at the site of ectopic. This can be minimized if care is taken to remove all floating chorionic tissue during salpingostomy. The simplest way of following up patients who have undergone salpingostomy is performing a sensitive pregnancy test a week after surgery. If the pregnancy test is positive, β-hCG is to be measured. Those with hCG >1000 mIU/ml, a week after surgery are probably at risk. The patient is given Inj. Methotrexate 1 mg/kg body weight if β-hCG and ultrasound scan suggest persistent ectopic.

Segmental Excision

Segmental excision containing ectopic is preferable for an isthmic pregnancy and an eroded or partially ruptured ampullary ectopic. It may also be resorted to when bleeding from the salpingostomy site cannot be controlled.

Technique

1. Grasp the tube with an atraumatic grasper at the site of ectopic.
2. Use a bipolar forceps to coagulate the tube proximal and distal to the ectopic. Divide the coagulated area with scissors.
3. Then coagulate and divide the mesosalpinx of the tube containing the ectopic in small serial steps till the segment is separated.
4. Remove the ectopic and clean the pelvis as already described.
5. Check the patency of the other tube if further child-bearing is anticipated.

Salpingectomy

Salpingectomy is done when the tube is ruptured, damaged or when the patient needs sterilization. It is also an option when there is recurrence of ectopic on the same tube.

1. Grasp the tube near the proximal end with a grasper introduced through the ipsilateral port. The tube is kept under tension. Coagulate the tube close to the cornua with a bipolar obliquely including mesosalpinx (Figs 26.28 and 26.29).

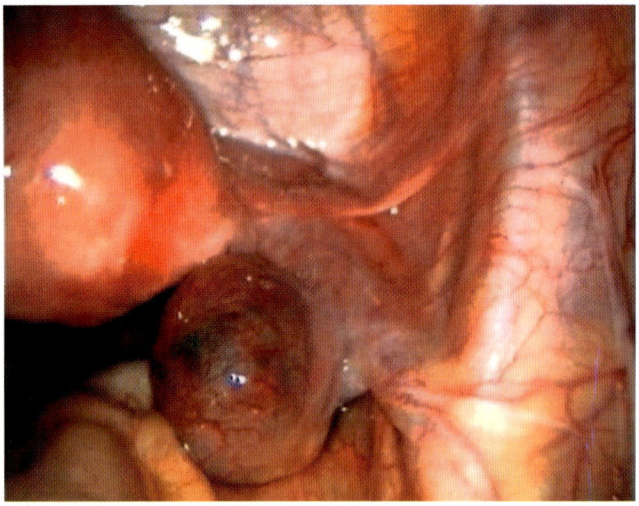

Fig. 26.28: Laparoscopy depicting an ampullary ectopic pregnancy distorting the tube

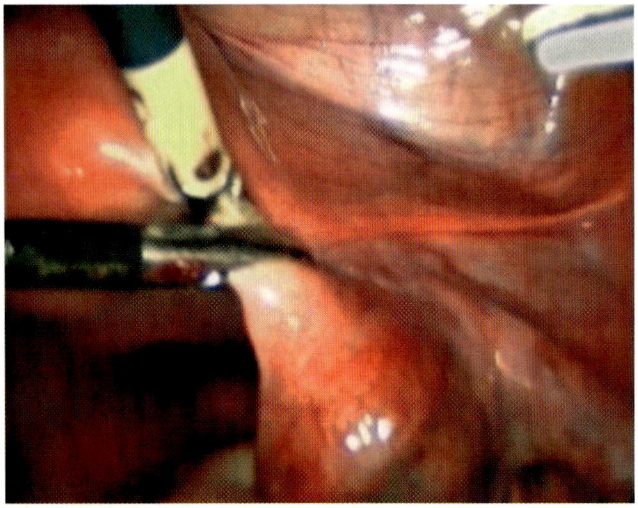

Fig. 26.29: Coagulation and division of tube from the medial end

2. Divide the coagulated area with scissors in small steps (Fig. 26.30).
3. Continue alternate coagulation and division till salpingectomy is completed (Fig. 26.31).

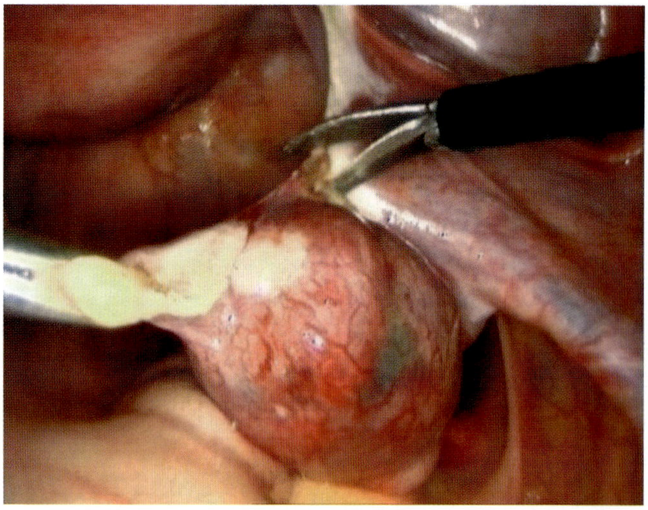

Fig. 26.30: Division of tube with scissors from medial end

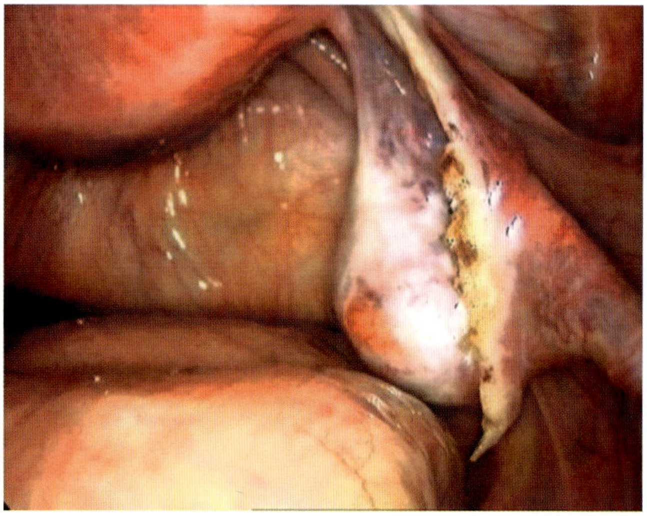

Fig. 26.31: After surgery (salpingectomy)

4. A 5 mm telescope is introduced through the left secondary portal. The light source and camera are then connected to this telescope. The 10 mm telescope in the umbilical port is replaced with a 10 mm claw forceps and the tissue is retrieved viewing through the 5 mm telescope.
5. Lavage the upper abdomen in reverse Trendelenburg position to remove collected blood in the sub-diaphragmatic space.
6. Check the whole length of salpingectomy site for hemostasis.

Chronic Ectopic

Occasional cases of ectopic pregnancy are diagnosed when a pelvic hemetocele has already formed. The hematocele will be covered with omental and rectosigmoid adhesions.

Instruments

Since the fleshy clots cannot be removed with 5 mm instruments, the following additional 10 mm instruments are required.

- 10 mm spoon forceps
- 10 mm suction cannula

Technique

Clean the pelvis with a 5 mm suction irrigation. Suck out all fluid blood if present. Release the omental or small bowel adhesions covering the hematocele by blunt dissection. Do an adhesiolysis by blunt dissection with a 5 mm suction irrigation cannula and identify the tubes and ovaries. The tube containing ectopic is usually a ruptured one. Remove all fleshy clots with a 10 mm spoon or 10 mm suction cannula. The organized blood clot might have formed a pseudosac in the POD. It is slowly peeled off with a 10 mm spoon forceps. Salpingectomy of the tube containing ectopic is now performed after releasing the tube from the ovary and other structures.

Difficulties

Poor visibility is one of the most common difficulties encountered. It is due to the poor lighting of the peritoneal cavity. Since the pelvis contains lots of blood clots, it absorbs light. First try to suck out all the fluid and wash the peritoneum with irrigating fluid so that clean peritoneum can reflect enough light. Increasing the intensity of light or increasing the gain of the camera can further improve the lighting condition. Sometimes sucking the organized clots with 10 mm cannula is difficult because it sucks out bowel and tubal fimbria also. If the 10 mm cannula has a side port with stop cock, it can be opened to release the bowel. In the absence of a side port, the suction tube needs to be detached to release the vacuum.

Reproductive Outcome

A meta-analysis of 9 studies involving 2,635 patients compared the reproductive outcome of salpingostomy versus salpingectomy.[3] This included 528 patients in the conservative group and 1246 patients in the salpingectomy group desiring fertility. The rate of subsequent intrauterine pregnancy was 53% in conservative group and 49.3% in the salpingectomy group. The recurrent ectopic rates were 14.8% and 9.9%, respectively. Another meta-analysis reported better reproductive outcome after conservative surgery in women with solitary patent tube. Among the 176 women attempting to conceive, there were 54.5% intrauterine pregnancies and 20.5% recurrent ectopic.[3]

Many other factors influence the subsequent fertility rate, apart from the type of surgical approach. History of infertility was found to be associated with decreased fertility rate.[4] Some studies have found that the status of the contralateral tube at the time of surgery is related directly to the subsequent fertility, regardless of the surgical modality used.[5] Silva et al reported prior tubal damage to be associated significantly with decreased pregnancy rate; 79% pregnancy rate in group without prior damage and 42% in the group with prior tubal damage.

Majority of spontaneous pregnancies after surgical treatment of ectopic pregnancy occur in the first 18 months.

26.8.2 Ovarian Cysts

Laparoscopic surgery has become the gold standard for the evaluation and treatment of benign adnexal cystic masses. The majority of women in the reproductive age group have benign adnexal masses. One of the major benefits of laparoscopic approach to adnexal masses is avoiding over treatment and unnecessary laparotomy. Most adnexal masses are benign. Malignancy rate is 7 to 13% among premenopausal and 8 to 45% among postmenopausal women.[6] The incidence of unsuspected ovarian cancer at laparoscopy has been shown to be only 0.04% by Nezhat et al[7] and in a 1990 survey of the American Association of Gynecologic Laparoscopists.[8] In reproductive-age women, the outcome of laparoscopically managed cysts which are less than 10 cm in size has been uniformly favorable. Decision for laparoscopic treatment of adnexal masses is taken based on the patient's age, pelvic examination, sonographic imaging and serum markers.

Intraoperative Evaluation

Treatment of benign-appearing adnexal masses must follow a protocol of cytologic examination of pelvis and cyst fluid, frozen section of a biopsy specimen and removal of the mass for histologic examination. Aspirating a cyst and vaporizing or coagulating the capsule is not acceptable alternatives. Clinical examination and the results of the preoperative work-up often indicate the benign or malignant nature.

After the upper abdomen and pelvis are examined, the cyst contents are aspirated. Once the capsule is opened, the interior of the capsule is examined and suspicious areas are biopsied and then the tissue is sent for frozen section if available. The entire cyst capsule is removed to search for an early carcinoma that may escape gross detection. Whether to do an oophorectomy or cystectomy depends on the patient's age and the characteristics of the mass. If malignancy were to be detected, immediate surgical staging should be performed by laparotomy.

Ovarian Cystectomy

Ovarian cystectomy consists of removal of the intact cyst with limited trauma to the residual ovarian tissue. Alternatively, the cyst fluid can be drained to minimize spillage and facilitate removal. The intact removal of a cyst greater than 5 cm is difficult laparoscopically. Aspiration before removal of large cysts is more practical. It is accomplished by the passage of a 5 mm trocar and sleeve (Fig. 26.32). The trocar is placed into the cyst and then replaced with the suction-irrigator (Fig. 26.33). The aspirate is sent for cytologic examination and the ovary is freed from adhesions to the lateral pelvic wall, uterus, or bowel. The cyst and pelvis are irrigated continuously, especially if the cyst is a benign cystic teratoma, mucinous cystadenoma, or an endometrioma. The most dependant portion of the cyst wall is opened and the internal surface is inspected. If excrescences or papillae are found, biopsy and frozen section should be done.

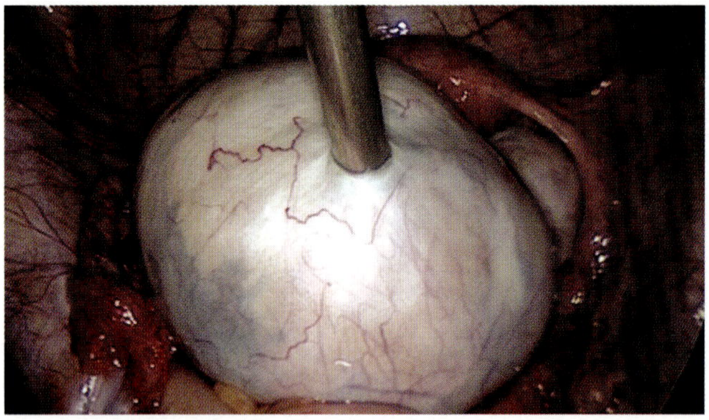

Fig. 26.32: Cyst puncture with 5 mm trocar

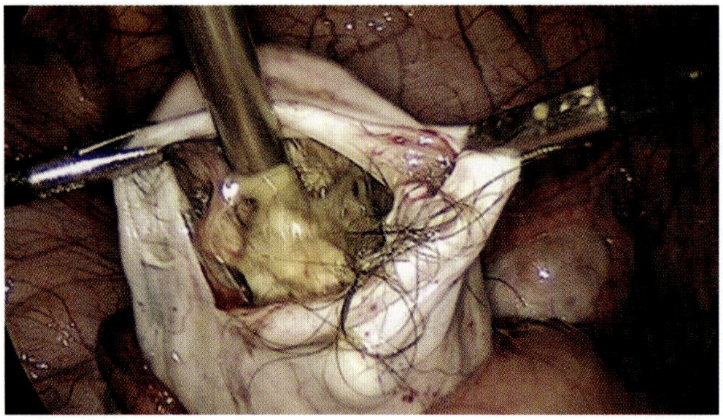

Fig. 26.33: Cyst aspiration with 5 mm suction irrigation cannula

If the cyst wall cannot be identified, the edge of the ovarian incision can be "freshened" with scissors and the resulting clean edge reveals the different layers. If this does not free the capsule, the base of the cyst is grasped and traction is applied to the cyst with counter traction to the ovary (Fig. 26.34). The entire cyst or portions of the wall may be adherent to the ovary, requiring sharp dissection to free it completely. Teratomas often can be excised intact, but if the cyst ruptures, the resulting contamination is greater than if the cyst were opened and aspirated. The atraumatic development of the plane between the cyst wall and the ovarian tissue is an important first step. Occasionally enucleation may be difficult if the opening is made at the thinnest portion of the cyst. In these cases an elliptical incision is made on the ovarian tissue surrounding the thinned out area. The graspers are now used to separate the cyst along with the thinned out ovarian tissue from the ovary. This technique is also very useful when multiple small cysts are present.

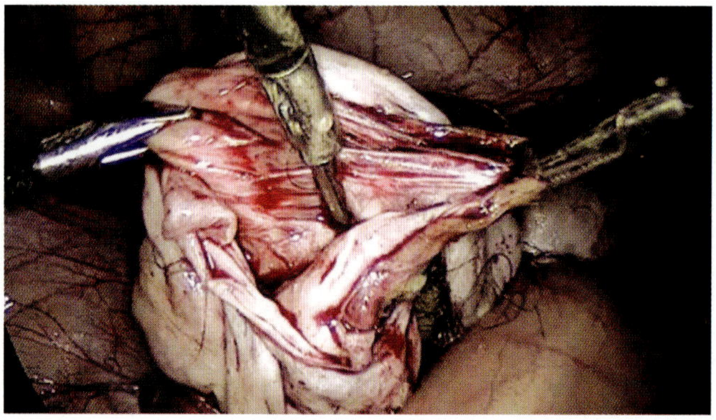

Fig. 26.34: Cyst enucleation with traction and counter-traction

Usually there will not be any active bleeding from the ovary except for generalized ooze. Coagulation will not be needed at all. If there is obvious bleeding, look near the ovarian ligaments or the hilum of ovary to identify the bleeder, which can be controlled by bipolar coagulation. The ovary is now reconstructed. It rarely requires suturing. The edges of the ovary are held together in a manner which gives the best shape for the ovary and exposes the healthy ovarian surface to the fimbrial end of the tube (Fig. 26.35). If the dead space cannot be compressed by this maneuver, the ovary is rolled on itself and kept pressed against the pelvic sidewall for few minutes. The peritoneal cavity is now lavaged with several liters of warm Ringer lactate. The upper abdomen, especially the subdiaphragmatic space is washed in a reverse Trendelenburg position. The ovary is now inspected for complete hemostasis.

In majority of the situations, the ovary can be reconstructed by just pressing the edges together for a few minutes, taking the advantages of natural fibrin formed at

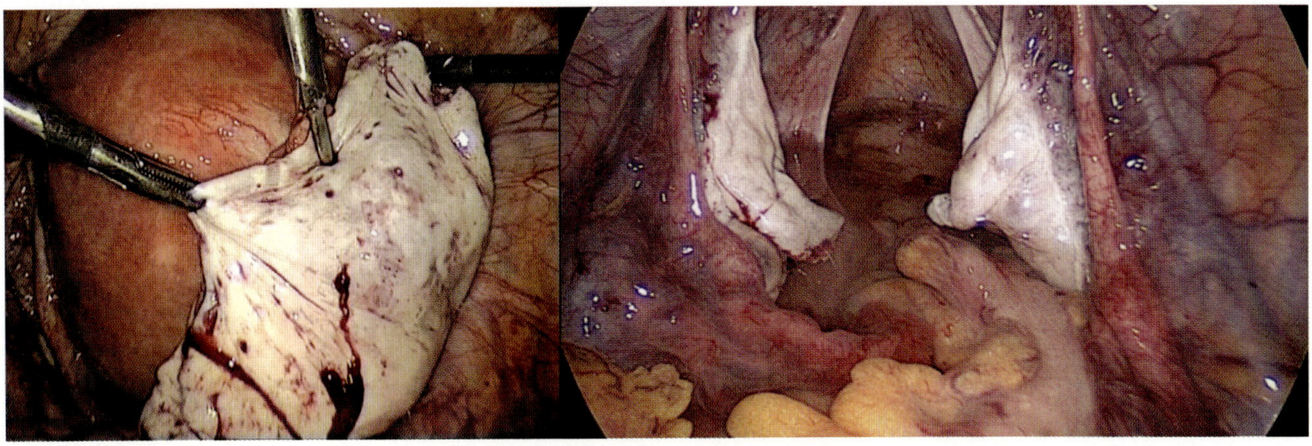

Fig. 26.35: Ovary reconstruction

the oozing surface. In occasional cases, the ovarian tissue will be partly torn from the ovarian ligament during enucleation. In these cases, a running suture taken through the inner edge of the ovary including the ovarian ligaments with 3-0 vicryl will reconstruct the ovary. It is always better to use the minimum number of sutures.

Tissue Removal

Small cysts can be removed through a 10 mm trocar by grasping with a spoon forceps or claw forceps. Larger cysts can be cut with scissors to make it into a ribbon shape and then removed.

Alternatively the cyst can be put inside an endobag (Fig. 26.36). It is then pulled out along with the 10 mm trocar, after enlarging the trocar wound. Tissue is removed from the endobag before retrieving from the wound to reduce the bulk. It is more convenient to retrieve through a colpotomy.

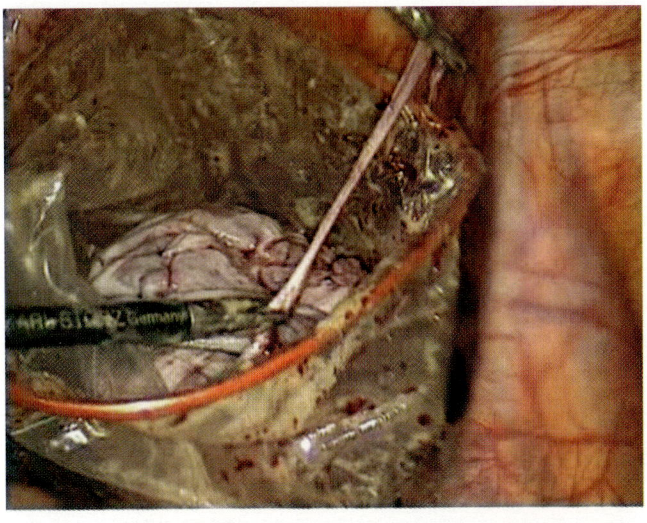

Fig. 26.36: Specimen removal in endobag

Large Ovarian Cysts

Occasionally a clear cyst in a young patient may extend up to or above the umbilicus. If the clinical and ultrasound criteria are suggestive of a benign lesion, a laparoscopic approach may be attempted. Trocar introduction is always difficult, unless the cyst is decompressed. In such cases primary trocar entry is done with an endotip and the cystic mass and peritoneal cavity are inspected for any signs of malignancy. The cyst is then decompressed and oophorectomy is performed. If any signs suspicious of malignancy are found, the procedure can be immediately converted to a laparotomy.

Salpingo-oophorectomy

Oophorectomy is usually performed for an ovarian cyst when the adnexa are not salvageable. If the cyst is adherent, complete ovariolysis is done before attempting oophorectomy. The ureters are identified at the pelvic brim and the distance between the infundibulopelvic ligament and ureters is assessed. The ovary is grasped near the infundibulopelvic ligament and pulled medially with a grasper passed through the contralateral port. A bipolar forceps passed through the ipsilateral port coagulates the stretched infundibulopelvic ligament close to the ovary. Watch for the blanching of tissue and make sure it does not extend to the ureters. The bipolar is removed and a curved scissor is used to incise the peritoneum over the coagulated area to skeletonize the vessels. The bipolar forceps is again introduced and the bare ovarian vessels are coagulated thoroughly. The pedicle is then transected in small steps and any bleeder is immediately coagulated. These steps of alternate coagulation and transection are continued till the cornual end is reached. The ovarian ligament and cornual end of fallopian tube is then divided after coagulation. Alternatively the ovarian ligament and fallopian tube can be divided first, and then proceed to the infundibulopelvic ligament.

The tissue removal technique is same as that for a cystectomy specimen. The peritoneal cavity is then thoroughly lavaged with Ringer's lactate. All the vessels in the pedicles are then reinspected for complete hemostasis.

Paraovarian Cysts

Although the risk of malignancy is low, the paraovarian cysts also should be screened like an ovarian cyst. The paraovarian cyst is punctured with a trocar between the vessels in the mesosalpinx away from the fimbrial end. The decompression of the cyst allows less traumatic enucleation of the cyst. If the cyst is very thick, enucleation from the broad ligament is comparatively easy. The cyst is held firmly with a grasper passed through the contralateral port. The broad ligament is separated from the cyst with a suction irrigation probe. Any fibrous attachments to the ovary are divided with scissors after coagulating with bipolar. After complete enucleation, the edges of the broad ligament are kept pressed with a non-toothed grasper for a few minutes.

26.8.3 Laparoscopic Myomectomy

Myomas are the commonest benign tumor in women. 25% of women over the age of 35 have myomas. Majority of the myomas are asymptomatic. The common indications for treatment are menorrhagia, pelvic pain, pressure on adjacent organs, infertility and habitual abortion. The role of myomas in producing infertility and habitual abortion is not proven. Treatment options for symptomatic myomas are myomectomy or hysterectomy. An increasing number of myomectomies are now being performed laparoscopically. But there are definite limitations for this procedure. Very large myomas or multiple myomas wherein the uterine size is more than 18 weeks are difficult to be operated upon laparoscopically.

Preoperative Investigations

Preoperative evaluation should include assessment of the hematocrit. Clinical assessment of the size and number of myomas are made. Abdominal and transvaginal ultrasound is done to localize and confirm the size of myomas. Myomas more than 4 or 5 in number are difficult to remove laparoscopically.

Hysteroscopy is always done before starting laparoscopy to exclude a submucous myoma. Submucous myomas that project more than 50% into the uterine cavity are removed hysteroscopically.

Instruments

A few special laparoscopic instruments are required for different types of myomectomy. Myoma screws are needed for enucleating myomas. Good sturdy needle holders are needed for suturing. Morcellation requires 12 or 15 mm morcellators.

Procedure

The primary trocar is introduced above the umbilicus if the uterus is more than the size corresponding to 14 weeks of pregnancy. The trocar may be introduced by open laparoscopy if there is not enough space to pass the Veress needle. After introduction of the telescope, a decision is made whether to proceed with a complete laparoscopic myomectomy or a minilap myomectomy, depending on the size and number of myomas. Multiple large myomas are handled by minilap myomectomy. Three 5 mm secondary trocars are now inserted. It may be placed at a higher level than the usual Pfannensteil incision depending on the size of the myomas.

Intramural Myomas

Dilute vasopressin (vasopressin 20 units in 50 cc normal saline) is injected into the serosa and myometrium over the proposed site of myomectomy. An unipolar diathermy needle is used for making the incision over the most protuberant portion of the myoma (Figs 26.37 and 26.38).

A vertical mid line incision is preferred for most myomas. The advantage is lesser amount of bleeding and the greater ease of suturing laparoscopically. The incision is made deep to the myoma cutting the capsule and exposing the myoma (Fig. 26.39). This is necessary to get the correct plane of enucleation. A pure cutting or blended current can be used for making the incision. Blended current produces more smoke. A fine tip unipolar needle produces less smoke. The correct technique is to activate the electrode before touching

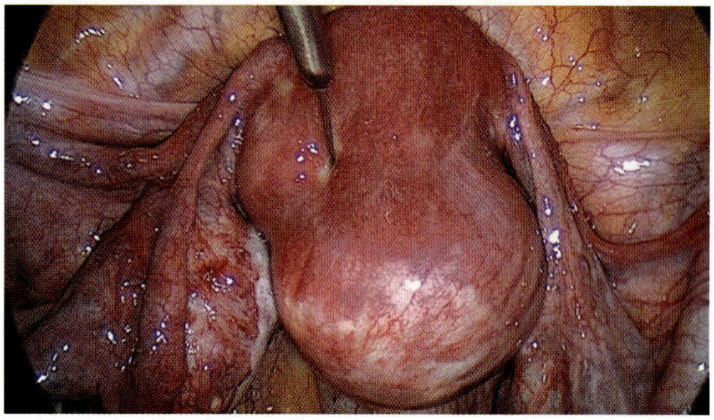

Fig. 26.37: Injection of vasopressin

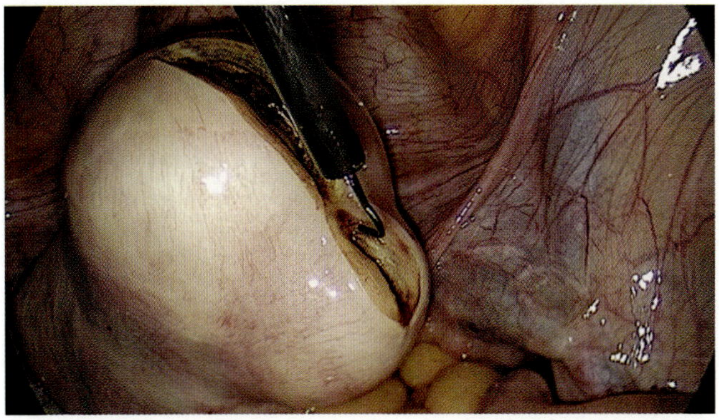

Fig. 26.38: Incision of myometrium with hook electrode

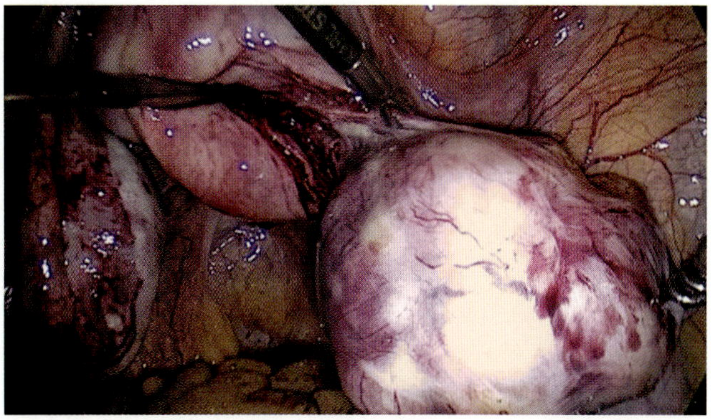

Fig. 26.40: Coagulation of vessels in psuedocapsule

the tissue, so that a small spark can be used for making the incision. Any spurting bleeder can be picked up with a fine tipped insulated grasper and coagulated with unipolar current. Suction irrigation is used to pin point the bleeder.

The myoma is now firmly fixed with a myoma screw. A 5 mm grasper is now used to grasp the myometrium and the pseudocapsule for counter traction (Fig. 26.39).

The myoma is enucleated by traction on the myoma screw and counter traction with the 5 mm grasper. The enucleation is done close to the myoma inside the pseudocapsule to minimize the bleeding. The myoma screw and 5 mm grasper are released and regrasped frequently so that traction and countertraction can be applied to attain enucleation in small steps with minimum injury to the vessels on the pseudocapsule. Any obvious bleeder is coagulated with a unipolar or bipolar forceps. Towards the end of enucleation the vessels that were actually surrounding the capsule are now seen as a vascular pedicle which is coagulated and divided (Fig. 26.40).

The myoma bed is now inspected and any spurting bleeders are identified and coagulated. The aim is not to attain complete hemostasis, which is difficult to attain because most of these bleeders have already retracted into the myometrium. A good technique is to attain hemostasis before completely detaching the myoma from its bed. The myometrium is sutured before morcellation of the myoma. It is preferable to have an intracorporeal suture with 1-0 polyglycolic acid for the myometrial approximation. A needle holder introduced from the right portal grasps the needle and is passed through the myometrium. The tail of the thread is kept in good vision on the right side. The long end is now brought near the tail with the right needle holder and wound twice around a steady grasper from the left portal. The grasper from the left portal grasps the tail of the thread and both instruments are pulled apart to form the first double half knot.

The long end of the thread is held with a grasper from the left portal and twisted around the needle holder from the right portal. The right needle holder grasps the tail end of the thread and both instruments are pulled apart to complete the knot (Fig. 26.41). Further sutures are inserted at a distance of 1.5 cm to completely approximate the myometrial defect (Fig. 26.42).

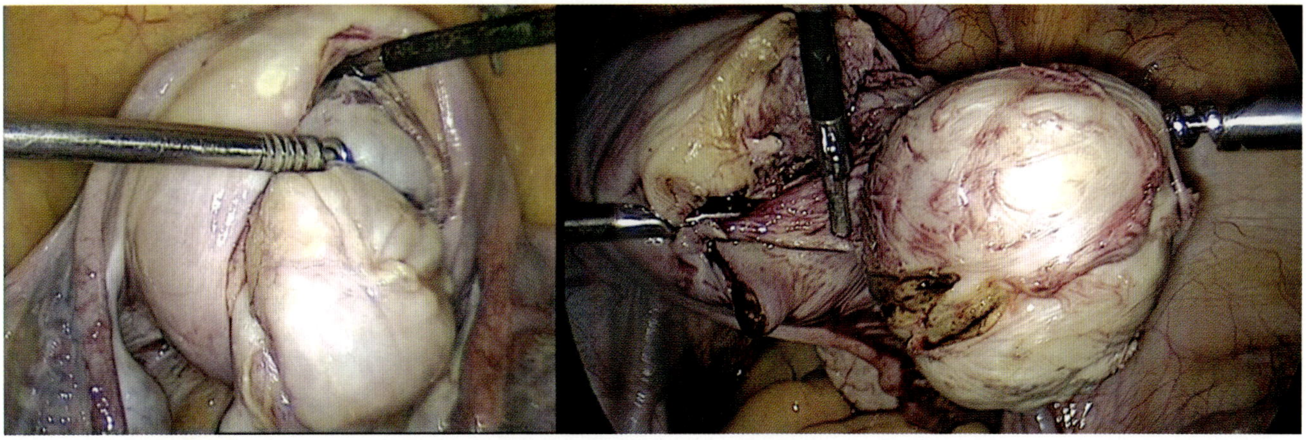

Fig. 26.39: Myoma enucleation

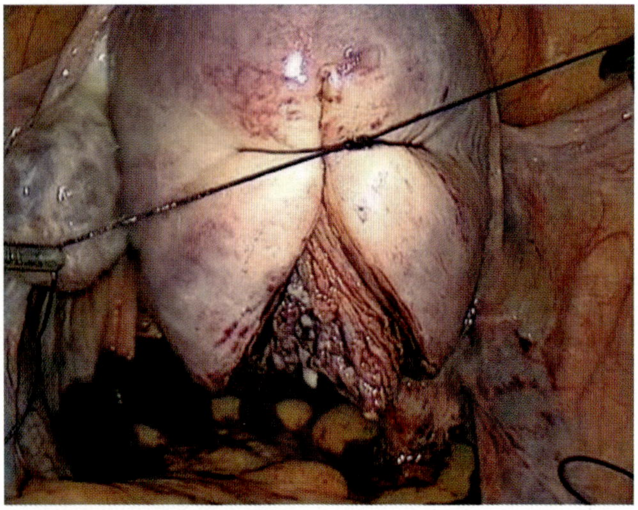

Fig. 26.41: Intracorporeal suturing

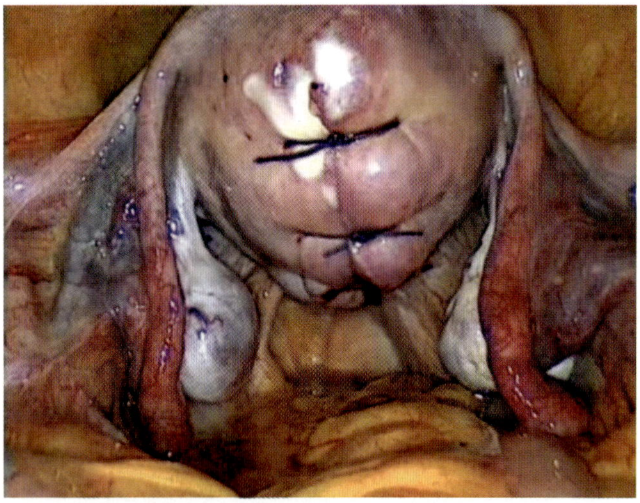

Fig. 26.42: Intracorporeal suturing completed

Pedunculated Myomas

Smaller pedunculated myomas are the easiest ones to remove. If the pedicle is small, it can be coagulated with a bipolar and then transected with a scissors. Pedunculated myomas with broader pedicles can be coagulated with bipolar in small steps and then divided with scissors (Fig. 26.43). Suturing is not required for these very superficial myomas.

Broad Ligament Myomas

Majority of broad ligament myomas are removed by a posterior incision unlike at laparotomy where division of round ligament and removal by anterior route is preferred. An oblique incision is made in the broad ligament parallel to the vessels. A myoma screw is now inserted and traction is applied slowly while a grasper connected to a unipolar diathermy is used for retracting the broad ligament. Any

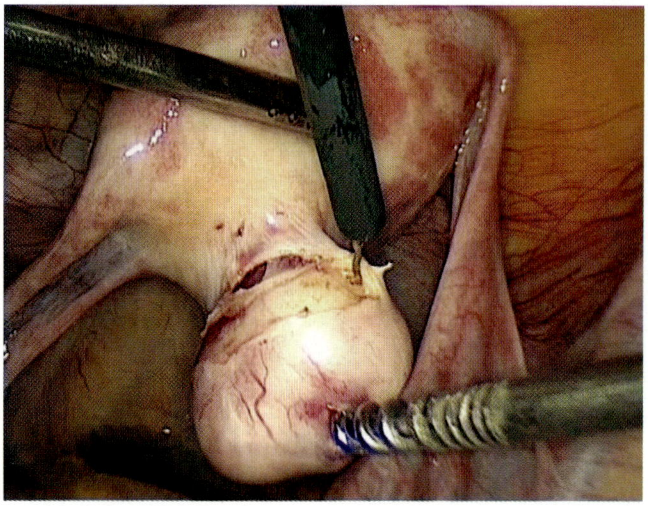

Fig. 26.43: Excision of pedunculated myoma

bleeding vessels are coagulated. After complete enucleation, the broad ligament is inspected for complete hemostasis. A suction drain is put through one of the secondary portals and observed.

Tissue Removal

Removal of the myoma from the abdomen is the most tedious part of the surgery. Myomas more than 1 cm has to be cut into smaller pieces before removal. Larger myomas need motorized morcellation or removal by colpotomy. A colpotomy is an excellent method for removal of myomas. The anatomic relationship between the rectum and the POD is first confirmed. A wet sponge on holder or a CCL extractor is placed behind the cervix to bulge the posterior fornix. The uterus is anteverted to clearly identify the bulging POD laparoscopically. A unipolar electrode is used to incise the bulging fornix till the sponge is visible. A 10 mm claw forceps is now inserted through this wound and visualized laparoscopically. The jaws are opened and the myoma is fed into the open jaws by another grasper. The myoma is now pulled out through colpotomy wound. If the myoma is large, it is morcellated vaginally with a knife till it comes out completely. The colpotomy is now closed with a few interrupted sutures. The peritoneal cavity is then thoroughly lavaged.

Minilap Myomectomy

Larger and multiple myomas are easily removed by a mini-laparotomy incision. It is an easy technique and less experienced endoscopic surgeon can easily perform this type of myomectomy safely. After initial evaluation the myomectomy incision site is selected and incised with a unipolar needle laparoscopically. It is important to make the incision well away from the fallopian tube and the uterine vessels so that if the incision gets extended, these structures are not injured.

The myoma is then partially enucleated laparoscopicaly as described earlier and it is grasped with a 10 mm myoma screw or claw forceps introduced through the trocar placed in the suprapubic region near the midline. The endoscope can now be kept away temporarily. The 10 mm trocar wound is extended to 3-4 cm and the myoma is directly grasped with towel clips. The myoma is now morcellated with a surgical knife removing small pieces at a time.

When the major diameter of myoma has been enucleated, the morcellation becomes very easy. Before completely enucleating the myoma, all attached vessels on the capsule are meticulously coagulated. The myometrial wound is now grasped with the allis forceps before completely detaching the myoma. The whole myometrial wound can be brought out of the minilap incision and myometrium is sutured in layers with 1-0 dexon or vicryl. Laparoscopic inspection is done and the peritoneal cavity thoroughly lavaged with Ringer's lactate.

26.8.4 Laparoscopic Hysterectomy

Laparoscopic hysterectomy was first performed in 1989 and has become one of the procedures that may be offered to women with significant gynecologic symptoms. Hysterectomy is the second most common major operation second only to cesarean section. Ninety percent of hysterectomies are performed electively for abnormal bleeding or other non-life-threatening indications. The major indications for abdominal hysterectomy are fibroids (40%), abnormal bleeding (10%) and endometriosis (13%).[9]

Women with intractable symptoms that affect their lives and who have not had benefit from other therapies may benefit from hysterectomy. The Maine Women's Health Study found that most women who had a hysterectomy performed for moderate or severe non-life-threatening symptoms were "very much satisfied" with the results of surgery and reported an improvement in the quality of life.[10] It does seem that for women who have significant symptoms, hysterectomy may provide relief, especially if other treatments have failed. As new developments prove successful, it is likely that the need for hysterectomy will decrease.

Laparoscopic Hysterectomy Compared with Abdominal and Vaginal Hysterectomy

For women who require a hysterectomy, the appropriate route of surgery is determined by anatomic considerations, the type of pathology expected, patient preference and physician experience and training. Seventy-five percent of all hysterectomies performed in the United States are abdominal hysterectomies. Laparoscopic hysterectomy has been suggested as an alternative to abdominal hysterectomy for most indications.

Most studies comparing the outcomes of laparoscopic hysterectomy with abdominal hysterectomy have been single-institution studies with small numbers of women, and few have been randomized. One well-designed prospective, randomized study analyzed outcomes from abdominal, vaginal, and laparoscopic hysterectomy performed by 43 gynecologists at 28 centers in the United Kingdom and South Africa.[11] Compared with abdominal hysterectomy, the rate of major complications including hemorrhage, bowel or ureter injury and return to the operating room were slightly more common in the laparoscopic hysterectomy group (11% versus 6%, 95% confidence interval, 0.9-9.1%). Intra-operative conversion from the laparoscopic to the abdominal approach occurred in 29 of the 584 women (4.9%). In this study, pain scores and quality of life measures, including sexual activity and physical and mental functioning were improved for all women having a hysterectomy but were significantly better for women having a laparoscopic hysterectomy.

Few studies have examined the long-term results of laparoscopic hysterectomy. A retrospective cohort study of 150 women who underwent laparoscopy-assisted vaginal hysterectomy and 146 who had abdominal hysterectomy found no difference after 8 years of follow-up in rates of vaginal vault prolapse, cystocele, rectocele, postcoital spotting, or cuff granulation. Although not blinded, this study suggests that similar long-term results may be expected for the two procedures.[12]

The ability to perform a vaginal hysterectomy on an outpatient basis with good patient acceptance has been established.[13] Therefore, if a vaginal hysterectomy is technically feasible for a patient, there is no added benefit with laparoscopic assistance.

Preoperative Preparation

Patients are evaluated as for any major abdominal surgery. No special bowel preparation is given except a laxative on the previous night. Prophylactic antibiotics are given.

A good uterine manipulator is required in addition to the regular laparoscopic instruments. The Clermont Ferrand uterine manipulator has a fornix bulger and vaginal blocker in addition to the ability to antevert and retrovert the uterus.

Technique

Laparoscopic hysterectomy is performed under general anesthesia with the patient in the low lithotomy position. A plain or indwelling catheter is introduced in the bladder. Clermont Ferrand uterine elevator (Karl Storz) is introduced in to the uterus after dilating the cervix.

One 10 mm trocar is introduced intraumbilically and two 5 mm trocars are inserted lateral to the inferior epigastric vessels. A third 5 mm trocar is introduced in the midline 5 cm above the symphysis pubis. A higher position is used for the secondary trocars if the uterus is enlarged. The pelvic organs are thoroughly inspected. The ureters are identified on both sides. A routine dissection of the ureter is not necessary. Any adhesions obscuring the view are lysed.

The round ligaments are grasped with an atraumatic grasper and kept stretched by simultaneous pushing of the uterus with a manipulator to the opposite side. The round ligament is coagulated with bipolar at the outer third (Fig. 26.44). It is divided in small snips with scissors (Fig. 26.45).

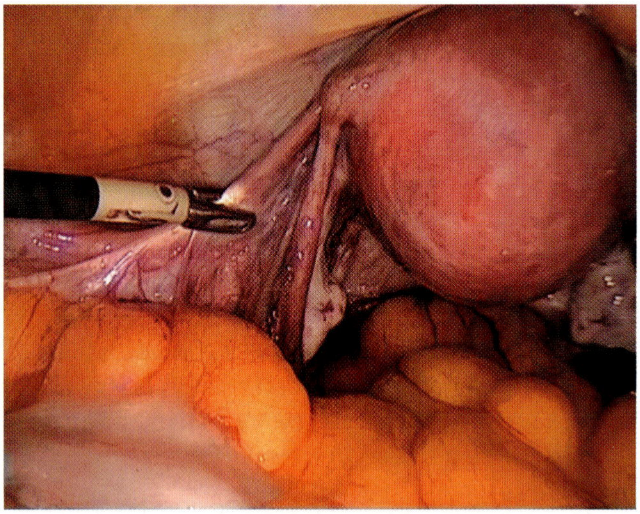

Fig. 26.44: Left round ligament coagulation with bipolar forceps

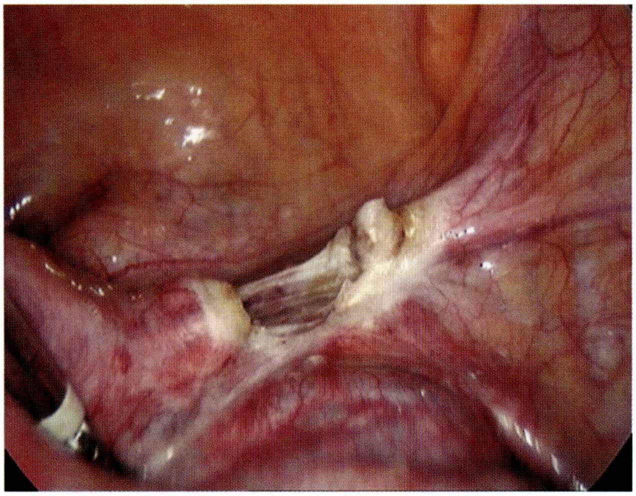

Fig. 26.45: Round ligament divided

If adnexa removal is contemplated, the tube and ovary are pulled to the opposite side with a grasper introduced through the contralateral port. The infundibulopelvic ligament is then coagulated close to the ovary and divided with the scissors; first incising the peritoneum followed by further coagulation (Fig. 26.46). Alternate coagulation and division in small steps is carried out till it reaches the already divided round ligament.

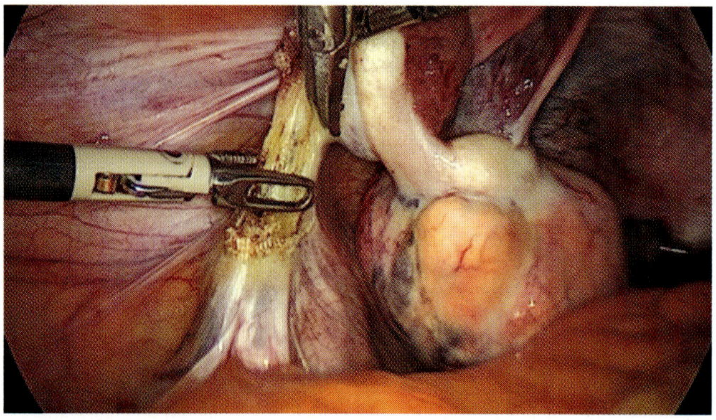

Fig. 26.46: Coagulation of infundibulopelvic ligament. Stretching the infundibulopelvic ligament will increase the distance between the ureter and the site of coagulation

If the adnexa are to be retained, the ovarian ligament and the fallopian tube are coagulated and divided in small steps as described above. The posterior half of broad ligament on both sides is divided with curved scissors and any oozing area is coagulated. The direction of division is towards the uterosacral ligament.

The loose uterovesical fold of peritoneum is now identified. It is then divided in the center with a unipolar hook electrode and then extended laterally (Fig. 26.47).

The fornix bulger is pushed into the anterior fornix to identify the vaginal limit. The bladder is now pushed down by sharp dissection in the center. The bladder pillars are

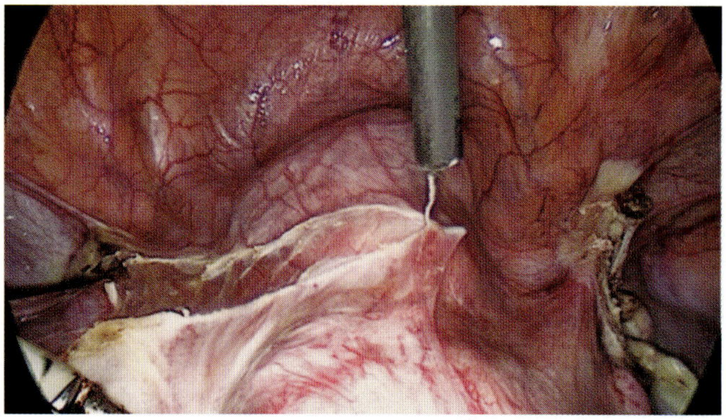

Fig. 26.47: Uterovesical fold opened with unipolar hook electrode

divided with a hook electrode to complete the bladder dissection.

The posterior leaf of broad ligament is then incised to skeletonize the uterine vessels. The skeletonized uterine vessels are coagulated with bipolar forceps (Fig. 26.48). The coagulated vessels are divided in small steps. Alternate coagulation and division is needed before completely transecting the uterine vessels (Fig. 26.49)

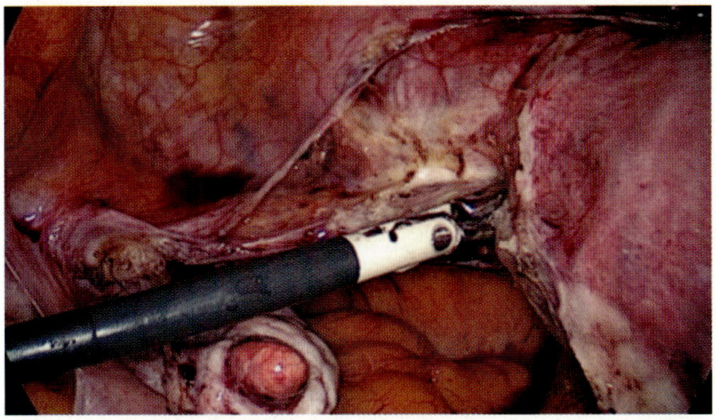

Fig. 26.48: Coagulation of uterine vessels

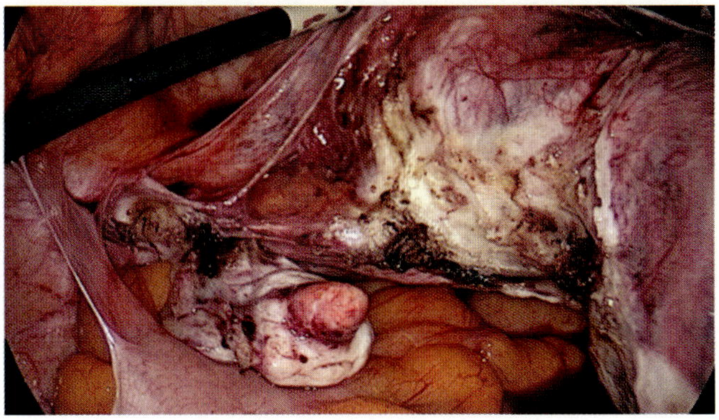

Fig. 26.49: Uterine vessels divided

The anterior fornix is outlined with the fornix bulger of the uterine manipulator. An incision is made between the bladder and cervix with a unipolar hook electrode (Fig. 26.50). The vagina is blocked with the silicon fins of the uterine manipulator to avoid leakage of gas.

The incision is now extended laterally and posteriorly to divide the cardinal and uterosacral ligaments. The uterosacral ligament is divided above the level of arch of uterosacrals. It is repeated on the other side to complete the separation of uterus from vagina (Fig. 26.51).

The uterus is now removed vaginally if normal size and morcellated if the size of uterus is bigger. The vagina is closed with 1-0 polysorb/vicryl laparoscopically after

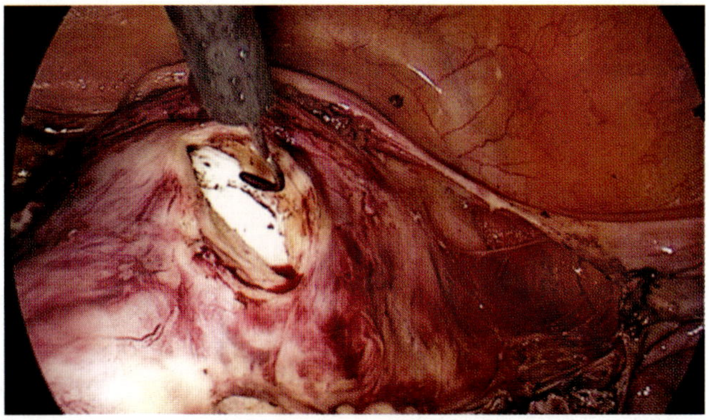

Fig. 26.50: Opening of anterior fornix

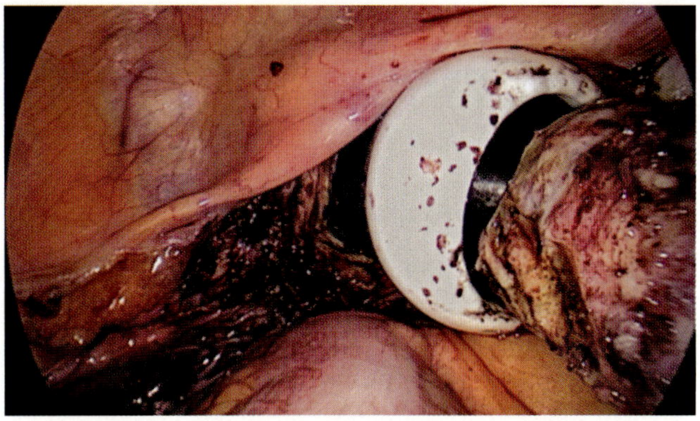

Fig. 26.51: Uterus completely separated from vagina

blocking the vagina with the specimen of the uterus or by a vaginal plug. The vaginal cuff angles on both sides are sutured incorporating the cardinal and uterosacral ligaments. The central part of the vagina is closed with one or two interrupted sutures (Fig. 26.52). Alternatively, the vaginal cuff can be closed using a vaginal approach.

The peritoneal cavity is lavaged with saline and complete hemostasis is ensured. A cystoscopy is done in cases where the bladder dissection was difficult.

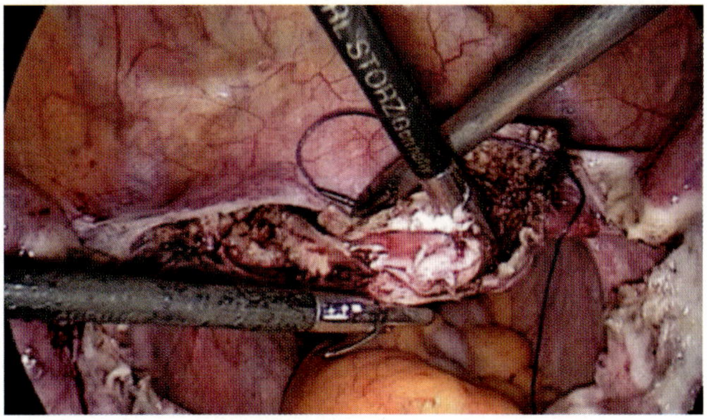

Fig. 26.52: Suturing the vault angle

Risks and Possible Complications

The risk of serious complications from abdominal or vaginal hysterectomy has been reported in a number of studies. For women aged 35 to 44 years who have a hysterectomy for benign conditions, the risk of dying is about 3 per 10,000 women, and for women of all ages the risk of dying is 6 per 10,000. The largest reported study to examine complications resulting from laparoscopic hysterectomy reported on 3928 women who had surgery at local, central, and university hospitals in Finland.[14] Major complications occurred in 88 women (2.2%). No major vascular injuries occurred, but one woman (0.002%) died from a massive pulmonary embolus following surgery. Although most studies were not randomized or adjusted for patient health status or pathology, injury to the bladder (1.8% versus 0.4%), ureter (0.3% versus 0%), and bowel (0.4% versus 0%) was more common with laparoscopic than abdominal procedures.

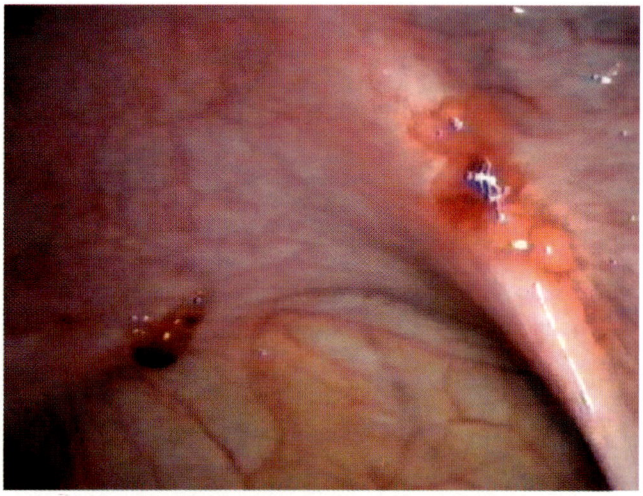

Fig. 26.53: Early endometriosis–Red lesions

26.8.5 Endometriosis

Endometriosis is a progressive and often debilitating disease affecting 10-15% of women during their reproductive period. Patients with endometriosis usually present with infertility or pelvic pain. The diagnosis is a visual one either by laparoscopy or at laparotomy. Treatment depends on the age of the woman, extent of disease, severity of symptoms and desire for fertility. Endometriosis is most often treated surgically than medically. Conservative surgery although not curative is associated with much lower recurrence rates than with medical therapy. It is effective in relieving pain and improves fertility rates associated with moderate to severe disease. Laparoscopic surgery has become the treatment of choice for endometriosis.

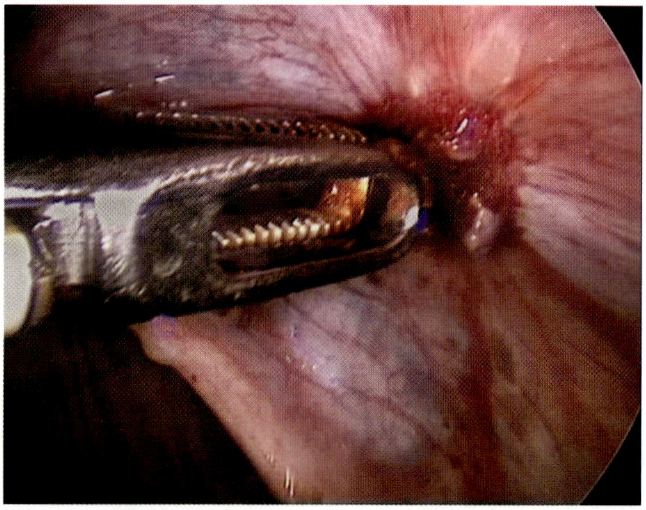

Fig. 26.54: Coagulation of endometrial implants

Endometrial Implants

Early endometriosis appears as red, white or black lesions (ASRM classification of endometriosis, 1996). The red lesions are either flame like lesions or clear vesicles (Figs 26.53 and 26.54). White lesions appear as either opacities or peritoneal defects. Black lesions can be black or blue in appearance. There is considerable controversy regarding the usefulness of treatment of minimal disease in enhancing fertility. A multicenter study has shown an improved pregnancy rate following laparoscopic ablation of endometrial implants compared with diagnostic laparoscopy. So, once a diagnostic laparoscopy is performed for confirmation of endometriosis, it is better to treat it simultaneously.

Laparoscopy is performed with a 5 mm telescope. Superficial endometrial implants can be coagulated with bipolar forceps. Irrigating the coagulated areas will help to identify the non-treated areas. Implants on the uterosacrals usually appear as puckered areas. These areas are first probed and washed with suction irrigation to drain any small collections of chocolate material. Fleshy and infiltrating implants require excision. A small incision is made at the margin of the implants with scissors and the suction irrigator introduced inside and fluid pushed into lift up the implants. The implant is grasped and excised with scissors without injuring the deeper tissues. Any bleeder is coagulated with bipolar.

Severe Endometriosis

The uterus is retroverted and retroflexed in most cases of severe endometriosis due to the uterine adhesions to the uterosacrals and the rectosigmoid. The ovaries will be adherent to ovarian fossa and pelvic sidewall with or without endometriotic cysts. There can be varying degrees of tubo-ovarian adhesions. The aim of surgery is to establish a near normal tubo-ovarian anatomy as well as to remove the endometriotic lesions.

Good uterine anteversion is a must for any good endometriosis surgery. The manipulator is inserted in the uterus at the beginning of the surgery. The introduction of manipulator is also important. In a retroverted uterus, the manipulator is passed with the tip pointing downwards and then rotated 180 degrees to antevert the uterus. The patient's buttocks should be well beyond the edge of the table to allow downward movement of the uterine manipulator. After initial inspection of pelvis and upper abdomen, the uterus is anteverted as far as possible without injuring it.

Any tubo-ovarian adhesions are released by blunt and sharp dissection. The ovaries are usually adherent to ovarian fossa and pelvic sidewall with or without endometriotic cysts. The adherent ovary is now grasped with an atraumatic grasper and using the suction irrigator it is gently freed from the uterus, uterosacrals and ovarian fossa. The flowing irrigating fluid always shows the clear cleavage plane. The pressure of the fluid opens up the natural planes of cleavage. Always start from the lateral most part of the adherent area, guided by the ovary so that the broad ligament is not opened up unnecessarily.

Different techniques have been suggested to excise deep endometriotic nodules. The uterus is usually retroflexed due to uterosacral adhesions and scarring. This is corrected by sharp incision with scissors and mechanical pressure with irrigation cannula and counter traction with a blunt grasper. The adherent rectum falls down during this maneuver. A probe in the rectum and another sponge on holder in posterior vaginal fornix help to delineate the POD anatomy. The fibrosed tissue behind the cervix and on the uterosacrals is excised with sharp scissors. The rectum is also mobilized and the scarred endometriosis on the wall is excised with minimal damage. At times the endometriosis infiltrates the vagina wall completely and bluish nodules will be visible in the vagina. In such cases an incision is made around these nodules vaginally and then excision of cul-de-sac nodule is performed laparoscopically. The defect in the vagina is then closed with sutures.

There are other techniques where the fibrotic endometriotic nodule is excised enbloc from posterior cervix first and then from the rectal wall or *vice versa*.[15] Endometriotic nodules in the rectal mucosa if present is excised completely and the defect sutured. Very rarely a laparoscopic segmental bowel resection with stapled anastomosis can be considered.

Endometriomas

Endometriomas can be extraovarian or intraovarian in origin. Extraovarian endometriomas are more common. Smaller cysts will not have cyst lining and peeling it off will destroy the normal ovarian tissue. They are managed by coagulating the endometrial implants inside the cyst. Larger endometriomas will have a true lining, which can be peeled off with the least damage to the ovary. When such a cyst is peeled off, it will be thin and will have a smooth surface.

Small Endometriomas

The adherent endometriotic cyst is released from the uterosacrals and pelvic sidewall by blunt dissection. Invariably the content of the cyst drains out. It is sucked from the pelvis and any remaining chocolate material is sucked out from the opened cyst. The inside of the cyst is now thoroughly washed by suction irrigation, and the opening is enlarged to inspect the cavity. The fibrosed edge of the cyst is excised. The endometriotic implants inside the cyst are identified and then coagulated with bipolar forceps.

Large Endometriomas (Enucleation)

Large endometriomas needs decompression before cystectomy (Fig. 26.55). One of the secondary trocar directly punctures the cyst away from the fimbrial end of the tube. The trocar is replaced with the suction irrigator and the chocolate material is sucked out. It is repeatedly lavaged with Ringer's lactate till the aspirate is clear. The adherent endometriotic cyst is released from the uterosacrals and pelvic sidewall by the blunt dissection. POD adhesions are released completely and superficial implants are coagulated.

The cyst cavity is now inspected by enlarging the punctured hole. A decision is made at this point whether or not to proceed with enucleation of the cyst lining. A small portion of the edge of the cyst is torn to identify the two layers clearly. The cyst lining is grasped with atraumatic forceps for better grip from the contralateral port. The ovarian tissue is grasped from the ipsilateral port with a second atraumatic forceps. By pulling them in opposite directions, the cyst lining is peeled off as far as possible. Both forceps are now released, but one at a time, then re-grasped near the cleavage line on the cyst and ovarian tissue respectively. They are then pulled apart and these steps are repeated till the enucleation is complete (Fig. 26.56). Dissection with scissors is rarely required.

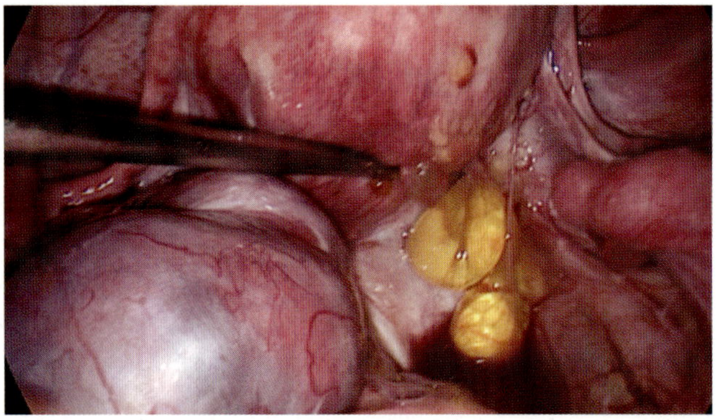

Fig. 26.55 Endometrioma of the left ovary

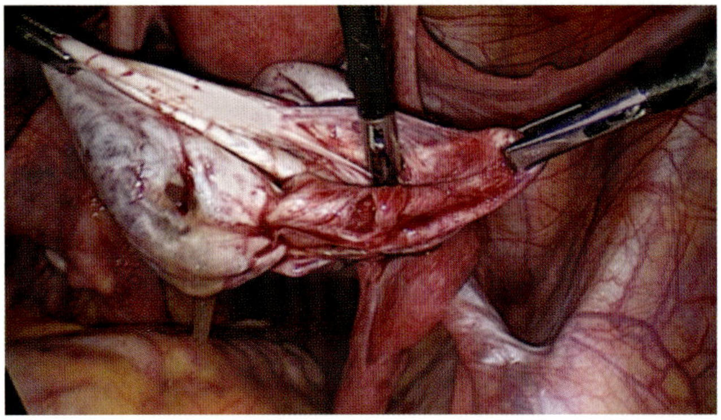

Fig. 26.56: Enucleation of endometrioma

After enucleation of the cyst lining, any active bleeder in the ovarian bed is looked for and if present is coagulated with, bipolar. The ovary is reconstructed holding the edge together with a grasper for 3-5 minutes. The aim of reconstruction is to give the ovary a natural shape with good ovarian surface for the fimbria to move around.

Suturing of the ovaries is avoided as it produces more adhesions.

26.8.6 Tubal Anastomosis

Microsurgical tubal anastomosis is the gold standard for reversal of sterilization. It gives an intrauterine pregnancy rate of 60-80% and a very low ectopic pregnancy rate of 1-6%.[16] The success rate mainly depends on the type of sterilization; Fallope rings and clips give a higher success rate than Pomeroy's and other techniques.[17] Two other prognostic factors associated with success of the procedure were tubal length and type of anastomosis. The isthmo-isthmic anastomosis gives a better result than the isthmo-ampullary anastomosis.[18] A tubal length of more than 5 cm is a good prognostic factor. The pregnancy rate decreased by 50% if the length of tube was 3-4 cm and no patient with tubal length less than 3 cm became pregnant.

Patients with poor prognostic factors are better treated by IVF. But the probability of conception is less than 10% in women over 40 years of age.[19] Trimbos-Kemper reported an overall intrauterine pregnancy rate of 45% following reversal of sterilization in women over 40 years of age.[20] The mean interval of surgery to pregnancy was 5.5 months. Therefore microsurgical reversal of sterilization is a better procedure than IVF in women over 40 years.

There have been several recent reports of successful tubal anastomosis performed at laparoscopy.[21] The development of new laparoscopic equipment such as the high definition camera with high resolution monitor and advanced instrumentation has made it possible to view even the very small tubal lumen and to use 7-0 or 8-0 intracorporeal sutures.

Equipment and Instruments

A magnification of 20 to 40 times is essential for identifying healthy mucosa and muscularis before anastomosis can be performed. This magnification can be achieved by using a high definition camera with zoom facility and a 20 inch video monitor.

Microinstruments are essential for effective laparoscopic suturing 3 mm needle holders and graspers with sandblasted tips to reduce glare, atraumatic terminal serrations, jaw apposition without slippage of fine sutures and a sensitive handle design are available.

7-0 or 8-0 polypropylene or nylon sutures with easily penetrable needles are ideal for tubal anastomosis.

Procedure

Four types of anastomoses are possible: Isthmo-isthmic, isthmo-ampullary, ampullary-ampullary, and tubo-cornual. The lumen size is very small in isthmo-isthmic anastomosis, but a thick muscularis allows a technically easier anastomosis and good pregnancy outcome. Luminal disparity is a technical problem in isthmic-ampullary anastomosis. In ampullary-ampullary anastomosis, the thin muscularis and prolapse of mucosal folds can be a problem. Tubocornual anastomosis is technically the most difficult tubal surgery.

It is very important to prepare the tube in two layers for a good anastomosis. Inclusion of any scarred portion in anastomosis can lead to poor healing. The site of sterilization is identified and held with a fine grasper. A circular incision is made on the proximal stump about half a centimeter from the probable site of transection with scissors or a fine unipolar needle. Dilute vasopressin is injected into the mesosalpinx to reduce bleeding. The proximal stump is cut with scissors 5 mm distal to the prepared seromuscular layer. Chromopertubation is done through the cervix to check the patency of the proximal stump (Fig. 26.57). The distal segment is also prepared in 2 layers in a similar manner. The patency of the segment is also checked by chromopertubation from the proximal end.

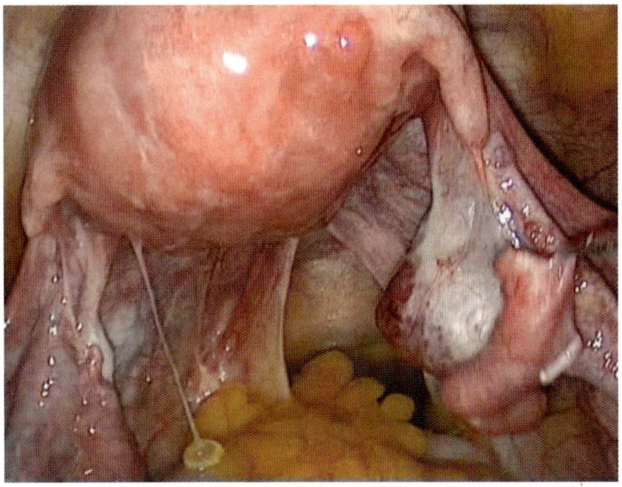

Fig. 26.57: Site of tubectomy

The mesosalpinx is approximated first with a 6-0 prolene suture. The anastomosis is then done by four 7-0/8-0 prolene sutures. The first suture is at 6 o' clock position (Fig. 26.58). The sutures may be taken through the lumen ignoring the mucosa. The 12 o' clock suture is then taken and tied last for proper placement of the other sutures (Fig. 26.59). Three and 9 o' clock sutures are then taken and tied. The serosa is then approximated with two or three interrupted 7-0 sutures and chromopertubation is done to check the patency (Fig. 26.60).

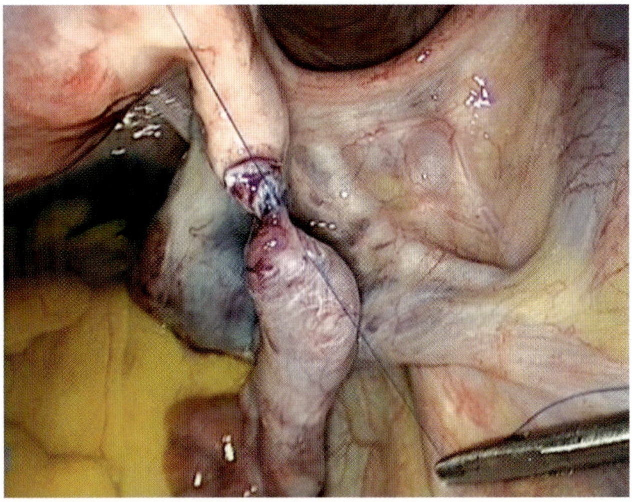

Fig. 26.58: 6 o' clock suture is taken from outside in on the proximal stump and inside out on the distal stump

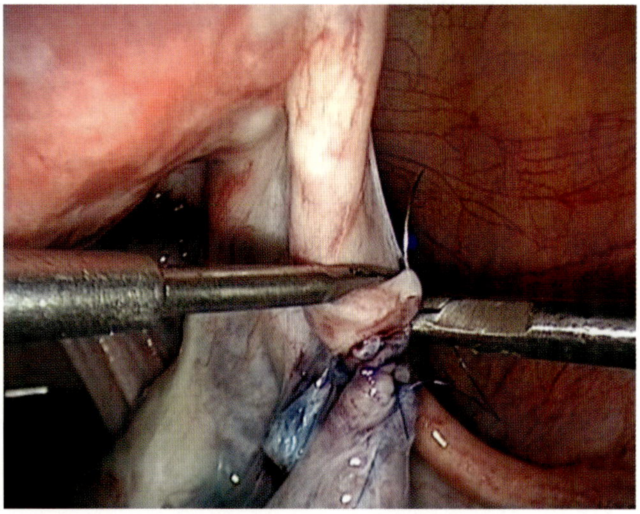

Fig. 26.59: 12 o' clock suture

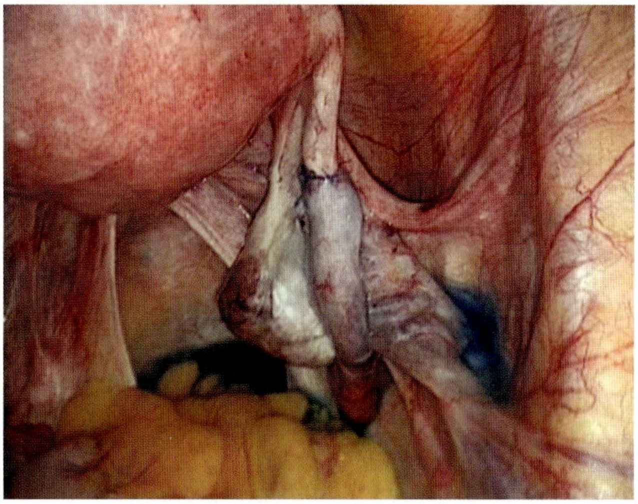

Fig. 26.60: Chromotubation

26.8.7 Laparoscopic Presacral Neurectomy

Dysmenorrhea is a very common gynecological complaint and medical treatment is often very successful. However there is a 20-25% failure rate and surgery has been an option for cases of dysmenorrhea that fail to respond to medical therapy. Presacral neurectomy is the usual procedure performed for intractable dysmenorrhea. It is usually performed along with conservative management of endometriosis for pelvic pain. Laparoscopic presacral neurectomy has been developed to provide an outpatient surgical treatment of pelvic pain which is central in location.

Principle

Pain impulses from the cervix, uterine corpus and the proximal fallopian tubes are transmitted through afferent sympathetic nerve fibers traversing cephalad from the central pelvis. These small, scattered, nerve fibers form the inferior hypogastric plexus and coalesce into the intermediate hypogastric plexus at approximately the level of the upper sacral and lower lumbar vertebral regions. The intermediate hypogastric plexus is composed of two or three separate trunks lying on the body of L5 vertebra. These nerve fibers further coalesce into the superior hypogastric plexus, which continues up and over the bifurcation of the aorta.

In presacral neurectomy, the structures resected are the superior and upper intermediate hypogastric plexus. A presacral neurectomy is neither presacral in location nor a neurectomy, because it is performed at the level of L4-L5 and it severs a nerve plexus rather than a single nerve.

Technique

Any pelvic abnormalities are treated laparoscopically. The patient is then given a steep Trendelenburg position and the sigmoid colon is displaced to the left side. The aortic bifurcation, the common iliac arteries and veins, the ureters, and the sacral promontory are identified. A transverse incision is made over the peritoneum 2-3 cm above the angle of the sacral promontory. The right common iliac vessels mark the right margin of the dissection, the left margin by the edge of sigmoid mesentery and left common iliac vein. The left ureter is hidden by the sigmoid mesentery.

A window is created by hook electrode or harmonic Ace through the retroperitoneal areolar tissue over L5 vertebra. The intervening tissue of the superior hypogastric plexus is grasped, elevated and transected with a unipolar hook or harmonic Ace (Fig. 26.61). All the remaining retroperitoneal neural and lymphatic tissues are removed laying the sacral promontory bare except for any presacral vessels. Closure of peritoneum is not necessary.

Intraoperative complications related to presacral neurectomy are rare. Injury to left common iliac vein is possible. Nezhat in his long-term follow-up of 67 patients had more than 50% pain relief in 83.1% of patients.[22] Only a minority of patients reported a worsening of constipation and urinary symptoms. Diarrhea and dyspareunia also improved in a large proportion of patients.

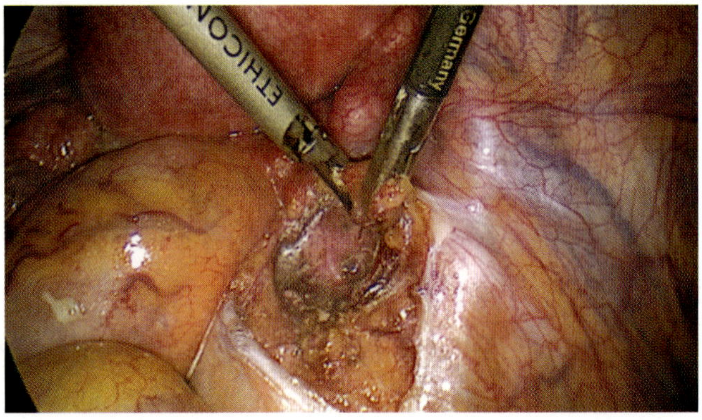

Fig. 26.61: Excision of presacral nerve plexus

REFERENCES

1. Nezhat C, Nezhat F. Conservative management of ectopic gestation. Fertil Steril.1990;53:382.
2. Lundorrf P, Halslin M , Shoblom P, Lindblom B. Persistent trophoblast after conservative treatment of tubal pregnancy - Prediction and detection Obstet Gynecol 1991;77:129.
3. Dubuisson JB, Aubriot FX, Foulot H, Bruel D, de Joliniere JVB, Mandelbrot L. Reproductive outcome after laparoscopic salpingectomy for tubal pregnancy. Fertil Steril 1990;53:1004-7.
4. Pouly JL, Chapron C, Manhes H, Canis M, Wattiez A, Bruhat MA: Multifactorial analysis of fertility after conservative laparoscopic treatment of ectopic pregnancy in a series of 223 patients. Fertil Steril 1991;56:453-60.
5. Silva PD, Schaper AM, Rooney B. Reproductive outcome after 143 laparoscopic procedures for ectopic pregnancy. Obstet Gynecol 1993;81:710-5.
6. Parker WH, Berek JS. Laparoscopic management of adnexal masses. Obstet Gynecol Clin N Am 1994;21:79-92.
7. Nezhat F, Nezhat CH, Welander CE, Benigno B. Four ovarian cancers diagnosed during laparoscopic management of 1011 women with adnexal masses. Am J Obstet Gynecol 1992;167: 790-6.
8. Hulka JT, Parker WH, Surrey MW. American Association of Gynecologic Laparoscopists survey of management of ovarian masses in 1990. J Reprod Med 1992;37:599-602.
9. Martin DC, Batt RE. Retrocervical, rectovaginal pouch, and rectovaginal septum endometriosis. J Am Assoc Gynecol Laparosc 2001;8:12-7.
10. Hughes EG, Fedorkow DM, Collins JA. A quantitative overview of controlled trials in endometriosis-associated infertility. Fertil Steril 1993;59:963-70.
11. Garry R, Fountain J, Mason S, Hawe J, Napp V, Abbott J, et al. The eVALuate study: two parallel randomised trials, one comparing laparoscopic with abdominal hysterectomy, the other comparing laparoscopic with vaginal hysterectomy. BMJ 2004;328(7432):129-36.
12. Shen C, Wu M, Lu C, Huang E, Chang H, Huang F, et al. Short and long-term clinical results of laparoscopic-assisted vaginal hysterectomy and total abdominal hysterectomy. J Am Assoc Gynecol Laparosc 2003;10: 49-54.
13. Stovall T, Summitt R, Bran D, Ling F. Outpatient vaginal hysterectomy: a pilot study. Obstet Gynecol 1992;80:145-9.
14. Harkki-Siren P, Sjoberg J, Kurki T. Major complications of laparoscopy: a follow-up Finnish study. Obstet Gynecol 1999; 94:94-8.

15. Redwine DB. Laparoscopic en bloc resection for treatment of the obliterated cul-de-sac in endometriosis. J Reprod Med 1992;37:695-8.
16. Gomel V. Microsurgical reversal of female sterilization: a reappraisal. Fertil Steril 1980;33:87-97.
17. Yoon TK, Sung HR, Kang HG, Cha SH, Lee CN, Cha KY. Laparoscopic tubal anastomosis: Fertility outcome in 202 cases. Fertil Steril 1999;72,1121-6.
18. Rock JA, Guzic DS, Katz E. Tubal anastomosis: pregnancy success following reversal of Falope ring or monopolar cautery sterilization. Fertil Steril 1987;48:13-17.
19. Tan SL, Royston P, Campbell S, et al. Cumulative conception and childbirth rates after in vitro fertilization. Lancet1992; 339:1390-4.
20. Trimbos-Kemper TC. Reversal of sterilization in women over the age of 40 years: a multicenter survey in the Netherlands. Fertil Steril 1990;53:575-7.
21. Nezhat CH, Siedman DS, Nezhat F, Nezhat C. Primary care update. Obstet Gyns 1998:1;5(4):197.
22. Feste JR, Wilson EE. Presacral neurectomy. J Reprod Med 1990;35:625-30.

27 Hysteroscopy

Paul PG, Sejal Naik, Madhu KN

27.1 INTRODUCTION

Hysteroscopy is an endoscopic procedure that allows direct visualization of the uterine cavity and the cervical canal and thus serves for the diagnosis of intrauterine pathology (diagnostic hysteroscopy) as well as for surgical intervention (operative hysteroscopy). Although hysteroscopic procedure was first described by Pantaleoni in 1869, advances in hysteroscopy had to wait another century for technical innovations before the technique became feasible in clinical practice.

27.2 ADVANTAGES OF HYSTEROSCOPY

1. It is possible to do an office hysteroscopy as an outpatient procedure without need of anesthesia or cervical dilatation.
2. It is minimally invasive without incisions.
3. Surgical correction of uterine malformations, intrauterine adhesions, submucous myomas which were formerly were limited to conventional surgery have now become a domain of hysteroscopic surgery.
4. Endometrial ablation or resection is considered an acceptable alternative to hysterectomy for the treatment of abnormal uterine bleeding.

27.3 INDICATIONS

1. Infertility evaluation
2. Evaluation of abnormal uterine bleeding
3. Diagnosis and management of mullerian abnormalities in recurrent pregnancy loss
4. Endometrial biopsy for suspected Koch's infection, endometrial carcinoma
5. Diagnosis and management of Asherman's syndrome

6. Misplaced IUD or foreign body
7. Proximal tubal block
8. Sterilization

27.4 CONTRAINDICATIONS

1. Suspected intrauterine pregnancy
2. Active cervicovaginal or pelvic infection
3. Active uterine bleeding

27.5 EQUIPMENT FOR HYSTEROSCOPY

Diagnostic and operative hysteroscopes are available.

27.5.1 Telescope and Sheath

A diagnostic hysteroscope consists of a telescope and a sheath for distension media. An operating hysteroscope system is comprised of

- Rigid telescope
- Inner sheath for influx of distension media
- Outer sheath for efflux of distension media
- Operative channel/working element to use operative instruments/electrodes.

Telescopes are available in different diameters (2-4 mm) and with a variety of viewing capabilities (0°, 12°, 30°, 70°). Operative hysteroscopy requires external sheath diameter ranging between 3.5 and 7 mm to allow for passage of telescope, operative instruments and liquid distention media.

Bettochi (Figs 27.1 and 27.2) (Karl Storz™,4 mm diameter, 30°) is the most popular hysteroscope for hysteroscopy. It can be used for diagnosis as well as for performing minor operative procedures without dilating the cervix.

The Versascope system (Johnson and Johnson™) is a hysteroscope having a telescope of 1.8 mm diameter with an operative sheath of diameter 3.5 mm and rotatable proximal collar.

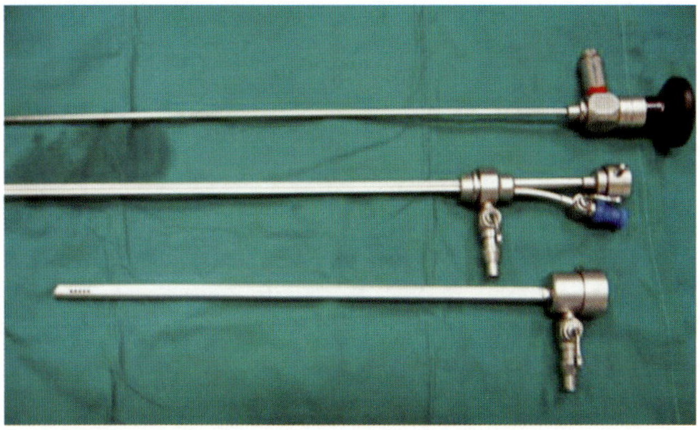

Fig. 27.1: Bettocchi hysteroscope—telescope 2.9 mm, inflow with operating channel and outer sheath

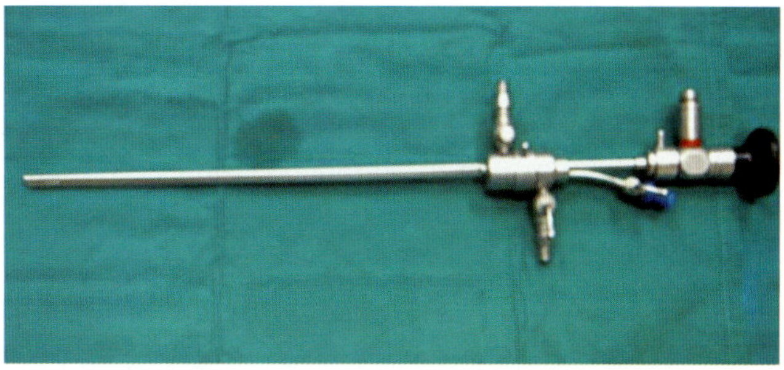

Fig. 27.2: Bettocchi hysteroscope-assembled

Resectoscope was originally designed for transurethral resection of prostate. In gynecological surgery, a modified one is used (Figs 27.3 and 27.4). The size of the whole assembly is 26 French. It has a continuous flow outer sheath, inner sheath with insulated ceramic tip, working element (Iglesias-type element) for one handed operation with spring action. A passive handle (working element remains inside the sheath at rest) is preferred in gynecological surgeries where a 4 mm Hopkins telescope with 12° or 30° is used. Due to its larger size, besides giving general anesthesia, one needs to dilate the cervix. It is designed to use for monopolar diathermy. Bipolar resectoscopes have recently become available. They allow the use of saline solution as distension medium.

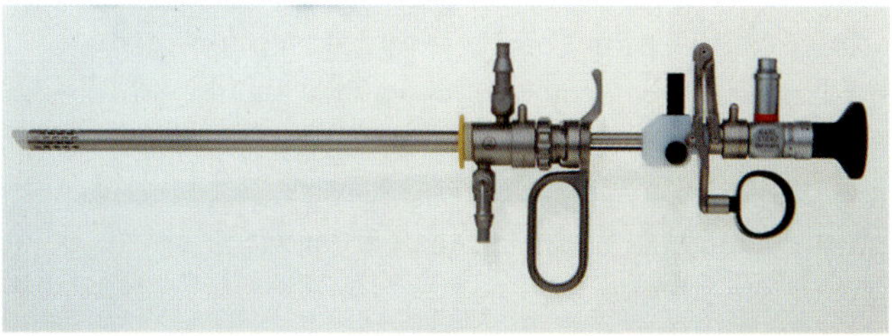

Fig. 27.3: Resectoscope (Karl Storz)

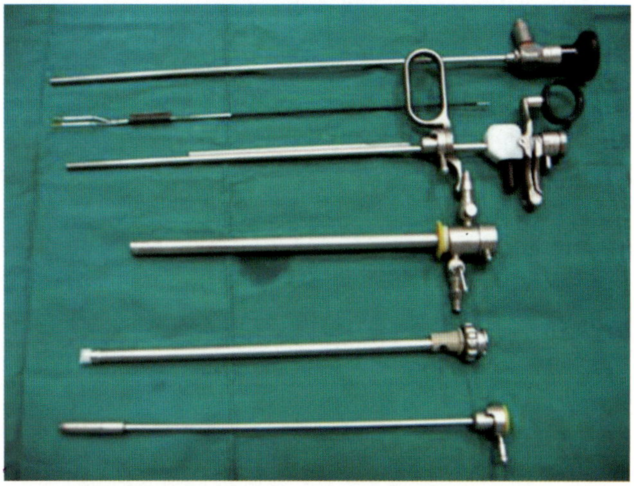

Fig. 27.4: Resectoscope—telescope, electrode, working element, sheaths and obturator (*Karl Storz*)

Electrodes: Different types of electrodes are available for different purposes. It may be cutting loop, ball, barrel, knife or vaportrode.

Ancillary equipment: The light source (halogen or xenon), CCD camera (Single/3chip/HD), recording device and electrosurgical unit are the same as used in laparoscopy.

27.5.2 Distension Media

The uterine cavity is a potential space which has to be distended for visualization as well as executing surgical procedures. Distention media can be gas or liquid.

Gaseous

Gaseous media can be used only for visualizing uterine cavity. Carbon dioxide (CO_2) is used exclusively for diagnostic/office hysteroscopy. It has refractive index same as air, giving a clear view. The disadvantage is distortion of view in the presence of blood or mucus. It needs an electronic hysteroflator for safe delivery of gas at correct flow rate (30-60 ml/min) and pressure (100-120 mm Hg). Due to these disadvantages, carbon dioxide is presently not used.

Liquid

Visualization of the uterine cavity needs sufficient distention which can be achieved by liquid distention media. The medium used for operative procedures should not transmit electric current as monopolar cautery is the usual energy source used for operative hysteroscopy. But when bipolar electrocautery is used, the distention medium can be an electrolyte solution.

- **Glycine** 1.5% is a non-electrolyte solution and can be used during monopolar electrosurgery.
- **High molecular weight liquid media (hyskon):** It is 32% dextran high viscosity solution but with limitations to its use like dextran allergy. It is rarely used now.
- **Low molecular weight liquid media** include electrolytic and non-electrolytic solutions: For diagnostic purpose electrolyte solutions like saline or ringer lactate and less frequently 5% and 10% dextrose are enough. For mechanical surgeries with scissors or forceps saline can be made use of. With the evolution of bipolar resectoscope, saline distention medium can be used while performing hysteroscopic electrosurgery.

27.5.3 Fluid Delivery System

Fluid delivery system with the ability to control flow and pressure is needed to distend the uterine cavity. The different types of fluid delivery systems are:

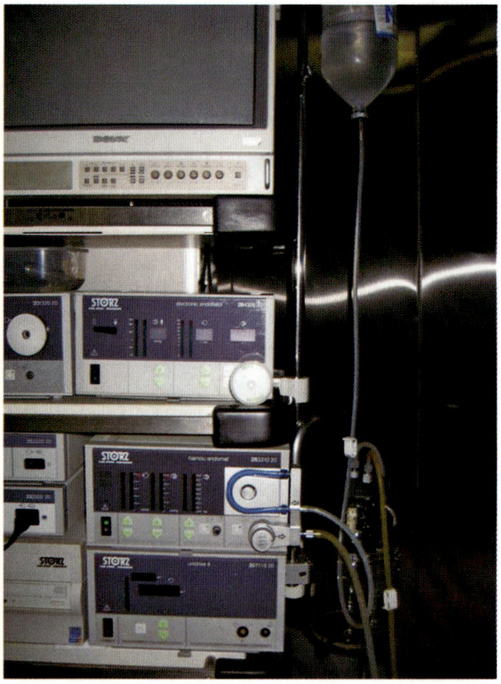

Fig. 27.5: Endomat with irrigation (*Karl Storz*)

- **Gravity fall system:** Fluid bag suspended at a height of about 90-100 cm above the level of the patient can achieve a pressure of about 70 mm Hg.
- A pressure cuff similar to that of a sphygmomanometer can be inflated around the bag to achieve a higher pressure of about 80-120 mm Hg.
- **Electronic suction and irrigation pump (Fig. 27.5):** The ideal fluid delivery system for operative hysteroscopy is an irrigation pump where the pressure and flow are electronically controlled. The irrigation pressure and volume can be set at desired level and maintained. A pressure of 90-110 mm Hg and a flow rate of 200 ml/minute and suction of 0.25 bar are usually selected.

27.6 PROCEDURE OF DIAGNOSTIC HYSTEROSCOPY

For diagnostic hysteroscopy as well as for most minor procedures general anesthesia is not necessary. Nonsteroidal anti-inflammatory drugs and mild sedatives can be used for pre-medication. If anesthesia is required, paracervical or intracervical block may be sufficient.

Before introducing the hysteroscope, irrigation system is connected and fluid is let in so that it fills the tubing and air bubbles are removed. After preparation of vagina with povidone-iodine, the cervix is caught with volsellum forceps and the hysteroscope assembly is gently inserted through the external os with the light cable position at 6 o'clock.

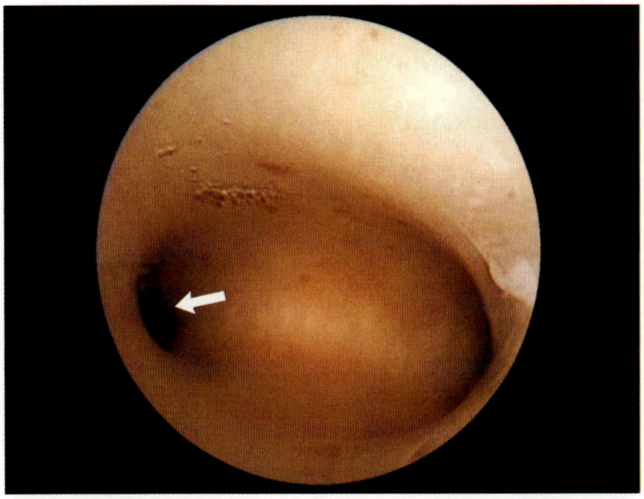

Fig. 27.6: Normal uterine cavity. The ostium is shown (arrow) on the right side

The hysteroscope is gently moved forward keeping the endocervical canal at 6 o' clock position eccentrically. When a 30° telescope is used, this position is needed to keep the telescope in the centre. The endocervical canal is inspected first followed by examination of fundus, anterior, posterior and lateral walls and both ostia by rotating the telescope (Fig. 27.6).

Precautions: There should be no air bubbles when using liquid as distention media, since presence of air bubbles can hampers vision. Pressure should be below 100 mm Hg to minimize pain.

27.7 OPERATIVE HYSTEROSCOPY

27.7.1 Hysteroscopic Lysis of Intrauterine Adhesions

Asherman described 'amenorrhea traumatica' as amenorrhea secondary to intrauterine adhesions following curettage for incomplete or missed abortion and postpartum hemorrhage. This condition is thus termed 'Asherman's syndrome'. Endometritis rarely causes adhesions except tuberculosis. Denudation of basalis layer and exposure of the muscularis layer produce adhesions by coaptation of the opposing uterine walls. This can cause hypomenorrhea, amenorrhea, infertility, ectopic pregnancy, recurrent pregnancy loss, preterm labor, abnormal placentation and fetal demise. It is demonstrated on HSG as single or multiple filling defects of variable size. They are seen as irregular, angulated filling defects with very sharp contours. Hysteroscopy can confirm and classify these adhesions according to the classification of the European Society for Gynecological Endoscopy (ESGE) which is based upon the grade and extent of intrauterine adhesions (Table 27.1).

Table 27.1: European Society for Gynecological Endoscopy (ESGE) classification of intrauterine adhesions

1. Thin or filmy adhesions
a. Easily ruptured by hysteroscope sheath alone
b. Cornual areas normal
2. Singular dense adhesion
a. Connecting separate area of the uterine cavity
b. Visualization of both ostia normal
c. Cannot be broken by hysteroscope sheath
2A. Occluding adhesions only in the region of the internal os. Upper uterine cavity normal
3. Multiple dense adhesions
a. Connecting separate areas of the uterine cavity
b. Unilateral obliteration of ostial areas of the tubes
4. Extensive dense adhesion with (partial) occlusion of the uterine cavity
a. Both tubal ostial areas (partially) occluded
5. Extensive endometrial scarring and fibrosis
a. In combination with grade 1 or grade 2 adhesions
b. With amenorrhea or pronounced hypomenorrhea
6. Extensive endometrial scarring and fibrosis
a. In combination with grade 3 or grade 4
b. Adhesions
c. With amenorrhea

The hysteroscopic semi-rigid scissors is used to divide adhesions at midpoint allowing the cut edges to retract. Thick vascular and dense adhesions are incised using electrosurgery (Collin's) knife or bipolar electrodes for which resectoscope is necessary.

Postoperative balloon catheter or plastic IUCDs can be used in case of severe adhesions to avoid reformation of adhesions. Estrogen is usually prescribed for 1-3 months to stimulate the endometrial lining.

Result of hysteroscopic adhesiolysis depend upon the type and extent of adhesions. The worst prognosis is for those due to genital tuberculosis. Hysteroscopic adhesiolysis restore normal menstruation in 80% cases. Pregnancy outcome reported was 64.1% (term deliveries) in one recent study.[1]

27.7.2 Fallopian Tube (Proximal) Cannulation

Tubal disease accounts for 25-35% of infertility in women.[2] Proximal tubal obstruction accounts for 10-25% of tubal factor. Tubal obstruction can be due to chronic salpingitis, salpingitis isthmica nodosa (SIN), intratubal endometriosis, amorphous material (e.g. mucus plugs or spasm). Most of the proximal tubal obstructions are thought to be caused by inflammatory process or endometriosis which leads to local fibrosis. In one report, only in 7 out of 18 cases, the surgically resected segment of the occluded tube showed an organic pathology.[3] In the rest of the cases the tubes appeared normal or with moderate fibrosis or inflammation. Hence a surgical correction is not warranted in majority of proximal tubal blocks. This principle is the basis for tubal cannulation. The traditional treatment for this condition is uterotubal implan-tation or tubocornual anastomosis. The term pregnancy rate reported for uterotubal implantation is as low as 11-15%.[4]

Development of a minimally invasive technique for correction of proximal tubal block began with interest in transcervical tubal sterilization. Since then, a variety of instruments and techniques have been developed for cannulation of the fallopian tube. Fallopian tubal cannulation can be done by hysteroscopic, fluoroscopic or ultrasonic techniques.

Tubal cannulation by hysteroscopic control offers a number of advantages over other techniques. Firstly, the guidance of the tubal catheter into the tubal ostia is simple because it is done under direct vision. Secondly, since it is done under laparoscopic guidance, the presence of distal tubal disease can be diagnosed and treated simultaneously. Hence it offers a one-step evaluation and treatment in infertile patient with proximal obstruction.

Procedure: A 5 mm Bettochi hysteroscope with a 5 Fr. operating channel is usually used. Novy's cannula with the obturator is then introduced through operating channel. Obturator is then removed and the guide wire introduced. The tip of the Novy's cannula is advanced near the ostium under constant visualization. The cannula is then railroaded over the guide-wire and introduced into the proximal part of the intramural portion. Guide-wire is then advanced for about 1-1.5 cm to negotiate the cornual block (Fig. 27.7). Simultaneous laparoscopy can help in negotiating the guidewire by lifting the tube with a grasper (Fig. 27.8). Chromopertubation can also be done to check for the success of the procedure. The procedure is repeated on the other side.

Novy's cannulation set is designed for single use. A urological catheter like Terumo guide-wire (Radifocus guide wire M diameter 0.89 mm) can be used as inner catheter with the Novy's outer catheter.

Advantages

1. As a therapeutic procedure
2. Differentiation between the spasm of tube, true pathological block and the functional block

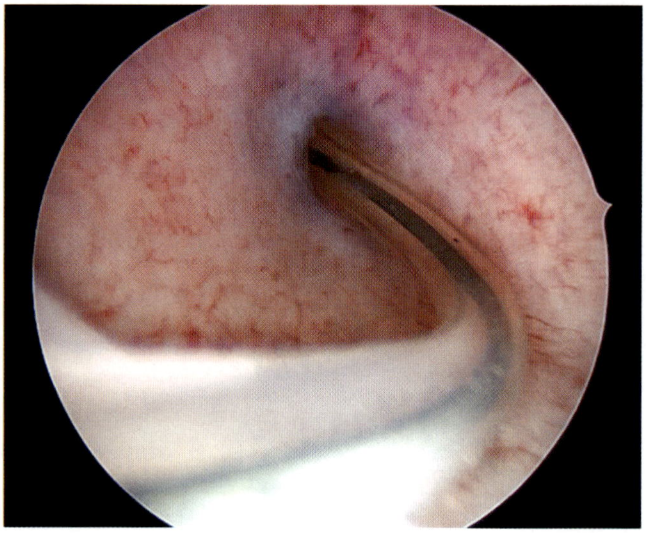

Fig. 27.7: Hysteroscopic cannulation—Guidewire with outer cannula

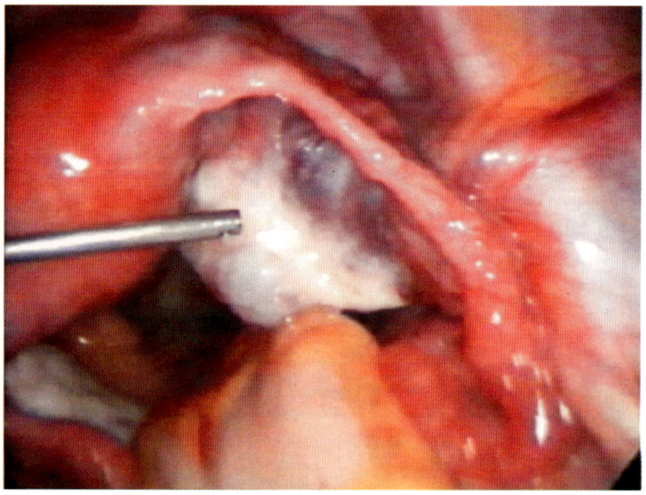

Fig. 27.8: Guide wire is seen in the isthmic portion of the tube

3. Low rate of complications
4. Low cost
5. Valuable information about the proximal and distal tubes

In a report published by the author about hysteroscopic cannulation in 31 patients (58 tubes) of proximal tubal obstruction,[5] at least one tube could be cannulated in 26 patients (83.9%). Associated distal tubal disease was present in 3 cases. 9 patients conceived after hysteroscopic cannulation. Five of these patients had associated pathologies. There were no ectopic pregnancies. Hysteroscopic cannulation was performed in 164 cases subsequently with similar results.

Complications: Perforation is reported in up to 10% of attempted procedures. Use of appropriate flexible catheter

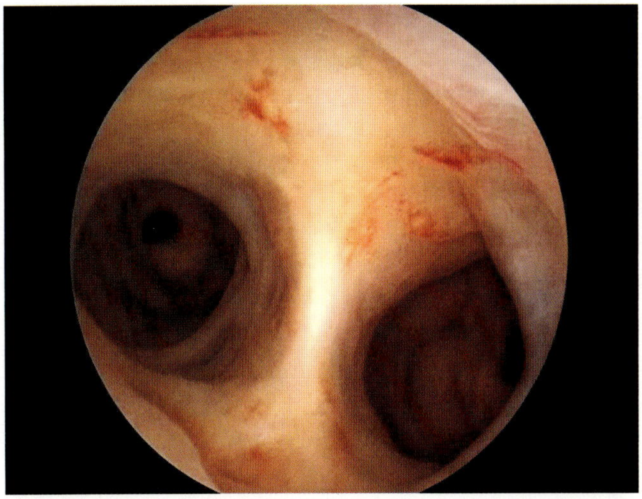

Fig. 27.9: Subseptate uterus

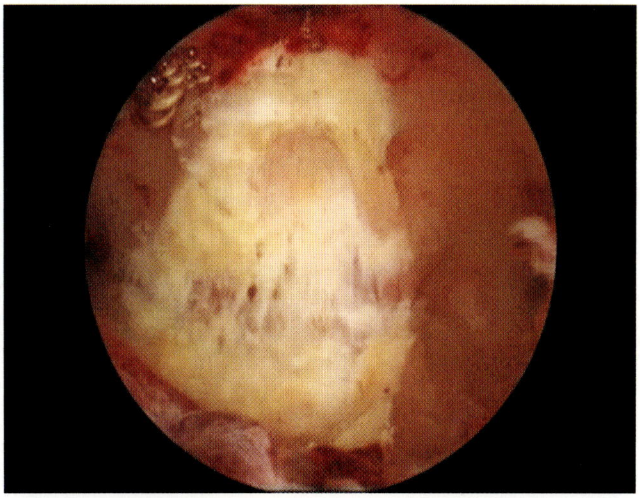

Fig. 27.12: Septum division completed. Note that both ostia are seen in the same field

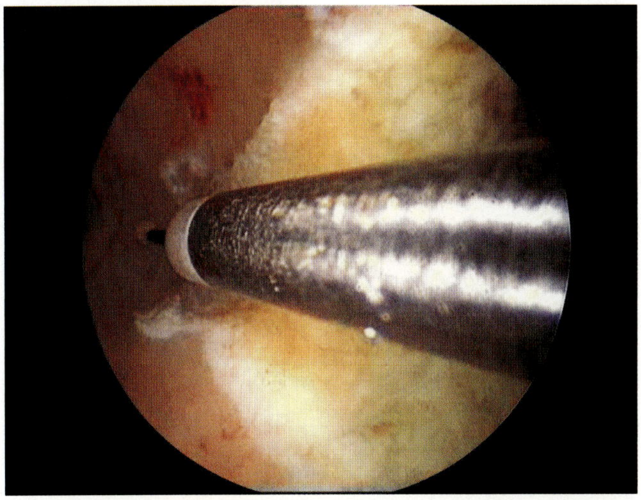

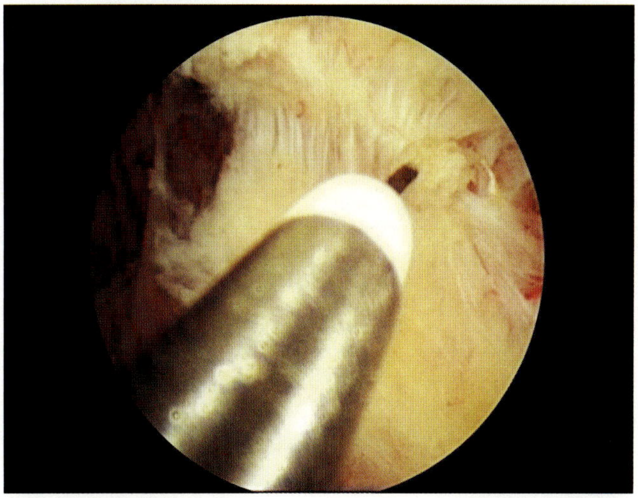

Figs 27.10 and 27.11: Septum division with Bettochi hysteroscope and bipolar electrode

may decrease the risk of perforation. When perforation occurs, it is left to heal spontaneously. Infection is rare.

27.7.3 Uterine Septum Resection (Figs 27.9 to 27.12)

The role of uterine septa as a cause for infertility is controversial. Uterine septum accounts for 25% of reproductive failure. Recurrent pregnancy loss may be the result of a poor blood supply to the septum, leading to poor implantation dynamics. Many recent reports advocate septum incision in infertility patients especially for those planned for ART.

The extent and thickness of the septum and differentiation from bicornuate uterus can be made with a fair degree of accuracy with 4D ultrasound. However, the septum should be confirmed by hysterolaparoscopy at the start of the procedure. Bettocchi hysterosope with 5 French operating channel is sufficient for septum division instead of a resectoscope. The septum is divided systematically from below upwards starting from the midpoint by side to side movement preferably using bipolar electrode. It is continued until both the uterotubal openings can be seen simultaneously and the cavity is near normal. A panoramic view from the internal os is useful for this decision. Intrauterine pressure of the distending fluid can be decreased to know whether arterial bleeding occurs for which hemostasis should be achieved using coagulation current. The final goal is to form a satisfactory uterine cavity.

Preoperative danazol or LHRH antagonist treatment is used for thinning the endometrium before the resection. Performing the procedure immediately after menses helps achieve the same goal. Follow-up examination can be performed one to two months after the operation. The take home baby rate obtained by various authors ranges from 70-80%, which is very similar to the results of traditional laparotomic metroplasty proposed by Tomkins, Te Linde and Jones.[6]

Advantages

1. An outpatient procedure without hospitalization
2. No scar on abdomen and uterine wall
3. No reduction in the volume of the uterine cavity
4. Result similar to traditional surgery

Complications: Perforation especially when extensive resection is done. These can be avoided by simultaneous laparoscopic control or ultrasonography guidance. Post-operative synechiae formation is rare.

27.7.4 Endometrial Polyp

Dilatation and curettage alone can detect endometrial polyps in only 43% of cases.[7] Polyps may be sessile or pedunculated and rarely include areas of neoplastic growth (Fig. 27.13). Scissors or electrocautery can be used for removal of polyp (Fig. 27.14). Fundal polyps are more difficult to remove as the pedicle cannot be easily visualized.

27.7.5 Hysteroscopic Myomectomy

Menorrhagia, infertility and dysmenorrhea can be caused by myomas protruding into the uterine cavity due to the anatomical distortion of the cavity. Hysteroscopic myomectomy is reported to improve pregnancy rate among women with submucous myoma.

European Society of Gynecological Endoscopy (ESGE) has classified intramural myoma into:

Grade 0: Pedunculated myoma or myoma limited within the cavity or has small base.

Grade 1: (Fig. 27.15) Myoma with partial intramural development, with more than 50% of intracavitary component. Angle of protrusion between the myoma and the uterine wall < 90°.

Grade 2: (Fig. 27.16) Predominantly intramural myoma with cavitary component < 50%. Angle of protrusion between the myoma and the uterine wall > 90°.

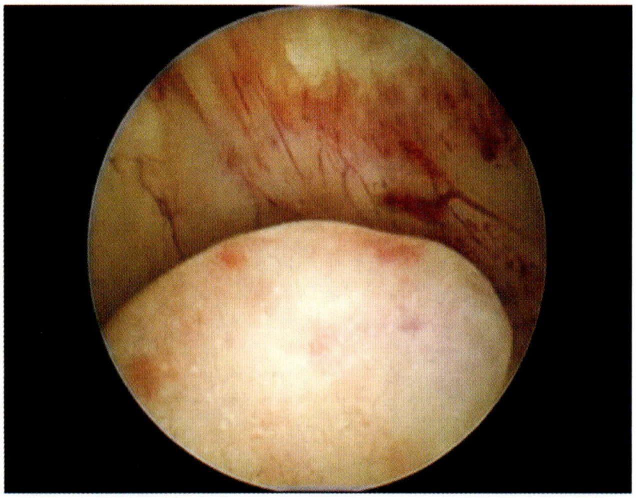

Fig. 27.13: Endometrial polyp

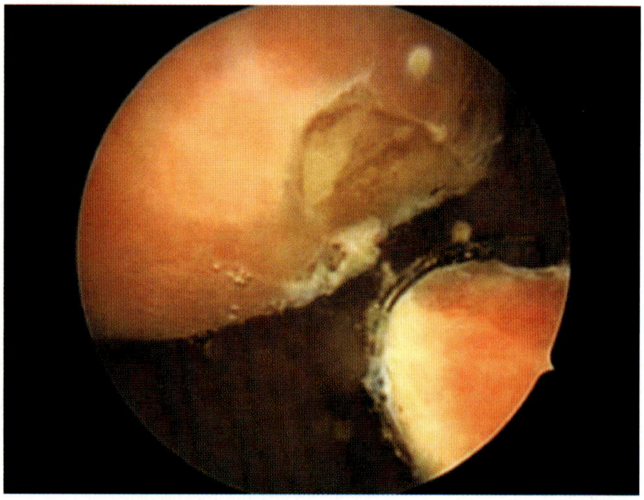

Fig. 27.15: Submucous myoma GradeI—Resection with loop electrode

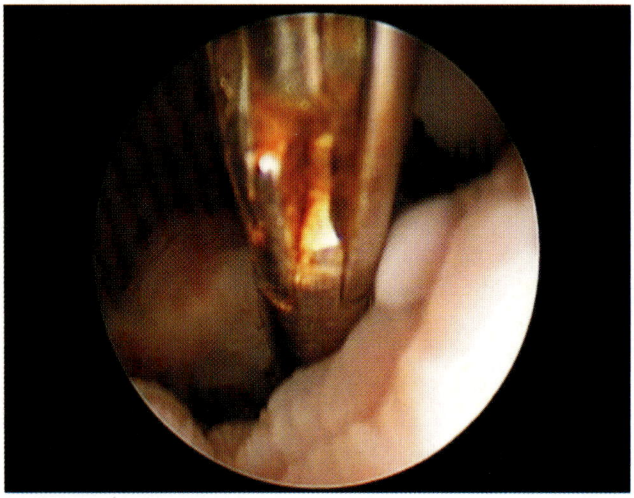

Fig. 27.14: Polypectomy

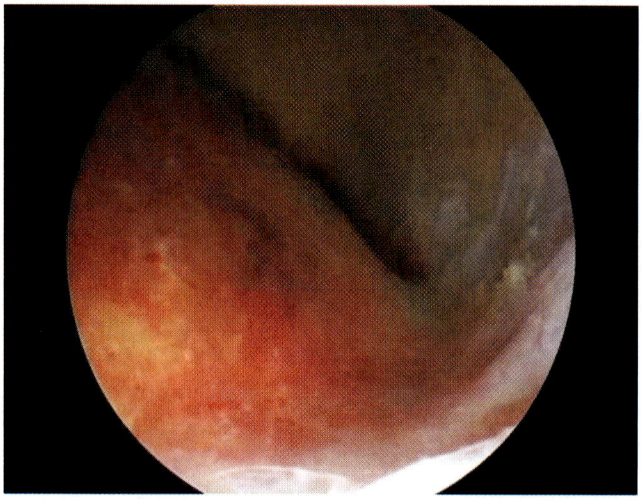

Fig. 27.16: Submucous myoma grade 2

Preoperative assessment: An accurate transvaginal ultrasound examination is mandatory. It may give a clue to the intramural extent of the myoma. Hysteroscopy is the gold standard for diagnosis.

Procedure (Figs 27.17 to 27.19): The standard monopolar resectoscope is commonly used. Newer bipolar resectoscope with saline is safer. Several fiber optic lasers like KTP, argon and Nd:YAG lasers are also available but few centers use it[8] because of the expense of the equipment and expertise needed.

Pedunculated and grade 1 submucous myomas are suitable for hysteroscopic resection. Grade 2 myomas may need second stage myomectomy. The loop is placed behind the myoma to be resected, power applied and the loop is drawn towards the internal os. Forward movement of the active loop is usually avoided to prevent perforation. This step is repeated till the complete myoma is resected. The resected pieces can interfere with visibility and has to be removed periodically. Once myometrium is seen, the procedure can be considered complete in that area. Once the resection is completed, any active bleeders have to be coagulated.[9]

The administration of GnRH analog preoperatively helps reducing the size and vascularity of the fibroid. Some data suggest that reduction in the size of uterine cavity and change in myoma quality can make the procedure technically more difficult.[10]

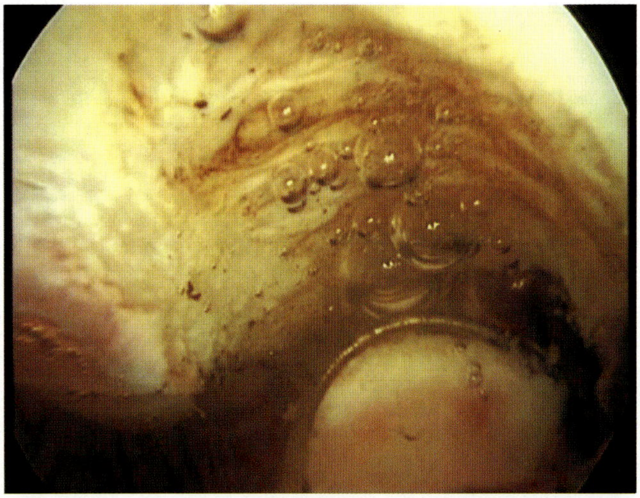

Fig. 27.17

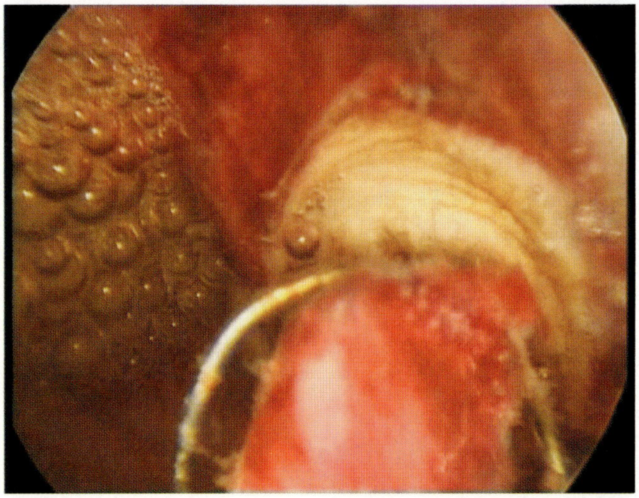

Fig. 27.18

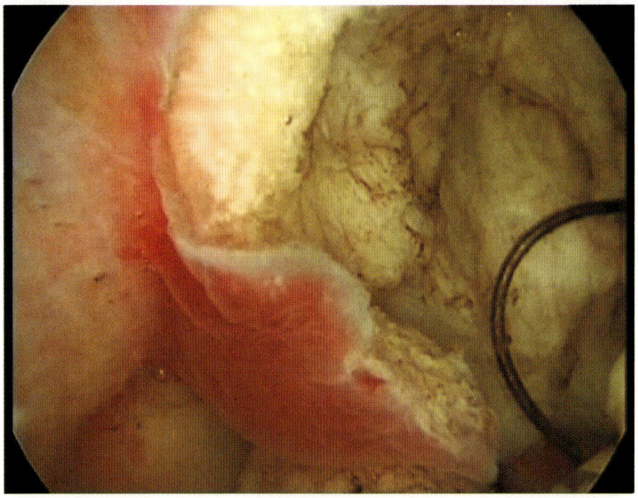

Fig. 27.19

Figs 27.17 to 27.19: Submucous myoma resection

27.7.6 Hysteroscopic Endometrial Ablation

Endometrial ablation involves destroying the full extent of endometrium as an alternative to hysterectomy for the treatment of abnormal uterine bleeding. Since endometrium has an extraordinary power of regeneration it is essential to remove the full thickness of the endometrium along with the superficial myometrium which includes the deep basal glands from which the endometrium regenerates.

Endometrial ablation is less invasive than hysterectomy and causes less morbidity. Endometrial ablation has become an acceptable alternative to hysterectomy for women who have completed family in whom endometrial atypia as well as carcinoma are ruled out.

Indications

1. Menorrhagia not responding to conservative management
2. Normal uterine cavity
3. Normal endometrial histology
4. Family completed

Contraindications

1. Premalignant or malignant endometrial histology
2. Multiple fibroids
3. Uterine size larger than 12 cm

Technique

A 26 French resectoscope is used for this procedure with glycine as distending medium. The entire thickness of endometrium is resected with loop electrode (Figs 27.20 to 27.22). The fundus and cornua are usually coagulated with ball electrode (Figs 27.23 and 27.24). The entire procedure can also be done with ball electrode. Cervical canal is excluded to prevent hematometra.

This is done under regional or general anesthesia as a day care procedure.

Postoperatively bleeding might last for 2-4 days and the patient can have discharge per vaginum lasting for 4-5 weeks. 30-40% of patients will have amenorrhea and the rest have normal or lighter period. Successful TCRE (85%) cause irreversible sterility. Hence, the procedure should be limited to those who do not wish further child bearing.

Complications

The majority of perforations (1%) attributed to the procedure occur during dilation of the uterus or insertion of hysteroscope. Perforation during resection is reported to be much less (0.1%). Significant bleeding which occurs rarely (0.5%) can be controlled by insertion of a Foley catheter followed by distention of the bulb. Volume overload, infection (2%), failure (2-5%) and hematometra (1-2%) are other complications.[11]

Endometrial samples retrieved during procedure should be sent for histopathological examination.

27.7.7 Hysteroscopic Removal of Intrauterine Devices or Foreign Bodies

Intrauterine devices may be misplaced in as many as 5% of cases.[12] A 4-7 mm hysteroscope with grasping forceps can be used for extraction of the IUD under GA or paracervical block. The IUD can be grasped with a toothed grasper under hysteroscopic guidance and pulled out together. Hysteroscopy is particularly useful in removal of fragmented devices.[13]

Different kinds of foreign bodies such as fragments of IUD and broken tip of hook electrode, unabsorbed thread, residual placenta, adherent placenta, residual fetal bone after MTP, etc. can be removed. These may cause uterine bleeding, amenorrhea, infertility, discharge and abdominal pain.

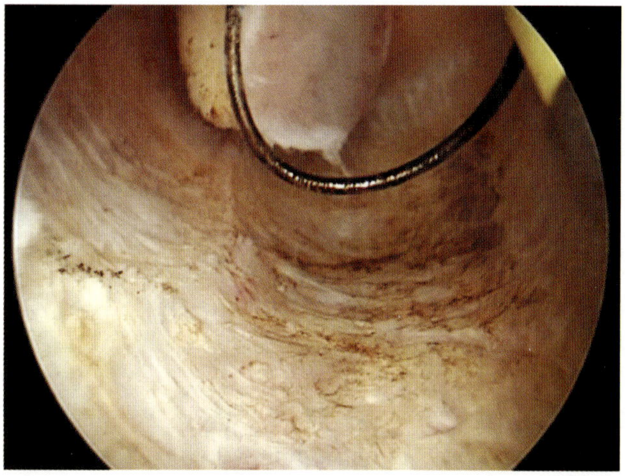

Fig. 27.21

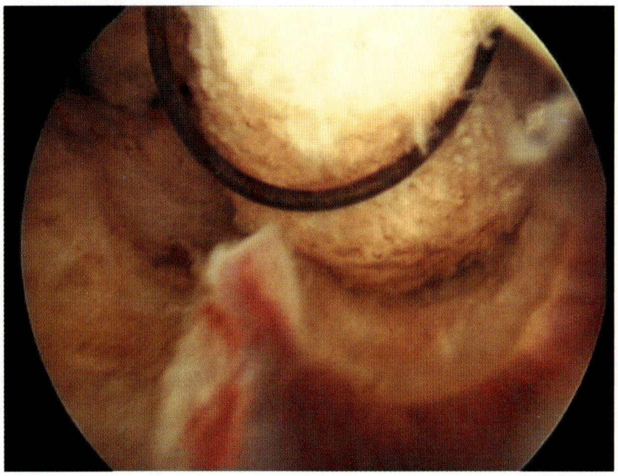

Fig. 27.20

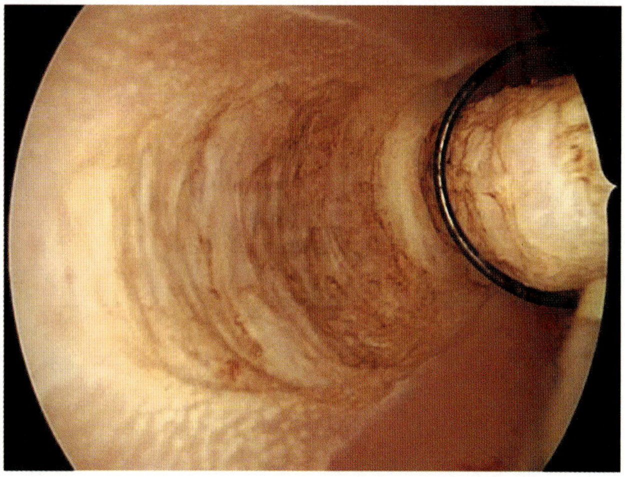

Fig. 27.22

Figs 27.20 to 27.22: Resection of endometrium

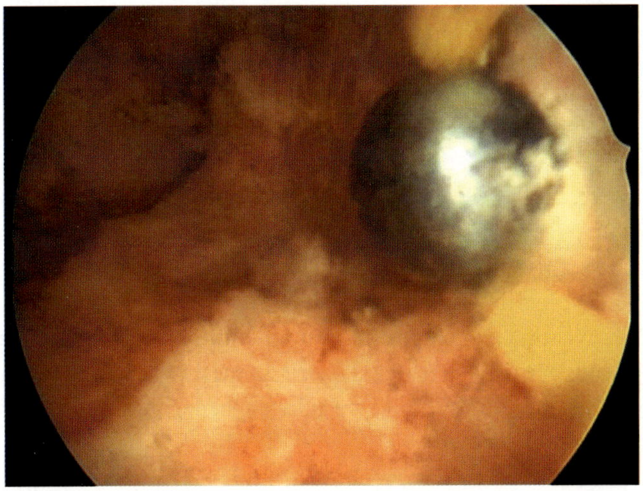

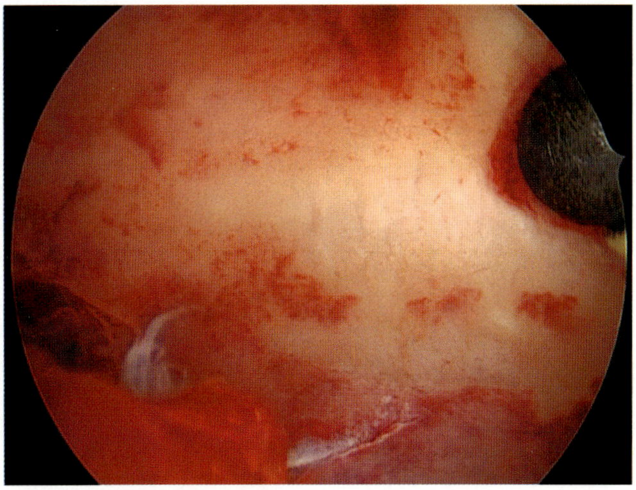

Figs 27.23 and 27.24: Coagulation with ball electrode

27.7.8 Hysteroscopic Sterilization

Transcervical sterilization is a safe, simple and highly effective alternative to transabdominal procedures for sterilization.

The less controllable destructive techniques involving the intrauterine or intratubal injection of sclerosing agents, tissue adhesives, elecrocoagulation or cryosurgery were associated with side effects related to tissue destruction such as abnormal uterine bleeding, discharge, infection and pelvic pain.

The microinsert, previously known as STOP (Selective tubal occlusion procedure), consists of a flexible stainless steel inner coil, a dynamic outer coil made of nickel-titanium alloy and a layer of polyethylene terephthalate (PET) fibers running along the inner coil.

The essure permanent birth control device is a dynamically expanding microinsert which is placed in the proximal section of the fallopian tube using a hysteroscopic approach for cannulating the tubes.[14] This device achieves sterilization through mechnical occlusion of the tube by inducing a local fibrous tissue in-growth from the surrounding tubal walls. Over a 3 month period the tissue in-growth completely occludes the tubal lumen. For the first three months after the procedure the woman should be advised alternative method of contraception.

Essure Device

The device can be delivered through a 4-7 mm hysteroscope with 5 French operating channel. Optimal positioning of the insert occurs when 3-8 mm of the proximal end of the microinsert is visible at the ostium. The guide wire attached to the device's inner coil aids placement. When released from the delivery catheter, the outer coil of the insert expands to span the intramural and proximal isthmic portion of the fallopian tube. This expansion serves to anchor the microinsert in the tubal lumen. Permanent placement of the microinsert is achieved upon subsequent fibrous tissue ingrowth.[15]

Ninety six percent of the women had achieved occlusion of lumen within 3 months of follow-up and 99% of women within 6 months. And it is well tolerated by up to 96% of women. The correct placement of device may not be achieved in up to 12% of women and can be advised alternative methods.[14]

27.8 COMPLICATIONS OF HYSTEROSCOPY

Complications occur when contraindications are ignored or when the procedure has been incorrectly performed on well chosen patients. They are not common and no serious complications were reported in many large series. The incidence of complications reported by Jansen is as low as 0.13% for diagnostic and 0.28% for operative hysteroscopies.[16]

Patient position:

- Nerve injuries: Brachial plexus injury, pressure on peroneal nerve
- DVT: Result from prolonged compression of calves.
- Electrical burns: If any part of patient is in contact with metal parts of the table.[17] Use of bipolar electrode obviates electrical burns.

Distention media related complications are specific to hysteroscopic surgery.

- *CO_2*: Cardiac arrhythmia and rarely gas embolism
  Saline: Electric burns if electric current is used. Fluid

overload with distending medium was reported in 0.2% of hysteroscopic procedures in a multicentric study. It is commonly seen during submucous myoma resection. It can be treated by diuretics, oxygen, central venous line and if necessary cardiac stimulants. The single most important factor in preventing fluid over load is to avoid intrauterine pressure above 100-110 mm Hg during the procedure.

- *Glycine*: Fluid overload presents as nausea and vertigo, hyponatremia, transient hypertension followed by hypotension, confusion and disorientation. This can be treated by hypertonic saline, diuretics and monitoring of serum electrolyte levels. Excessive overload may produce elevated blood ammonium levels leading to encephalopathy requiring hemodialysis and rarely death.[18,19]

27.8.1 Intraoperative Complications

Traumatic injuries are more common during operative hysteroscopy. Cervical lacerations due to tenaculum injury or dilatation have been reported. Perforation of the cervix and uterus is the most common complication with an incidence of 14 per 1000 cases. The risk of perforation during dilatation or insertion of hysteroscope is more in acutely anteflexed or retroflexed uterus and in stenotic cervix.[20] It can be avoided by inserting the hysteroscope under vision. Laparoscopy should be done if perforation or bleeding are suspected.

Large perforations usually occur with forceps, scissors, resectoscope or electrosurgical instruments. Perforations commonly occur during resection of synechia or septum. One in 100 perforation has been reported during division of uterine septum.[21] Concomitant laparoscopy is mandatory to prevent or immediately detect perforation. Thermal injuries to bowel, bladder or large vessels can also occur.[17,22,23]

Primary hemorrhage is the second most common complication of hysteroscopy and is reported to occur in 2.5% of the patients.[20] Major degree of hemorrhage can occur during resection or ablation due to deep resection of the myometrium or resecting close to the endocervix. Resection of myoma on the lateral wall near the uterine artery can also cause bleeding due to injury to branches of the uterine artery. Individual bleeding vessels should be coagulated separately. If bleeding continues, the operation should be abandoned and Foley catheter should be inserted into the cavity and the bulb inflated. This procedure usually controls the bleeding and the catheter can be removed after 6 hours. Vasopressin (20 U in 20 ml saline) may be injected into the cervix to arrest bleeding from the lower uterine segment. If facilities are available for uterine artery embolization it can be tried before considering hysterectomy if bleeding still continues.

Gas embolism is a rare but devastating complication of hysteroscopy. Brooks has reviewed 7 cases of air embolism with 5 fatalities.[24] First recognizable change of gas embolism is decrease in end-tidal CO_2. This is followed by hypoxia, tachycardia, tachypnea, hypotension followed by bradycardia and cardiovascular collapse. Auscultation over the precordium reveals typical mill wheel murmur. Following steps should be taken when gas embolism is diagnosed:

- Remove hysteroscope to discontinue insufflation, make sure vagina is closed or occluded with a wet sponge.
- Turn patient to left side to elevate and keep gas in the right side of the heart, decreasing the chance of paradoxic embolus.
- Consider precordial thumps to break up air pocket.
- Administer intravenous bolus of normal saline.
- Consider echocardiography to identify and possibly aspirate gas from the right side of the heart.

Transfer of the patient to an intensive care unit is mandatory because pulmonary edema and adult respiratory distress syndrome are likely sequelae of air embolism.

27.8.2 Postoperative and Late Complications

1. **Infection:** Infection is rare (0.8-2%) after diagnostic hysteroscopy.[25-27] The most common infections are uncomplicated cystitis, endometritis, or parametritis. The operation is better avoided in the presence of STD, vaginal discharge or recurrent acute PID. Prophylactic antibiotics may decrease the risk of postoperative infection.
2. **Endometrial cancer after endometrial ablation:** Functional islands of viable endometrial tissue can persist after endometrial ablation. Recently Valle and Baggish surveyed 6 cases of endometrial cancer diagnosed 5 months to 5 years after endometrial ablation.[28] Most of these patients had multiple risk factors, most notably endometrial hyperplasia. Women with multiple risk factors for endometrial cancer should be counseled for hysterectomy rather than endometrial ablation. Patients should be followed up with trans-vaginal sonography to detect residual endometrium after endometrial ablation. Any abnormal bleeding must be investigated with hysteroscopy and directed biopsies.
3. **Hematometra:** This may occur due to intrauterine adhesion behind which there is active endometrium,

which undergoes cyclical bleeding producing a small localized haematometra. Patients present with cyclical pain and could be diagnosed with TVS. Drainage may be performed by repeat hysteroscopy. Postoperative hematometra has been reported to occur in 1-2% of all endometrial ablation.[29]

4. **Uterine rupture during pregnancy:** Uterine rupture during pregnancy has been reported after operative hysteroscopic procedure like myoma resection, septum incision, and adhesiolysis.[30] Precipitating events include mechanical or electrosurgical perforation.

REFERENCES

1. Enlan X. The Reproductive Outcome of Hysteroscopic Adhesiolysis for 85 Women with Asherman's syndrome. J Minimal Invasive Gynecol 2007;14:41-42.
2. Musich J, Berman S. Surgical management of tubal obstruction at the uterotubal junction. Fertil steril 1983;40:423-40.
3. Sulak P, Letterie G, Coddington C,Woodward J, Klein T. Histology of proximal tubal occlusion. Fertil steril 1987;48:437-40.
4. Rock J, Katayama K, Martin E. Preganancy outcome following uterotubal implantation: A comparison of reamer and sharp corneal wedge excision techniques. Fertil 1979;31:634-40.
5. Paul P.G, Jeevanraj Rani J. Hysteroscopic cannulation for Proximal tubal Obstruction. J. Obstet Gyecol society of India 1998;48:65-67.
6. Porcu G, Carvello L, D'Ercole C, Cohen D, Rogern V, De Mongolfier R, Blanc B. Hysteroscopic metroplasty for septate uterus and repetitive abortions: Reproductive outcome. European Journal of Obstetrics and Gynecology and Reproductive Biology 2000;88:81-84.
7. Gebauer G, Hafner A, Siebzehnrubl E, Lang N. Role of hysteroscopy in detection and extraction of endometrial polyps: Results of a prospective study. Am J Obstet Gynecol 2001;184:59-63.
8. Donnez J, Gillerot S, Bourgonjon D, et al. Neodymium:YAG laser hysteroscopy in large submucous fibroids. Fertil Steril 1990;54:999-1003.
9. Donnez J, Jadoul P, Smets M, Squifflet J. Hysteroscopic myomectomy: Atlas of operative laparoscopy and hysteroscopy 2007;515-26.
10. Hallez JP. Single stage total hysteroscopic myomectomies: indications, techniques and results. Fertil Steril 1995;63: 703-08.
11. BJ van Herendael. Endometrial resection. Atlas of operative laparoscopy and hysteroscopy 2007;527-32.
12. Trivedi S, Goel M, Jain S. Hysteroscopic management of intrauterine devices with lost strings. The British journal of family planning 2000;26:229-30.
13. Xia E, Duan H, Huang X, Zheng J, Yu D, Cheng L. Hysteroscopic removal of foreign bodies and its method of monitoring. China medical journal 2003;116:125-28.
14. Kerin J, Cooper J, Price T, Bruno J, Enrique C, Daniel C, Charles C. Hysteroscopic sterilization using a micro-insert device: Results of a multicentre Phase II study. Human Reproduction 2003;18:1223-30.
15. J Greenberg. Hysteroscopic sterilization: History and current methods. Review Obstet Gynecol 2008;1:113-21.
16. Jansen FW, Vredevoogd, et al. Complications of hysteroscopy: A prospective, multicenter study. Obstet Gynecol 2000;96:266-70.
17. Kivneck S, Kanter MH. Bowel injury from rollerball ablation of the endometrium. Obstet Gynecol 1992;79:833.
18. Arieff Al, Ayus JC. Endometrial Ablation Complicated by fatal hyponatremic encephalopathy. JAMA 1993;270:1230-32.
19. Baggish MS, Brill Al Rosensweig B, et al. Fatal acute glycine and sorbitol toxicity during operative hysteroscopy. J Gynecol surg 1993;9:137-43.
20. Hulka JF, Peterson JA, Philips JM, et al. Operative hysteroscopy: AAGL 1993 membership survey. J Am Assoc Gynecol Laparosc 1995;2:131-32.
21. Hassiakos Ok, Zourlas PA. Tranascervical division of uterine septum. Obstet Gynecol survey 1990;45:165-73.
22. Perry CP, Daniel JF, Gimpelson RJ. Bowel injury from Nd:yag endometrial ablation. J Gynecol Surg 1990;6:199-203.2.
23. Sullivan B, Kenney P, Seibel M. Hysteroscopic resection of fibroid with thermal injury to sigmoid. Obstet Gynecol 1992;80:546-47.
24. Brooks PG. Venous air embolism during operative hysteroscopy. J Am Assoc Gynecol Laparosc 1997;4:399-402.
25. Loffer FD. Endometrial ablation - where do we stand? Gynecol Endosc 1992;2:1-5.
26. Loffer FD. Removing intrauterine lesions: Myomectomy and polypectomy. In Bieber EJ , Loffer FD (eds). The Gynecologic Resectoscope . Cambridge , Blackwell Scientific Publications 1994:168-94.
27. Salat - Baroux J, Hamou JE, Maillard G, et al. Complications from microhysteroscopy. In Siegler AM, Lindemann J (Eds): Hysteroscopy: Principles and Practice. Philadelphia Jb Lippincott 1984;1:12-17.
28. Valle RF, Baggish MS. Endometrial carcinoma after endometrial ablation: High-risk factors predicting its occurrence. Am J Obstet Gynecol 1998;179:569-72.
29. Whitlaw NL, Garry R, Sutton CJ. Pregnancy following endometrial ablation: Two case reports. Gynaecologic Endoscopy 1992;1:129-32.
30. Deaton JL, Maier D, Andreoli J. Spontaneous uterine rupture during pregnancy after treatment of Asherman's syndrome. Am J Obstet Gynecol 1989;160:1053-54.

Index

D

E

U

V

W

Y

Z